PREFACE

Given the requirement to maintain certification within the specialty of Physical Medicine and Rehabilitation, concise compendiums of the curriculum of PM&R are an asset. The proliferation of PM&R journal and book publications testifies to the growth of the specialty in regard to our workforce as well as our clinical knowledge base. It is likely that the board certification and recertification examinations will undergo modification over the next several years. Therefore the format and possibly content specifications of these examinations may change as well with the development of sub specialization certification in our field. Therefore it is prudent to conceptualize the curriculum of PM&R as a living and dynamic one. It is anticipated that this publication will need to model itself after this conceptual curriculum. The format and content edition is derived from the ABPM&R outline certification booklets. The review book does not reproduce the outline contents in a rigid construct. The structure of the review book contents and format are intended to survey the curriculum contents of PM&R in a coherent and meaningful manner. The review book will likely be of value as well to PM&R residents preparing for their written and oral certification examinations. It is not a substitute for earnest and dedicated learning through patient management and appropriate reading and teaching references.

The implementation of a computer based examination for recertification and the progressive growth of clinical knowledge in the field of Physical Medicine and Rehabilitation necessitate a revised edition in the Pearls of Wisdom publication. Pensive scrutiny and review of the original manuscript has yielded a publication with enhanced organization, content and comprehensiveness. It will serve as an excellent reference tool for board certification examination preparation for residents and candidates requiring recertification. The following amendments should be noted. A section on pulmonary rehabilitation has been added, the section devoted to neuromuscular diseases has been greatly expanded. Additional material has been incorporated to the sections on musculoskeletal and neurological rehabilitation to further strengthen the educational value of the chapters included in these sections. Previous chapters have been reassigned to CD-R format. These chapters include: 1) The review of anatomy and physiology germane to PM&R 2) The principles of clinical evaluation and diagnostic approaches to impairment and disability 3) research, statistics and functional outcome measures. The editor has an electronic file of the full text articles and reference books utilized in the preparation of the manuscript. Readers wishing to access these files may contact the editor in chief. Given the large file size however, most e-mail services will not accommodate the delivery. Therefore copies can be distributed through CD-R for an extra charge or through Windows messenger® on high-speed internet access free.

The Association of Academic Physiatrists (AAP) has published in appendix 5 of the Directory of the PM&R residency Training Programs a compendium of books in PM&R. The Directory may be accessed as follows: http://www.physiatry.org. The book bibliography that I have compiled is more thorough and current in its references. Additional AAP resources included on the AAP web page education site is "The Essential Articles in PM&R report". This bibliographic report includes articles germane to PM&R published during 1980-2003. This repository was utilized in updating the second edition manuscript. On a cautionary note, these articles are of historical educational value and do not necessarily reflect the current consensus and evidence with regard to epidemiology, pathogenesis, diagnostic accuracy or therapeutic efficacy. For more up to date clinical guidelines of evidence-based medicine, one may access the National Guidelines Clearing house (http://www.guideline.gov). Another helpful resource is The Cochrane Collaboration: Cochrane Reviews. This is a repository of evidenced based reviews covering the broad spectrum of the biomedical sciences. Online access is available through academic institutions or through Wiley Interscience. **This book is not intended to serve as a primary learning tool for residency or fellowship training. It is not intended to replace personal or group based formal preparation for the Part I and II of the American Board of PM&R certification examinations.**

DEDICATION

This book is dedicated to my parents Beatrice and Sidney Kaplan and my uncle Stanley Kaplan who inspired within me the delight of teaching. I also wish to thank the residents of the Harvard Medical School Department of PM&R who challenged me to develop a didactic curriculum and bestowed upon me the honor of teacher of the year in 2000.

I also wish to thank the academic and clinical staff at Northwestern University Feinberg School of Medicine, Rehabilitation Institute of Chicago, and the Mount Sinai School of Medicine Department of Rehabilitation Medicine.

EDITOR-IN-CHIEF:

Robert J. Kaplan, MD
Assistant Professor of Physical Medicine and Rehabilitation
Mount Sinai School of Medicine Department of PM&R
Staff Physiatrist Mount Sinai Hospital
New York, NY

TABLE OF CONTENTS

CARDIOVASCULAR

○ **To what degree does cardiovascular disease (CAD) contribute to morbidity and mortality in the United States?**

Cardiovascular disease is the leading cause of morbidity and mortality in the United States, responsible for almost 50 percent of all deaths. Coronary disease, the major category of cardiovascular disease, is clinically manifest as stable angina pectoris, unstable angina pectoris, myocardial infarction, silent myocardial ischemia, and sudden death. More than 13.5 million Americans have a history of myocardial infarction or experience angina pectoris. Nearly 1.5 million Americans sustain myocardial infarction each year, of which almost 500,000 are fatal.

○ **What are the recent prevalence rates for cardiovascular disease in the United States?**

Coronary heart disease 13,200,000
Myocardial infarction (heart attack) 7,800,000
Angina pectoris (chest pain) 6,800,000
Congestive heart failure 5,000,000

○ **What are the demographics of potential cardiac rehabilitation candidates?**

In 2001 an estimated 6,188,000 inpatient cardiovascular operations and procedures were performed in the United States; 3.6 million were performed on males and 2.6 million were performed on females.

In 2001 an estimated 1,051,000-angioplasty procedures, 516,000 bypass procedures, 1,314,000 diagnostic cardiac catheterizations, 46,000 implantable defibrillators and 177,000 pacemaker procedures were performed in the United States. 928,000 is a conservative estimate for the number of people with acute coronary syndrome (ACS) discharged from hospitals in 2001. Hospital Discharges for Cardiovascular Diseases United States: 1970-2001.

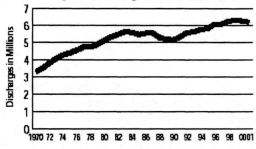

○ **What are the target populations for cardiac rehabilitation?**

Target populations for participation in cardiac rehabilitation Programs

Ischemic heart disease
Post-MI, coronary artery bypass graft, percutaneous
transluminal coronary angioplasty
Stable angina
Other heart conditions
Compensated heart failure
Controlled dysrhythmias
Automatic implanted cardioverter-defibrillate/pacemaker
Post-valve replacement
Cardiomyopathy
Myocardial aneurysm resection
Pre- and post-heart transplant
Congenital heart defects
Other chromic diseases
Stroke
Peripheral vascular disease
High risk of developing CVD
CVD, Cardiovascular disease; MI, myocardial infarction.

○   **What are irreversible risk factors for coronary artery disease (CAD)?**

Male gender, Family history of premature CAD (before age 55 in a parent or sibling), Past history of CAD, Past history of occlusive peripheral vascular disease, Past history of cerebrovascular disease, and Age.

○   **What are reversible actors from CAD?**

Cigarette smoking, Hypertension, Low high-density-lipoprotein cholesterol [<0.9 mmol/L (35 mg/dL)], Hypercholesterolemia [>5.20 mmol/L (200 mg/dL)], High lipoprotein A, Abdominal obesity, Hypertriglyceridemia [>2.8 mmol/L (250 mg/dL)], Hyperinsulinemia, Diabetes mellitus, Sedentary lifestyle.

○   **What role does risk modification play in comorbid diabetes mellitus?**

Close control of diabetes is an important part of the care of individuals with heart disease. Good control of blood glucose levels decreases the risk of cardiac disease by slowing the development of atherosclerosis and secondary conditions such as nephrogenic hypertension. Exercise training can also help to improve diabetic control. The exact benefits of exercise training in combination with good glucose control are still being elucidated.

○   **What role does risk modification play in comorbid hypertension?**

Control of hypertension is also important in the care of individuals with cardiac disease. Although control of hypertension is clearly beneficial in the prevention of stroke, the data for heart disease are more mixed. In patients with normal electrocardiograms, hypertensive control is especially useful. Two of the most important factors in the control of hypertension are reducing salt intake and increasing exercise to improve conditioning. Numerous pharmacologic agents are available for the control of hypertension, but a clear benefit with the use of one type of agent over another has not been demonstrated, except in some special situations.

○   **What role does risk modification play in comorbid hypercholesterolemia?**

The American Heart Association (AHA) recommendations are that the total amount of calories from fat in the diet should not exceed 30%. Control of cholesterol can be achieved through a three-step program, as outlined in the National Cholesterol Education Program (NCEP) guidelines. Phase I is an adoption of nutritional guidelines, lifestyle changes, and general improvement in health habits. Phase II involves the addition of fiber supplements and possibly nicotinic acid. Phase III includes lipid-lowering drugs. Lipid-lowering programs can retard the progression of CAD. With the addition of physical activity, HDL cholesterol concentration can rise 5% to 16%, but the data on the lowering of low-density-lipoprotein (LDL) cholesterol are still controversial.

○   **What role does risk modification play in the comorbid condition of obesity in cardiac rehabilitation?**

Weight loss is an integral part of any cardiac rehabilitation program for individuals who are overweight. The benefits to the loss of weight include decreased blood pressure, improved lipid profile, and improved ability to perform exercise.

○   **What is the role of cigarette smoking as a risk factor for coronary heart disease?**

Cigarette smoking is one of the greatest single modifiable risk factors for cardiac disease. The 10-year mortality in individuals with angiographically demonstrated CAD or MI who stopped smoking is decreased by more than 30%. Smoking causes accelerated atherosclerosis and is a contributor to hypertension. Exercising alone does not contribute to decreased smoking and smokers tend to be less compliant in cardiac rehabilitation programs. However, a program of cardiac rehabilitation coupled with counseling for smoking cessation can decrease smoking. Because smoking cessation is important for survival, it is crucial to include counseling as part of a complete cardiac rehabilitation program.

○   **How does myocardial infarction alter normal cardiac physiology?**

Myocardial Infarction (MI) will decrease the ejection fraction of the heart, and thus reduce the stroke volume (SV) and cardiac output. Ischemic heart disease will cause the maximum heart rate to be lowered, and will lower the MVO_2 and VO_2max that can be achieved, and may decrease the SV if the ventricle becomes stiff during the ischemic episode.

○   **How does valvular heart disease alter normal cardiac physiology?**

Valvular heart disease will decrease the maximum cardiac output, either through tight stenotic valves as in aortic stenosis, or through regurgitation as is seen in mitral insufficiency. The end result of the valve disease is a decreased MVO_2 and VO_2max and increased VO_2 at any level of submaximal exercise.

○   **How does cardiac disease alter normal cardiac physiology?**

CHF leads to lower VO_2 lower SV, higher resting heart rates, and decreased cardiac output. Arrhythmias will decrease the cardiac output through decreased SV and increased heart rates.

○   **How does cardiac transplantation alter normal cardiac physiology?**

Cardiac transplantation will correct many of the abnormalities seen with CHF that usually precede the transplantation, but a persistently high heart rate and a limited ability to increase SV can limit the exercise response.

○   **What are the sensitivities and specificities for the available cardiac exercise tests?**

	SENSITIVITY	SPECIFICITY
Stress ECG	68%	77%
Thallium-201	84%	87%
Quantified thallium	89%	89%
SPECT thallium	90%	89%
Tc-99 sestamibi	89%	90%
SPECT Tc-99 sestamibi	90%	93%
Dipyridamole thallium-201	85%	87%
Stress echo	80%	90%
During exercise	93%	86%
Dobutamine	89%	85%
PET scan	95%	95%
History and physical examination	79%	83%

○   **What are the outcomes of cardiac rehabilitation with CAD?**

Improvement in exercise tolerance.
Improvement in symptoms.
Improvement in blood lipid levels.
Reduction in cigarette smoking.
Improvement in psychosocial well-being and reduction of stress.
Reduction in mortality.

○   **What are the phases of cardiac rehabilitation after myocardial infarction?**

Cardiac rehabilitation is best viewed as being divided into four stages or phases. The first phase is the acute phase, which is the in-hospital period immediately following the MI and leading up to discharge. Rehabilitation during this phase includes early mobilization. The second phase is the convalescent phase, which is done at home and continues the program started in phase I, until the myocardial scar has matured. The third phase is the training phase initiated after healing is completed; the patient must be safe to begin the aerobic conditioning that is characteristic of phase III. The final phase is devoted to the maintenance of the aerobic conditioning gains made in phase III, through a program of regular exercise. Risk factor modifications are taught and re-emphasized throughout all phases.

○ **What is the treatment plan and progression of physical activity in the first phase of cardiac rehabilitation?**

As soon as medically stable, patients are encouraged to be sitting out of bed and in a chair, usually by day 1 or 2 (steps 1–5). By day 2 or 3, short-distance ambulation can be initiated, and bathroom privileges are full (steps 6–9). Around day 4 or 5, the patient is introduced to the home exercise program, and climbing stairs and increasing the duration of ambulation are encouraged (steps 10–13). After successful completion of a low-level exercise tolerance test (ETT) for risk stratification on day 5 or 6, the patient completes learning the home program and is discharged (step 14). During this mobilization program, it is usually recommended that cardiac monitoring be performed under the supervision of a trained physical, occupational therapist, or nurse. The post-MI heart rate rise with activity should be kept to within 20 bpm of base line, and the systolic blood pressure rise within 20 mm Hg of baseline. Any decrease of systolic blood pressure of 10 mm Hg or more should be considered worrisome and the exercise halted. The major goal of phase 1 is to condition the patient to perform activities up to 4 METs, which is within the range of most daily activities at home after discharge.

THE STEPS OF STAGE I CARDIAC REHABILITATION MODIFIED FROM WEGNER

STEP ACTIVITY

1 Passive ROM, ankle pumps, introduction to the program, self-feeding.
2 As above, also dangle at side of bed.
3 Active-assisted ROM, sitting upright in a chair, light recreation, use of bedside commode.
4 Increased sitting time, light activities with minimal resistance, patient education.
5 Light activities with moderate resistance, unlimited sitting, seated ADLs.
6 Increased resistance, walking to bathroom, standing ADLs, up to 1-h-long group meetings.
7 Walking up to 100 ft, standing warm-up exercises.
8 Increased walking, walk down stairs (not up), continued education.
9 Increased exercise program, review energy conservation and pacing techniques.
10 Increase exercise with light weights and ambulation, begin education on home exercise program.
11 Increased duration of activities.
12 Walk down two flights of stairs; continue to increase resistance in exercises.
13 Continue activities, education, and home exercise program teaching.
14 Walk up and down two flights of stairs, complete instruction in home exercise program and in energy conservation and pacing techniques.

○ **What are the elements of the second phase of cardiac rehabilitation after myocardial infarction?**

During the convalescent phase the scar over the infarction is allowed to mature. Because there is vulnerability to myocardial rupture, arrhythmia, and sudden death if overexertion occurs during this time, the patient's exercise intensity is limited to a target heart rate that is known to be safe. The target heart rate is determined during a low-level ETT per-formed prior to discharge and at the end of phase I. This exercise test is usually performed to a level of approximately 70% of maximum heart rate or a MET level of 5. For a person 40 years or older this generally represents a maximum heart rate of 130 bpm or 5 METs, and for an individual younger than 40 years, 140 bpm or 7 METs. A Borg rating of perceived exertion of 7 (modified scale) or 15 (old scale) can also be used to determine the maximum tolerated exercise. The program can consist of six phase II monitored sessions of 1 hour each, with a home exercise program over 6 weeks for the uncomplicated patient. At the end of the 6-week healing period, a full-level ETT can be performed, and then the third or training phase of cardiac rehabilitation can be started.

○ **What are examples of different heart rate formulas that a patient may use in a cardiac rehabilitation program?**

1. Age-Adjusted Method: The most commonly known way to determine your training zones. We have all seen this one:
220-age = MHR (maximum heart rate)
2. Karvonen Formula: The Karvonen formula is similar to the percentage of maximal heart rate. The difference is that the Karvonen formula incorporates the resting heart rate. The formula is ((MHR– RHR) x % intensity) + RHR = Training Zone

O   **What is the Borg Scale?**

BORG SCALE	PERCEIVED EXERTION	MODIFIED BORG SCALE	PERCEIVED EXERTION
---	---	0.0	Nothing at all
---	---	0.5	Very, very weak
---	---	1.0	Very weak
---	---	1.5	---
---	---	2.0	Weak (light
6	---	2.5	---
7	Very, very light	3.0	Moderate
8	---	3.5	---
9	Very light	4.0	Somewhat strong
10	---	4.5	---
11	Fairly light	5.0	Strong (heavy effort)
12	---	5.5	---
13	Somewhat hard	6.0	---
14	---	6.5	---
15	Hard	7.0	Very strong
16	---	7.5	---
17	Very hard	8.0	---
18	---	8.5	---
19	Very, very hard	9.0	---
20	---	9.5	---
---	---	10	Very, very strong
---	---	>10	Maximal

O   **What elements comprise the third phase of cardiac rehabilitation?**

The training phase of the cardiac rehabilitation program is started after performance of the symptom-limited full-level ETT. The heart rate maximum obtained by this test is the one used to determine the maximum exertion to be performed by the patient during aerobic training. In patients who are low risk, a program designed to achieve 85% of the maximum heart rate is safe. Gradation of the program to lower target heart rates needs to be tailored to the individual patient based on the results of the ETT and the reason for cessation of exercise. For patients with life-threatening arrhythmias or chest pain, a lower target heart rate should be chosen. Even a target heart rate at 65% to 75% of maximum can be safe and effective in a regular program, and target rates as low as 60% can still yield a training benefit.

O   **What elements constitute the fourth or maintenance phase of cardiac rehabilitation?**

Although often the least discussed, the maintenance phase of a cardiac conditioning program is the most important part. The actual exercises need to be integrated into the patient's lifestyle and interests to ensure compliance. The secondary prevention measures also need to be integrated into the patient's lifestyle. The ongoing exercises should be performed at the target heart rate for at least 30 minutes three times a week, if at a moderate level of intensity. If at a low level of intensity, exercises need to be performed five times a week. During the maintenance phase, electrocardiographic monitoring is not necessary.

O   **Does cardiac rehabilitation reduce morbidity and mortality in patients' after MI?**

Meta-analysis of the randomized controlled trials of exercise rehabilitation in patients following myocardial infarction establishes a reduction in mortality approximating 25 percent at 3-year follow up. This reduction in mortality approaches that resulting from pharmacologic management of patients following myocardial infarction with beta-blocking drugs or patients with left ventricular systolic dysfunction with angiotensin-converting enzyme (ACE) inhibitor therapy. The reduction in cardiovascular mortality was 26 percent in multifactorial randomized trials of cardiac rehabilitation and 15 percent in trials that involved only an exercise intervention.

O   **What is the rationale for cardiac rehabilitation program with patients' after CABG?**

Because patients who undergo CABG often have not had a recent MI and have just been revascularized; they make excellent candidates for cardiac rehabilitation. Some patients have incomplete revascularization after CABG and can still be subject to ischemia. The initiation of a cardiac rehabilitation program also allows for the initiation of an education program to help modify risk factors. Both supervised and unsupervised home programs are of benefit in preventing recurrent cardiac disease. These improvements include improved cardiac conditioning, decreased immobility post surgery, improved sense of well being, and improved lipid status.

O   **What are the elements of the first stage of cardiac rehabilitation program for a patent s/p CABG?**

Cardiac rehabilitation after CABG can be thought of in two stages: the immediate postoperative period and the later maintenance stage. The initial period has three parts: 1) intensive mobilization in the immediate postoperative period, 2) progressive ambulation and daily exercises, and 3) discharge planning and exercise prescription for the maintenance stage. Mobilization in the intensive care unit on postoperative day 1 includes sitting upright, active leg exercises, and mobilization out of bed. The second through fifth days include progressive ambulation and daily exercise. Initial ambulation with supervision for distances of 150 to 200 feet is followed by gradually increasing the distance, with most patients beginning independent ambulation by the third day. In the last few days prior to discharge, the patient and physicians develop a program that can be self-monitored at home and allows for gradual progression to previous levels of activity.

O   **What are the elements of cardiac rehabilitation for a patient s/p CABG in the second stage?**

The second stage of a program for a post-CABG patient is usually conducted at home or on an outpatient basis for most patients. High-risk patients or those who need other intensive interventions may require an inpatient rehabilitation setting. The home and outpatient rehabilitation patients are regularly supervised by their physicians.

O   **What types of programs are available for the patient s/p CABG in the second stage of rehabilitation?**

Patients can be in one of three types of programs: low, moderate, or high intensity. A low-intensity program is a progressive walking program with energy expenditures in the area of 2 to 4 metabolic equivalents (METs) and a target heart rate at 65% to 75% of the maximum heart rate. A moderate-intensity program is a progressive walk to walk-jog program with energy expenditures of 3 to 6.5 METs and a target heart rate 70% to 80% of the maximum heart rate. A high-intensity program is a progression from walk-jog to jogging with expenditures of 5 to 8.5 METs and a target heart rate 75% to 85% of the maximum heart rate. A level of exercise that equals a rating of perceived exertion (RPE) of 13 is a level of training that can be prescribed safely for the outpatient setting.

O   **What are the elements of cardiac rehabilitation for the patient s/p percutaneous transluminal coronary angioplasty?**

The rehabilitation of patients after percutaneous transluminal coronary angioplasty (PTCA) is essentially the same as that after CABG. PTCA patients tend to be younger and have disease limited to only one or two vessels. The exercise recommendations should be similar to those for the post-CABG patient population.

O   **What are the unique features of altered physiology in the cardiac transplant patient?**

The physiology of the transplant patient is somewhat different from that of the normal cardiac patient. Because of the loss of vagal inhibition to the SA node, the resting heart rate of the denervated heart is usually near 100 bpm. The resting tachycardia implies a small SV, and therefore, in response to light exercise, cardiac output can be increased via the Frank-Starling mechanism. With increased exercise, the circulating catecholamine-induced chronotropic and inotropic responses increase cardiac output. Therefore, because of loss of direct sympathetic innervation of the transplanted heart, patients have a blunted heart rate response to an incremental exercise test, with peak heart rates 20% to 25% lower than those seen in matched controls.

O   **What are the exercise physiology characteristics of the cardiac transplant patient?**

At submaximal exercise levels, perceived exertion, minute ventilation, and the ventilatory equivalent for oxygen are all higher than in normal individuals, while oxygen uptake is the same, implying an earlier onset of anaerobic metabolism. At maximum effort, transplant patients demonstrate lower work capacity, cardiac output, heart rate, systolic blood pressure, and oxygen uptake, while resting heart rate and systolic blood pressure are higher than those in normal individuals. Resting and exertional diastolic blood pressures are higher after cardiac transplantation than in normal individuals.

O   **What are the treatment plan components for the patient with cardiac transplant?**

In the initial postoperative period, sitting upright, lower-extremity exercises, and mobilization from the bed are encouraged. Patients are then encouraged to start ambulating, as with post-CABG patients. At the time of discharge, after patients have learned self-monitoring, they are encouraged to increase ambulation to 1 mile. The program then consists of progressively increasing distances for ambulation, with the pace designed to be at a level at 60% to 70% of peak effort for 30 to 60 minutes three to five times weekly. The RPE, using the old Borg scale, should be maintained at 13 or 14, with the level of activity increasing incrementally to stay at this level.

O   **What are the reported rehabilitation outcomes for the cardiac transplant patient?**

The outcomes of rehabilitation in the cardiac transplant population have been generally favorable. Patients usually achieve increased work output and improved exercise tolerance. Some transplant patients can even resume competitive-level athletics. Regarding areas of general well-being and quality of life, in a recent survey transplant recipients reported a quality of life at the level of cardiac arrest survivors and post-MI patients, but less than that for normal individuals. There were also significant musculoskeletal complaints in this group of patients. It is hoped that the use of an exercise-conditioning program in combination with reduction of other cardiac risk factors will help prevent accelerated atherosclerosis. The mechanism of this disease process is not known, but may be related to immunosuppressive drug therapy.

O   **What are the characteristics of severity grades in valvular stenosis?**

SEVERITY OF STENOSIS	MEAN VALVE GRADIENT (MM HG)	VALVE AREA (CM²)
Aortic valve		
Mild	<25	>1.2
Moderate	25-50	0.7-1.2
Severe	>50	<0.7
Mitral valve		
Mild	<5	>1.5
Moderate	5-10	1.0-1.5
Severe	>10	<1.0

Adapted from AMA *Guides to the evaluation of permanent impairment,* ed 4, Chicago, 1993, American Medical Association.

O   **What are the potential benefits of cardiac rehabilitation for the patient with cardiac valvular disease?**

In patients with valvular heart disease, the major problem is often deconditioning and Congestive heart failure (CHF), as in the transplant population. After surgical correction, the patient's cardiac fitness improves as measured by improved VO_2 training can increase physical work capacity by 60%, decrease the RPE, and decrease the rate pressure product (RPP) by 15%. The training program is similar to that followed for the post-CABG patient.

O   **What are the characteristic exercise responses in patients with CHF?**

Exercise in heart failure patients can cause a drop in ejection fraction, a decrease in systolic volume (SV), exertional hypotension, and syncope. In the worst cases, cardiac output may not increase sufficiently to generate a dynamic exercise response at all. Low endurance and fatigue are also problems encountered with this population, with some experiencing fatigue for hours to days after achieving a high aerobic workload. In addition, there may be concomitant factors such as atrial fibrillation, fluid overload, or medication noncompliance that decrease exercise tolerance.

O   **What benefits are obtainable through cardiac rehabilitation for the patient with CHF?**

There is a documented benefit from exercise in this patient population. A gradual program of increasing the heart rate above the resting rate can be safe and increases oxygen extraction efficiency. Exercise duration can increase by as much as 18% to 34% and peak oxygen uptake can increase by 18% to 25%. Patients who have participated in cardiac rehabilitation programs have lower heart rates at rest and during submaximal exercise, raised anaerobic thresholds, and increased maximal workloads. The improved ability to sustain activity at a low MET level can mean the difference between independent living and dependency for a patient with heart failure.

○   **What clinical evaluation should the CHF undergo prior to cardiac rehabilitation?**

The evaluation of the CHF patient consists of a graded ETT and may include measurements of left ventricular ejection fraction by multiple gated acquisition scanning or echocardiography during exercise. Unstable angina, decompensated CHF, and unstable arrhythmias are contraindications to cardiac rehabilitation.

○   **What points are worthy to emphasize in a cardiac rehabilitation program for a patient with CHF?**

Prolonged warm-up and cool down periods are appropriate since these patients can increase the duration of exercise but are unable to tolerate more than a limited workload. Dynamic exercise is preferable to isometric exercise, and the target heart rate should be 10 bpm below any significant end point, such as exertional hypotension, significant dyspnea, or sustained arrhythmia seen in the pre-training exercise test. The exercise program is best done under supervision initially, until the patient is able to monitor himself or herself and prevent complications during exercise. Patients with severe left ventricular dysfunction will need to be followed by telemetry during the warm-up, exercise, and cool down. Clinical status and progress can be monitored by measurements of body weight, blood pressure, and heart rate response to exercise.

○   **What are the different classes of risk stratification for patients with cardiac disease and exercise tolerance and safety?**

Classification for Exercise Training for Patients With Coronary Artery Disease, Based on AHA and ACSM Standards

Class and Description (Subclass)	Population	Exercise Recommendations
A. Apparently healthy(A-1)	Young patients	Can engage in moderate and vigorous exercise without exercise testing or prior medical exam
(A-2)	Older persons	May participate in moderate activity without prior medical exam or symptom-limited exercise test
(A-3)	Patients with <2 CV risk factors and normal exercise tests	
B. Known stable CAD, low risk for vigorous exercise but slightly higher than for apparently healthy persons	Clinically stable patients with CAD, valvular heart disease, congenital heart disease, cardiomyopathy, or exercise test abnormalities that do not meet class C criteria	Should have medical exam and a maximal exercise test before participating in moderate or vigorous exercise; data from a medical exam done within 1 yr. acceptable unless clinical status has changed
C. Moderate-to-high risk of cardiac complications during exercise, or those who are unable to self-regulate activity or understand the recommended activity level	Persons with CAD, acquired valvular disease, congenital heart disease, cardiomyopathy, exercise test abnormalities not directly related to ischemia, previous ventricular fibrillation or cardiac arrest not occurring with acute ischemic event or cardiac procedure, complex ventricular arrhythmias that are uncontrolled at mild-to-moderate work intensity with medication, 3-vessel or left main CAD, or ejection fraction <30%	Same as for class B
D. Unstable disease with activity restriction	Patients with unstable ischemia, uncompensated heart failure, uncontrolled arrhythmias, severe and symptomatic aortic stenosis, HCM or cardiomyopathy from recent myocarditis, severe pulmonary hypertension, or other conditions that could be aggravated by exercise (eg, resting systolic BP >200 or resting diastolic BP >110 mm Hg, active	No activity recommended for conditioning

or suspected pericarditis)

AHA = American Heart Association; ACSM = American College of Sports Medicine; CV = cardiovascular; CAD = coronary artery disease; HCM = hypertrophic cardiomyopathy; BP = blood pressure

○   **What are the different classes of functional capacity for risk stratification of exercise in cardiac disease?**

Functional Capacity (revised New York Classification scheme)	Objective Assessment
Class I. Patients with cardiac disease but without resulting limitation of physical activity. Ordinary physical activity does not cause undue fatigue, palpitation, dyspnea, or anginal pain.	**A.** No objective evidence of cardiovascular disease.
Class II. Patients with cardiac disease resulting in slight limitation of physical activity. They are comfortable at rest. Ordinary physical activity results in fatigue, palpitation, dyspnea, or anginal pain.	**B.** Objective evidence of minimal cardiovascular disease.
Class III. Patients with cardiac disease resulting in marked limitation of physical activity. They are comfortable at rest. Less than ordinary activity causes fatigue, palpitation, dyspnea, or anginal pain.	**C.** Objective evidence of moderately severe cardiovascular disease.
Class IV. Patients with cardiac disease resulting in inability to carry on any physical activity without discomfort. Symptoms of heart failure or the anginal syndrome may be present even at rest. If any physical activity is undertaken, discomfort is increased.	**D.** Objective evidence of severe cardiovascular disease.

○   **What is the risk of cardiac arrhythmia associated with cardiac rehabilitation?**

The risk of death from cardiac arrhythmia during rehabilitation exercises is very low. From 1980 to 1984, one arrest per 112,000 patient-hours of exercise was reported.

○   **Which patients are at an increased risk for arrhythmia in cardiac rehabilitation?**

Acute infarctions within 6 weeks.
Active ischemia by angina or exercise testing.
Significant left ventricular dysfunction (LVEF<30%).
History of sustained ventricular tachycardia.
History of sustained life-threatening supraventricular arrhythmia.
History of sudden death, not yet stabilized on medical therapy.
Initial therapy of patient with automatic implantable cardioverter defibrillator (AICD).
Initial therapy of a patient with adaptive cardiac pacemaker.

○   **What are the metabolic equivalents for common functional, recreational and labor related activities?**

Energy Requirements for Selected Physical Activities

Activity	Workload in METs
Calisthenics, walking (3-3.5 mph), noncompetitive softball, badminton (social doubles), archery, fly fishing, horseback riding (trot), small-boat sailing, household activities: mopping, window cleaning, stocking shelves, packing or unpacking light or medium objects, plumbing, raking leaves	3-4
Walking (3.5-4 mph), social dancing, golf (carrying bag), table tennis, badminton (singles), tennis (doubles), noncompetitive baseball, calisthenics (moderate), swimming (light), rowing or canoeing (3 mph), gardening, light carpentry, painting, using power saw on hardwood, pushing a power mower or cart	4-5
Walking (4-5 mph), tennis (singles), scuba diving (warm water), competitive badminton, heavy calisthenics, water skiing, cross-country hiking, moderate swimming, dancing (rhumba, square), snow shoveling, hand lawn mowing, splitting hard wood, carrying or lifting weights (20-29 kg [45-64 lb]), exterior carpentry, backpacking (2.2 kg [5 lb])	5-7
Heavy labor, handball, squash, running (6-7 mph)	>9

MET = metabolic equivalent (3.5 mL O_2/kg/min)

O   **What is the Haskell classification for cardiac impairment?**

	PEAK METS	ACTIVITY
Very Heavy	>6	Climb stairs
Medium	4-6	Carry 50 lbs
Light	2-4	Carry 20 lbs
Sedentary	<2	Sit/carry 10 lbs

Adapted from Haskell, W, et al: Task Force II: determination of
occupational working capacity in patients with ischemic heart disease.
JACC 1989; 14:1027.

O   **What impairment ratings are utilized by the AMA for cardiac disease based on exertion?**

$\dot{V}O_2$MAX	PEAK METS	ACTIVITY
>25	>7	None
20-25	5-7	Mild to moderate
15-20	2.5-5	Severe
<15	<2.5	Total

Adapted from AMA *Guides to the evaluation of permanent impairment,*
ed 4, Chicago, 1993, American Medical Association.

O   **What is the likelihood of a patient s/p MI returning to work?**

After an MI, 49% to 93% of patients return to work.

O   **What factors determine the likelihood of return to work?**

A study of 1252 employed patients with CAD reports that approximately 20% of patients did not return to work after
coronary revascularization via coronary bypass or coronary angioplasty. No difference was shown in the rate of return to
work for those treated medically versus those having undergone a revascularization procedure. Demographic and
socioeconomic factors accounted for almost half of the influence for return to work outcome, physical and emotional
functioning were responsible for 29%, and medical factors represented only 20% of the predictors in this model. Importantly,
the patient's perception about his or her activity status was highly predictive of return to work status.

O   **Summarize the multidisciplinary approach to cardiac rehabilitation.**

Initial evaluation
Take medical history and perform physical examination
Measure risk factors
Obtain electrocardiograms at rest and during exercise
Provide vocational counseling
Determine level of risk
Goal: formulation of preventive plan in collaboration with primary care physician
Management of lipid levels
Assess and modify diet, physical activity, and drug therapy
Primary goal: LDL cholesterol level <100 mg/dl
Secondary goals: HDL cholesterol level >45 mg/dl, triglyceride level <200 mg/dl
Management of hypertension
Measure blood pressure frequently at rest and during exercise
If resting systolic pressure is 130–139 mm Hg or diastolic pressure is 85–89 mm Hg, recommend lifestyle modifications,
  including exercise, weight management, sodium restriction, and moderation of alcohol intake; if patient has diabetes
  or chronic renal or heart failure, consider drug therapy
If resting systolic pressure is »140 mm Hg or diastolic pressure is »90 mm Hg, recommend drug therapy
Monitor effects of intervention in collaboration with primary care physician

Goal: blood pressure <140/90 mm Hg (or <130/85 mm Hg if patient has diabetes or chronic heart or renal failure)

Cessation of smoking

Document smoking status (never smoked, stopped smoking in remote past, stopped smoking recently, or currently smokes)

Determine patient's readiness to quit; if ready, pick date

Offer nicotine-replacement therapy, bupropion, or both

Offer behavioral advice and group or individual counseling

Goal: long-term abstinence

Weight reduction

Consider for patients with BMI >25 or waist circumference >100 cm (in men) or >90 cm (in women), particularly if associated with hypertension, hyperlipidemia, or insulin resistance or diabetes

Provide behavioral and nutritional counseling with follow-up to monitor progress in achieving goals

Goals: loss of 5–10% of body weight and modification of associated risk factors

Management of diabetes

Identify candidates on the basis of the medical history and base-line glucose test

Develop a regimen of dietary modification, weight control, and exercise combined with oral hypoglycemic agents and insulin therapy

Monitor glucose control before and after exercise sessions and communicate results to primary care physician

For newly detected diabetes, refer patient to primary care physician for evaluation and treatment

Goals: normalization of fasting plasma glucose level (80–110 mg/dl) or glycosylated hemoglobin level (<7.0%) and control of associated obesity, hypertension, and hyperlipidemia

Psychosocial management

Identify psychosocial problems such as depression, anxiety, social isolation, anger, and hostility by means of an interview, standardized questionnaires, or both

Provide individual or group counseling, or both, for patients with clinically significant psychosocial problems

Provide stress-reduction classes for all patients

Goal: absence of clinically significant psychosocial problems and acquisition of stress-management skills

Physical-activity counseling and exercise training

Assess current physical activity and exercise tolerance with monitored exercise stress test

Identify barriers to increased physical activity

Provide advice regarding increasing physical activity

Develop an individualized regimen of aerobic and resistance training, specifying frequency, intensity, duration, and types of exercise

Goals: increases in regular physical activity, strength, and physical functioning, expenditure of at least 1000 kcal per week in physical activity

Strength of evidence ratings for modification of various outcomes and cardiovascular disease risk-factors as a result of cardiac rehabilitation participation

Outcome	Strength of evidence*
Smoking cessation, relapse prevention	B
Improved lipid profile	A
Decreased blood pressure	B
Improved blood sugar control	B
Increased exercise capacity	A
Increased physical activity	B
Decreased body weight	B
Improved psychosocial well-being	A
Improved social functioning	B

* A, Evidence provided by well-designed, controlled trials with statistically significant results consistent across trials; B, evidence provided by observational studies or controlled trials with less consistent results; C, opinion of expert consensus due to a lack of controlled trials and/or consistent results.

PERIPHERAL VASCULAR DISEASE

○ **What clinical features suggest vascular insufficiency?**

The examiner should check for pitting edema and palpate calf muscles, observing for tenderness, firmness, and muscle tension. These findings may indicate DVT. With the patient in the supine position, both lower extremities should be elevated to approximately 60 degrees and observed for unusual pallor. The examiner should then sit the patient up, lower the feet into a dependent position, and observe for return of the usual color, which should occur within 10 seconds. The gradual appearance of rubor or dusky erythema suggests a compromise in arterial circulation. In the standing position, the examiner should inspect the saphenous system for varicosities, redness, or cords. Systolic blood pressure should be recorded in each arm and, using Doppler measurement, in each leg. From this, the ankle-arm index (AAI) can be calculated.

○ **What is the AAI and how does it compare to manual palpation of the arterial pulse?**

The AAI is determined by dividing the ankle pressures on each side by the higher of the two brachial pressures. An assessment of the reliability of palpation of pulses found that the sensitivity was at least 95% for palpation over the femoral pulse; but ranged from 33% to 60% for observers of varying experience feeling for the posterior tibial pulse; the rate of false-positive observations was 20%. Therefore, it was suggested that pulse palpation alone is an unreliable physical sign and should be combined with other objective measurements to guide clinical management.

○ **How does arterial occlusive disease compromise skeletal muscle circulation?**

The normal peripheral vascular system provides sufficient blood flow to deliver oxygen in adequate amounts to satisfy the requirements of lower extremity muscles during all activities. In the presence of peripheral vascular disease, the blood flow is compromised and the supply of oxygen to the muscles during exercise is not equal to the demand. Intermittent claudication is a result of muscle ischemia and in turn, can occur in response to any condition capable of compromising the arterial blood supply to muscles. While the most common cause of arterial obstruction is atherosclerosis and arteriosclerosis obliterans, other causes include emboli, thrombi, fibromuscular dysplasia, and external compression. Occlusions may occur at one or more points along the iliac, superficial femoral, popliteal, or distal arteries.

○ **What are the factors that determine the onset, progression and manifestations of ischemia?**

In order for a reduction in blood flow to take place, a 75% narrowing of cross-sectional diameter of a vessel must be present. This serves to explain why slowly progressive atherosclerotic arterial disease does not usually manifest itself clinically until later in life when the critical threshold of 75% stenosis has been reached. It should be noted that the physiologic severity of a lesion depends on various factors including absolute vessel diameter and eccentricity, lesion length, presence of multiple lesions in the same vessel, and existence of collateral flow. Therefore, measurement of the reduction in the luminal diameter (in percent) caused by stenosis does not accurately predict blood flow. While lesser degrees of narrowing as measured on Doppler studies are often noted not to be "hemodynamically significant," this does not serve to exclude the possibility of acute embolization of distal vessels by atherosclerotic plaques resulting in obstruction and gangrene.

○ **What hemodynamic properties and rheological properties of the vascular system are relevant to arterial occlusive disease?**

The total peripheral resistance in blood flow is partially determined by its rheologic properties (i.e., fluidity). Consequently, blood flow through diseased arteries can also be affected by factors impacting on rheology, which include viscosity, hematocrit, red blood cell deformability, and red blood cell aggregation. Energy losses in flowing blood occur as a result of friction (viscous losses) or changes in velocity or direction (inertial losses).

○ **What role do metabolic phenomena play in the onset of skeletal muscle ischemia and claudication?**

The metabolic phenomena at the level of the muscle cell play an important role in the development of ischemic symptoms and in the response to interventions. When ischemia occurs and blood flow to the muscles diminishes, metabolic waste products accumulate. The local buildup of these substances produces pain and usually causes the patient to rest until the oxygen demand has again diminished and metabolic waste products are washed from the system. Immediately after treadmill testing, levels of lactate and hypoxanthine are noted to be significantly elevated in the bloodstream, returning to pre exercise levels within 30 minutes (lactate) and 60 minutes (hypoxanthine). Improved exercise tolerance can occur without changes in muscle blood flow during activity. This suggests that beneficial changes are occurring within the muscle itself, to adapt to a decreased blood flow.

○   **Have animal model studies of skeletal muscles ischemia elucidated mechanisms of claudication?**

Results of animal studies suggested that the peripheral adaptations within active muscle cells include 1) a redistribution of blood flow, 2) enhanced capillary density, and 3) an increase in mitochondrial content. Despite limited blood flow, improvements in muscle metabolism may facilitate the extraction of oxygen and substrates and permit increased exercise capacity. Biopsy samples of ischemic muscles have shown a significant reduction in total plasma carnitine concentration, and treatments with carnitine supplements have restored normal levels along with improvements in exercise performance.

○   **Are there metabolic studies in humans to correlate arterial occlusive disease and claudication?**

Increases in maximum walking distance after training have been correlated to the enzyme activity of cytochrome-c oxidase in patients with peripheral arterial insufficiency. This metabolic adaptation reverses itself after arterial reconstructive surgery but the increased oxidative capacity can persist with a therapeutic program of surgery and training.

○   **How is the AAI useful in evaluating the patient with arterial occlusive disease?**

The AAI, or ankle-brachial index (ABI), is a quantitative technique widely used to determine the presence and severity of peripheral arterial disease. It is a prognostic indicator for mortality due to atherosclerotic disease in older men and women. Normally, systolic pressures should be higher in the lower extremities than in the upper extremities. When there is arterial occlusive disease in the lower extremities, pressures distal to the occlusion will be decreased.

○   . **What stratification exists for arterial occlusive disease based on the AAI?**

Some analyses proposed a stratification of severity, with mild disease corresponding to an AAI of 0.90 to 0.71, moderate disease having an AAI of 0.70 to 0.51, and severe disease corresponding to an AAI of 0.50 or less. High ankle pressures and a normal AAI sometimes occur despite advanced arterial disease, as a result of a loss of compressibility of lower-extremity arteries. This occurs particularly in diabetics with arteriosclerotic disease. Measurement of the AAI is useful in identifying those at high risk for mortality due to atherosclerotic heart disease who may benefit from aggressive therapy. Because AAI measurement is a simple procedure, it is suggested that it could be a useful component in geriatric screening programs.

○   **What is the role of B- mode ultrasound and Doppler imaging in arterial occlusive disease?**

Serial noninvasive testing is useful in assessing arterial obstructive disease and arterial bypass grafts and in diagnosing local vascular complications of arterial catheterization. Color flow imaging combines high resolution B-mode and Doppler imaging systems to provide simultaneous anatomic and physiologic information. B-mode ultrasonography provides a gray scale image of the blood vessels while Doppler probes permit analysis of flow patterns and velocity. Color flow Doppler and two-dimensional ultrasound have had an expanding role in the noninvasive evaluation of peripheral arterial diseases and can help to diagnose stenosis or occlusion by demonstrating absent, diminished, high velocity, and collateral flow. They can also visualize atherosclerotic plaque or thrombus, calcified plaque or vessel wall, and aneurysms, pseudoaneurysms, perivascular masses, arteriovenous fistulae, and arterial conduit occlusions.

○   **How do the signs and symptoms of arterial occlusive disease manifest over time?**

The signs and symptoms of peripheral arterial disease are stable in the majority of patients and can often improve, but the occlusive process is progressive in approximately 20% of patients, in whom complications ranging from intermittent claudication to rest pain, skin ulcerations, and gangrene will develop. Most patients with intermittent claudication are not at immediate risk for limb loss.

○ **What are the conservative treatment approaches in the patient with arterial occlusive disease?**

The primary goals of treatment in these individuals are to reduce risk factors and to improve exercise tolerance and functional capacity. These goals are generally achieved through education, exercise, and in some patients, drug therapy.

○ **What is the role of drug therapy in the patient with arterial occlusive disease?**

Drug therapy has primarily generally consisted of treatment with hemorheologic drugs (i.e., pentoxifylline & cilostazol) and antiplatelet agents (i.e., aspirin, ticlopidine, and dipyridamole). No drug has been clearly proved to be effective in the treatment of limb threatening ischemia. Various classes of vasodilators (adrenergic agents, direct-acting agents, calcium channel blockers, angiotensin-converting enzyme inhibitors, and prostaglandins) have been studied with respect to improvement of blood flow to ischemic areas and have been used in the treatment of obstructive arterial disease and vasospastic disorders. While heparin is used during vascular surgery or interventional radiologic procedures, the role of oral anticoagulants (i.e., warfarin) in the management of peripheral arterial disease has not been well established although they have been prescribed after distal bypass procedures.

○ **What aggressive interventions are available for refractory occlusive vascular disease?**

Other less widely utilized interventions include lumbar neurolytic sympathetic blockade, electrical spinal cord stimulation, ozone therapy, and hyperbaric oxygen. Patients with disabling claudication (inability to perform a job or normal daily life activities), rest pain, ulceration, gangrene, or Leriche syndrome (occlusion of the terminal aorta) should be considered for surgical revascularization (bypass) or angioplasty. Thrombolytic therapy, used for acute segmental arterial occlusion, has been successful in restoring distal pulses and improving the AAI in selected patients. The risk of complications, however, is significant and complications include thromboembolic events, arterial dissection, and major hemorrhage, with mortality rates as high as 25%.

○ **What is the role of exercise in the management of arterial occlusive vascular disease?**

Exercise programs have been designed to be carried out both in supervised cardiovascular treatment settings using endurance training equipment and in unsupervised home and community settings, emphasizing walking and simple independently performed exercises. Various functional benefits have been established and include increased pain tolerance, increase in walking distance, increase in walking time, and increase in duration of exercise tolerance, and improved motivation.

○ **What evidence of efficacy exists regarding the therapeutic role of exercise?**

Based on a meta-analysis of exercise rehabilitation programs aimed at reducing claudication pain in patients with peripheral arterial disease, Gardner and Poehlman concluded that the optimal exercise program for improving claudication pain distances uses intermittent walking to near maximal pain during a program of at least 6 months' duration. Gardner et al suggested that stair climbing might offer an advantage over treadmill walking for patients with claudication, noting that similar metabolic, claudication, and peripheral hemodynamic measurements are obtained with less demand on the cardiovascular system.

○ **What possible mechanisms may account for the benefits of exercise?**

Several possible mechanisms for increased walking ability that were proposed in earlier literature included development of increased collateral blood flow, redistribution of available flow, change in walking pattern, increased pain tolerance, and metabolic adaptation in leg muscles. While some more recent work continued to suggest enhanced blood flow to muscle resulting from physical training, studies have not provided consistent and significant evidence for these mechanisms.

○ **What is the pathophysiological mechanism of venous insufficiency and its clinical presentation?**

DVT is considered the most common cause of chronic insufficiency of the deep venous system in the lower extremities. This condition is frequently referred to as *post-phlebitic syndrome*. Thrombosis and phlebitis in the deep venous system can result in destruction of the normal valvular mechanisms and lead to valvular incompetence, calf pump dysfunction, venous hypertension, and reflux. When there is incompetence of the perforating draining veins of the lower leg, blood flow from the deep venous system backs up into the skin and subcutaneous tissue, causing edema and, if persistent and severe enough, ulceration. Hemosiderin deposits from stagnant blood result in the brown hyperpigmented appearance. The clinical manifestations of chronic venous insufficiency includes swelling, pain, complaints of heaviness in the legs, dilated superficial veins, skin changes, and ulceration.

O   **What are the most common conservative treatment approaches for chronic venous insufficiency?**

The primary treatment for chronic venous insufficiency is compression therapy. Stockings exerting 40 mm Hg of pressure at the ankle are associated with a reduction in ambulatory venous pressure, which may in turn lead to clinical prevention or improvement of the various sequelae associated with chronic venous hypertension. A frequent pitfall in the use of elastic compression stockings is the difficulty many patients encounter in donning them, particularly patients who are older, debilitated, and arthritic. Such patients should be evaluated and supplied with appropriate assistive devices or the patient's caregiver should be instructed in assisting with the application of the stockings. Walking and gentle exercises are helpful in enlarging and maintaining venous collaterals. Tipping of the bed into a head-down position reduces edema and muscle compartment tension at night.

O   **What treatments are available for refractory chronic venous insufficiency?**

Surgical treatment is indicated when severe stasis symptoms persist despite conservative therapy and also may be considered in younger patients and those requiring a rapid recovery and return to normal activities. Venous ligation and, when necessary, sclerotherapy have been used successfully in an outpatient setting in a young group of working patients who were able to return to work rapidly following treatment.

O   **What is the origin of most chronic leg ulcers?**

The majorities of chronic leg ulcers are venous in origin and tend to occur in older individuals with a history of DVT or an associated condition. The goal in treatment of a venous ulcer is rapid and permanent re-epithelialization of the ulcer bed. Early treatment will improve outcome. Management may be surgical or nonsurgical and can include wound débridement, electrical stimulation, compression therapy, exercise, leg elevation at rest, and paste gauze boots (Unna boot).

O   **Describe a protocol for the evaluation and management of chronic venous leg ulcers:**

Assessment for infection and the extent of edema.
5 to 7 days of bed rest, when necessary, to resolve the edema.
Short-term intravenous or oral antibiotic treatment for cellulitis with dry gauze dressings changed every 12 hours;
Avoidance of topical agents;
Fitting with below-knee 30- to 40-mm Hg elastic compression stockings when edema or cellulitis has resolved (two pairs);
Wound care throughout the course of therapy consisting of daily washing with soap and water and covering with dry gauze dressing held in place with the compression stocking;
Topical corticosteroids applied to the surrounding areas of significant stasis dermatitis but not to the ulcer itself.
Continued ambulatory compression therapy once the ulcer has healed.

O   **What other types of compression devices are available to manage venous insufficiency?**

Various other forms of elastic compression devices are available. The CircAid® is a compression orthosis that produces rigid compression, is easy to apply, and is adaptable to a reduction in edema. The orthosis is designed with multiple, pliable, rigid, adjustable compression bands that wrap around the leg from the ankle to the knee and are held in place with Velcro tape.

O   **What is the rationale for the Unna boot?**

(Unna boot) have been used as treatment for venous ulcers. The Unna boot as a functional substitute for the failing muscle pump in chronic venous insufficiency; it is a non-invasive ambulatory method of controlling edema and treating ulcers. The Unna Boot, an inelastic bandage impregnated with zinc oxide, provides physical support to improve the function of the calf muscle pump. It needs to be changed only once or twice weekly, an important consideration in patient compliance. Zinc oxide is slowly solubilized, and may correct local zinc deficiency. In addition it may directly enhance re-epithelization and decrease inflammation and bacterial growth.

○   **What problems are associated with Unna boots?**

The Unna Boot, however, does not adapt to decreased edema and may induce allergic contact dermatitis. As many as 4% of the leg ulcer patients demonstrate patch test sensitivity to the former. Even so, the Unna Boot, gauze, and elastic wrap compression bandage remain in common use.

○   **What is the rationale for the use of hydrocolloid dressings?**

The development of occlusive dressings is based on principles of wound healing. In an initial inflammatory phase, macrophages; digest microorganisms and nonviable tissue. Epithelial cells at the ulcer's edge, and sometimes at islands within the ulcer, proliferate and begin to migrate to cover the gap. When new blood vessels, macrophages, fibroblasts, and loose connective tissue proliferate, the wound is said to be forming granulation tissue or "granulating." Numerous cytokines, including growth factors, prostaglandins, interleukins, and colony stimulating factors improve granulation tissue, tensile strength, and re-epithelialization. Developers of topical treatments and occlusive dressings have acted to enhance what our bodies have provided.

○   **What evidence supports the use of hydrocolloid dressings?**

Hydrocolloid dressings such as Duoderm® appear to decrease trauma to granulation tissue during dressing changes, and they decrease the risk of both contamination and pain. Duoderm® CGF hydroactive (HD) dressing with compression has been reported to result in faster ulcer healing rates as compared with the Unna boot during initial therapy (the first 4 weeks), and possibly over a 12-week treatment period. However, occlusive hydrocolloid dressings are also associated with an increased rate in infectious complications.

○   **What other topical agents have been utilized?**

Calcium alginate dressings appear particularly easy to use and quite capable of absorbing copious amounts of exudates. Lyophilized type I collagen is more helpful than hydrocolloid dressings in venous leg ulcers. It is posited that the collagen recruits platelets and macrophages that produce growth factors that activate the wound healing cascade. Superior re-epithelialization with dressings of cultured keratinocytes adhering to a collagen film has been observed

○   **What is the role for Trental® or Pletal® in treating chronic venous ulcers?**

Numerous reports have cited pentoxifylline and cilostazol as a valuable adjunct to venous leg ulcer therapy. Although these studies report improved healing, one study found that Doppler continuous wave ultrasound studies were not improved over controls. One beneficial program is 200 mg intravenously daily and 400 mg orally three times daily for 7 days, followed by 400 mg orally three times daily for another 60 days. Local inflammation in venous ulcers causes accumulation of neutrophils in capillaries and interstitial fluid. Pentoxifylline probably works by decreasing the plasma fibrinogen level and enhancing neutrophil motility.

○   **What is the role of intermittent compression pump therapy?**

Another treatment modality is the use of a sequential compression pump. Whether or not pumps increase oxygen tension is debated. Although expensive, these pumps me quite helpful for elderly or inactive patients with calf pump inadequacy. The sequential compression pumps are usually used for 1 hour daily at pressure less than diastolic, and a ratio of 90 seconds on to 30 seconds off.

○   **What is the recurrence rate of venous ulcers?**

Venous ulcers have a recurrence rate of nearly 70% and once healing is accomplished, compression stockings should be used on a permanent basis along with elevation and frequent lower-extremity motion.

○   **What is the role for surgery in chronic refractory venous ulcer therapy?**

The value of surgery on the veins themselves has been debated. Ligation of the communicating veins and saphenous vein stripping has been reported to accomplish healing in only 25% of the cases. When valvuloplasty was also done, the healing rate incased to 87%. Adjunctive use of an elastic stocking and sequential compression reduces postoperative edema and improves the long-term prognosis. Surgical correction of venous incompetence prevents reflux and restores the normal vasodilator response to exercise. With tissue oxygenation thus maintained, the ulcers heal at the maximum rate. It would appear that communicating vein ligation, saphenous vein stripping, and valvuloplasty offer an aggressive alternative in refractory venous ulcers.

○   **Is there a role for topical antibiotic therapy in venous leg ulcer care?**

Topical antibiotic administration probably does little to alter bacterial counts, and they interfere with epithelial migration. Silver nitrate compresses (0.25%), which dry exudates and precipitate bacterial proteins, are probably more effective than topical antibiotics. Allergic sensitization is a major problem in leg ulcers. Not only are local eruptions common, but widespread systemic reactions can occur. Neomycin, a potent antibiotic sensitizer, induces sensitivity when applied to ulcers in 30% of patients. Other topical sensitizers in leg ulcers include EDTA, lanolin, nitrofurazone, parabens, and vitamin E cream. Topical antibiotics should probably not be used, and any topical treatment of leg ulcers should be considered with extreme caution.

○   **How does the clinician differentiate leg ulcers?**

Clinical Differentiation of Arterial, Venous, and Neuropathic Ulcers

	Arterial Ulcers	**Venous Ulcers**	**Neuropathic Ulcer**
Location	Lower one third of leg, toe, feet, interdigital spaces	Typically just proximal to medial malleolus of ankle	Plantar surface of foot be neath metatarsal head
Pedal Pulses	Diminished or absent	Usually present	Diminished or absent
Appearance	Irregular shape	Irregular shape	Punched out shape
	Edges smooth, well defined	Good granulation	Good granulation
	Minimal to no granulation	Usually shallow	Callus around ulcer
	Usually deep	Marked edema	Intact skin shiny
		Intact skin dark, fibrotic	Lack of sensations
Pain	Severe pain	Minimal to moderate pain	No pain
	Increased with ambulation	Increased with ambulation	
	Decreased with rest	Decreased with elevation	

HYPERTENSION

○ **What are the mechanisms by which hypertension responds to therapeutic exercise?**

The mechanisms by which exercise training lowers BP are unclear. Possibilities include:

Decrease in plasma norepinephrine levels
Increase in circulating vasodilator substances
Amelioration of hyperinsulinemia
Alteration in renal function

○ **What is the initial response to heavy resistance exercise training?**

The cardiovascular responses to a single session of resistance exercise differ from those for endurance exercise in several fundamental ways. In particular, heavy resistance exercise elicits a pressor response that involves only moderate increases in heart rate and cardiac output, relative to those seen with dynamic exercise, but a greater elevation in systolic and diastolic BP. With the exception of circuit weight training, chronic strength or resistive training has not consistently been shown to lower resting BR.

○ **What recommendations have been established by the JNC on HTN?**

Blood Pressure Stage (mm Hg)	Risk Group A No major risk factors No TOD/CCD	Risk Group B At least one major risk factor, not including DM No TOD/CCD	Risk Group C TOD/CCD and/or DM, with or without other risk factors
High-Normal BP 130-139/85-89	Lifestyle Modification	Lifestyle Modification	Medication Lifestyle Modification
Stage 1 HTN 140-159/90-99	Lifestyle Modification (up to 12 mo)	Lifestyle Modification (up to 6 mo)	Medication Lifestyle Modification
Stage 2, 3 HTN 160/100	Medication Lifestyle Modification	Medication Lifestyle Modification	Medication Lifestyle Modification

TOD=Target organ damage; CCD=Clinical cardiovascular disease.

○ **What physiological response occurs with a single episode of dynamic exercise?**

A single session of dynamic exercise usually evokes a normal rise in systolic BP from baseline levels in unmedicated persons with hypertension, although the response may be exaggerated or diminished in certain individuals. However, because of an elevated baseline level, the absolute level of systolic BP attained during dynamic exercise is usually higher in persons with hypertension. In addition, their diastolic BP may not change, or may even slightly rise, during dynamic exercise, probably as a result of an impaired vasodilatory response.

○ **What are the physiological effects of an ongoing dynamic exercise program in patients with hypertension?**

Recent studies have documented a 10 to 20 mm Hg reduction in systolic BP during the initial 1 to 3 hours following 30 to 45 minutes of moderate intensity dynamic exercise in persons with hypertension. This response, which may persist for up to 9 hours, appears to be mediated by a transient decrease in stroke volume rather than peripheral vasodilation.

○ **What effects have been documented with endurance exercise training with regards to hemodynamics?**

Existing evidence indicates that endurance exercise training reduces the magnitude of rise in BP that can be expected over time in persons at increased risk for developing hypertension. Longitudinal studies further show that endurance training may elicit an average reduction of about 10 mmHg in both systolic and diastolic BP in persons with stage 1 or 2 hypertension. Both the Joint National Committee and ACSM (1993) advocate regular aerobic exercise as a preventive strategy to reduce the incidence of high BP, and indicate that exercise training can be effectively used as definitive or adjunctive therapy for hypertension. More recently the ACSM reasserted the role of therapeutic exercise as a central element in the management of hypertension. The new guideline entitled Exercise and Hypertension replaces ACSM's 1993 Position Stand, Physical Activity, Physical Fitness, and Hypertension.

○ **What is the influence of antihypertensives on the therapeutic exercise response?**

Beta-blockers and, to a lesser degree, the calcium antagonists diltiazem and verapamil reduce the heart rate response to submaximal and maximal exercise. In contrast, dihydropyridine-derivative calcium antagonists and direct vasodilators may increase the heart rate response to submaximal exercise. With the exception of beta-blockers, most antihypertensive agents do not substantially alter the systolic BP response to a single session of dynamic exercise, however, they do lower the resting BP and therefore the absolute level attained. Antihypertensive agents that reduce total peripheral resistance by vasodilation may predispose to postexercise hypotension. This potential adverse effect can usually be prevented by avoidance of abrupt cessation of exercise and use of a longer cool down period. Diuretics may result in serum potassium derangements and thereby accentuate the risk for exercise induced dysrhythmias.

○ **Summarize the guidelines for the clinical evaluation and exercise recommendations for key different patient populations with hypertension.**

Program Element	Adolescent	Obese	Diabetic	Adult Onset	Elderly
Patient selection and evaluation	Prescribe antihypertensive medication to reduce baseline resting pressure Switch to an endurance sport; heavy-resistance sports are contraindicated	Look for associated diseases: diabetes, mellitus, ischemic heart disease, peripheral vascular disease Emphasize weight loss as the first priority Prescribe a walking program as tolerated to lose some weight before testing	Exclude silent MI Look for associated diseases: lipid disorders, retinopathy, peripheral neuropathy, peripheral vascular disease, renal insufficiency, depressed left ventricular function Control blood glucose Modify drugs and diet to avoid exercise-induced hypoglycemia	Address individualized risk factors; query for other comorbid diseases; query family history	Give precautions for falls Check for musculoskeletal diseases: osteoarthritis, osteoporosis, herniated disk, fractures Look for associated and underlying diseases, especially neurologic or cardiovascular disorders
Exercise testing and monitoring	GXT with Bruce protocol to gauge magnitude of BP response during exercise and rate of recovery	GXT with a modified Naughton protocol	GXT with a modified Naughton protocol Rule out asymptomatic ischemic heart disease Radionuclide imaging if needed	For patients without risk factors, begin with a walking program without a maximal GXT For others, GXT with a modified Naughton protocol	GXT with a modified Naughton protocol
Exercise type	Aerobic activities: jogging, biking, swimming Circuit weight training	Aerobic, low-impact activities: walking until weight loss is 10%-15%, then biking, step-climbing, swimming, treadmill walking	Aerobic, low-impact activities: walking, biking, swimming	Aerobic activities: jogging; if more than 40 yr. old, low-impact exercise: walking, swimming, biking	Aerobic, low-impact activities: walking, biking, swimming, tai chi
Frequency	6-7 days/wk	5 days/wk (minimum)	5 days/wk (minimum)	5 days/wk (minimum)	2-5 days/wk (minimum)
Intensity	Up to 85% of maximum HRR or 85% of maximal heart rates	Start at 50%-60% maximum HRR and lowly increase to 70%; within 6 wk, work at 85% HRR or from	Start at 50%-60% maximum HRR and slowly increase to 70%; within 6 wk, work at 85% HRR or from 50%-90% of maximal	Start at 50%-60% maximum HRR and slowly increase to 70%; within 6 wk, work at 85% HRR or from 50%-90% of maximal heart rate	Start at 50%-60% maximum HRR and slowly increase to 70%; within 6 wk, work at 85% HRR or from 50%-90% of maximal heart rate

		50%-90% of maximal heart rate	heart rate		
Duration	45-50 min/day	20-30 min/day of continuous activity for first 3 wk, then 30-45 min/day for next 4 to 6 wk, and 60 min/day as maintenance	20-30 min/day of continuous activity for first 3 wk, then 30-45 min/day for next 4 to 6 wk, and 60 min/day as maintenance	20-30 min/day of continuous activity for first 3 wks, then 30-45 min/day for the next 4-6 wk, then 30-45 min/day for next 4-6 wk, and 60 min/day as maintenance	Duration depends on intensity of the activity: lower intensity for longer periods, can start with 20-30 min/day of continuous activity for first 3 wk, then 30-45 min/day for next 4-6 wk, and 60 min/day as maintenance

MI = myocardial infarction; GXT = graded exercise test; BP = blood pressure; HRR = heart resting rate

LYMPHATICS AND LYMPHEDEMA

○ **What is the function of the lymphatic system?**

The function of the lymphatic system is to collect fluid as well as protein, red blood cells, bacteria, and other particles that are too large to drain through small venules. Lymph is transported from lymphatic capillaries through afferent vessels to regional lymph nodes, and then trans-ported through the thoracic duct to the subclavian vein, or through other lymphovenous communications to the peripheral vessels. Lymph channels normally achieve central flow through the combined effect of lymphatic valves, muscular contractions, respiration, and arterial pulsation.

○ **What is lymphedema?**

Lymphedema results from an excessive accumulation of fluid associated with disruption or compromise of the lymph channels. The lymphatics normally protect against bacterial invasion; thus, limbs with lymphedema are at increased risk of infection.

○ **How do clinicians classify lymphedema?**

Lymphedema has been classified based on etiology, severity, time of onset, and anatomic features. Primary lymphedema is congenital and results from agenesis (complete failure to develop) or aplasia (poor development) of the lymphatic system. Primary lymphedema is typically noted in young females and characterized by diffuse swelling of the lower extremities. Lymphedema praecox generally occurs in females in the second or third decade of life and lymphedema tarda is characterized by onset after age 3. Hyperplasia can also result in a small percentage of cases of primary lymphedema. Secondary lymphedema is acquired and may occur in association with malignancy, radiation, trauma, surgical excision, inflammation or infection, parasitic invasion (filariasis), sarcoidosis, paralysis, and acquired immuno deficiency syndrome.

○ **What are the basic features of lymphedema treatment?**

Treatment should be multidisciplinary and include both hygienic and mechanical components.

○ **What is the association between lymphedema and breast cancer in women?**

Breast cancer affects one in nine women in the United States. Modified radical mastectomy with corresponding lymphadenectomy and radiation results in clinically symptomatic lymphedema in a significant portion of the postmastectomy patients, with reported incidence ranging from 5.5% to 80.0%. The diagnosis can usually be made 6 weeks after breast cancer surgery, when postsurgical swelling has subsided.

○ **What are treatment goals in lymphedema management?**

Goals of treatment include relief of pain and discomfort, restoration of normal movement and body image, and psychosocial adjustment. Patient education, skin hygiene, and avoidance of injury are of primary importance.

○ **What physical interventions are recommended?**

Elevation is recommended to reduce edema. Additionally, compression garments, elastic bandaging, massage, manual lymph drainage, and therapeutic exercises can reduce edema and the feeling of heaviness in the arm. Pneumatic compression pumps have shown some evidence of success but remain controversial.

○ **What is sub contraction high voltage stimulation?**

Subcontracting high voltage electrical stimulation in the rat increased lymphatic uptake of labeled protein; it has been suggested that this modality has the potential to reduce edema. In one clinical trial, however, electrically stimulated lymphatic drainage did not demonstrate any benefit over treatment with an elastic sleeve. A combination of techniques to treat lymphedema has been referred to as manual lymphatic therapy. This includes skin hygiene, a special lymphatic massage, compression bandaging, compression garments, and exercises.

O   **What is the rationale for intermittent compression therapy?**

Intermittent pneumatic compression is used in the treatment of lymphedema as well as the treatment of edema associated with venous insufficiency, venous ulceration, postoperative or posttraumatic edema, and prevention of DVT. While devices that apply intermittent compression of uniform strength (single chamber) are available, those that produce sequential gradient compression (multi-chamber graded) have received the most attention.

O   **How do single vs. multiple chamber intermittent pneumatic compression therapy compare?**

Theoretically, the disadvantage of a single-chamber device is related to high pressure exerted proximally and distally, potentially forcing fluid into the distal portion of the extremity. In a comparison of multi chamber to single-chamber devices in the treatment of lymphedema, the multi chamber device decreased edema faster both in the upper and in the lower extremities, with treatment times of 2 hours with the multi chamber device and 6 hours with the single chamber device.

O   **Is there evidence of the efficacy for the use of intermittent pneumatic compression therapy in lymphedema?**

In the treatment of lymphedema of the lower extremity, favorable outcomes were reported using a protocol consisting of 2 to 3 days of hospitalization with daily 6 to 8 hour treatment with sequential high-pressure intermittent pneumatic compression using the Lymphapress device, followed by the use of custom two-way stretch elastic stocking.

O   **What maintenance therapy is recommended for the treatment of lymphedema?**

Once reduction in limb size is achieved through pneumatic compression, elevation, and other methods, maintenance of limb size largely depends on the use of external support devices. Over the counter graduated elastic support stockings are sufficient in some patients but when there is severe edema or an unusual leg shape, custom-made stockings are necessary. Compression categories for elastic stockings include 20 to 30, 30 to 40, 40 to 50, and 50 to 60 mm Hg. Treatment of lymphedema generally requires a pressure of at least 40 to 50 mm Hg. Lower pressure compression stockings can be useful in cases of venous insufficiency, particularly when the use of high pressure compression stockings is limited by arthritis or arterial occlusive disease.

O   **Why are women with breast cancer at risk for lymphedema?**

Any dissection of axillary lymphatics and nodes places a woman at risk for edema of the arm. Axillary surgery and Radiation can lead to lymphedema, which may be caused by direct damage to axillary lymphatics. Fibrosis of the axilla secondary to surgery and/or radiation causes venous and lymphatic obstruction by compressing major vascular trunks and blocking regeneration of lymphatic and venous collaterals. Additional radiation therapy, trauma, and infections are other causative factors.

O   **What is late arm edema?**

Development of late arm edema is associated with age, extensive cancer within the axilla, extent of axillary dissection, and dose and techniques for administration of radiation. Nearly 33% of patients aged greater than 55 years and 25% of patients with more than 15 nodes dissected developed 2 cm or greater difference in the circumference of their arms by 3 years. Late breast edema, after axillary dissection performed in conjunction with breast-preservation surgery, is less common, so always consider the presence of an infection or recurrent cancer as possible causes for late edema.

O   **What does the evaluation of late arm edema entail?**

Perform a medical assessment to determine the cause of swelling. Rule out or treat infection, venous thrombosis, or cancer recurrence. Prescribe antibiotics if development of edema is acute. Make serial measurements of both arms with the olecranon as reference point. Assess shoulder, arm, and hand strength; sensory changes; color; turgor; pulses; and mobility. Long-standing lymphedema can rarely lead to lymphangiosarcoma, a highly aggressive tumor with poor survival despite forequarter amputation.

O   **What are the necessary components to conservative management of lymphedema?**

Conservative management of lymphedema should include preventive and mechanical modalities as needed. Pharmacologic means include antibiotic prophylaxis to prevent and treat cellulitis and lymphangitis. Drugs such as anticoagulants, hyaluronidase, pyridoxine, benzopyrones and others have been used but have no proven therapeutic value. Preventive care should emphasize identification of patients at highest risk of lymphedema. Comorbid illnesses such as hypertension, heart disease, and diabetes and kidney disease can contribute to edema also. Patients should understand lymphatic drainage, pathology leading to lymphedema, signs, symptoms and complications of lymphedema.

O   **What are the self-care instructions given to women with lymphedema?**

Proper nutrition with balanced nutrition, higher protein and lower salt intake
Weight management
When possible, arm should be elevated above the level of heart
Home exercise program
ROM exercises
Exercises and techniques to improve venous drainage
The importance of gravitational drainage
Static resistance exercises and positional changes need to be incorporated into daily activities, including positioning for sleep
No heavy lifting with involved arm, typically less than 15 lbs.
Injury and infection should be avoided
No venipuncture or finger sticks on the involved side
Skin breaks should be cleaned with mild soap and water, followed by antibacterial ointment use
Long sleeve shirts and bug-repellents for prevention of bug bites
Use of gloves during gardening
Use of electric razor for shaving
Good nail care, including not cutting the cuticles
Gauze wrapping instead of tape use
Physician should be notified with rashes, erythema, swelling, pain, increased warmth or with localized infection
Daily cleaning and lubrication of skin
Avoid constrictive pressure on arm
No blood pressure cuff
No constrictive bands
Follow up with physician regularly and with sudden change in arm circumference, as well as evidence of infection

O   **What is manual lymph drainage (MLD)?**

MLD is a superficial massage that has been shown to facilitate resorption of the large protein molecules found in lymph fluid, and increase the frequency of lymph vessel contraction thus increasing lymph circulation.

O   **What is complex lymphedema therapy (CLT)?**

Complex lymphedema therapy is used to treat peripheral lymphedema. This therapy consists of manual compression, external compressive bandaging and specific therapy exercises, including manual and massage techniques. The basic concept of CLT is to maximize central lymphatic drainage. This is accomplished by opening collateral vessels to channel peripheral lymph into normally functioning lymphatics. Reduction of fluid, relief of discomfort, restoration of function, decreased incidence of infection, and the ability to manage the lymphedema either independently or with the assistance of a caregiver are the goals of treatment.

O   **What is appropriate counseling to offer women with lymphedema?**

Counsel patient regarding the permanent nature of the condition and how to prevent progression. It is important to remember that with increased interstitial protein, progressive fibrosis and "chronic inflammation" can ensue. Although time consuming, particularly in its initial phases, treatment is associated with improved body image and function, thus increasing quality of life (QOL). Arm swelling has been associated with greater psychiatric morbidity, as reflected by anxiety, depression, and poorer adjustment to breast cancer. Consider psychological intervention when lymphedema is obvious to the casual observer.

PULMONARY REHABILITATION

O   **To what degree does chronic obstructive pulmonary disease (COPD) contribute to morbidity and mortality?**

An estimated 15 million to 25 million Americans suffer from chronic obstructive pulmonary disease (COPD), a term that includes emphysema and chronic bronchitis. The impact of COPD is major: Not only is it responsible for 200,000 deaths yearly, but in men over 40 it ranks second only to coronary heart disease as a cause of disability.

O   **How does the pathophysiology of COPD limit exercise and activity tolerance?**

In most individuals, cardiac response or muscle endurance, not lung function, is the limiting factor in exercise capacity. The normal lung can move a tremendous volume of oxygen, more than enough to satisfy the demands of physical exertion. But the increased airway resistance and hyperinflation that characterize COPD dramatically raise a patient's metabolic cost of breathing. In pulmonary patients, up to 40% of total oxygen intake during low-level exercise is devoted to the respiratory muscles, compared to 10% to 15% in healthy persons.

O   **What are the consequences of respiratory disease in general?**

Types of Secondary Morbidity	Mechanism(s)
Peripheral muscle dysfunction	Deconditioning, steroid myopathy, ICU neuropathy, malnutrition, decreased lean body mass, fatigue, effects of hypoxemia, acid-base disturbance, electrolyte abnormalities
Respiratory muscle dysfunction	Mechanical disadvantage secondary to hyperinflation, malnutrition, diaphragmatic fatigue, steroid myopathy, electrolyte abnormalities
Nutritional abnormality	Obesity, cachexia, decreased lean body mass
Cardiac impairment	Deconditioning, car pulmonale
Skeletal disease	Osteoporosis, kyphoscoliosis
Sensory deficits (impaired vision, hearing, etc.)	Medications (e.g., steroids, diuretics, antibiotics)
Psychosocial	Anxiety, depression, guilt, panic, dependency, cognitive deficit, sleep disturbance, sexual dysfunction

O   **What non-COPD indications are there for pulmonary rehabilitation?**

NON-COPD INDICATIONS FOR PULMONARY REHABILITATION

Asthma
Chest wall disease
Cystic fibrosis
Interstitial lung disease, including post-ARDS pulmonary fibrosis
Lung cancer
Selected neuromuscular diseases
Perioperative states (e.g., thoracic, abdominal surgery)
Postpolio syndrome
Pre-lung and post-lung transplantation
Pre-lung and post-lung volume reduction surgery

O   **What are the goals of pulmonary rehabilitation?**

Practical goals of pulmonary rehabilitation programs

Reduce work of breathing
Improve pulmonary function
Normalize arterial blood gases
Alleviate dyspnea
Increase efficiency of energy use
Correct poor nutrition
Improve exercise performance and activities of daily

living
Restore a positive outlook
Improve emotional state
Decrease health-related costs
Lengthen survival

○   **What efficacy has been demonstrated for pulmonary rehabilitation programs?**

Outcomes of pulmonary rehabilitation in patients with advanced COPD (chronic obstructive pulmonary disease)

Outcome	Source of data
Large and significant increase in exercise endurance	Well-controlled, randomized studies
Modest increase in exercise work capacity	Well-controlled, randomized studies
Changes in biochemical muscle enzymes (the effects of which are controversial)	Well-controlled, randomized studies and well-designed controlled trials in small numbers of patients
Significant reduction of dyspnea	Well-controlled, randomized studies
Improved quality of life	Well-controlled, randomized studies
Reduced health-related costs	Multiple time series

○   **What are the key elements that comprise a clinical evaluation and exercise prescription for the COPD patient?**

Evaluation
Assess cardiac risk
Assess exercise capacity with the Naughton protocol using a treadmill or stationary cycle, starting at a low workload and increasing extremely slowly, and monitoring desaturation with a pulse oximeter
Determine appropriate exercise levels to prevent arrhythmias or hypoxia in cardiac-impaired patients
Determine the amount of supplemental oxygen needed during exercise
Determine need for bronchodilators during exercise
Assess side effects of beta-agonist inhalers or aminophylline derivatives during exercise
Supervised Exercise
Direct patient to a supervised rehabilitation program if disease is significant
Set a goal of eventually graduating to independent exercise (many patients can do this in about 6 weeks)
Independent Exercise
Suggest an appropriate training mode: stationary cycling, bicycling, treadmill walking, outdoor walking, stair climbing, or arm ergometry
Set a goal of 60% to 80% of maximum heart rate for 20 to 30 minutes, 3 days a week (but build on individual ability)
Expect a 70% to 80% increase over initial work capacity within 6 weeks
Provide active encouragement and reassurance (especially at first) to overcome anxiety associated with dyspnea
Exercise Aids
Oxygen supplementation
Bronchodilators (adrenergic agonists, anticholinergic derivatives, leukotriene inhibitors)

Mucolytics
Corticosteroids (inhaled or oral)
Monitoring

○ **How can the specific exercise prescription accommodate the specific exercise limitations in COPD?**

Specific Exercise Limitation	Thresholds Influencing Intensity Range	Focus of Exercise Prescription
Physical deconditioning (i.e., premature lactic acidosis)	Lactic acidosis (metabolic threshold)	**Reconditioning exercise** Target intensity should be above metabolic threshold
Ventilatory limitation (e.g., VEmax > MVV)	Dyspnea	**Increase ventilatory capacity**
	Hypoxemia Lactic acidosis (metabolic acidosis) Offer ventilatory assistance Hypoventilation	Improve respiratory system mechanics (PFTs) Increase respiratory muscle strength **Reduce ventilatory requirement** Prevent desaturation with supplemental oxygen Mitigate lactic acidosis through reconditioning
Ventilatory inefficiency (e.g., dynamic hyperinflation in COPD or high VD/VT)	Bronchospasm or airway collapse	**Relieve expiratory airflow obstruction**
	Tachypnea Hypoventilation	Optimize bronchodilator therapy **Reduce respiratory rate** Teach breathing techniques Teach panic control
Gas exchange failure (i.e., hypoxemia or hypercapnia)	Desaturation Respiratory acidosis	**Prevent hypoxemia and hypoventilation** Use supplemental oxygen Offer assisted ventilation
Cardiovascular limitations (e.g., myocardial ischemia, hypertension, pulmonary vascular disease)	Angina	**Cardiovascular monitoring**
	Hypertension Dysrhythmia	ECG telemetry BP during exercise Adjust intensity range for safety Adjust cardiovascular medications
Symptomatic limitations	Dyspnea Anxiety Fear	**Psychotherapy** Desensitization Mastery Panic control

○ **What are the educational components of pulmonary rehabilitation?**

COMMON TOPICS ADDRESSED IN EDUCATIONAL COMPONENT
Anatomy and physiology of the lung
Pathophysiology of lung disease
Airway management
Breathing training strategies
Energy conservation and work simplification techniques
Medications
Self-management skills
Benefits of exercise and safety guidelines
Oxygen therapy
Environmental irritant avoidance
Respiratory and chest therapy techniques
Symptom management
Psychological factors-coping, anxiety, panic control
Stress management

End of life planning
Smoking cessation
Travel/leisure/sexuality
Nutrition

○ **What is ventilatory therapy?**

This includes controlled breathing techniques (diaphragmatic breathing, pursed-lip breathing, and forward-bending exercises) and chest physical therapy (postural drainage, chest percussion, and vibration). The controlled breathing exercises help decrease dyspnea, and chest drainage enhances removal of secretions. Benefits include less dyspnea and anxiety, fewer panic attacks, and improved sense of well-being.

○ **What is breathing training?**

This helps control respiratory rate and breathing patterns, thus decreasing air trapping. It also attempts to decrease the work of breathing and improve the position and function of the respiratory muscles. The easiest of these maneuvers is pursed-lip breathing. Patients inhale through the nose and exhale for 4 and 6 seconds through lips pursed in a whistling or kissing position. The exact mechanism by which this decreases dyspnea is unknown. It does not seem to change functional residual capacity or oxygen uptake, but it does decrease respiratory frequency and increase tidal volume.

○ **What is the role of forward bending posture?**

Forward bending posture has been shown to decrease dyspnea in some patients with severe COPD, both at rest and during exercise. The best explanation is that increased gastric pressure during forward bending allows better diaphragmatic contraction. These changes can also be seen in the supine and Trendelenburg positions.

○ **What is diaphragmatic breathing?**

Diaphragmatic breathing changes the breathing pattern from one where the rib cage muscles are the predominant pressure generators to a more normal one, where the pressures are generated with the diaphragm.

○ **How is it taught?**

The technique can be taught by having the supine patient place a hand on the abdomen and breathe in. With proper diaphragmatic breathing, the hand moves up on inspiration. The patient then exhales with pursed lips and is encouraged to use the abdominal muscles to return the diaphragm to a more lengthened, resting position. After using diaphragmatic breathing in the supine position, the patient is encouraged to try it while standing. Diaphragmatic breathing is most helpful when used for at least 20 minutes two or three times daily.

○ **What is the physiological response to diaphragmatic breathing?**

Although most patients report improvement in dyspnea and clinical perception of symptoms with diaphragmatic breathing, little or no change occurs in oxygen uptake and resting lung volume. Respiratory rate and minute ventilation usually fall and tidal volume increases.

○ **What is chest physical therapy?**

This approach includes postural drainage, chest percussion, vibration, and directed cough. The goal is to remove airway secretions and decrease airflow resistance and bronchopulmonary infection. The single most important criterion for chest physical therapy is the presence of sputum production. Postural drainage uses gravity to help clear the individual lung segments. Chest percussion also assists drainage but should be used with care in patients with osteoporosis or bone problems.

○ **Compare directed and controlled cough?**

Although cough is effective for removing excess mucus from the larger airways, patients with COPD often have impaired cough mechanisms. Maximum expiratory flow is reduced, ciliary beat is impaired, and the mucus itself has abnormal viscoelastic properties. Directed cough is preferred, and cough spasms should be avoided because of risks of dyspnea, fatigue, and increased obstruction. With controlled coughs, patients are instructed to inhale deeply, hold their breath for a few seconds, and then cough two or three times with the mouth open. They are also taught to tighten the upper abdominal muscles to assist in the cough.

○   **What effect does chest physical therapy have on pulmonary function?**

Pulmonary function does not improve with any of these techniques. Nonetheless, studies show that programs using postural drainage, percussion, vibration, and cough increase the clearance of inhaled radiotracers and increase sputum volume and weight.

○   **What is ventilatory muscle training?**

Specific respiratory muscle training can improve strength and endurance. Because inspiratory muscles tend to be weakened in patients with COPD, the role of respiratory muscle training in these patients has been viewed with great interest. Strength training has limited clinical significance.

○   **Is ventilatory muscle training efficacious?**

In controlled trials, endurance training has increased the time that ventilatory muscles can tolerate a known load. Some data show a significant increase in strength and a decrease in dyspnea during inspiratory load and exercise. In studies where exercise performance was evaluated, the increase in walking distance proved to be minimal. While ventilatory muscle training with resistive breathing improves muscle strength and endurance, it has marginal effects on overall exercise performance. Whether this effort results in decreased morbidity or mortality or offers any other clinical advantage is not clear.

MUSCULOSKELETAL MEDICINE

○ **What is rheumatoid arthritis (RA)?**

Rheumatoid arthritis (RA) is a chronic systemic inflammatory disease of unknown cause that primarily affects the peripheral joints in a symmetric pattern. Constitutional symptoms, including fatigue, malaise, and morning stiffness, are common. Extra-articular involvement of organs such as the skin, heart, lungs, and eyes can be significant. RA causes joint destruction and thus often leads to considerable morbidity and mortality.

○ **What is the incidence of rheumatoid arthritis?**

The worldwide incidence of RA is approximately 3 cases per 10,000 population, and the prevalence rate is approximately 1%. The prevalence of definite RA among adults in the USA has been estimated to be approximately 10 per 1000, with an overall prevalence of 7 per 1000 for men and 16 per 1000 for women RA affects all populations, although a few groups have much higher prevalence rates (eg, 5-6% in some Native American groups) and some have lower rates (eg, black persons from the Caribbean region). First-degree relatives of patients with RA have an increased frequency of disease (approximately 2-3%).

○ **What are the gender and age profiles for RA?**

Women are affected approximately 3 times more often than men. Sex differences diminish in older age groups. Although RA can occur at any age, the incidence increases with advancing age. Sex differences diminish in older age groups. The peak incidence of RA occurs in individuals aged 40-60 years.

○ **Is there a difference in extraarticular disease activity pattern between males and females?**

It also should be noted that characteristics other than distribution of articular lesions have reportedly differed between men and women with rheumatoid arthritis. For example, male patients with the disease have been found to have more severe joint destruction, a higher prevalence of rheumatoid nodules, and frequent vasculitis and pulmonary involvement.

○ **What is the pathophysiology of RA?**

RA has an unknown cause. Although an infectious etiology has been speculated (eg, *Mycoplasma* organisms, Epstein-Barr virus, parvovirus, rubella), no organism has been proven responsible. RA is associated with a number of autoimmune responses, but whether autoimmunity is a secondary or primary event is still unknown.

○ **What genetic factors contribute to RA?**

RA has a significant genetic component, and the so-called shared epitope of the HLA-DR4/DR1 cluster is present in up to 90% of patients with RA, although it is also present in more than 40% of controls.

○ **What cellular and humoral mechanisms play key roles in the pathogenesis of RA?**

Major cellular roles are played by CD4 T cells, mononuclear phagocytes, fibroblasts, osteoclasts, and neutrophils, while B-lymphocytes produce autoantibodies (i.e., rheumatoid factors [RFs]). Abnormal production of numerous cytokines, chemokines, and other inflammatory mediators (eg, tumor necrosis factor alpha [TNF-alpha, interleukin (IL)–1, IL-6, transforming growth factor beta, IL-8, fibroblast growth factor, platelet-derived growth factor) have been demonstrated in patients with RA.

○ **Is the difference between RA and other inflammatory arthropathies solely based on immune mediators such as cytokines?**

The major difference between RA and other forms of inflammatory arthritis, such as psoriatic arthritis, does not lie in their cytokine patterns but rather in the highly destructive potential of the RA synovial membrane and in the local and systemic autoimmunity. Synovial cell hyperplasia and endothelial cell activation are early events in the pathologic process that progresses to uncontrolled inflammation and consequent cartilage and bone destruction.

○   **What are the revised criteria for the diagnosis of rheumatoid arthritis (RA)?**

1988 Revised American Rheumatism Association Criteria for Classification of Rheumatoid Arthritis [*]

Criterion	Definition
1. Morning stiffness	Morning stiffness in and around the joints lasting at least 1 hr before maximal improvement
2. Arthritis of three or more joint areas	At least three joint areas simultaneously having soft tissue swelling or fluid (not bony overgrowth alone) observed by a physician (the 14 possible joint areas are [right or left] PIP, MCP, wrist, elbow, knee, ankle, and MTP joints)
3. Arthritis of hand joints	At least one joint area swollen as above in wrist, MCP, or PIP joint
4. Symmetric arthritis	Simultaneous involvement of the same joint areas (as in criterion 2) on both sides of the body (bilateral involvement of PIP, MCP, or MTP joints is acceptable without absolute symmetry)
5. Rheumatoid nodules	Subcutaneous nodules over bony prominences or extensor surfaces, or in juxta-articular regions, observed by a physician
6. Serum rheumatoid factor	Demonstration of abnormal amounts of serum "rheumatoid factor" by any method that has been positive in less than 5 percent of normal control subjects
7. Radiographic changes	Changes typical of RA on PA hand and wrist radiographs, which must include erosions or unequivocal bony decalcification localized to or most marked adjacent to the involved joints (osteoarthritis changes alone do not qualify)

Abbreviations: MCP, Metacarpophalangeal; MTP, metatarsophalangeal; PA, posteroanterior; PIP, proximal interphalangeal; RA, rheumatoid arthritis.

*For classification purposes, a patient is said to have RA if he or she has satisfied at least four of the seven criteria. Criteria 1 through 4 must be present for at least 6 weeks. Patients with two clinical diagnoses are not excluded. Designation as classic, definite, or probable rheumatoid arthritis is not to be made.

○   **Compare the characteristics of RA in younger and older patients**

Characteristics of rheumatoid arthritis in younger versus older patients

Younger patients	Older patients
Female preponderance	Women and men equally affected
Insidious onset	Acute onset
Small joints of hands and feet affected	Large proximal joints affected
Fewer systemic manifestations	More systemic manifestations, including elevated acute phase reactants
Rheumatoid factor test usually positive	Rheumatoid factor test usually negative

○   **Compare RA with JRA**

Similarities and differences between RA and JRA/JIA

Feature	RA	JRA/JIA
Classification criteria	Single disease with different manifestations	Phenotypically and genetically distinct subtypes
Gender	Females > males	Females > males except in systemic arthritis
Age of onset	Puberty plus; peak 4th to 5th decade	Polyarticular: throughout childhood; peak 1-3 years of age
		Pauciarticular: early childhood; peak 1-2 years of age
		Systemic: throughout childhood; no peak
Extended multiplex families	Present	Very rare
Family history of other autoimmune disorders	Present	Present
Typical ocular involvement	Keratoconjunctivitis sicca	Chronic anterior uveitis

Prevalence	10/1000	0.86/1000
Ethnic distribution	Reported in all populations	EOPA is rare in non-Caucasians
HLA association	*HLA DRB1*0401, 0404, 0101* in Caucasians	EOPA: HLA-A2, -DR5, -DR8, *-DPB1*0201*. (HLA-DR4 is protective)
		Late pauciarticular: HLA-B27
		Polyarticular: HLA-DR1, -DR4
Shared epitope	Defined; amino acid positions 67-74 of third hypervariable region	Not described
Growth/developmental issues	Rare	Common
Pathophysiology	Th1-mediated disease	Th1-mediated disease (Pauciarticular: Also Th2-mediated)
Autoantibodies	IgM RF common	IgM RF rare
Natural history	Majority have long-term disability	Fewer than half have long-term disability

EOPA, early-onset pauciarticular arthritis; HLA, human leukocyte antigen; JIA, juvenile idiopathic arthritis; JRA, juvenile rheumatoid arthritis; RA, rheumatoid arthritis; RF, rheumatoid factor; Th, T helper.

O **What are the different clinical courses of rheumatoid arthritis?**

There are now believed to be 3 characteristic clinical courses of RA: course I, monocyclic; course II, polycyclic; and course III, progressive. In a given patient, it is not possible to predict the future course of the disease at its outset. However, in the presence of subcutaneous nodules, high titer of RhF, and erosive x-ray changes, rapid progression and destructive changes are inevitable.

Course I monocyclic	Course II polycyclic	Course III progressive
Approximately one third of all patients who develop RA undergo complete and permanent remission within 2 years of disease onset, with or without treatment. The course is benign and self-limiting.	This is a slow, progressive course with moderate activity interspersed with short episodes of acute arthritis. Periods of acute activity become more sustained with the passage of time. This is also known as the palindromic type of RA, and it affects around 40% of patients.	This course affects approximately 20% of patients. It represents an unrelenting, progressive, and destructive form of RA with deformity, disfigurement, and even death.

O **What prodromal symptoms are common in RA?**

Various prodromal symptoms have been noted in rheumatoid arthritis, including fatigue, anorexia, weight loss, malaise, and muscular pain and stiffness.

O **What are the typical symptoms and signs of articular involvement?**

Articular involvement becomes manifest as pain that is aggravated on motion, swelling, stiffness, and limitation of movement. Redness, a clinical feature that may be associated with joint inflammation, is extremely rare in rheumatoid arthritis. Periarticular soft tissue swelling that is fusiform or spindle-shaped in configuration due to increased intra articular fluid, synovial hypertrophy, and thickening of adjacent soft tissues is accentuated by atrophy of contiguous muscles.

O **What joints are commonly involved in RA?**

The most typically affected joints are the proximal interphalangeal and metacarpophalangeal joints of the hand, the wrist, the metatarsophalangeal joints of the foot, the knee, the joints of the shoulder, the ankle, and to a lesser extent, the hip; any joint can be involved, however, including the temporomandibular and cricoarytenoid articulations. Symmetry is the hallmark of joint alteration in this disease; in most patients, a remarkable degree of symmetry is demonstrated in the distribution of the arthritis on both sides of the body.

O **Can RA present as a mono- or pauciarticular disease?**

Initially, monoarticular or pauciarticular abnormalities can be noted that do not obey the rule of symmetry. The reported frequency of monoarthritis in rheumatoid arthritis has varied from approximately 5 to 20 per cent of cases. It may persist for weeks or months; the knee and the wrist are the two articulations that are the most frequent sites of monoarthritis...In general, a monoarticular or pauciarticular distribution in rheumatoid arthritis will soon become symmetric.

○   **What factors are useful for differentiating RA from OA?**

Factors Useful for Differentiating Early Rheumatoid Arthritis from Osteoarthrosis (Osteoarthritis)		
	Rheumatoid Arthritis	**Osteoarthritis**
Age at onset	Childhood and adults, peak incidence in 50s	Increases with age
Predisposing factors	HLA-DR4, -DR1	Trauma, congenital abnormalities (e.g., shallow acetabulum)
Symptoms, early	Morning stiffness	Pain increases through the day and with use
Joints involved	Metacarpophalangeal joints, wrists, proximal interphalangeal joints most often; distal interphalangeal joints almost never	Distal interphalangeal joints (Heberden's nodes), weight-bearing joints (hips, knees)
Physical findings	Soft tissue swelling, warmth	Bony osteophytes, minimal soft tissue swelling early
Radiologic findings	Periarticular osteopenia, marginal erosions	Subchondral sclerosis, osteophytes
Laboratory findings	Increased erythrocyte sedimentation rate, rheumatoid factor, anemia, leukocytosis	Normal

○   **What is the utility of the rheumatoid factor?**

RF testing may be appropriate in patients suspected of having rheumatoid arthritis. The test is most useful when there is a moderate level of suspicion for rheumatoid arthritis. If clinical suspicion is low (i.e., absence of joint inflammation), RF testing is unlikely to be helpful because of the high incidence of false-positive results in the general population. Even when clinical suspicion is high, 20 percent of patients with rheumatoid arthritis are seronegative. Furthermore, up to 40 percent of patients with rheumatoid arthritis may be seronegative early in the course of the disease.

○   **Does RF testing have any prognostic value?**

In patients with rheumatoid arthritis, the RF titer generally correlates with extra-articular manifestations and disease severity. RF testing may have prognostic value in these patients. However, RF titers are not helpful in following disease progression. Once a patient has a positive RF result, repeating the test is of no value.

○   **What is the specificity and sensitivity of the RF?**

The rheumatoid factor test is used most often to diagnose rheumatoid arthritis. In an unselected population, its sensitivity is 80% and specificity 95% for this disease.

○   **Summarize other conditions that may yield a false positive RF.**

Conditions Associated with a Positive Rheumatoid Factor Test

Rheumatic conditions (prevalence)

Rheumatoid arthritis (50 to 90%)
Systemic lupus erythematosus (15 to 35%)
Sjögren's syndrome (75 to 95%)
Systemic sclerosis (20 to 30%)
Cryoglobulinemia (40 to 100%)

Mixed connective tissue disease (50 to 60%)

Nonrheumatic conditions

Aging
Infection: bacterial endocarditis, liver disease, tuberculosis, syphilis, viral infections (especially mumps, rubella and influenza), parasitic diseases
Pulmonary disease: sarcoidosis, interstitial pulmonary fibrosis, silicosis, asbestosis
Miscellaneous diseases: primary biliary cirrhosis, malignancy (especially leukemia and colon cancer)

○ **What value does the ESR offer in patients with RA?**

The ESR is a means for staging rheumatoid arthritis, rather than a major diagnostic criterion. The ESR value tends to correlate with clinical disease activity and to parallel such symptoms as morning stiffness and fatigue, although joint examination is far more useful in assessing synovitis. The sensitivity of an elevated ESR value is approximately 50 percent in patients with signs of rheumatoid arthritis. However, the specificity of an elevated ESR is quite low, limiting its use as a diagnostic test.

○ **What role does C- reactive protein play in RA diagnosis?**

The C-reactive protein concentration is another marker of systemic inflammation used to evaluate systemic rheumatic diseases, especially rheumatoid arthritis. Some rheumatologists believe the C-reactive protein concentration is more useful than the ESR because it may be less affected by other conditions, but the higher cost and longer time requirement for obtaining results have limited its popularity.

○ **What is the Anti-CCP Antibodies (Anti-Cyclic Citrullinated Peptide Antibodies) assay?**

The test is as sensitive as standard rheumatoid factor testing but more specific for rheumatoid arthritis (RA). Anti-CCP antibodies may predict those patients with "undifferentiated arthritis" who will likely go on to develop rheumatoid arthritis (93% of positives versus 25% of negatives). If positive in a patient with RA, it increases likelihood of erosive type disease i.e. a more aggressive form of the disease.

○ **When will this test be utilized in the RA patient?**

This test will be utilized early on in patients with arthritic symptoms since it is highly correlated with a diagnosis of rheumatoid arthritis. A positive result should spur the treating physician to possibly start more aggressive type therapy early on in the course of the illness to avoid the potential for erosive arthritis.

○ **What differences in RA manifestations are seen in patients with underlying neurological disease?**

A striking asymmetry or even unilateral involvement has been described in patients with poliomyelitis, meningioma, encephalitis, neurovascular syphilis, strokes, and cerebral palsy. Joints are spared on the paralyzed side, and the degree of protection demonstrates a rough correlation with the extent of paralysis. The protective effect on the affected side is less if a neurologic deficit develops in a patient who already has RA.

○ **Where are subcutaneous nodules found in patients with RA?**

Subcutaneous nodules are evident in approximately one fourth of patients with rheumatoid arthritis. They appear at pressure points, especially the juxta-articular regions of the elbow. Other tendinous and soft tissue locations commonly reveal similar nodules, and these lesions may be demonstrated in distant body sites, including the lungs, pleurae, vocal cords, larynx, scalp, sclerae, peritoneum, and abdominal wall.

○ **What patterns of muscle weakness and atrophy occur in patients with RA?**

Muscular weakness and atrophy can be prominent in patients with rheumatoid arthritis. These muscular abnormalities can relate to disuse or inflammatory changes. With regard to the inflammatory myopathy, three patterns of cellular infiltration have been defined: arteritis, polymyositis, and focal nodular myositis. None of these patterns is specific for rheumatoid arthritis, and the relationship among them is not clear. A second form of myopathy results from denervation atrophy of muscle fibers. This type of myopathy is a consequence of the peripheral neuropathy seen in the disease. Miscellaneous forms of myopathy result from muscle disuse, dystrophy-like changes, and corticosteroid therapy.

○   **What types of peripheral neuropathies are encountered in RA?**

Peripheral neuropathies in this disease are of several types. A mild or severe sensory and motor neuropathy has been noted. Its manifestations include a symmetric distribution, involvement of upper or lower extremities, a "stocking" distribution of sensory impairment, and wrist and foot drop. Vasculitis with or without toxic or metabolic factors may be responsible for this complication.

○   **What entrapment neuropathies have been described in RA?**

Entrapment or compressive neuropathies also are observed. These neuropathies, which relate to mechanical irritation of a specific peripheral nerve at a vulnerable anatomic site (within fibrous or osseofibrous canals), can affect the median nerve (carpal tunnel syndrome, , and anterior interosseous syndrome), ulnar nerve (cubital canal syndrome, canal of Guyon syndrome, and double crush syndrome), and radial nerve (posterior interosseous syndrome) in the upper extremity; and the sciatic nerve (tibial or common peroneal entrapment by a Baker's cyst), common peroneal nerve (pressure palsy), and posterior tibial nerve (tarsal tunnel syndrome, medial plantar syndrome, lateral plantar syndrome) in the lower extremity.

○   **What metabolic bone disturbances are encountered in RA patients?**

Osteopenia is a well-recognized manifestation of rheumatoid arthritis. In almost all patients, such osteopenia relates to osteoporosis, the severity of which is influenced by the age and sex of the patient, the duration of the disease, the extent of immobilization, and the administration of corticosteroids. In addition, osteomalacia related to inadequate intake of vitamin D, malabsorption, and lack of sunshine and hypercalcemia with secondary hyperparathyroidism are two additional mechanisms that may contribute to osteopenia.

○   **What pathological findings occur in the hands in patients with RA?**

The joints of the hand are affected in almost all persons with rheumatoid arthritis. Metacarpophalangeal and proximal interphalangeal joint alterations predominate. On clinical examination, fusiform soft tissue swelling is associated with tenderness elicited by firm pressure at these locations. Clinical (as well as radiologic) evidence of distal interphalangeal joint disease is less frequent and rarely is severe; however, the diagnosis of rheumatoid arthritis cannot be eliminated by the finding of involvement of the distal interphalangeal joints. Swelling on the volar aspect of the digits reflects the inflammatory changes in the flexor tendon sheaths.

○   **What findings occur in long standing disease?**

In long-standing disease, swan-neck deformities (hyperextension at proximal interphalangeal joints and flexion at distal interphalangeal joints), boutonnière deformities (flexion at proximal interphalangeal joints and hyperextension at distal interphalangeal joints), and hitchhiker's or Z-shaped deformity of the thumb (flexion at the metacarpophalangeal joint and hyperextension at the interphalangeal joint) can be observed. The articulations themselves become relatively fixed in position due to fibrous (or less commonly, bony) fusion.

○   **Can spontaneous rupture of tendons occur in RA?**

Spontaneous rupture of extensor tendons of the digits is a well-recognized complication of this disease. As at other sites, factors that appear important in the pathogenesis of these tendinous ruptures include abnormal stress, intrinsic tendon abnormality, tenosynovitis, and injury from adjacent osseous structures. Attrition and rupture of flexor tendons in the hand also are observed in rheumatoid arthritis.

○   **What radiographic findings are evident in advanced RA of the hand?**

With further destruction of cartilage and bone, the articular space may be obliterated completely. Erosion of central portions of the joint can lead to apparently enclosed radiolucent defects, cysts, or pseudocysts. In most instances, radiographs obtained in multiple projections will reveal that these defects communicate with the articular cavity, corresponding to sites of transchondral extension of pannus. The cysts usually are distributed symmetrically and most often are located about the proximal interphalangeal and metacarpophalangeal joints (as well as in the wrists and feet).

O **What are characteristic findings on radiographs of the hand in patients with RA?**

The pathological articular/periarticular changes in RA relate to synovial hypertrophy, accumulation of intra-articular fluid, soft tissue edema, and osteochondral destruction in the vicinity of inflammatory pannus, are most evident at specific target sites in the hand in rheumatoid arthritis. The second and third metacarpophalangeal joints and the third proximal interphalangeal joint may reveal the earliest abnormalities. Subsequently fusiform soft tissue swelling, periarticular osteoporosis, concentric loss of articular space, and marginal erosions become evident at many or all of the proximal interphalangeal and metacarpophalangeal joints.

O **Where do marginal erosions occur in the hands of patients with RA?**

The marginal erosions, which occur at the osseous surfaces that do not possess protective cartilage, appear at the radial and ulnar aspects of the articulation. At both proximal interphalangeal and metacarpophalangeal joint locations, the erosions are larger on the proximal bone that constitutes the articulation (the metacarpal head at the metacarpophalangeal joint; the proximal phalanx at the proximal interphalangeal joint) because the unprotected areas are more extensive at these sites. Marginal erosions about the distal interphalangeal joints generally are small compared with those of the more proximal digital joints, although any distal interphalangeal joint can reveal focal marginal defects. The erosions at these articulations may be more common if coexisting osteoarthritis is present.

O **What is the boutonnière deformity?**

The peculiar anatomy of the three-joint system of the digits (metacarpophalangeal, proximal interphalangeal and distal interphalangeal articulations) influences the pattern of joint deformity that may accompany rheumatoid arthritis. A collapse deformity (buckling) of this system can lead to hyperextension of one joint and reciprocal flexion of the contiguous articulation. In normal situations, the balanced tendon mechanism and ligamentous restriction prevent collapse deformity of the digits, but in rheumatoid arthritis, the vulnerable balance is compromised by the direct effect of this disease on articulations, tendons, and ligaments. Flexion of the proximal interphalangeal joint combined with hyperextension at the distal interphalangeal joint produces the boutonnière deformity of the digit.

O **What is the swan neck deformity?**

Swan-neck deformity consists of hyperextension of the proximal interphalangeal joint and flexion of the distal interphalangeal joint.

O **What MCP joint anomalies have been described in RA?**

A variety of metacarpophalangeal articular deformities and deviations appear in the rheumatoid hand, including ulnar drift, extensor tendon subluxation, and palmar subluxation and flexion of the joint.

O **What is the frequency of ulnar deviation in RA?**

The reported frequency of ulnar deviation at the metacarpophalangeal joints in rheumatoid arthritis varies according to the population being studied and the techniques used to investigate the patients. In a typical population, ulnar drift has been recorded in 27 per cent of patients. In patients with more chronic disease, radiographs outline ulnar deviation in 47 percent of hands in patients with rheumatoid arthritis.

O **What is the pathogenesis of the ulnar deviation process in RA?**

The pathogenesis of ulnar drift is complex and not fully understood. An inflammatory synovitis of the metacarpophalangeal joint with a rise in intra-articular pressure appears to be the initial factor in the development of this deformity; stabilization at this articulation is sacrificed by destruction of ligamentous, capsular, and muscular tissues. Instability and ulnar deviation of extensor tendons may be another primary factor or an aggravating factor in the production of ulnar deviation. An additional contributing factor, metacarpal volar descent, results from ligamentous laxity of the fourth and fifth carpometacarpal joints. Gravity and lateral pressure on the hand produced during everyday maneuvers have been described as causes of ulnar deviation.

O   **What thumb malalignments occur in RA?**

The malalignments that are most frequently encountered in the thumb in rheumatoid arthritis are collapse deformities (boutonnière deformity) related to disturbance of function at the first metacarpophalangeal joint; swan-neck deformity, related to disturbance of function at the first carpometacarpal joint; and instability, stiffness, or pain of the interphalangeal, metacarpophalangeal, and carpometacarpal joints.

O   **What clinical findings are observed in the wrist in more advanced cases of RA?**

The more advanced clinical features of the wrist in rheumatoid arthritis relate to dorsal subluxation of the distal portion of the ulna, the carpal tunnel syndrome attributable to synovitis in the carpal tunnel with dysesthesias along the course of the median nerve, and rupture of one or more extensor tendons. The pathogenesis of extensor tendon rupture of the wrist has been related to rheumatoid involvement of the inferior radioulnar compartment with the production of irregular osseous spikes that injure the adjacent tendon or hypermobility of the ulnar head.

O   **What pattern of wrist malalignment can accompany ulnar deviation of the hand?**

Imbalance of the muscles and the tendons contributes to radial deviation at the wrist, and imbalance of the tendons also may be associated with ulnar deviation at the metacarpophalangeal joints, producing the zigzag deformity of the hand.

O   **What clinical findings are encountered on examination of the elbow in patients with RA?**

Clinical symptoms and signs are variable but can lead to considerable disability due to limitation of both flexion and extension of the joint. Additional clinical manifestations include local pain and tenderness, swelling over the lateral aspect of the joint between the radial head and the olecranon, antecubital soft tissue masses related to synovial cysts with compression of adjacent nerves, and para olecranon nodules, synovial cysts, or bursitis.

O   **What soft tissue disorder most commonly occurs in the glenohumeral joint in patients with RA?**

Rotator cuff atrophy or tear is common in long-standing rheumatoid arthritis owing to the damaging effect of the inflamed synovial tissue on the under surface of the tendons adjacent to the greater tuberosity.

O   **What is the manifestation of this pathology on plain x-ray?**

This complication can be visualized radiographically as progressive elevation of the humeral head with respect to the glenoid cavity, narrowing of the space between the top of the humerus and the inferior surface of the acromion, sclerosis and cyst formation on adjacent portions of humeral head and acromion, reversal (or concavity) of the normal convex shape of the inferior acromion, and accentuation of cystic and sclerotic changes on the superolateral aspect of the head of the humerus owing to abutment of this surface against the acromion on abduction of the shoulder.

O   **What forefoot pathology is encountered in the patient with RA?**

Clinical abnormalities of the forefoot are especially common in rheumatoid arthritis (80 to 90 per cent of patients) and may be the initial manifestation of the disease (10 to 20 per cent of patients). The metatarsophalangeal joints of the lateral digits are affected most frequently. Intermittent or constant pain, tenderness, and soft tissue swelling can be prominent findings, even in the early stage of the disease. With more long-standing arthritis, a shuffling gait and characteristic deformities appear.

O   **What common forefoot deformities are encountered in the patient with RA?**

1. Forefoot spread (spreading of the metatarsal bones due to changes in the deep transverse ligaments).

2. Hallux valgus.

3. Fibular deviation of the first to fourth digits (lateral deviation of the toes at the metatarsophalangeal joints).

4. Hammer toe (acute flexion of the distal or proximal interphalangeal joints, or both, with the distal phalanx pointing directly downward).

5. "Cock-up" toe (hyperextension of the toe at the metatarsophalangeal joint with subluxation of the phalanx above the metatarsal head).

6. Painful callosities are evident beneath the metatarsal heads (especially the second and third) and distal phalanges.

○   **What additional findings may be observed in the rheumatoid forefoot?**

Additional findings in rheumatoid arthritis include insufficiency (stress) fractures, peripheral neuropathy, tendon injury and rupture, widespread edema, and hallux rigidus.

○   **What anomalies are encountered in the midfoot of a patient with RA?**

In the midfoot in rheumatoid arthritis, weakness of the muscles and stretching of the inflamed ligaments may be followed by postural deformities. The most frequent midtarsal deformity in this disease is pes planovalgus, which was noted in 50 per cent of the women and 40 per cent of the men in one series of patients with rheumatoid arthritis. This deformity may relate to rupture of an inflamed tibialis posterior tendon.

○   **What soft tissue disorders are encountered in the heel among patients with RA?**

Retrocalcaneal bursitis is characterized by a fluctuating mass that falls to the sides of the Achilles tendon; Achilles tendinitis is associated with pain, local tenderness to palpation, and a thickened or swollen tendinous structure; and plantar fasciitis can lead to redness, swelling, and tenderness of the plantar surface of the calcaneus. In rheumatoid arthritis, retrocalcaneal bursitis is more frequent than Achilles tendinitis or plantar fasciitis.

○   **How does the frequency of ankle involvement in RA compare to the hand and knee and foot?**

The frequency of clinical and radiologic abnormalities in the ankle in rheumatoid arthritis is lower than that in the knee and the articulations of the hand, wrist, and foot.

○   **How does the frequency of hip involvement compare to the knee in RA?**

The hip is less frequently involved early in RA than in juvenile RA. Hip joint involvement must be ascertained by a careful clinical examination. Pain on the lateral aspect of the hip is often a manifestation of trochanteric bursitis rather than synovitis. About half the patients with well-established RA have radiographic evidence of hip disease.

○   **When the hip is involved what pattern of altered joint function is observed?**

Pain, tenderness, shortening of the limb, gait abnormalities, and decreased range of motion, particularly internal rotation, extension, and abduction, are the observed clinical manifestations. Soft tissue swelling on the anterior aspect of the joint and over the greater trochanter (due to bursitis) can be evident in as many as 15 per cent of patients with rheumatoid arthritis.

○   **What is acetabular protrusion?**

Acetabular protrusion, which is defined as inward movement of the acetabular line so that the distance between this line and the laterally located ilioischial line is 3 mm or more in men and 6 mm or more in women, is particularly characteristic of rheumatoid arthritis. Protrusio acetabuli has been noted in up to 14 per cent of rheumatoid arthritis patients with hip disease, especially elderly women with long-standing arthritis. The deformity commonly is bilateral and associated with subchondral cystic lesions, osseous collapse of the acetabular roof and femoral head, and osteoporosis. It progresses more rapidly in patients who bear their weight on these joints and are physically active and in those who are receiving corticosteroid medication.

○   **What are the manifestations of rheumatoid arthritis in the knee joint?**

In contrast to the hips, synovial inflammation and proliferation in the knees are readily demonstrated on physical examination. Early in knee disease, often within a week after the onset of symptoms, quadriceps atrophy is noticeable and leads to the application of more force than usual through the patella to the femoral surface. Another early manifestation of knee disease in RA is a loss of full extension, a functional loss that can become a fixed flexion contracture unless corrective measures are undertaken.

O   **What is the significance of knee joint malalignment?**

Many patients have a genu varum or valgus that precedes the onset of RA. In these individuals, it is the medial or lateral compartment that bears the most stress from the malalignment that is first symptomatic and is likely to have radiographic evidence of erosion of bone and thinning of cartilage.

O   **Why do patients with rheumatoid arthritis develop a Baker's cyst?**

Flexion of the knee that has a moderate to large effusion markedly increases the intraarticular pressure. This may cause an outpouching of posterior components of the joint, producing a popliteal or Baker's cyst. Jayson and Dixon have demonstrated that fluid from the anterior compartments of the knee may enter a popliteal cyst but does not readily return. This one-way valve may generate pressures so high in the popliteal space that it may rupture down into the calf or, less often, superiorly into the posterior thigh. Rupture occurs posteriorly between the medial head of the gastrocnemius and the tendinous insertion of the biceps.

O   **What secondary problems can arise from involvement of the cervical spine in RA?**

Approximately 60 to 80 per cent of rheumatoid arthritis patients develop symptoms and signs related to cervical spine abnormalities at some time during their illness. Pain is the most common clinical manifestation of cervical spine involvement. It may be brief or sustained in duration. In patients with atlantoaxial subluxation, pain may be expressed in the temporal and retro-orbital region; occipital pain is considered to arise from level C2-C3 or below. Weakness and abnormal mobility also can be evident. Neurologic manifestations include paresthesias, paresis, and muscle wasting; in some instances, quadriplegia and death occur.

O   **What are the findings associated with atlantoaxial subluxation in the patient with RA?**

The consensus of prior reports on anterior atlantoaxial subluxation in rheumatoid patients indicates a frequency of 20 to 25 per cent. This frequency rises with increasing severity of the disease, although in patients with significant odontoid erosions, an abnormally wide gap between the atlas and odontoid process may indicate not a lax or disrupted transverse ligament but rather an increased incongruity of apposing osseous surfaces. In postmortem studies, anterior subluxation has been noted in 11 to 46 per cent of cases of rheumatoid arthritis.

O   **What is the pathogenesis of atlantoaxial subluxation in RA?**

The pathogenesis of anterior atlantoaxial subluxation relates to the presence of transverse ligament laxity due to synovial inflammation and hyperemia of the adjacent articulations, especially that between the posterior surface of the odontoid process and the anterior surface of the ligament.

O   **What is the prognosis for patients with RA?**

Many studies of survival and prognosis in RA patients have been published in the last three decades; in almost all, an average shortening of lifespan by 3–18 years has been observed. The decreased survival of RA patients is important; severely disabled patients have a similar prognosis to 3-vessel coronary artery disease or stage IV Hodgkin's disease.

O   **What effect does the degree of disability have on prognosis and mortality in RA?**

Increased mortality and morbidity were observed in patients with severe dysfunction, as assessed by responses to a questionnaire (HAQ) on activities of daily living, modified walking time and the button test. The differences between these patients and patients with values indicating good functional capacity were highly significant. Patients with poor functional capacity had at least a three-fold relative risk of mortality over the next 9 years, with survival over the next 5 years of less than 50%. This relative risk was not explained by other baseline variables, such as age, duration of disease or other disease features.

○   **What is the rate of disability in the RA patient population?**

Functional status declines progressively with the progression of the disease; after 15 years about 60% of patients are disabled, and by 30 years 90% are disabled.

○   **What instruments are utilized to assess quality of life and function in patients with RA?**

There are various ways to estimate functional capacity based on joint mobility or the ability to perform certain tasks as evaluated by an observer. The most widespread methods currently used consist of specific questionnaires for rheumatic disease such as the HAQ or its abbreviated form, the Modified Health Assessment Questionnaire (MHAQ), or the Arthritis Impact Measurement Scale (AIMS). They are based on the patient's own opinion about his or her disease. These questionnaires are standardized instruments of proven validity and reliability. They evaluate those health dimensions that are most affected by RA, particularly disability, especially in relation to physical function, and pain.

○   **What morbidity and disability occurs in association with RA?**

Daily living activities are impaired in most patients. Spontaneous clinical remission is uncommon (approximately 5-10%). After 5 years of disease, approximately 33% of patients will not be working; after 10 years, approximately half will have substantial functional disability. Although work disability is associated with more severe joint swelling, radiographic joint damage or an elevated level of ESR and rheumatoid factor, it is more likely to be associated with age, occupation, education and functional disability than with these traditional measures of disease status.

○   **How does the mortality for RA patients differ from the normal (unaffected) population?**

Life expectancy for patients with RA is shortened by 5-10 years, although those who respond to therapy may have lower mortality rates. Overall, the frequencies of various attributable acute causes of death in patients with RA do not differ from those in the general population, although patients with RA are more likely to have their acute cause of death attributed to infection, renal disease, respiratory disease or gastrointestinal disease

○   **What factors are associated with increased morbidity and mortality?**

Increased mortality rates are associated with poor functional status, age, male sex, socioeconomic factors (eg, level of education), positive RF findings, extra-articular disease, elevated acute phase response (erythrocyte sedimentation rate [ESR], C-reactive protein [CRP]), and increased clinical severity (eg, more involved joints). Mortality is increased by causes such as infections, cardiovascular disease, renal disease, GI bleeding, and lymphoproliferative disorders; these events may be directly due to the disease and its complications (eg, vasculitis, amyloidosis) or to therapy-induced adverse effects.

○   **Is DMARD administration associated with better functional outcomes in patients with RA?**

Eight clinical trials between 1994-2000 provided evidence based on HAQ scores. The cumulative evidence supports a beneficial effect of DMARDs in terms of slowing functional disability in RA.

○   **Is DMARD administration associated with reduced mortality in patients with RA?**

Three clinical trials between 1991-2000 provided evidence that mortality rates were reduced. The studies referred to above included patients with both early and advanced RA prior to therapy, but they nonetheless suggest that active and effective treatment with DMARDs is associated with a longer life expectancy than expected.

○   **What pharmacotherapeutic agents have been recently added to the armamentarium for the patient with RA?**

New Drugs for the Treatment of Rheumatoid Arthritis.

Drug	Primary Action	Route of Administration	Usual Dose	Half-Life

Leflunomide	Inhibits pyrimidine synthesis	Oral	Loading dose of 100 mg daily for 3 days, then 20 mg daily	2 Wk
Etanercept	Binds TNF-*a* and TNF-*b*	Subcutaneous injection	25 mg twice/wk or 50 mg once/wk	4 Days
Adalimumab	Human anti–TNF-*a* antibody	Subcutaneous injection	40 mg every second wk	2 Wk
Infliximab	Chimeric anti–TNF-*a* antibody	Intravenous infusion	3 mg/kg of body weight at 0, 2, and 6 wk, then every 8 wk; For incomplete response, maintenance dose may be gradually increased to a maximum of 10 mg/kg	9 Days
Anakinra	Interleukin-1–receptor antagonist	Subcutaneous injection	100 mg daily	6 Hr

○ What are the monitoring guidelines for these agents?

Monitoring Recommendations.

Drug	Monitoring Recommendation
Leflunomide	Obtain a complete blood count and alanine aminotransferase measurements at baseline and then monthly until stable. Usual clinical practice is to repeat these tests at intervals of 2 to 3 mo.
Etanercept	Be clinically alert for tuberculosis, histoplasmosis, and other infections.
Adalimumab	Same as for etanercept.
Infliximab	Same as for etanercept.
Anakinra	Obtain a complete blood count at baseline, monthly for 3 mo, and every 3 mo thereafter.

○ How are the more traditional DMARDs administered and monitored?

Disease-modifying antirheumatic drugs (DMARDs)

Generic (brand)	Usual dose range for arthritis	Cost Brand (generic)	Baseline evaluation	Clinical and lab monitoring
Azathioprine (Imuran)	2.5 mg/kg/d	166.80 (157.28)	CBC, platelets, SCr, LFTs	CBC, platelets q 1-2 weeks w/dose changes, then q 1-3 months, sx of myelosuppression
Cyclophosphamide (Cytoxan)	50-100 mg/d	129.50 (111.89)	CBC, platelets, U/A, SCr, LFTs	CBC, platelets q 1-2 weeks w/dose changes, then q 1-3 months, U/A q 6-12 months after cessation, sx of myelosuppression, hematuria
Cyclosporine, oral (Neoral, Sandimmune) Oral solution (Sangcya)	2.5-4 mg/kg/d	288.64 320.76, 364.25 311.03	CBC, SCr, uric acid, LFTs, BP	SCr q 2 weeks until dose stable, then monthly; periodic CBC potassium LFTs, edema, BP q 2 weeks until dosage stable then monthly
Gold Salts-Auranofin (Ridaura)	3 mg bid or 6 mg qd	135.20	CBC, platelets, U/A	CBC, platelets, U/A q 4-12 weeks, sx of myelosuppression edema, rash, diarrhea
Aurothioglucose (Solganal)	50 mg/wk	63.85		
Hydroxychloroquine sulfate (Plaquenil)	200 to 400 mg/d	44.01 (34.82)	If over age 40 or has previous eye disease	Funduscopic and visual fields q 6-12 months
Methotrexate, oral (Rheumatrex)	10-25 mg/week	71.48 (60.16)	CBC, chest X-ray, hepatitis B/C serology (high-risk pts), LFTs, albumin, SCr	CBC, platelets, LFTs, albumin, SCr q 4-8 weeks, sx of myelosuppression, shortness of breath, NV, lymph node swelling
Methotrexate, injectable	10-25 mg/week	22.52		
Minocycline (Minocin)	50-200 mg/day	64.83 (38.95)		
Sulfasalazine (Azulfidine)	2-3 grams/day	37.08 (29.27)	CBC, LFTS (high-risk pts), G6PD	CBC q 2-4 weeks for first 3 months, then q 3 months, sx of myelosuppression, photo sensitivity, rash

O **What are the revised classes of functional status of RA published by the ACR?**

The classification of global functional status was reviewed in 1991 by the American College of Rheumatology. The four revised classes are:

1. Able to perform usual activities of daily living (self care, vocational, avocational)
2. Able to perform usual self care and vocational activities, but limited in avocational activities
3. Able to perform usual self care activities, but limited in vocational and avocational activities
4. Limited in ability to perform usual self care activities, vocational and avocational activities

O **What is the role of exercise therapy in RA?**

In general, exercise routines can be categorized as passive, active, or active assisted. Active exercise is further classified as isotonic, isometric, or isokinetic. A usual regimen will be customized to a specific patient's needs and will include combinations of different types of exercises, performed either on land or in an aquatic medium (hydrotherapy). Stretching routines and recreational activity are also emphasized in such programs.

O **What evidence is there for deconditioning in RA patients?**

Evidence of deconditioning in the RA patient population exists (25% reduction and low isometric biceps and quadriceps muscle strength-between 33-52% lower). Other studies relate that RA patients had 30-45% the quadriceps strength of normals. Although endurance of muscle was measured isokinetically, it was not significantly less than normals. RA patients on low-dose corticosteroids (5-10 mg/day) have been reported to show significantly less quadriceps strength by isokinetic testing than those who received no steroid. In addition, the mean walking speed was significantly less in those receiving steroid therapy. Stamina of arthritis is also diminished as confirmed by the observation that maximum workload levels for class II RA patients are less than very sedentary controls.

O **What recommendations can be given to patients with RA regarding dynamic resistance exercise training?**

It is recommended that patients with non-acute RA receive isometric strengthening exercises of key muscle groups: quadriceps, tibialis posterior, hip abductors, forearm extensors, biceps brachii, and deltoid. Isotonic strengthening with low arc, low weight, and low repetitions should follow, provided joint alignment is reasonably well preserved. Isotonic exercise in a pool for strength and endurance is highly recommended.

O **What recommendations are appropriate with regard to stretching exercise?**

Stretching and ROM can also be done in a pool. If endurance is low, which is likely in functional class II and functional class III RA, and the joints are not acute, endurance training by ergometry or swimming is recommended provided previous strengthening with isometrics and isotonic exercise has been done.

O **What recommendations are appropriate regarding recreational exercise?**

Recreational exercise is encouraged when inflammation has abated. Adaptive handles for sports equipment may be helpful. Running, jogging, and aerobics are not recommended for patients who have lower extremity involvement of hip, knee, or ankle.

O **What is the clinical evidence supporting the efficacy and safety of therapeutic exercise in patients with RA?**

A Cochrane review of randomized controlled trials (RCTs) using dynamic exercise therapy to treat RA suggested that dynamic exercise therapy is effective at increasing aerobic capacity and muscle strength (Van den Ende et al., 2002). The majority of studies included in this review showed a positive effect of dynamic exercise therapy in reducing impairments, e.g. aerobic capacity, muscle strength or joint mobility, but only a small, not significant improvement in functional ability assessed by validated questionnaires. This discrepancy might be explained by methodological consequences related to assessing functional ability. RCTs published after the latest update of this review suggest that significant functional gains may be achieved. No detrimental effects on disease activity and pain were observed.

O   **What effects are noted with the application of heat to diarthroidal joints?**

Normal intra-articular temperature is reported to be lower than body temperature. Skin and joint temperature is increased by 34°C to 37.5°C in patients with active arthritis. When joint temperature is increased from 30.5°C to 36°C, as it is in active RA, the collagenase enzyme from a rheumatoid synovium is four times as active with lysis of cartilage. Increasing joint temperatures could contribute to perpetuating inflammation and joint destruction. However, Mainardi and associates found no increase in joint destruction and inflammatory activity in the hand in RA with the use of superficial heat.

O   **What therapeutic value can the application of cold achieve?**

Recent studies indicate that cold air and ice decrease joint temperature in inflammatory arthritis patients. Some clinical studies have shown more relief of pain with ice in patients with RA than with deep heat by diathermy. Ice also causes more prolonged relief of pain then superficial heat in RA patients. Other investigations found the increase of knee joint ROM to be the same with either ice or superficial beat applied daily for 5 days, with a 9-day interval between the two treatments.

O   **What is the evidence supporting the role of thermal agents in RA symptom management**

The Cochrane database review on thermotherapy in RA has shown neither positive nor detrimental effects of heat therapy on important outcomes or on joint destruction in RA patients. The reviewers conclude that thermotherapy can be used as needed by patients with RA, especially wax baths as a palliative therapy and an adjunct therapy combined with exercises. However, these conclusions are limited by the poor methodological quality of the trials available and the large number of borderline values. This review has shown that thermotherapy can be used as an adjunct and palliative therapy. No harmful side effects were reported.

O   **What evidence is there to support the role of ultrasound as a modality in the symptom management of RA?**

Ultrasound in combination with the following treatment modalities: exercises, faradic current and wax baths is not supported and cannot be recommended. Ultrasound alone can, however, be used on the hand to increase grip strength, and to a lesser extent and based on borderline results, increase wrist dorsal flexion, decrease morning stiffness, and reduce the number of swollen and painful joints. No harmful side effects were reported with ultrasound treatment. It is important to note that these conclusions are limited by the methodological considerations of poor quality of the trials, the low number of clinical trials (two), and the small sample size of the included studies.

O   **What modalities should be considered during an acute flare?**

In treating the acutely inflamed or early subacute joint, the goal is pain relief. One is careful not to use interventions that may perpetuate inflammation. The use of cold seems most logical because it can decrease the pain threshold, can relax surrounding spastic muscles, and is associated with decreased joint temperature, collagenase, and cell count in the joint fluid.

O   **What modalities should be considered in the subacute flare of RA?**

Later in the subacute period, when inflammatory pain is subsiding and stiffness is present, and the patient may have lost some ROM, either cold or superficial heat with TENS is appropriate before starting active-assistive ROM and isometric exercise. When inflammation has fully subsided, superficial heat for pain is appropriate. If tight periarticular structures remain, ultrasound or cold and TENS followed by stretching to increase joint ROM is suitable. Transcutaneous electrical nerve stimulation has been reported to relieve joint pain in RA and pain in RA neuropathy.

O   **What orthoses interventions for the ankle/foot may be appropriate in patients with RA?**

A well designed orthotic can correct common calcaneal eversion and subtalar pronation. An ankle-foot orthosis can be used to immobilize an ankle with chronic effusion and structural pathology, reducing pain and improving gait.

O   **What considerations for shoe wear are given in the RA patient?**

Critical areas in shoe structure are those that can cause possible compression, specifically the toe box, heel counter, and vamp. A softer material for shoe fabrication is needed to accommodate abnormal foot anatomy. Shoes should have high and broad toe boxes, wide vamps, and non-constraining heel counters to maximize inner shoe volumes and decrease metatarsal apposition. The sole of the shoe can be modified by the use of 1) a metatarsal bar to relieve pressure on the painful metatarsals; 2) a built up lateral or medial under surface to create a valgus or varus moment on the ankle; or 3) a rocker sole to alleviate metatarsal pressure, and make the push-off phase of gait more comfortable and efficient.

○ **What considerations should be given for a genu varus or valgus deformities in RA?**

If a valgus knee deformity exists, an ankle-foot orthotic to decrease the pronation moment at the subtalar joint may be helpful. Additionally, building up the medial aspect of the foot creates a varus moment at the ankle and a varus moment at the knee. This orthotic intervention is most successful if the medial knee compartment is relatively intact.

○ **What therapeutic interventions can be considered for the RA patient with swan neck deformities?**

Regarding therapeutic interventions, the use of heated paraffin may loosen soft-tissue elements and provide analgesia. Digital massage may reduce edema and the risk of fibrous tissue development. "Ring splints," used principally over the PIP joint, are designed to create a flexion moment at the PIP joint, reversing the passive flexion moment at the DIP joint and offsetting MCP joint flexion deformity. Stretching should focus on elongation of the intrinsic muscles, promoting MCP extension and PIP flexion.

○ **What therapeutic interventions can be considered for the boutonnière deformity?**

Digital massage and paraffin may be useful therapy. Stretching exercises should encourage MCP flexion, PIP extension, and DIP flexion. Intrinsic muscle strengthening may provide some assistance with PIP extension and MCP flexion. Orthotics should promote an extension moment at the PIP joint to create a DIP flexion moment or attempt to provide a DIP flexion moment with three points of pressure and reversal of PIP joint flexion. The latter is more difficult because the forcing of the DIP joint into flexion strongly inhibits the extensor mechanism and PIP and MCP extension becomes limited.

○ **What therapeutic interventions can be considered for ulnar MCP joint deviation?**

The application of serial casting may prove beneficial by preventing ligamentous stretching and placing the joint at rest. This process is not intended to correct but to maintain. Casting an affected joint, however, may trigger more proximal or distal joint inflammation. Therefore, careful monitoring for MCP joint overuse must occur. Other physical modalities include paraffin, edema massage, and ultrasound. Orthotics may be used to provide relief when the joint is at rest. However, functional splinting is often difficult to self-apply and can be quite bulky. In some cases, patients are aided by wrist or hand splints that focus on MCP radial return.

○ **What is the clinical evidence of efficacy for splints and orthosis in the symptomatic management of RA?**

It appears, though, that working wrist splints do not have short or long-term detrimental effects for grip strength or range of motion (ROM), nor is there any clear indication that they provide pain relief. However, ready-made elastic wrist gauntlets are relatively inexpensive and, since they may provide pain relief for some patients in some activities, it seems reasonable to try patients with these orthoses until further data becomes available.

○ **What is the clinical evidence supporting the role of orthotics and shoe wear in RA patients?**

There is preliminary evidence to support the use of extra-depth shoes, with or without semi-rigid insoles, to relieve pain on walking and weight bearing. Supported insoles appear to limit progression of hallux valgus angle but do not decrease pain or enhance function. The potential of orthotics to provide pain relief for varying periods of time in certain patients, and at a relatively low cost, tends to support the current practice of recommending that patients try out various splints/orthoses in different activities in order to determine whether these splints are helpful to them.

○ **What is the evidence statement with regard to the efficacy of patient education in RA?**

For the outcome measures included in the Cochrane database analysis there was a small beneficial effect of patient education at first follow-up for pain (4%), disability (10%), joint counts (9%), patient global assessment (12%), psychological status

(5%) and depression (12%). At final follow-up (3-18 months) no significant effects were found in the main analyses, only a trend for scores on disability favoring patient education. Detailed results are provided below for each outcome.

○ **What role does "relative rest" play in managing RA?**

Rest improves synovitis in RA and is recommended during the acute flares of the disease. Patients with RA are often tired, and energy conservation behaviors, consisting of interspersing physically active periods with short rest periods once or twice daily, have been shown to be effective in increasing total amounts of physical activity as compared with standard occupational therapy without tiring the patient. Some patients find it helpful to integrate various relaxation techniques into their daily routine, and balancing work and rest could permit RA patients to go on working for longer periods. The amount of rest necessary must be determined individually and depends on the stage and the activity of RA. Such behavior-changing interventions are easier for outpatients, and could favor a better adaptation to the disease.

○ **What are joint protection techniques?**

The aim of joint protection is to reduce loading through vulnerable joints. The elements of joint protection are thus:

1. Prevent preventable contractures and decline in muscle efficiency,
2. Prevent potential joint damage by the use of ergonomic and bioengineering principles and reduce joint loads,
3. Make such changes in life-style as are necessary to effect the above,
4. Use technical aids and/or orthoses to help achieve these aims.

○ **Is there a role for cognitive behavioral intervention in RA?**

Psychological interventions can be integrated into management of RA patients. Psychological factors are implicated in pain perception, and the intensity of pain is in part related to patients' beliefs in their ability to cope with or control the effects of their disease. Cognitive behavioral therapies can produce significant reductions in RA patients' self-reported pain, functional disabilities or joint involvement. Psychological therapy can improve patients' self-esteem and social behavior.

○ **What is the clinical evidence in support of occupational therapy interventions in the patient with RA?**

There is strong evidence for the efficacy of instruction of joint protection on functional ability. Studies that evaluated comprehensive OT showed limited evidence for the effectiveness on functional ability. Studies that evaluated splint interventions reported indicative findings for the effectiveness on pain. These results are encouraging for the occupational therapy practice as an important part in the treatment of patients with rheumatoid arthritis.

OSTEOARTHRITIS

○   **What is the epidemiology of osteoarthritis (OA)?**

Osteoarthritis is the most common of all joint diseases and one of the most frequent causes of physical impairment. It is a universal disorder, affecting both sexes and all races; Nevertheless, there are considerable differences in its rate of occurrence in different ethnic groups, in the different genders within any group, and in the different joints of individuals. Reports of the prevalence of osteoarthritis vary, depending on the age distribution of the population studied, the method of evaluation, and the diagnostic criteria used.

○   **How is osteoarthritis classified?**

Classification of Osteoarthritis
I. Primary (idiopathic)
A. Localized (principal site)
1. Hip (superolateral, superomedial, medial, inferoposterior)
2. Knee (medial, lateral, patellofemoral)
3. Spinal apophyseal
4. Hand (interphalangeal, base of thumb)
5. Foot (first metatarsophalangeal joint, midfoot, hindfoot)
6. Other (shoulder, elbow, wrist, ankle)
B. Generalized
1. Hands (Heberden's nodes)
2. Hands and knees; spinal apophyseal (generalized osteoarthritis)
II. Secondary
A. Dysplastic
1. Chondrodysplasias
2. Epiphyseal dysplasias
3. Congenital joint displacement
4. Developmental disorders (Perthes' disease, epiphysiolysis)
B. Post-traumatic
1. Acute
2. Repetitive
3. Postoperative
C. Structural failure
1. Osteonecrosis
2. Osteochondritis
D. Postinflammatory
1. Infection
2. Inflammatory arthropathies
E. Endocrine and metabolic
1. Acromegaly
2. Ochronosis
3. Hemochromatosis
4. Crystal deposition disorders
F. Connective tissue
1. Hypermobility syndromes
2. Mucopolysaccharidoses

O   **What are the risk factors for osteoarthritis?**

Multiple risk factors have been linked to osteoarthritis in epidemiology studies including:

Age
Gender
Obesity
Lack of osteoporosis
Occupation
Sports activities
Previous injury
Muscle weakness
Proprioceptive deficits
Genetic elements
Acromegaly
Calcium crystal deposition disease

O   **What is the pathogenesis of osteoarthritis?**

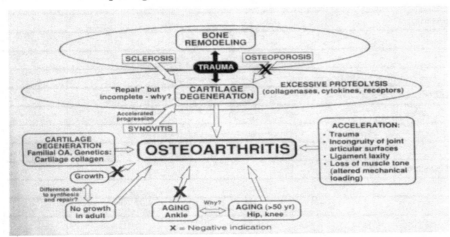

The pathogenesis is multifactorial but, may be divided into local and systemic factors.
The local processes are:

1) excessive breakdown of articular cartilage matrix elements
2) inefficient repair mechanisms in articular cartilage matrix elements
3) Compromise of subchondral bone secondary to 1 and 2
4) Impaired mechanisms of subchondral bone repair

O   **What are the characteristics of osteoarthritic chondrocytes?**

Characteristics of osteoarthritic (OA) chondrocytes*
Increased functions
Type II collagen and aggrecan synthesis (early OA)
Cell proliferation (chondron formation)
Catabolic cytokine production
Proteinases (MMPs, aggrecanase, PA, cathepsins)
IL-1 receptor type I
IGFBP-3
Apoptosis, NOS, COX-2
Expression of collagen types VI, III, X, IIA
Decreased functions
Type II collagen and aggrecan synthesis (late OA)
IL-1 receptor antagonist
Response to IGF-1
MMPs matrix metalloproteinases; PA plasminogen activator; IL-1 interleukin-1; IGFBP-3 insulin-like growth factor binding protein 3; NOS nitric oxide synthase; COX-2 cyclooxygenase 2; IGF-1 insulin-like growth factor 1.

O   **What are the ACR criteria for the diagnosis of hip, knee and hand OA?**

American College of Rheumatology clinical criteria for the classification of hip, knee and hand osteoarthritis.

Hip
Hip pain for most days in the previous month hip internal rotation 5 158 AND pain on internal rotation AND morning stiffness of the hip 4 60 minutes AND age 4 50 years

Knee
Knee pain age 5 40 years AND morning stiffness 4 30 minutes AND crepitus on active joint motion

Hand
Hand pain, aching or stiffness for most days of the prior month hard tissue enlargement of 5 2 of 10 selected joints[a] AND soft-tissue swelling of 5 3 MCP joints AND (hard-tissue enlargement of 5 1 DIP joint OR deformity of 5 1 of 10 selected joints)

[a]2nd and 3rd DIP, 2nd and 3rd PIP, 1st CMC joints of both hands.

O   What patterns of OA occur based on occupational profile?

Occupation	Involved Joints	Risk of OA
Miners	Elbow, knee, spine	Increased
Pneumatic drillers	Shoulder, elbow, wrist, MCPs	Increased/none
Dockworkers	Intervertebral disks, DIPs, elbow, knee	Increased
Cotton mill workers	Hand	Increased
Diamond workers	Hand	Increased
Shipyard laborers	Knees	Increased
Foundry workers	Lumbar spine	Increased
Seamstresses	Hand	Increased
Textile workers	Hand	Increased
Manual laborers	MCPs	Increased
Occupations requiring knee bending	Knee	Increased
Farmers	Hip, knee	Increased

O   What OA patterns are encountered related to sport activity?

Sport	Site (Joint)	Risk
Ballet	Talus	Probably increased
	Ankle	
	Cervical spine	
	Hip	
	Knee	
	Metatarsophalangeal	
Baseball	Elbow	
	Shoulder	
Boxing	Hand (carpometacarpal joints)	
Cricket	Finger	
Cycling	Finger	
	Feet	Probably increased
	Ankle	
	Knee	
	Spine	
	Shoulder	
	Elbow	

Sport	Site (Joint)	Risk
	Wrist	
	Hip	
	Knee	
	Ankle	
Martial arts	Spine	
	Knee	
	Ankle	
	Spine	
Rugby	Knee	
Running	Knee	Small
	Hip	
	Ankle	
Soccer	Ankle-foot	Probably increased
	Hip	
	Knee	
	Talus	
	Talofibular	
Weight lifting	Cervical spine	
	Elbow	Probably increased
	Knee	

○   **What are the monoarticular and pauciarticular clinical patterns of OA?**

The occurrence of monoarticular osteoarthritis in a young adult is often secondary to a congenital abnormality or previous trauma. A pauciarticular form of OA is common in middle age and usually affects the large, weight-bearing joints of the lower extremities.

○   **What is the polyarticular clinical pattern of OA?**

Polyarticular or generalized OA is the most common form, typically affecting middle-aged or elderly women. The presence of Heberden's and Bouchard's nodes and involvement of the first carpometacarpal joint are common in these patients; the knees, hips, metatarsophalangeal joints and spine may also be involved. The onset of the arthritis may be heralded by an initial, inflammatory phase. Erosive, inflammatory OA is a variant of this polyarticular form that follows a more aggressive course and frequently results in joint deformities.

○   **What are the central pathological features of OA?**

The central pathologic features are focal areas of fibrillation, loss of volume, and destruction of the articular cartilage. The underlying bone is generally sclerotic, and may form cysts. At the joint margin, growth of fibrocartilage and bone leads to chondrophytes and osteophytic lipping. There is a variable, patchy synovitis, and fibrotic thickening of the joint capsule.

○   **What are common radiological findings in OA?**

Loss of interbone distance reflects extensive loss of cartilage volume, and if this is severe, the bony pathology will be apparent in the form of subchondral sclerosis, bony cysts and osteophytes visible on a radiograph.

○   **What is the Kellgren and Lawrence grading system for OA radiography?**

Radiographic grading scheme for osteoarthritis

Grade	Criteria
0	Normal
1	Doubtful narrowing of joint space, possible osteophyte development
2	Definite osteophytes, absent or questionable narrowing of joint space
3	Moderate osteophytes, definite narrowing, some sclerosis, possible joint deformity
4	Large osteophytes, marked narrowing, severe sclerosis, definite joint deformity

Adapted from Kellgren and Lawrence.

○ What are common symptoms and signs of OA?

The commonest clinical sequelae is pain, most often related to joint use, but sometimes occurring at rest and at night. Stiffening or gelling of joints in the morning and after any extended period of inactivity usually occurs, but is relieved within minutes rather than hours. The range of movement is often restricted, with pain at the end of the range. On palpation there is usually firm swelling of the affected joints and palpable crepitus on movement. In severe cases the integrity of the joint may become disrupted, with loss of bone as well as cartilage, and instability of the joint.

○ How do patients with OA describe their pain?

In a detailed study of pain reporting by 500 patients with peripheral joint OA, Cushnaghan confirmed previous reports that use related pain was the most frequently described symptom. The pain related to activity usually starts within seconds or minutes of onset of joint use, but may continue for hours after the activity has ceased. Some patients describe discrete, stabbing pains coinciding precisely with certain movements or with weight bearing; others describe a poorly localized, constant ache or pain brought on by activity. Whereas nearly all symptomatic patients with OA have use-related pain, only some 50% or less describe rest pain, and about 30% report night pain.

○ What are the subjective characteristics of stiffness in OA?

The most characteristic feature of joint stiffness in OA is the phenomenon of 'gelling' after inactivity. This appears to be a problem of getting the joint to move after a period of rest, and although it may be severe, it usually only lasts for a few minutes. Patients may talk about having to 'work the joint in' after a rest period or first thing in the morning. Longer periods of stiffness in the morning occur in some patients, but in contrast to that of RA, it rarely lasts longer than about 30 minutes and is usually confined to a small number of affected joints.

○ What may account for crepitus in OA?

Course crepitations are usually felt on movement of an osteoarthritic joint. Along with 'bony' swelling of the affected joint, crepitus stands out as one of the best signs in the clinical differentiation of OA from other disorders. In advanced OA the crepitus may be clearly audible, as well as palpable, loud cracks emanating from a hip or knee joint on walking, for example. The noise is probably due to the roughening of the joint surface and outgrowths at the rim of the joint interfering with the normally smooth movement between the joint surfaces. 'Cavitation' or the formation of gas bubbles within the synovial fluid may also contribute. The crepitus of OA can usually be felt through much of the total range of movement, distinguishing it from the occasional 'cracking' of a normal joint. It also has a much coarser feel than the fine crepitus that can be caused by tenosynovitis and other inflammatory disorders.

○ What are the most common patterns of knee OA?

Isolated medial compartment, or medial plus patellofemoral disease are the commonest combinations. Maximum evidence of cartilage damage is usually found on the lateral facet of the patella in patellofemoral OA, and on the tibial plateau area least well protected by the menisci in tibiofemoral disease. Whereas the medial tibiofemoral compartment usually has the most loss of articular cartilage, osteophytosis is often more extensive in the lateral compartment.

○ How does knee OA present clinically?

Pain on walking, stiffness of the joint and difficulty with steps and stairs are the major symptoms. The physical signs depend on the distribution and severity of the OA within the joint. Wasting of the quadriceps muscle, bony swelling, and tenderness on and around the joint line, painful limitation of full flexion and course crepitus are the usual signs. Medial compartment disease often results in a varus deformity, a very common finding in knee OA. In patellofemoral OA, anterior crepitus, abnormal movement and tracking of the patella, and tenderness on patella compression occur.

O What anatomical patterns of hip OA are described?

Three different patterns of distribution of OA of the hip joint are described. The superior pole pattern is commonest, and often results in superolateral migration of the femoral head. Medial pole disease is less common, but similarly, can sometimes result in medial migration and protrusio acetabulae. The concentric pattern, in which the whole of the joint appears to be involved, has been linked with the existence of OA at other joint sites more strongly than the other anatomic patterns. Involvement of the postero-inferior portion of the joint can occur, and may be missed unless a lateral radiograph is taken.

O What have biomechanical studies of the hip revealed with regards to the development of OA?

Biomechanical studies have shown that the forces through the hip joint are a product of body weight and abduction forces. The superior pole of the hip is the main area of contact on weight bearing, and the most susceptible area to OA.

O How does hip OA present with symptoms?

Pain on walking is the major symptom. It may be felt in the buttock region, in the groin, in the front of the thigh, or in the knee, causing potential problems with diagnosis. Inactivity stiffness and a reduced range of motion are common and patients frequently have difficulty bending to put shoes, socks and stockings on.

O What exam findings are found in hip OA?

On examination there is a reduced range of passive movement, with pain at the end of the range; internal rotation is usually the most compromised movement. Crepitus may be audible in severe cases, but cannot be palpated. Tenderness in the groin, over the front of the joint, is common, and there may be a secondary trochanteric bursitis causing lateral tenderness as well. In advanced cases leg shortening can develop due to the migration of the femoral head, referred to above. Muscle wasting around the joint is usually present in advanced disease. These features result in the typical 'antalgic' (coxalgic) gait and the 'Trendelenburg' sign in which the pelvis dips down when the patient tries to stand on the affected leg.

O What is the pattern most commonly encountered in the hand for OA?

OA predominantly affects the distal (DIP) joint more than proximal (PIP), and the joints at the base of the thumb. The metacarpophalangeal joints and joints of the wrist are involved less often and less severely.

O What clinical findings of IP joint OA are remarkable?

The hallmarks of interphalangeal joint OA are the 'Heberden's (DIP joints) and Bouchard's (PIP joints) nodes'. These firm swellings, maximal on the superolateral aspect of the joints, are the most striking and characteristic clinical finding. They are often tender and sometimes red. Cysts may form as they first grow, and if punctured, these cysts exude a thick, colorless jelly, rich in hyaluronan. Later in the evolution of the condition, lateral instability often develops. Loss of flexion also develops, with occasional interphalangeal joint fusion. Consequent disabilities can include difficulties with activities requiring fine finger movements.

O What are the clinical characteristics of 1st CMC joint OA?

Thumb base disease causes pain and tenderness, which may be poorly localized 'around the wrist'. Tenderness over the base of the first metacarpal, with pain and crepitus on moving that bone, often occur. In more severe disease an adduction deformity of the metacarpal develops. Combined with the bony swelling this causes the classical appearance of 'squaring' of the thumb base. It may be accompanied by hyperextension of the proximal phalanx. An effusion is occasionally palpable. Difficulty with pinch grip and bottle/jar tops is frequent complaints.

O   **What do hand radiographs reveal in OA?**

Radiographs of thumb joint and interphalangeal joint OA show the typical features, including loss of joint space, osteophytosis, sclerosis and cysts. In addition, in severe cases there may be loss of cortical integrity over the surface of the joint, in which case the condition may be labeled 'erosive' OA.

O   **What pattern of OA is encountered in the spine?**

Apophyseal joint OA is similar to OA elsewhere, and disc degeneration is accompanied by osteophytic lipping of the vertebrae. The variable degree of new bone formation is a major factor determining the consequences of spinal OA. The association between apophyseal joint OA and disc degeneration probably reflects their biomechanical relationship. Any change in the anatomy of one of these joints will put abnormal stresses on the other. The distribution of spinal osteophytes probably indicates where these stresses are maximal.

O   **Which MTP joint is most often involved in OA?**

The first metatarsophalangeal joint is the prime site of OA changes in the forefoot.

O   **What is hallux rigidus?**

Osteoarthritis of the first metatarsophalangeal joint (hallux rigidus) is very commonly may be detected in adolescents or young adults, as well as in middle-aged and elderly persons, and appears to be more common in men. The condition may lead to painful restriction of dorsiflexion of the great toe. The cause of hallux rigidus is unknown. Radiographic evaluation reveals joint space loss, bone sclerosis, and osteophytes, particularly on the dorsal aspect of the metatarsal head.

O   **What is hallux valgus?**

An additional common lesion of the first metatarsophalangeal joint is termed hallux valgus. The early and essential intrinsic lesion of this condition may be stretching of the ligaments about the metatarsophalangeal joint that attach the medial sesamoid and basal phalanx to the metatarsal bone, with erosion of the ridge that separates the grooves for the sesamoids on the metatarsal head.

O   **Summarize the categories of treatment approaches for OA**

Non-pharmacological	*Pharmacological*	*Surgical*
Patient education	NSAIDs*	Joint replacement
Cognitive Behavioral therapy	Analgesics	Osteotomy
Exercise	Opioids	Arthroscopic debridement
Footwear, including insoles	SYSADOA*	Lavage
Assistive device	Sex hormones	
Balanotherapy	Topical (periarticular) treatment	
Patellar tape	Intra-articular steroids	
Knee orthoses	Intra-articular hyaluronic acid	
Diet		
Vitamins		
Minerals		

*NSAIDs = non-steroidal anti-inflammatory drugs; SYSADOA = symptomatic slow acting drugs for osteoarthritis (chondroprotective agents)

O   **Summarize the pharmacotherapy guidelines espoused by the ACR.**

Pharmacologic therapy for patients with osteoarthritis*
Oral
Acetaminophen
COX-2–specific inhibitor
Nonselective NSAID plus misoprostol or a proton pump
Inhibitor†
Nonacetylated salicylate
Other pure analgesics

Tramadol
Opioids
Intraarticular
Glucocorticoids
Hyaluronan
Topical
Capsaicin
Methylsalicylate
* The choice of agent(s) should be individualized for each patient as
noted in the text. COX-2 cyclooxygenase 2; NSAID nonsteroidal
antiinflammatory drug.
† Misoprostol and proton pump inhibitors are recommended in patients who are at increased
risk for upper gastrointestinal adverse events.

O   What is the efficacy of acetaminophen compared to NSAIDs?

The efficacy of acetaminophen has been demonstrated to be superior to placebo in relief of pain due to OA, but is less effective than NSAIDs. The American College of Rheumatology treatment guidelines for OA support the use of NSAIDs in conjunction with nonpharmacologic measures for some acetaminophen naive patients, particularly those with more severe pain.

O   Are certain NSAIDs more efficacious than others?

The Cochrane database systematic review found no evidence of superiority of a given NSAID compared to another. The COX-2 selective agents appear to have equal efficacy when compared to the non-selective COX inhibitors.

O   What topical therapies are available and efficacious in OA?

Topical capsaicin cream, which depletes sensory nerve endings of the peptide substance P, may reduce joint pain and tenderness when applied topically to treat OA of the knee and hand. Topical NSAIDs have been widely used in Europe and shown to be efficacious in both soft tissue disorders as well as joint disorders.

O   What therapeutic exercises are appropriate for hip OA?

Muscle strengthening exercises focus on the hip and lower back, particularly the hip abductors and extensors. Active hip abductor strengthening exercises include side lying leg lifts, prone "skateboard" abduction exercises, and standing abduction exercises. Weights are added according to what the patient can tolerate. Exercise in the pool is an efficient method to increase strength, range of motion, and endurance in a pain-free environment. Hip extensors can be strengthened in the supine or standing position. Stretching exercises, particularly in abduction and extension, are exceedingly important. Patients should lay prone daily for a few minutes to stretch the hip flexors. Trunk strengthening and stretching exercises, use of shoe orthotics, and functional gait training are also important.

O   What adaptive equipment may be beneficial for hip OA?

Adaptive equipment including long-handled sponges, reachers, sock donners, elevated toilet seats, grab bars, shower bench, and seat cushions may ease some functional tasks.

O   What education strategies are appropriate for hip OA?

Educating the OA patient about energy conservation and joint protection completes the prescription. Under-standing the hip joint as a simple lever system can direct the prescription of techniques to prevent abnormally high forces being distributed through the hip. For example, the loss of 1 lb of body weight translates to a 3-1b reduction in force distributed by the abductors. Use of a cane in the opposite hand acts to reduce the force generated by the abductors. Similarly, when reaching down to pick up an item, patients should support their weight on the contralateral hand (for instance, on a dresser) and lift with the ipsilateral hand. Heavy loads should be carried with two hands if possible, otherwise by the ipsilateral hand.

O   What therapeutic exercises are appropriate for OA of the knee?

Therapeutic exercise regimes that are common practice include muscle strengthening and aerobic activity. Studies evaluating the efficacy of muscle strengthening exercises in participants with OA of the knee and hip have shown to have positive results. Participants were reported to having improved muscle strength decreased pain decreased stiffness and overall improved function. Aerobic exercise has also been shown to have beneficial results for people with OA of the hip and knee. Studies have investigated aerobic exercise modes such as walking, running, cycling, aquatics, and aerobic dance. Participants have reported the following improvements: 1) increased aerobic capacity 2) decreased depression and anxiety 3) increased physical activity 4) decreased fatigue 5) increased muscular strength and flexibility 6) decreased pain 7) and increased functional status. It was also found that these benefits were achieved without an increase in pain or further exacerbation of arthritic symptoms.

○ **What orthoses are appropriate for knee OA?**

The general purpose of knee bracing is to improve the proprioception and stability. For unicompartmental osteoarthritis there are special valgisation and varisation braces to unload the pathologic compartment and to reduce the adduction moment. Knee orthoses are available specifically for patellofemoral disorders. The designs vary, however doughnut cut out orthoses have been most often prescribed. Similarly therapeutic patellofemoral taping may also aid in the reduction of pain and enhancement of function. Lateral heel and sole wedges are effective in managing the symptoms of medial compartment OA. It is unclear however, whether these wedges are more effective than unloading braces or pharmacotherapy.

○ **What is the efficacy of chondroprotective agents (nutraceuticals) in the management of knee OA?**

There is good evidence that glucosamine is both effective and safe in treating osteoarthritis based on the Cochrane systematic database reviews. Efficacy of chondroitin sulfate appears less convincing. The long-term effectiveness and toxicity of glucosamine therapy and chondroitin sulfate in OA remains unclear. As well, it is not known whether different glucosamine or chondroitin sulfate preparations prepared by different manufacturers are equally effective in the therapy of OA.

○ **What is the efficacy of PEMF and ultrasound in the management of OA?**

There is little consistent clinical evidence to support the use of these modalities in the management of OA Systematic reviews have concluded that there was no benefit of ultrasound therapy for pain relief, range of motion or functional status.

○ **What is the efficacy of local cryotherapy compared to thermotherapy in OA?**

In systematic reviews ice massage showed a significant benefit in improving ROM and function, in the treatment of knee OA. The effectiveness of ice on relieving pain is unclear. The application of an ice pack did not relieve pain any better than a control, although when applied using massage ice had a significant benefit on pain relief compared with control. Application of cold packs resulted in significant reduction in knee edema when compared with control or heat.

○ **What is the efficacy of TENS in knee OA?**

Active TENS and 'acupuncture like' TENS (AL-TENS) treatment for at least four weeks effectively reduced pain. Knee stiffness also improved significantly.

○ **What is the clinical efficacy for viscosupplementation therapy?**

The preponderance of evidence supports intraarticular injections of hyaluronic acid derivatives being more efficacious than intraarticular placebo. However, the magnitude of the benefit is modest. A series of three or five injections of hylan GF-20 or Hyalgan, respectively, may be beneficial to some patients with knee OA and have an acceptable safety profile.

○ **What is the efficacy of intraarticular corticosteroid injections in the management of knee OA?**

Intraarticular corticosteroid injections may be appropriate in patients with OA who have one or several joints that are painful despite the use of NSAIDs and in patients with monoarticular or pauciarticular inflammatory osteoarthritis in whom NSAIDs are contraindicated. Intraarticular corticosteroids slow cartilage catabolism and osteophyte formation in animals; they are also effective for short-term pain relief and can increase quadriceps strength after knee injection. Repeated corticosteroid injections over a period up to two years appear to be safe, and may provide more relief than saline injections. There is no strong evidence that corticosteroid injections are superior to viscosupplementation therapy in the management of knee OA.

MIXED CONNECTIVE TISSUE DISEASES

○   **What is Systemic lupus erythematosus (SLE)?**

Systemic lupus erythematosus (SLE) is a chronic inflammatory disease of unknown cause which can affect the skin, joints, kidneys, lungs, nervous system, serous membranes and/or other organs of the body. Immunologic abnormalities, especially the production of a number of antinuclear antibodies, are another prominent feature of the disease. The clinical course of SLE is variable and may be characterized by periods of remissions and chronic or acute relapses. Women, especially in their 20s and 30s, are affected more frequently than men.

○   **What is the incidence of SLE?**

The incidence is 14.6-50.8 cases per 100,000 people.

○   **What is the mortality profile for patients with SLE?**

With full access to medical care, overall survival for SLE is 85% at 5 years and 63% at 15 years.

○   **What is the most common presentation of SLE?**

The most common pattern is a mixture of constitutional complaints with skin, musculoskeletal, mild hematologic and serologic involvement.

○   **What are the ACR criteria for the Classification of Systemic Lupus Erythematosus (SLE)?**

Criterion	Definition
1. Malar rash	Fixed erythema, flat or raised, over the malar eminences, tending to spare the nasolabial folds
2. Discoid rash	Erythematous raised patches with adherent keratotic scaling and follicular plugging; atrophic scarring may occur in older lesions
3. Photosensitivity	Skin rash as a result of unusual reaction to sunlight, by patient history or physician observation
4. Oral ulcers	Oral or nasopharyngeal ulceration, usually painless, observed by physician
5. Arthritis	Nonerosive arthritis involving 2 or more peripheral joints, characterized by tenderness, swelling, or effusion
6. Serositis	a) Pleuritis--convincing history of pleuritic pain or rubbing heard by a physician or evidence of pleural effusion OR b) Pericarditis--documented by ECG or rub or evidence of pericardial effusion
7. Renal disorder	a) Persistent proteinuria greater than 0.5 grams per day or grater than 3+ if quantitation not performed OR b) Cellular casts--may be red cell, hemoglobin, granular, tubular, or mixed
8. Neurologic disorder	a) Seizures--in the absence of offending drugs or known metabolic derangements; e.g., uremia, ketoacidosis, or electrolyte imbalance OR b) Psychosis--in the absence of offending drugs or known metabolic derangements, e.g., uremia, ketoacidosis, or electrolyte imbalance
9. Hematologic disorder	a) Hemolytic anemia--with reticulocytosis OR b) Leukopenia--less than 4,000/mm^3 total on 2 or more occasions OR c) Lymphopenia--less than 1,500/mm^3 on 2 or more occasions OR d) Thrombocytopenia--less than 100,000/mm^3 in the absence of offending drugs
10. Immunologic disorder	a) Positive LE cell preparation OR b) Anti-DNA: antibody to native DNA in abnormal titer OR c) Anti-Sm: presence of antibody to Sm nuclear antigen OR d) False positive serologic test for syphilis known to be positive for at least 6 months and confirmed by *Treponema pallidum* immobilization or fluorescent treponemal antibody absorption test
11. Antinuclear antibody	An abnormal titer of antinuclear antibody by immunofluorescence or an equivalent assay at any point in time and in the absence of drugs known to be associated with "drug-induced lupus" syndrome

○   **What is the most frequent complaint in SLE?**

Fatigue is the most common complaint, and occasionally the most debilitating. It occurs in 80 to 100 percent of patients, even when no other features of active disease are present. Fatigue is strongly associated with diminished exercise tolerance.

❍ What are the most common musculoskeletal symptoms in SLE?

Musculoskeletal symptoms, particularly arthralgia, myalgia, and arthritis, represent the most common presenting complaints in SLE. Arthritis tends to be migratory and asymmetrical. It can affect any joint, but the small joints of the hands, wrists, and knees are involved most frequently. Arthritis classically is nonerosive and usually nondeforming. Soft tissue swelling is common, and effusions, when they occur, usually are mildly inflammatory. However, as many as 10% of patients develop hand deformities due to chronic arthritis and tendinitis, called Jaccoud arthropathy, which mimic the changes observed in rheumatoid arthritis.

❍ What are the neurological manifestations associated with SLE?

Among the neurologic manifestations of SLE, the most common are the organic encephalopathies (35-75% of case series), which basically comprise all potential variations of acute confusion, lethargy, or coma; chronic dementias; depression, mania, or other affective disturbances; or psychosis.

❍ What is the risk for epilepsy in SLE?

Seizures occur in 15-20% of patients with SLE and may result from cerebral vasculitis (ischemic or hemorrhagic manifestations), cardiac embolism, opportunistic infection, drug intoxication, or associated metabolic derangements.

❍ What cranial neuropathies occur in SLE?

Cranial nerve abnormalities (most prominently, optic neuritis) occur in 10% of patients with SLE. Oculomotor nerve palsies and all other cranial neuropathies have been reported.

❍ What is the risk of stroke in the SLE patient?

Stroke is clinically evident in 5-10% of most series and may involve small, medium, or large vessels by a variety of mechanisms. Subacute evolution or any premonitory symptoms suggest a thrombotic or vasculitic mechanism, whereas an abrupt onset with maximum deficit initially supports an embolic mechanism.

❍ What are the spinal cord manifestations of SLE?

Spinal cord involvement is rare but devastating. Transverse myelitis, subacute-to-chronic demyelinating syndromes, and abrupt vascular occlusive events (eg, spinal artery thrombosis) have been described.

❍ What peripheral neurological disorders are associated with SLE?

Peripheral neuropathy occurs in as many as 18% of patients. A sensory or sensorimotor predominantly distal polyneuropathy is most common; Myositis is clinically apparent as proximal weakness and myalgias in 3-5% of patients but, if assiduously sought, may be found in as many as 50%.

❍ Summarize the serological tests used in SLE and mixed connective tissue diseases (MCTD).

Autoantibodies Detected in Patients with Connective Tissue Diseases

Autoantibody	Disease (frequency of autoantibody)	Cost ($)*	Comments
RF	Rheumatoid arthritis (80%), other connective tissue diseases (see Table 1)	15	Sensitive but not specific for rheumatoid arthritis; correlates with prognosis of disease severity (not disease activity)

ANA	Systemic lupus erythematosus (99%), drug-induced lupus (100%), other connective tissue diseases (see Table 2)	30	Sensitive but not specific for connective tissue diseases; correlates poorly with disease activity
Anti-dsDNA	Systemic lupus erythematosus (60%)	30	Specific but not sensitive for systemic lupus erythematosus; correlates with lupus nephritis and disease activity
Anti-ssDNA	Infrequent	200†	Nonspecific and of little clinical utility
Anti-histone	Drug-induced lupus (90%), systemic lupus erythematosus (50%)		Sensitive but not specific for drug-induced lupus
Anti-Sm	Systemic lupus erythematosus (20 to 30%)		Specific but not sensitive for systemic lupus erythematosus
Anti-U1 snRNP	Systemic lupus erythematosus (30 to 40%), mixed connective tissue disease (100%)		Associated with disease activity in systemic lupus erythematosus
Anti-Ro (anti-SS-A)	Sjögren's syndrome (75%), systemic lupus erythematosus (40%)		Associated with photosensitive skin rash, pulmonary disease and lymphopenia in systemic lupus erythematosus
Anti-La (anti-SS-B)	Sjögren's syndrome (40%), systemic lupus erythematosus (10 to 15%)		Associated with late-onset systemic lupus erythematosus, secondary Sjögren's syndrome and neonatal lupus syndrome
Anti-ribosome	Systemic lupus erythematosus (10 to 20%)	30	Highly specific but not sensitive for systemic lupus erythematosus; associated with lupus psychosis
Anti-centromere	Scleroderma (22 to 36%)	30	Associated with CREST syndrome and Raynaud's phenomenon
Anti-topoisomerase I (anti-Scl-70)	Scleroderma (22 to 40%)	40	Highly specific but not sensitive for scleroderma
Anti-Jo1	Polymyositis and dermatomyositis (30%)	40	Associated with pulmonary fibrosis and Raynaud's phenomenon
c-ANCA	Wegener's granulomatosis (>90%)	30	Highly specific and sensitive for Wegener's granulomatosis; correlates with disease activity
p-ANCA	Wegener's granulomatosis (10%), microscopic polyangiitis, glomerulonephritis	30	Sensitivity and specificity quite low in Wegener's granulomatosis

O   What are appropriate rehabilitation strategies for the patient with SLE?

SLE is a chronic inflammatory disease that can affect any organ in the body. The most frequently involved sites are the skin, joints, pleuro-pericardium, kidneys, and central nervous system. Its course is varied in severity and duration. The rehabilitation team is often consulted with respect to a number of functional problems. Fatigue is a common problem and is partly due to the chronic inflammatory process, but it also can be secondary to a disturbed sleep-wake process or myositis. The use of prednisone influences this also. Treatment may include an energy conservation-training program teaching that physical activity is interrupted by rest. Naps are taken during the day, and sleep can be promoted by the use of relaxation tapes.

O   How can arthralgias be symptomatically managed?

Pain is common in the small joints of the hands and feet because of arthralgias and arthritis. Joint pain also can result from avascular necrosis of bone. Joint deformity is also seen. Control of joint pain has been successful with acupuncture and acupressure techniques, heat, cold, and TENS. These techniques are more effective in treating arthralgias than in treating avascular necrosis, which requires un weighting of the lower extremity, which, when unsuccessful, requires joint replacement to control symptoms.

O   What therapeutic interventions are considered for patients with renal or cardiopulmonary involvement?

Patients with renal disease often have diminished stamina and fatigue. Improvement will occur with good blood pressure control and management of edema. In patients with nephrotic syndrome and significant edema, care must be taken to position the limb in the most functional position to minimize contracture; compression pumps and garments can be used to help with and maintain the reduction of limb edema. Precautions must be taken for patients with cardiac failure. They must be compressed slowly or not at all because they may not tolerate any additional fluid load resulting from compression.

○ **Do patients with SLE demonstrate evidence of deconditioning?**

Patients with SLE have been shown to have decreased aerobic capacity. An aerobic exercise program has been shown to increase endurance by 20%.

○ **What psychosocial interventions may be used for the disabled SLE patient?**

The patient with SLE has to overcome major obstacles to successfully cope with this multifaceted illness. Support groups and family have been shown to be helpful in increasing compliance and are an essential component in the rehabilitation process.

○ **What is progressive systemic sclerosis (PSS)/Scleroderma?**

Scleroderma is a systemic disease that affects many organ systems. It is most obvious in the skin; however, the gastrointestinal tract, the respiratory, renal, cardiovascular, and genitourinary systems, as well as numerous vascular structures, are involved frequently. The symptoms result from progressive tissue fibrosis and occlusion of the microvasculature by excessive production and deposition of types I and III collagens.

○ **What is the incidence and prevalence of PSS?**

The estimated incidence is 19 cases per million population, and the prevalence is 240 cases per million population.

○ **What is the mortality profile for the PSS patient?**

Pulmonary hypertension and its complications are the most frequent causes of mortality. Survival time is averaged at 13 years from diagnosis, and survival is evaluated best based on the disease type (I, II, III). Type I, sclerodactyly only, has a 10-year survival rate of 71%. Type II with skin involvement proximal to the metacarpal-phalangeal joint and without trunk involvement has a 10-year survival rate of 58%. Type III with diffuse skin induration, including the trunk, has a 10-year survival rate of 21%.

○ **How is scleroderma classified by the ACR?**

Major criterion: Presence of symmetric sclerodermatous skin changes of the fingers plus involvement at any location proximal to the
Minor criteria: Sclerodactyly: symmetric thickening, tightening and induration of fingers.
The diagnosis of SSc is based on the presence of the major criterion **OR** two or more minor criteria. The sensitivity of these criteria is 97% and the specificity 98%.

○ **What are indicators for poor prognosis in PSS?**

INDICATORS FOR POOR PROGNOSIS
Advanced age at presentation   Male sex   Black American race   Diffuse cutaneous involvement. Patients with diffuse disease has a 10 year survival rate of about 20%   • Rapidity of development of skin involvement.   • Presence of significant renal of pulmonary disease.   • Presence of anti-Scl 70 antibodies.

○ **What musculoskeletal pathology occurs in PSS?**

Patients may present with generalized arthralgias and morning stiffness that may mimic other systemic autoimmune diseases. Clinically apparent synovitis is uncommon. Tendon friction rubs can occur and are correlated more strongly with diffuse than limited scleroderma and are a bad prognostic factor. The cause of the tendon friction rubs is unknown and may be due to low-grade tenosynovitis or edema of the tendon. Flexion contractures occur most often at the hands, including the metacarpophalangeal joints (MCPs), PIPs, and, occasionally, DIPs, and also at the wrists, but can occur elsewhere.

○   **What other musculoskeletal problems are described in the PSS?**

Acro-osteolysis is also present in limited and diffuse scleroderma. These features can be seen on physical examination and on radiographs. Subcutaneous lesions (the calcinosis) often occur on extensor surfaces and areas that rub or have trauma. They can leak whitish discharge and rarely can be mistaken for tophi. Acro-osteolysis includes absorption of the distal fingertip (tuft) and can be very painful with loss of fingertip pulp and underlying phalangeal bone.

○   **What are the characteristics of myositis in patients with scleroderma?**

Myositis is more common in diffuse than limited scleroderma and is often accompanied by a decreased forced vital capacity. Myositis and myopathy can yield an elevated creatine kinase (CK) and proximal muscle weakness. Myositis has more inflammatory features on electromyogram (spontaneous fibrillations) accompanied by a more inflammatory biopsy. It also tends to produce a marked increase in the ESR.

○   **What peripheral nerve pathology is noted in PSS?**

Peripheral nerve entrapment may be a feature of scleroderma; the most common compression neuropathies are carpal tunnel syndrome (median nerve compression) and trigeminal neuropathy.

○   **What types of impairments does PSS give rise to?**

PSS gets its name from the fibrosis like changes that occur in skin and epithelial tissues of affected organs. In addition, heart, lung, kidney, GI tract, and small vessels also can be involved. Although there is no cure, treatment is thought to prolong life. The rehabilitation management depends on the extent and severity of the involvement. Skin involvement occurs in 90% of patients and is often accompanied by Raynaud's syndrome, a condition in which there is vasospasm of the digital arteries often leading to ulceration of the fingertips. Impact of the skin involvement produces characteristic effects.

○   **Describe the phase progression of ROM limitation in PSS.**

There is an early painless edematous phase, during which ROM may be limited but pain and weakness are not a problem. In a subsequent phase, the skin becomes tight and bound to deeper structures, the dermis becomes thin, and there is hair loss and decreased sweating. This period is associated with significant morbidity, with loss of joint motion, itching of the skin, and an overall decrease in functional level.

○   **What rehabilitation interventions are appropriate for patients with progressive systemic sclerosis?**

Rehabilitation interventions are directed at maintaining ROM, increasing skin elasticity, and preserving or increasing function. The techniques for accomplishing this include heat, paraffin, or ultrasound. The management of Raynaud's syndrome may require nothing more than education about hand protection in the cold and the use of warm mittens. For those who are significantly affected, there is evidence that temperature biofeedback is helpful in controlling vasospasm, although it has proved most effective in laboratory settings and less so in daily use. However, patients report feeling that they are more in control of their environment.

○   **What is the role of therapeutic exercise in PSS?**

Exercise to maintain ROM is essential and should be performed daily or twice daily. Strengthening exercise should be prescribed with caution and only after inflammatory myositis with abnormal levels of muscle enzymes has been ruled out. A variant of PSS, eosinophilic fasciitis, a syndrome that has tight skin as one of its features, may be precipitated by unusually strenuous exercise, reinforcing the concern that strengthening exercise should be used with caution and properly supervised.

○   **Describe the problems of pulmonary and esophageal pathology that can develop in patients with PSS and formulate therapeutic strategies to address them.**

Pulmonary involvement takes the form of pleuritis, interstitial fibrosis, and pulmonary hypertension. Symptoms include chest wall pain, pleurisy, and dyspnea. Educating the patient about breathing mechanics and practicing chest wall expansion may help improve ventilation. Transcutaneous electrical nerve stimulation may relieve chest wall pain. Energy conservation training and the use of adaptive equipment may increase functional independence. Weight loss, constipation, and dysphagia are GI symptoms that accompany PSS. The speech pathologist or occupational therapist may be helpful in demonstrating techniques that can improve mastication and swallowing.

SPONDYLOARTHROPATHIES

○ **What are the features of the most common spondyloarthropathies (SpAs)?**

Features of the Most Common Spondyloarthropathies

Features	Ankylosing spondylitis	Reactive arthritis (including Reiter's syndrome)	Psoriatic arthritis	IBD-associated spondyloarthropathy
Prevalence	0.1% to 0.2%	0.1%	0.2% to 0.4%	Rare
Age at onset	Late teens to early adulthood	Late teens to early adulthood	35 to 45 years	Any age
Male to female rate	3:1	5:1	1:1	1:1
HLA-B27	90% to 95%	80%	40%	30%
Sacroiliitis				
Frequency	100%	40% to 60%	40%	20%
Distribution	Symmetric	Asymmetric	Asymmetric	Symmetric
Syndesmophytes	Delicate, marginal	Bulky, nonmarginal	Bulky, nonmarginal	Delicate, marginal
Peripheral arthritis				
Frequency	Occasional	Common	Common	Common
Distribution	Asymmetric, lower limbs	Asymmetric, lower limbs	Asymmetric, any joint	Asymmetric, lower limbs
Enthesitis	Common	Very common	Very common	Occasional
Dactylitis	Uncommon	Common	Common	Uncommon
Skin lesions	None	Circinate balanitis, keratoderma blennorrhagicum	Psoriasis	Erythema nodosum, pyoderma gangrenosum
Nail changes	None	Onycholysis	Pitting, onycholysis	Clubbing
Ocular conditions	Acute anterior uveitis	Acute anterior uveitis, conjunctivitis	Chronic uveitis	Chronic uveitis
Oral conditions	Ulcers	Ulcers	Ulcers	Ulcers
Cardiac conditions	Aortic regurgitation, conduction defects	Aortic regurgitation, conduction defects	Aortic regurgitation, conduction defects	Aortic regurgitation
Pulmonary features	Upper lobe fibrosis	None	None	None
Gastrointestinal conditions	None	Diarrhea	None	Crohn's disease, ulcerative colitis
Renal conditions	Amyloidosis, IgA nephropathy	Amyloidosis	Amyloidosis	Nephrolithiasis
Genitourinary conditions	Prostatitis	Urethritis, cervicitis	None	None

○ **What is the incidence and prevalence of ankylosing spondylitis?**

Incidence of SpAs is 0.1-0.2% of the general population. The prevalence of AS is 0.1-0.2% overall but is higher in certain Native American populations and lower in African Americans.

○ **What are the New York and Rome criteria for AS?**

New York Criteria (1984)	Rome Criteria (1961)
Low back pain with inflammatory characteristics Limitation of lumbar spine motion in sagittal and frontal planes Decreased chest expansion Bilateral sacroiliitis grade 2 or higher Unilateral sacroiliitis grade 3 or higher	Low back pain and stiffness for >3 months which is not relieved by rest Pain and stiffness in the thoracic region Limited motion in the lumbar spine Limited chest expansion History of uveitis
Definite AS when the fourth or fifth criterion mentioned presents with any clinical criteria	**Diagnosis of AS when any clinical criteria present with bilateral sacroiliitis grade 2 or higher**

○ **What pattern of peripheral joint pathology is evident in AS?**

Enthesitis and synovitis account for some of the peripheral joint involvement. Peripheral joint disease occurs in 33% of patients, most commonly in the hips. Hip involvement usually occurs in the first 10 years of the disease course and typically is bilateral. Other joints may be involved, including the shoulder girdle (glenohumeral, acromioclavicular, and sternoclavicular joints), costovertebral joints, costosternal junctions, manubriosternal joints, symphysis pubis, and temporal mandibular joints.

○ **What are the laboratory findings in AS?**

The laboratory findings are less remarkable in AS than in RA and include increased erythrocyte sedimentation rate with mild normocytic, normochromic anemia and negative results for rheumatoid factor and antinuclear antibodies. HLA-B27 is positive in more than 90% of AS patients, 3% to 75% of Reiter syndrome patients, 50% of patients with psoriatic arthritis with spinal involvement, and 50% of colitic spondylitis patients. The diagnostic value of HLA-B27 for AS is limited by low specificity. It may be most useful in early or atypical AS and Reiter syndrome.

○ **What are the distinguishing findings of AS in imaging studies?**

Radiographic findings in AS remain the most important diagnostic and monitoring tools; initial abnormalities occur in sacroiliac joints and thoracolumbar and lumbosacral junctions. All parts of the axial skeleton and sites of enthesopathy may develop characteristic abnormalities with advanced disease. Computed tomography shows detailed images of the sacroiliac joints and may be useful to clarify uncertain diagnoses. Magnetic resonance imaging is not superior to plain radiography or computed tomography for detecting sacroiliitis, but is helpful in the evaluation of cauda equina syndrome and medullary compression in atlantoaxial instability.

○ **What is the differential diagnosis for sacroiliitis?**

The sacroiliitis of AS involves both sides of the sacroiliac joints, whereas osteitis condensans ilii involves only the iliac side and occurs more commonly in multiparous women. The sacroiliac joint is not usually involved in diffuse idiopathic skeletal hyperostosis. The vertical syndesmophytes and squaring of vertebrae in AS differentiate it from the large curved osteophytes and the paravertebral ossification of Reiter syndrome and psoriatic arthritis. Spotty involvement of the spine and absence of severe cervical spinal change are typical of Reiter syndrome and psoriatic arthritis. Spondylitis in inflammatory bowel disease resembles AS.

○ **What is the natural history for the spondyloarthropathies?**

A predictable pattern of AS emerges within the first 10 years of the disease. Fewer than 20% of patients with adult-onset AS deteriorate to a condition of significant disability. The life span of patients with AS is nearly normal. Deaths are usually attributable to cardiac involvement, cervical spinal fractures or subluxation, or amyloidosis.

○ **What are important prognosticators in the spondyloarthropathies?**

Early peripheral joint disease, iritis, pulmonary fibrosis, and persistently high erythrocyte sedimentation rates indicate a poor prognosis. Investigators found that patients with peripheral joint involvement performing heavy work tended to have prolonged sick leaves, whereas long-term disability was more frequent when work involved exposure to cold conditions and prolonged standing. Sedentary work and involvement in formal vocational rehabilitation programs lessened the incidence of long-term disability. Many patients with Reiter syndrome experience relapses, often after many symptom-free years. Approximately 20% to 50% develop chronic peripheral arthritis or progressive spondylitis. Severe disability usually occurs from arthritis of the foot and the ankle, aggressive axial involvement, or blindness.

O   **What DMARDs are considered for the management of peripheral joint pathology in AS?**

Sulfasalazine and methotrexate.

O   **What role do the biological agents have in the treatment of AS?**

Patients who are being considered for anti-TNF therapy should meet classification criteria for definite AS and have disease that has been active for at least a month. Active disease as indicated by both the Bath ankylosing spondylitis disease activity Index (BASDAI) score and a physician global assessment should be present to warrant anti-TNF therapy.

Univariate analysis the parameters which are predictive of a positive response to TNF blockers are	When analyzed using a multivariate model the predictors of a positive response to TNF blockers are
Younger age Shorter disease duration Good functional ability (as measured by the Bath Ankylosing Spondylitis Functional Index (BASFI)) Elevated ESR and CRP	Disease duration Better functional index (BASFI) Higher disease activity as measured by BASDAI Elevated CRP.

O   **What rehabilitation problems occur in the spondyloarthropathies?**

With axial involvement, a number of rehabilitation problems occur, including limitation of motion of the cervical and lumbar spines, paravertebral muscle spasm, and decreased chest expansion due to thoracic and costovertebral involvement. Loss of both cervical extension and lumbar lordosis is common. Visual impairment is associated with the former. Functional disability is proportional to loss of axial motion in the cervical region. In addition to back pain, which is frequently seen in this syndrome, feet and ankles are often the most symptomatic anatomic regions affected by arthritis. The entheses, including Achilles and posterior tibialis tendons, are involved. Reiter's syndrome is associated with fusion of the tarsal and metatarsal joints and Achilles tendon shortening.

O   **What are the key elements to incorporate in the rehabilitation program for a patient with a spondyloarthropathy?**

Key elements in a rehabilitation program include maintaining critical ROM, posture, and strength; relieving pain; and providing appropriate orthotics. An AROM program to maintain at least critical joint motion is prescribed (e.g., maintaining at least 75° of shoulder abduction, 10° of elbow flexion, 90° of wrist supination, 15° of hip flexion, 30° of knee flexion, and the ability to obtain neutral position at the ankle and functional grasp at the hand). In addition, encouraging good posture is extremely important, and a firm mattress or bed board should be recommended. The patient should rest in the prone position to encourage extension of the spine. Lying on the side is to be avoided because this encourages cervical and thoracic kyphosis. Use of good postural habits in walking and sitting is requisite.

O   **What evidence exists for the role of therapeutic exercise in patients with AS?**

Exercise studies in patients with AS have indicated benefit in terms of increased ROM and strength, and some studies have claimed long-term benefits provided that exercises are continued. Appropriate exercise should be prescribed to promote spinal extension and ROM of the neck, shoulders, and hips. Swimming is excellent for isotonic ROM and aerobic exercise and may require use of a mask and snorkel. Mirror devices for the car or prism glasses for reading are helpful for patients with limited neck motion, as are long handled reachers and shoehorns. All preventive and restorative rehabilitation strategies help ensure maximal function and psychological and vocational adjustment.

○   **If patients with AS undergo hip reconstructive surgery what complication is noted to be higher in this patient population?**

Patients with severe deforming disease, especially involving the hips and knees may benefit from total joint
replacement. However, the outcome of total hip arthroplasty may be compromised by heterotopic ossification and
reankylosis. Investigators have reported that 6% of patients with severe hip disease required total hip arthroplasty, with good
or excellent results in more than two-thirds of patients.

CRYSTALLINE ARTHROPATHIES

○ **What is the typical clinical presentation of pseudogout?**

This disease is characterized by acute or subacute self-limited attacks of arthritis involving one or several appendicular joints. The attacks, which range in duration from 1 day to several weeks, generally are less painful than attacks of gout and may be provoked by trauma, surgery, intraarticular injections, or medical illness. The knee is the most common site of acute arthritis, but other sites, such as the hip, shoulder, elbow, wrist, ankle, and acromioclavicular, talocalcaneal, and metatarsophalangeal joints, may be involved. Occasionally pain in the heel or spine may be the initial complaint. Inflammation may begin in one joint and spread to another.

○ **In which medical conditions is their an association of CPPD?**

DM, OA, hyperparathyroidism, Charcot arthropathy, gout

○ **What is chondrocalcinosis?**

Chondrocalcinosis is the deposition of calcium pyrophosphate crystals in cartilage. It may deposit in fibrocartilage or hyaline cartilage. Fibrocartilaginous calcification is most common in the menisci of the knee, triangular cartilage of the wrist, symphysis pubis, anulus fibrosus of the intervertebral disc, and acetabular and glenoid labra, although it may be observed at other sites, such as within the discs of the acromioclavicular and sternoclavicular joints. Fibrocartilaginous deposits appear as thick, shaggy, irregular radiodense areas, particularly within the central aspect of the joint cavity. Hyaline cartilage calcification may occur in many locations but is most common in the wrist, knee, elbow, and hip. These deposits are thin and linear and are parallel to and separated from the subjacent subchondral bone.

○ **What are the demographic characteristics of gout?**

Idiopathic gout occurs far more frequently in men than in women (20 to 1). The first attack of arthritis most frequently appears during the fifth decade of life in men and in the postmenopausal period in women, although it may occur at any age, having been described even in patients over the age of 100 years.

○ **What presentation characterizes acute gouty arthritis?**

Early in the course of gouty arthritis the disorder usually is monoarticular or oligoarticular, although occasionally it is polyarticular. Gout has predilection for the joints of the lower extremity, particularly the first metatarsophalangeal and intertarsal joints, ankles, and knees. The first metatarsophalangeal joint is the most common site of initial involvement and may eventually be altered in 75 to 90 per cent of patients with gout. The onset and severity of arthritis in acute gout often are dramatic, and the clinical findings of acute gout may simulate those of a septic arthritis. Pain, tenderness, and swelling occur within several hours and may persist for days to weeks.

○ **What pathological features develop later on in the course of gout?**

The interphalangeal and metacarpophalangeal joints of the fingers, wrists, and elbows often are abnormal in persons in whom the arthritis is of longer duration. Inflammatory changes in the spine, hip, shoulder, or sacroiliac joints are unusual and generally occur only in long-standing articular disease.

○ **What trends have been noted with regard to chronic tophaceous gout as a result of anti-hyperuricemic therapy?**

Although in the past 50 to 60 per cent of patients with gout developed clinical or radiographic evidence of deposits of monosodium urate (called tophi) prior to the advent of effective therapy for hyperuricemia, this frequency has now decreased sharply. Chronic gouty arthritis occurs in less than one half of patients who experience recurrent acute attacks.

○ **What are the characteristics of tophi?**

Tophi commonly occur in the synovium and subchondral bone and frequently are noted on the helix of the ear and in the subcutaneous and tendinous tissues of the elbow, hand, foot, knee, and forearm. These deposits may appear as irregular, hard masses and produce ulceration of the overlying skin with extrusion of chalky masses or urate crystals. In rare circumstances, such deposits in soft tissues occur in the absence of articular disease.

○ **Summarize the pharmacotherapy for acute gouty arthritis**

Systemic Therapy Options for Acute Gouty Arthritis.

Drug	Example Regimens	Major Considerations
Nonsteroidal antiinflammatory drugs		
Nonselective COX inhibitors		
Naproxen	750–1000 mg orally daily for 3 days, then 500–750 mg orally daily for 4–7 days (in 2 divided doses)	Potentially cost saving Avoid in patients with renal or hepatic failure and patients at risk for clinically significant gastrointestinal adverse effects, hemorrhage, congestive heart failure, or asthma
Sulindac	300–400 mg orally daily (in 2 divided doses) for 7–10 days	
Indomethacin	150–200 mg orally daily for 3 days, then 100 mg orally daily for 4–7 days (in 2–4 divided doses)	
Selective COX-2 inhibitors		
Celecoxib	400 mg orally on the first day, then 200 mg daily (in 2 divided doses) for 6–10 days	Use with caution in patients at risk for clinically significant gastrointestinal adverse effects, including active peptic ulcer; May increase risk of cardiovascular events
Systemic corticosteroids		
Prednisone	40–60 mg daily for 3 days, then decrease by 10–15 mg per day every 3 days until discontinuation	Avoid use if joint sepsis not excluded Avoid in patients subject to hyperglycemia
Methylprednisolone	100–150 mg per day for 1–2 days	
Triamcinolone acetonide	60 mg intramuscularly once	
Corticotropin	25 USP units subcutaneously for acute small joint monoarticular	Not universally available; Less effective in patients receiving long-term oral corticosteroid therapy
	40 USP units intramuscularly or intravenously once for involvement of larger joints or polyarticular	Risk of corticotropin hypersensitivity attenuated by the use of synthetic formulation
Colchicine	To curtail acute episodes of gout within the first few hours: 0.6 mg once every hour for up to 3 hr (maximum, 3 pills); after the acute attack, low-dose oral colchicine can be used as follows for prophylaxis against acute gout, particularly before the initiation of antihyperuricemic therapy: 0.6 mg orally twice daily in patients with creatinine clearance =50 ml/min 0.6 mg orally per day in patients with creatinine clearance of 35–49 ml/min 0.6 mg every 2–3 days in patients with creatinine clearance of 10–34 ml/min Avoid in patients with creatinine clearance <10 ml/min, patients receiving hemodialysis, patients with clinically significant hepatic or hepatobiliary dysfunction, and those with combined hepatic and renal disease Reduce the maintenance doses recommended above by half in patients =70 yr. of age	Potential severity of nausea, vomiting, diarrhea, and dehydration and efficacy and safety of other options generally render unnecessary the use of more extended dosing regimens of oral colchicine as a primary therapy Becomes less effective as primary treatment for acute gout after the first day of gouty arthritis Caution and dose reduction needed in patients with history of colchicine use Patients receiving long-term low-dose oral colchicine should be regularly monitored for weakness, potential elevation in creatine phosphokinase, and bone marrow suppression. Potential drug interactions with erythromycin, simvastatin, and cyclosporine can increase risk of colchicine-induced toxic effects Avoid intravenous colchicine

○ **How is allopurinol used as a prophylactic agent?**

Allopurinol is indicated in the presence of urate overproduction, either of endogenous origin or of dietary origin, or because of increased marrow cell turnover due to myeloproliferative disorders (so-called secondary gout). Allopurinol therapy should be initiated only after the acute attack of gout has entirely resolved. Administration to a patient with subsiding gout can cause severe exacerbation of the gout. It is wise to increase the dose of allopurinol slowly so that the full proposed dosage is reached only after 3–4 weeks. Concurrent colchicine prophylaxis (0.5 mg bid.) is also of value in preventing acute flare-ups during the institution of urate-lowering therapy. The requisite dose need be given once daily and should be adjusted to bring the serum urate concentration to less than 6.7mg/dl (0.4mmol/l). The maximum effect is seen between 4–14 days and results in a stable fall of the serum urate.

O   **What patterns of presentation are observed in patients with neuropathic arthropathy?**

The distribution of joint involvement depends on the underlying neuropathy. The following rule is a reasonable clinical guide: tabes dorsalis involves the larger joints of the lower limbs; syringomyelia the larger joints of the upper limbs and diabetes mellitus the joints of the foot.

O   **How does neuropathic arthropathy present in the knee?**

Although onset of neuropathic arthropathy may be gradual, it is often sudden occurring occasionally within a few hours (pseudo-inflammatory). The knee becomes warm and swollen with signs of joint effusion. Since there is relatively little pain and functional disability, the patients often do not seek medical consultation and the condition may regress within a few weeks. However, there is often a slowly or more rapidly progressive deterioration and the knee may become permanently symptomatic and swollen, with instability leading to valgum, varum or recurvatum deformities, enlargement of the articular bones and periarticular tissues. Although abnormalities are gross and the clinical picture even alarming, the joint is surprisingly painless. The patient is able to walk, although with a limp. On examination the range of motion is usually subnormal, but on occasion may even be excessive as a result of laxity and subluxation. Instability becomes permanent and deteriorates with time.

O   **How does neuropathic arthropathy present in other proximal limb joints?**

A more or less similar evolution of the condition may occur in other major limb joints (e.g. hip, ankles, shoulder, elbow or wrist). More than one joint may be affected in the individual patient. Mono- or oligoarticular involvement is most common, but polyarticular forms do occur. When the hip is affected it can often result in extensive joint destruction, shortening of the leg, severe loss of function and a limp on walking. Similarly, when the shoulder is involved the process may be highly destructive and finally result in a painless dangling arm.

O   **How does neuropathic arthropathy present in the tarsometatarsal joints?**

When the tarsometatarsal joints are affected there is edema of the dorsum of the foot and the condition may ultimately lead to bony deformities with dorsal prominence or plantar protrusion. Downward collapse of the tarsal bones may produce abnormal convexity of the volar surface.

O   **What are the features of involvement in the metatarsophalangeal joints?**

Localization of neuropathic arthropathy in the metatarsophalangeal joints may result in swelling and other signs of inflammation. Predominant localization in the first metatarsophalangeal joint occasionally mimics gout. The articular disorder is frequently accompanied by trophic skin lesions and ulcers in the sole of the foot. Chronic ulceration may be present predominantly in weight-bearing areas of the metatarsophalangeal joints (particularly the first and fifth), the heel and the lateral edge of the foot. These ulcers are often circular (round) and between a few millimeters and 1cm in diameter. The edges are protruding, sharp, atrophic, often grayish and usually do not cicatrize.

O   **What happens in long standing neurogenic arthropathy?**

The condition evolves with successive exacerbations characterized by signs of inflammation in the foot, the appearance or increase in cutaneous ulcers and an increase in articular deformities. Due to the relative painlessness, the condition is well tolerated. During the course of the disease the foot becomes further mutilated. The process may also affect the interphalangeal joints. The phalangeal bones of the toes may disappear and the tarsus and metatarsus telescope causing the foot to become shortened and the plantar arch to disappear. These may result in enlargement of the foot, which together with the other abnormalities, give rise to a so-called cubic foot. Skin and bone lesions often become infected and are difficult to manage.

O   **How does neuropathic arthropathy present in the spine?**

In the spine localization is most frequent in the lumbar region although the cervical and dorsal spine may also be involved. Involvement of the spine may lead to severe deformity (kyphosis, scoliosis) in the presence of normal mobility and relative absence of pain. Because of this paucity of symptoms, the condition is often first discovered during examination. Occasionally, signs of nerve root compression are present.

O   **How does neuropathic arthropathy present in patients with syringomyelia?**

This condition is more common in men than woman with onset between the ages of 20 to 40. The disease usually progresses slowly. Arthropathy may occur early after diagnosis of the neurologic disease and is present in as many as 25% of cases of syringomyelia. Joints affected are predominantly the shoulder, elbow and more rarely the wrist, fingers and cervical spine, usually unilaterally. Arthropathy is similar to that of tabes dorsalis, although the condition is almost exclusively found in the upper limbs. Neurologic manifestations are characteristic loss of sensitivity to temperature and pain, whereas tactile and postural sensitivity are preserved (so-called syringomyelic dissociation), associated with amyotrophic paralysis in the same region of the neck, or upper limb. Magnetic resonance imaging of the spinal cord is required for (or may reveal) the diagnosis of syringomyelia.

O   **How does neuropathic arthropathy present in DM?**

Sensory diabetic neuropathy (superficial and deep, distal hypoesthesia of the lower limb) complicates long-standing (poorly controlled) type I or type II diabetes mellitus, and has become the major cause of neuropathic arthropathy. It has been estimated that neuropathic arthropathy occurs in 0.1–0.5% of diabetic patients. The joint disease is most frequently unilateral, but may be bilateral. It occurs equally in both sexes, mostly after the age of 50 and is largely found in the foot, often associated with ulcers. The condition has been identified in the following joints: tarsal, tarsometatarsal and metatarsophalangeal. The tibiotarsal joint and knee are rarely affected.

O   **What other miscellaneous conditions can present with neuropathic arthropathy?**

A variety of other neurologic diseases affecting the spinal cord or peripheral nerves can lead to neuropathic arthropathy. These include spinal cord or peripheral nerve injury, intraspinal tumors, degenerative spinal disease, arachnoiditis, myelopathy of pernicious anemia, Charcot–Marie–Tooth disease, familial interstitial hypertrophic polyneuropathy of Dejerine and Sottas, congenital insensitivity to pain, hereditary dysautonomia, amyloidosis, and yaws.

O   **Illustrate the pathogenesis of neuropathic arthropathy**

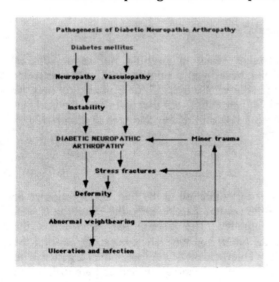

The pathogenesis of this condition is uncertain but it is probably due to a combination of mechanical and vascular factors resulting from diabetic peripheral neuropathy. Lack of proprioception secondary to peripheral neuropathy may result in ligamentous laxity, increased range of joint movement, instability, and damage by minor trauma, to which the relatively insensitive neuropathic foot is prone. An alternative theory suggests that automatic neuropathy results in vasomotor changes and the formation of arteriovenous shunts. These in turn result in reductions in effective skin and bone blood flow, despite the good and sometimes bounding foot pulses in these patients.

O   **What management strategies are utilized in neuropathic arthropathy?**

Immobilization of the joint is an important principle and should be done as soon as possible. In cases where the lower limb is involved, cessation of weight bearing is important. This is particularly mandatory during periods of apparent vasomotor disturbance. Joint immobilization and rest should last for between several weeks and three months and can lead to stabilization of the joint and improvement in the osteoarticular lesion. For neuropathic arthropathy of the lower limbs the following additional measures are indicated: use of an assistive device and accommodative footwear for joint protection.

Total contact casting, walking splints, felt foam padding, cutout sandals, short leg walkers (orthosis), wedged sandals, custom molded shoes can be fabricated to correct for limb joint abnormalities and/or subluxation. In cases of foot sole ulcers, rigorous hygiene is required: disinfection should be carried out cautiously to avoid the cytotoxic effects of these agents. Sterile bandaging and antibiotic treatment of superimposed infection should be assiduously pursued.

REGIONAL MUSCULOSKELETAL PAIN SYNDROMES:

ACUTE AND CHRONIC

○ **What does the stress strain curve depict?**

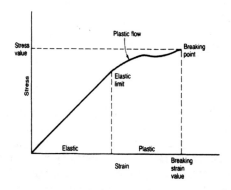

The stress strain curve is the fundamental principle that underlies the pathophysiological basis of both acute trauma and overuse injuries of the musculoskeletal system. Whether through the single application of external forces or the repetitive loading or impact of external forces the safety factor of the musculoskeletal system may be exceeded resulting in failure of its constituent tissues and subsequent injury and concomitant inflammatory reaction. The inflammatory reaction in the musculoskeletal system gives way to the connective tissue repair phase. The biomechanical properties of repairing tissues vary during the process. Until remodeling is complete the repair process itself is vulnerable to reinjury.

○ **What biomechanical feature is common to both athletic and occupational injuries?**

The ability to adapt to these repetitive demands depends on the magnitude of each load, the frequency of the repetitions, the duration of the cycles, the frequency of the rest periods, and the tolerance level and condition of the tissue being stressed. The smaller the individual load, the greater the number of load cycles that may be tolerated. Repeated loads that are within the physiologic range of repair create improved tolerance of the musculoskeletal system and the anticipated rewards of an exercise regimen; repeated overloading results in an inflammatory tissue response that produces weakening and fatigue of the involved body tissue, increased susceptibility to injury, and, with continued stress, injury.

○ **What kinds of loads are common in athletic and occupational injuries?**

Five major types of load exist: traction, compression, bending, twisting, and shearing. Traction loads result in muscle, tendon, or ligament rupture when the intrinsic tensile strength is exceeded. Compression loads typically are responsible for cartilaginous and osseous injuries. Bending loads usually are responsible for osseous fracture originating at the maximum point of tensile stress. Twisting (torsion) loads are responsible for osseous fracture or ligamentous rupture (i.e., a spiral fracture of the proximal portion of the humerus in a professional pitcher or an anterior cruciate ligament rupture in a skier or a football player). Shear stress loads typically are responsible for joint surface injuries (e.g., a tear of the knee menisci or osteochondral fracture).

○ **How does age affect the patterns of musculoskeletal injury?**

The injury varies according to the patient's age and the corresponding musculoskeletal development (i.e., elasticity and strength of the various components). Muscular strength and the elasticity of tendons and ligaments decrease after the age of approximately 30 years, and the strength of bone decreases after approximately 50 years of age; hence, the same athletic pursuit results in different injuries in the skeletally immature person, the young adolescent, the adult, and the elderly patient.

○ **What is the pattern of injury in the skeletally immature patient?**

In the skeletally immature patient, the physeal cartilage is weaker than the joint capsule; therefore, injuries through the growth plate (physis) or apophysis are more common.

O   **What type of injury pattern is encountered in the adolescent?**

Similarly, the physeal cartilage is weaker than the tendon and ligaments, and a violent rapid loading of a muscle, sufficient to produce a tendon rupture in an adult, typically will result in an apophyseal bony avulsion in the adolescent patient. The adolescent patient also is prone to chondral and osteochondral fractures (in comparison to the adult, who suffers stress fractures)

O   **What type of injury pattern is likely to occur in the older adult?**

The elderly patient is prone to tendon and ligament ruptures and osteoarthritis.

O   **What are the characteristic features of muscle injury?**

Muscle injuries account for approximately 10 to 30 per cent of all athletic/occupational injuries. The mildest injury is a muscle cramp from dehydration and minute muscle rupture, bleeding, or impaired circulation. Muscle soreness, pain, tenderness, and swelling can occur after strenuous training. Muscles are injured by both impact (direct) (e.g., football) and overloading (indirect) (e.g., running). A muscle rupture occurs from either distraction or compression. Distraction injuries result primarily from over stretching and affect the superficial parts of the muscles at their insertions and origins; these are discussed in the section on muscle strains. Compression injuries (muscle contusion) result from direct impact and affect primarily the deep parts of the muscles.

O   **What are the characteristics of musculotendinous junction injuries?**

The site of musculotendinous injury depends on the patient's age; musculotendinous junction injuries occur more commonly in the adolescent and adult, whereas tendon injuries are more common in the adult and elderly patient. The myotendinous junction is vulnerable when tension is applied quickly, when it is applied obliquely, when the muscle is maximally innervated and under tension before loading, or when the tendon is weak with respect to the muscle. The musculotendinous junction is especially vulnerable in those muscles that cross two joints (e.g., hamstrings, quadriceps, and gastrocnemius). Muscle strains typically localize to a single muscle within a group of synergists (e.g., the adductor longus, rectus femoris, and the medial head of the gastrocnemius).

O   **What are the pathological features of musculotendinous junction injuries?**

A myotendinous junction injury is characterized by inflammation and edema and, to a lesser extent, hemorrhage. When disruption occurs at the myotendinous junction, fluid may collect at the site of disruption and dissect along the epimysium and subcutis remote from the musculotendinous junction.

O   **How are muscle strains graded?**

Muscle strains are graded as follows: grade one (mild)—less than 50 per cent fiber disruption and no loss of strength or restriction of movement; grade two (moderate)—50 per cent disruption and partial loss of strength; and grade three (severe)—complete musculotendinous rupture, with or without muscle retraction and with loss of strength and function.

O   **What are the characteristics of ligament injuries?**

Ligaments attach bone to bone and are a frequent source of pain and instability in the young adult and adult athlete. Inflammation of the ligamentous attachment to bone from repeated stresses may produce bleeding, periosteal irritation, bone fragmentation, and traction enthesophyte. Ligament injuries occur in all joints but are most prevalent in the knees, ankles, elbows, and metacarpophalangeal joint of the thumb of athletes. Ligament strains are graded similarly 1-3.

O   **What diagnostic modalities aid in the diagnosis of ligament injuries?**

If guarding can be eliminated, stress films, with comparison to the opposite side, may confirm the existence of ligamentous laxity or joint instability. Although intraarticular ligaments can be evaluated arthrographically, MR imaging and ultrasound are noninvasive methods of visualizing both intra and extraarticular ligaments directly and distinguishing acute from chronic injury.

○   **What are the characteristics of bursae injury?**

A bursa is a sac formed by two layers of synovial tissue located at sites of friction between a bone and a tendon or superficial to a bone or tendon. Bursitis indicates inflammation and edema, usually as a result of repetitive trauma from friction or external pressure.

○   **What factors are responsible for nerve injuries?**

The peripheral nerves can be affected by direct trauma, repetitive motion and loading, muscular hypertrophy, ganglia, or irritation by posttraumatic bone excrescences. Decreased flexibility has been implicated in nerve entrapment syndromes in athletes. Acute denervation of muscle is not demonstrated reliably by MR imaging; subacute denervation has prolonged T1 and T2 values; and chronically denervated muscles show atrophy and fatty infiltration in T1-weighted images. Any and all peripheral nerves are at risk.

SHOULDER

○   **What is the association of scapula winging and serratus anterior dysfunction?**

Winging of the scapula can be demonstrated by asking the patient to do a push-up against the wall. It is indicative of serratus anterior weakness (as in long thoracic nerve palsy). Loss of muscle function results in a particular type of scapular winging. At rest with the arm at the side, the scapula as a whole is translocated medially with the inferior angle rotated medially. The affected side's shoulder appears somewhat "lower" because of the rotation. Such abnormalities are accentuated by having the patient abduct the arm and flex it anteriorly.

○   **What are the features associated with scapula winging from trapezius and rhomboid dysfunction?**

Scapular winging can result not only from serratus anterior dysfunction, but also from rhomboid and trapezius muscle weakness. Close inspection of the patient can help to distinguish clinically the type of scapular winging and hence which nerve is potentially injured. In trapezius palsy (spinal accessory nerve), the shoulder droops and winging is accentuated by arm abduction at the shoulder level. Rhomboid weakness is best demonstrated by slowly lowering the arms from the forward elevated position.

○   **Describe the apprehension test for the glenohumeral joint**

Apprehension test for anterior shoulder dislocation: A test designed to determine whether a patient has a history of anterior dislocations. With the patient supine, the examiner slowly abducts and externally rotates the patient's arm. The test is positive if the patient becomes apprehensive and resists further motion.

○   **What is the apprehension test for posterior dislocation?**

Apprehension test for posterior shoulder dislocation: A test designed to determine whether a patient has a history of posterior dislocations. With the patient supine, the examiner slowly flexes the patient's arm to 90° and the patient's elbow to 90°. The examiner then internally rotates the patient's arm. A posterior force is then applied to the patient's elbow. The test result is positive if the patient becomes apprehensive and resists further motion.

○   **Describe the clunk test.**

A test designed to determine the presence of a tear of the glenoid labrum. With the patient supine, the examiner places one hand on the posterior aspect of the shoulder over the humeral head. The examiner fully abducts the arm over the patient's head and then pushes anteriorly with the hand over the humeral head. The test is positive if a "clunk" or grinding is palpated. The test may also cause apprehension if anterior instability is present.

○ **Describe the drop arm test.**

A test designed to determine the presence of a torn rotator cuff. With the patient seated, the examiner abducts; the patient's shoulder to 90'. The test result is positive if the patient is unable to lower the arm slowly to the side in the same arc of movement or has severe pain when attempting to do so.

○ **Describe the Hawkins-Kennedy test.**

A test designed to identify supraspinatus tendinitis. The patient stands while the examiner flexes the arm to 90° and then forcibly internally rotates the shoulder. The test result is positive if pain is present during the maneuver.

○ **Describe the impingement test.**

A test designed to identify inflammation of tissues within the subacromial space. The patient's upper extremity is forcibly flexed forward by the examiner. The maneuver is thought to decrease the space between the head of the humerus and acromion process. The test result is positive if the patient reports pain.

○ **Describe Ludington's test.**

A test designed for determining whether there has been a rupture of the long head of the biceps tendon. The patient is seated and clasps both hands on top of the head, supporting the weight of the upper limbs. The patient then alternately contracts and relaxes the biceps muscles. The test result is positive if the examiner cannot palpate the long head of the biceps tendon of the affected arm during the contractions.

○ **Describe Speeds test.***

A test designed to determine whether bicipital tendonitis or subluxation are present. With the forearm supinated and elbow fully extended, the patient tries to flex the arm against resistance applied by the examiner. The test result is positive if the patient reports increased pain or instability in the area of the bicipital groove. See comment under Yergason's test.

○ **Describe the sulcus sign.**

A test designed to determine the presence of inferior instability. The patient stands with the arm by the side and the shoulder muscles relaxed. The examiner grasps the patient's forearm and pulls distally. The test result is positive if a space larger than one thumb width appears between the acromion and the humeral head.

○ **What is the supraspinatus test.**

A test designed to identify a tear in the supraspinatus tendon. The seated patient's upper limbs are positioned horizontally at 30° anterior to the frontal plane and internally rotated. The examiner applies a downward force on the patient's limbs. The test result is positive if pain and weakness are present on the involved side.

○ **Describe the transverse humeral ligament test.**

A test designed to identify a torn transverse humeral ligament. The examiner abducts and internally rotates the patient's shoulder. The examiner then palpates the bicipital groove while externally rotating the patient's shoulder. The test result is positive if the biceps tendon can be felt to "snap" in and out of the groove with shoulder external rotation.

○ **Describe Yergason's test.***

A test designed to identify tendonitis/subluxation of the long head of the biceps. The seated patient's arm is positioned at the side with the elbow flexed to 90°. Supination of the forearm against resistance produces pain or instability in the biceps tendon in the area of the bicipital groove. *Note that traditionally this test was solely intended for assessing instability of the long head of the biceps tendon in distinction to Speeds test which is intended for eliciting pain associated with long head of biceps tendinitis.

○ **What mechanical factors contribute to impingement of the supraspinatus tendon?**

The anatomical configuration of the shoulder joint is such that the cuff is subjected to stresses when the arm is in the elevated position. Impingement can occur as the supraspinatus tendon is compressed between the humeral head and the overlying anterior acromion, coracoacromial ligament and even the inferior border of the acromioclavicular joint. Impingement may be structural due to the presence of an acromial spur or degenerative acromioclavicular joint, but it may also be functional, due to superior migration of the humeral head during abduction and elevation.

○ **What mechanical factors contribute to rotator cuff tendinopathy in the younger athlete?**

Underlying glenohumeral instability is a frequent cause of rotator cuff tendinitis, particularly in the younger patient, as is eccentric overload in the throwing athlete, where the rotator cuff muscles act as decelerators of the throwing arm. As the rotator cuff becomes inflamed, thinned or torn, so its function as a humeral head depressor is compromised and superior migration of the humeral head can occur due to the unopposed action of the deltoid, giving rise to further impingement.

○ **What mechanical factors contribute to rotator cuff tendinopathy in the older worker?**

In the degenerative cuff with a complete tear this can eventually result in a cuff arthropathy with degenerative changes taking place at the subacromial and glenohumeral joints. The subacromial bursa lies between the rotator cuff tendons and the overlying acromial arch and becomes inflamed with this impingement. This is a reactive process and is usually a secondary phenomenon, although primary subacromial bursitis can result from trauma.

○ **How does the presentation of RTC disorders vary according to age group?**

Presentation depends to a degree on the age of the patient and the likely etiology. Tendinitis resulting from eccentric overload or glenohumeral instability in the young adult usually presents acutely following an activity such as throwing. In the middle-aged individual, onset may be more gradual, reflecting the underlying chronic changes seen in the involved tendon. The patient may present with aching and discomfort in the shoulder, pain on movement and a history of repetitive or strenuous upper limb activity. The elderly patient may present with no history of antecedent trauma or repetitive activity and there is usually a gradual history of increasing shoulder discomfort, night pain, pain with movement, and weakness if a degenerative tear is present

○ **What are the pain characteristics in RTC disorders?**

Patients frequently complain that they have difficulty with overhead activities. The pain at night usually occurs when rolling onto the affected side and is typically felt in the deltoid region rather than the point of the shoulder, although this can occur. Active movements may be restricted by pain and in the more severe or chronic cases a secondary capsulitis can develop, further restricting movement at the shoulder.

○ **What exam findings occur in RTC disorders?**

Findings on examination include a painful arc of abduction usually occurring between 70–120° abduction. When lowering from full abduction there is often a 'catch' of pain usually at midrange as impingement occurs. Passive motion tends to be full and pain-free if adequate muscle relaxation can be achieved. Point tenderness over the greater tuberosity can occur but is not always present and the diagnosis is confirmed by reproducing pain when resisting movement of the affected tendon and on impingement testing. In the older patient acromioclavicular joint involvement is often present and there may be early joint stiffness.

○ **What mechanisms are proposed in RTC disorders?**

Impingement has been shown to occur in forward flexion when the anterior margin of the acromion impinges on the supraspinatus tendon. The etiology is multifactorial. Four microtraumatic mechanisms of rotator cuff injury have been described, and several may occur simultaneously in the same patient. The mechanisms can be divided into primary impingement or secondary impingement pathology. In addition scapulothoracic dysfunction is postulated to be a contributing mechanism.

O   What is primary impingement?

The first is the classic impingement injury, now called primary impingement. Repetitive overhead activity results in impingement of the supraspinatus against the anterior, inferior aspect of the acromion and/or the coracoacromial ligament. The shape of the anterior slope of the acromion has been implicated in the development of primary impingement. Three distinct shapes have been described on the basis of a Y view or lateral radiograph of the scapula. Type I is a flat acromion, type II is curved, and type III is hooked. Although the cause-effect relationship between acromial shape and rotator cuff disorders is unclear, the occurrence of a full-thickness tear appears to correlate closely with a type II and especially a type III acromion.

O   What is secondary impingement?

The second microtraumatic mechanism is secondary impingement. Individuals who have shoulder instability as a result of congenital laxity, repetitive microtrauma (from participation in overhead sports), or macrotrauma place increased demands on the rotator cuff as it attempts to keep the humeral head centered in the glenoid. These demands are especially pronounced with overhead activities. Fatigue, intrinsic injury (tendinitis), and a partial under surface tear of the cuff may ensue. If the rotator cuff continues to fatigue, it may no longer center the humeral head in the glenoid, and dynamic cephalad migration of the humeral head in the glenoid occurs, resulting in secondary impingement of the rotator cuff under the coracoacromial arch.

O   What is a third mechanism contributing to impingement syndrome?

A third mechanism of microtrauma to the rotator cuff is tensile failure with throwing. During this repetitive eccentric loading, the rotator cuff is prone to overload, fatigue, tendinitis, and even a partial under surface tear. Again, as the rotator cuff fatigues, dynamic cephalad migration of the humeral head can occur, resulting in secondary impingement of the rotator cuff under the coracoacromial arch.

O   What is a fourth mechanism for impingement syndrome?

The fourth and final mechanism of microtrauma is internal or posterior superior glenoid impingement. This occurs with repetitive overhead activities, particularly in throwers, when the arm is abducted 90° and maximally externally rotated. In this position, the posterior inferior aspect of the supraspinatus is impinged between the greater tuberosity of the humeral head and the posterior superior labrum, producing fraying of the posterosuperior labrum and an under surface tear of the posterior aspect of the supraspinatus.

O   What is the Neer classification of the impingement syndrome?

The pathology of this impingement syndrome has been classified by Neer into three stages:
    Stage I, edema and hemorrhage of the tendon;
    Stage II, fibrosis of the subacromial bursa and tendinitis of the rotator cuff;
    Stage III, tendon degeneration, bony changes at the acromion and humeral head and eventual tendon rupture.
Generally, stage II occurs in patients aged 25–40 years, stage III in those aged over 40 years and stage I is the pathology found in those less than 25 years of age.

O   What imaging modalities are appropriate for RTC disorders?

Plain radiographs may show evidence of calcification in the rotator cuff tendons in chronic cases, and in long-standing cases there are changes suggestive of rotator cuff degeneration, i.e. cystic and sclerotic changes of the greater tuberosity insertion. Upward or superior migration of the humeral head also occurs. Diagnostic ultrasound and magnetic resonance imaging (MRI) can be used to demonstrate partial tears of the rotator cuff, although observer-dependence may present a problem with interpretation. Partial tears and tendinosis are best seen with MRI.

◯   **What pharmacotherapies are appropriate for rotator cuff disorders?**

Nonsteroidal antiinflammatory medication is appropriate in the acute phase for both its analgesic and antiinflammatory effects. Corticosteroid injection into an inflamed subacromial bursa provides rapid relief of inflammation. The injection must be correctly placed, however, because corticosteroid injected into musculotendinous-nous structures can weaken these structures and increase the risk of rupture.

◯   **What physical agents can be considered in RTC disorders?**

Cryotherapy, TENS, and ultrasound have all been used to expedite resolution of inflammation of the bursa and rotator cuff tendons. Gentle passive and active assisted range of motion may begin immediately. Particular attention should be paid to tightness of the external rotators with resultant limitation of internal rotation. Manual mobilization and cross-friction massage also help restore flexibility.

◯   **What role does surgical intervention have in rotator cuff disorders?**

Indications for surgery vary according to the age of the patient, stage of impingement or tendinitis, and the symptoms. The major indication for surgical intervention is pain, and in the presence of an intact rotator cuff, failure to respond to a conservative program within 1 year is a reasonable indication for surgery. This involves subacromial decompression and encompasses an anterior acromioplasty and resection of the coracoacromial ligament, both of which can be carried out arthroscopically. Any impingement due to acromioclavicular joint pathology must also be addressed at operation.

◯   **What therapeutic exercise strategies are appropriate initially for RTC disorders?**

Strengthening exercises begin isometrically. Static resistance exercises should be done in all planes and various angles that do not produce pain. During recovery, new connective tissue is laid down along lines of stress. Isometric exercises provide the appropriate physical environment in which fibroblasts can make healthy, organized connective tissue, yet avoid untoward force and movement on the healing tendon.

◯   **When is it appropriate to advance to dynamic resistance exercise therapy?**

Once full, pain-free range of motion is achieved, the athlete progresses to dynamic resistance strengthening exercises in all planes. External rotation should be strengthened preferentially over internal rotation to correct muscle imbalance. In addition to focusing on the rotator cuff itself, special emphasis is placed on fortifying the scapular stabilizers, which help to properly position the rotator cuff. Finally, once flexibility and strength have been regained, the patient must complete task-specific shoulder exercises prior to being allowed to return to work activity.

◯   **How do rotator cuff tears present clinically in the younger patient?**

In the young adult a partial tear can result from a fall or explosive shoulder movement and presents very much as a rotator cuff tendinitis, although onset is acute. Also, full active range of motion may be preserved. The acute complete rupture after trauma should be readily diagnosed. The mechanism of injury is usually a fall onto the outstretched arm, a hyperabduction injury or a fall onto the side of the shoulder. Bruising is often delayed and occurs in the upper arm, and there is an immediate loss of active abduction with weakness of abduction and external rotation.

◯   **How do rotator cuff tears present in older patients?**

Chronic full thickness tears are found in 7–27% of patients at autopsy, and many patients with a documented complete tear of the supraspinatus tendon have full active abduction, occasionally in the absence of pain. There may be no history of trauma and symptoms frequently become apparent with increased activity. The usual picture is one of pain on abduction and flexion with varying degrees of loss of active movement depending on the size of the tear. The patient may complain of weakness of abduction, flexion or external rotation depending on the tendon involved. There is a close association between dislocation of the shoulder in the patient over 40 years of age and partial or complete tears of the rotator cuff.

◯   **What exam findings are characteristic of RTC tears?**

Examination reveals many of the features of rotator cuff tendinitis but there is often an inability to maintain the arm in abduction when lowering from the elevated position, i.e. a positive 'drop-off' sign. Subacromial crepitus and pain on impingement testing are present. In advanced tears one may observe wasting of the infraspinatus, and to a lesser extent supraspinatus, muscle bellies, together with weakness of abduction, but more often weakness of external rotation reflects the size of the tear. Rupture of the long head of biceps tendon is frequently associated with chronic rotator cuff pathology.

O   What other imaging modalities are utilized for RTC tears?

Full thickness tears are readily demonstrated with single or double contrast arthrography, and although false negatives can occur, sensitivity approaches 90%. Partial tears can occasionally be seen. Estimation of the size of the defect using this technique is unreliable. Consequently MRI has largely replaced arthrography for the diagnosis of full and partial tears given its noninvasive safety and accuracy.

O   What are the advantages of arthroscopy in the diagnosis of rotator cuff pathology?

 Arthroscopy is now readily available as a means of establishing the diagnosis in the patient with shoulder pain who requires further assessment. It is particularly useful in the assessment of instability while at the same time allowing visualization of the rotator cuff, subacromial bursa, intra-articular bicipital tendon and glenoid labrum. It also has a role in the estimation of the size of a cuff tear prior to more definitive surgery.

O   What are surgical indications for the management of rotator cuff tears?

Surgeons normally reserve operative treatment of pathological rotator cuff conditions for failures of nonoperative treatment. It is imperative that nearly full motion be regained before surgical intervention to prevent severe postoperative stiffness. Surgery may be appropriate for an acute rotator cuff injury in a young patient with a massive avulsion or in an older patient (60 to 70 years of age) with a defined injury who is suddenly unable to externally rotate the arm against resistance. In clinical experience, these patients usually have an excellent return of both strength and function.

O   What surgical options are there for rotator cuff tears?

Orthopedic surgeons currently perform arthroscopic debridement of partial-thickness tears when they are found on intraarticular inspection during arthroscopic acromioplasty. When a lesion involves less than 50% of cuff thickness or is less than 1 cm in size, acromioplasty and debridement are sufficient treatment. When a tear is longer or thicker, elliptical excision of the diseased tendon and suturing to a trough in bone are indicated.

O   What postoperative rehabilitation is usually recommended?

After standard repair a Velpeau sling or a shoulder immobilizer is worn for 2 or 3 days, and then is removed for assisted exercises in flexion and external rotation to avoid adhesions, disuse atrophy, and disruption of the repairs. The repair is weakest at 3 weeks, and tendon strength is less than at the time of surgery for the first 3 months after surgery. Somewhat empirically we advance to isometric exercises of external rotation at 6 weeks, and at 12 weeks active motion is permitted. Patients are cautioned that overaggressive use of the extremity can lead to disruption of the repair for 6 to 12 months.

O   What is the etiology of bicipital tendon disorders?

Although frequently diagnosed, bicipital tendinitis is not often seen in isolation and usually occurs in association with rotator cuff tendinitis or impingement, or with glenohumeral instability. Primary involvement of the tendon is seen as an overuse injury in sports such as weight lifting where there is a repetitive stress placed upon the tendon, or after prolonged and repetitive carrying, e.g. of small children. The bicipital tendon acts as a secondary stabilizer of the humeral head and the translational movement seen with glenohumeral laxity can place increased stress upon the tendon leading to tendinitis. With chronic impingement or rotator cuff degeneration the biceps tendon may become fibrotic and attenuated and eventually rupture.

O   What symptoms and signs are evident with bicipital tendon disorders?

Pain is usually felt over the anterior aspect of the shoulder, often radiating into the biceps muscle with well localized tenderness over the tendon as it runs in the bicipital groove. Pain is felt with overhead activities and often with shoulder extension and elbow flexion. Examination may reveal features of impingement, rotator cuff tendinitis and instability, all of which are important in determining the etiology of bicipital tendinitis. Pain may be reproduced with resisted elbow flexion, supination and shoulder flexion and various provocation tests are described, although none appears to be consistently positive. Passive shoulder extension stretches the biceps and may be painful. Rupture of the tendon is evident when there is the characteristic deformity of the upper arm with bunching up of the lateral muscle belly of the biceps best seen with resisted elbow flexion and supination.

O   **How does acute rupture of the transverse ligament present?**

Acute rupture of the transverse humeral ligament can result in subluxation or dislocation of the tendon. This can present with symptoms similar to bicipital tendinitis but often a more specific complaint is made of catching and a clicking sensation at the shoulder. Clinical examination may demonstrate subluxation of the tendon, which is felt as the arm is passively moved through internal and external rotation while in the 90° abducted position.

O   **At which anatomical sites is the bicipital tendon vulnerable to injury?**

The tendon of the long head of biceps may be involved at several sites: its attachment to the superior glenoid labrum, which may be injured in a fall or throwing action; as it runs across the glenohumeral joint (intra-articular); or as it runs in the bicipital groove (extraarticular). The transverse humeral ligament stabilizes the tendon in the bicipital groove and if this mechanism is disrupted subluxation or dislocation of the tendon can result. This tends to occur as the arm is rotated in the abducted position. Also, the presence of a complete rotator cuff tear exposes the intra-articular portion of the bicipital tendon to the overlying acromion and further impingement.

O   **What imaging modalities are appropriate for bicipital tendon disorders?**

Special radiographic views demonstrate the bicipital groove, allowing assessment of its depth and the presence of any degenerative spurring. Filling of the synovial extension around the tendon is seen on arthrography and may be reduced in cases of chronic fibrosis. Computed tomographic arthrography can be used to demonstrate subluxation and dislocation of the tendon. Although MRI has proven to be equal in diagnostic accuracy. The tendon and any surrounding fluid can be seen well with diagnostic ultrasound, and this assists in the diagnosis of tears, both partial and complete, as well as tendinitis. Arthroscopy allows visualization of the intra-articular portion of the tendon and its labral attachment.

O   **What treatment approaches are appropriate for bicipital tendon disorders?**

It is necessary to establish whether the tendinitis is primary or secondary, since a failure to address any underlying rotator cuff pathology or instability will lead to a recurrence of symptoms. The principles of management are rest, and physical modalities, such as laser, coupled with NSAIDs as required. Corticosteroid injection is helpful in chronic cases but care should be taken not to inject the tendon itself. Since most cases of bicipital tendinitis are secondary, they usually settle as the primary condition is treated. The primary cases due to lifting or other activities respond to rest and simple antiinflammatory measures. Any conservative program must include range of motion exercises, stretches and, once symptoms have settled, a graduated eccentric and concentric biceps and rotator cuff strengthening program.

O   **When should surgical intervention be considered?**

In chronic resistant cases surgery can be considered and this may involve subacromial decompression in cases of impingement, or tenodesis when there is chronic thickening of the tendon in the groove. Rupture of the tendon is normally treated conservatively except in the occasional young patient where upper arm strength is critical to their sport or profession. Subluxation of the tendon is usually treated conservatively, although occasionally surgery is necessary.

O   **What is the definition of primary capsulitis of the glenohumeral joint (GHJ)?**

Primary capsulitis of the shoulder can be defined as a condition of unknown etiology in which there is a painful global restriction of glenohumeral movement in all planes, both active and passive, in the absence of joint degeneration sufficient to explain this restriction.

○   **What is the definition of secondary capsulitis of the GHJ?**

A condition known as secondary capsulitis exists in which is seen a similar clinical condition but in association with a clearly defined clinical disorder or precipitating event. Underlying diseases associated with this condition are diabetes mellitus, thyroid disease, pulmonary disorders such as tuberculosis or carcinoma, and cardiac disease or surgery. Myocardial infarct, cerebrovascular accident or shoulder trauma may precipitate the development of a shoulder capsulitis.

○   **What is the prevalence of adhesive capsulitis?**

The idiopathic form is uncommon. Good incidence and prevalence data are lacking, but one study estimated a 1-year incidence in patients seen in general practice ranges from 2/1,000 (7), to 2/100. The prevalence in an elderly population has been shown to be less than 1/100. The secondary form may be more common. Studies show up to 20% of diabetic patients may develop capsulitis, as do a similar percentage of neurosurgical inpatients.

○   **What are the demographics of adhesive capsulitis?**

Onset under the age of 40 years is rare, with the mean age of onset being in the sixth decade. Women are slightly more affected than men.

○   **Can the contralateral shoulder be involved?**

Involvement of the contralateral shoulder occurs in 6–17% of patients over the subsequent 5 years 20. It is commonly stated that recurrence in the same shoulder does not occur.

○   **What precipitates primary adhesive capsulitis?**

There is a frequent history of minor shoulder strain or injury prior to the onset of symptoms but whether this represents a true strain of the shoulder or simply the earliest awareness of pain is unclear.

○   **What is the natural history of adhesive capsulitis?**

The natural history of this condition has been assessed by various authors and it appears that there are three phases in its development and progression. The shoulder moves from being simply painful, to being painful and stiff and eventually to being less painful but profoundly stiff. This last stage appears to be self-limiting and recovery is gradual and spontaneous. These stages have been termed painful, adhesive and resolution.

○   **What is the duration of the stages of adhesive capsulitis?**

The duration of each stage in the overall condition varies considerably, but approximate durations are 3–8 months for the painful phase, 4–6 months for the adhesive phase and 1–3 years for the resolution phase.

○   **What is the extent of the recovery?**

The extent of recovery is variable, with quoted figures of 33–61% of patients having a clinically detectable limitation of shoulder movement, and although many remain asymptomatic 7–15% of patients may have a persisting functional disability. Up to half of patients will have mild but detectable loss of external rotation and abduction that persists for years. The extent to which the duration of the painful and adhesive phases determine the degree of residual disability remains controversial.

○   **What are the characteristics of the painful phase?**

This is characterized by the insidious onset of symptoms, usually in the form of pain on shoulder movement and background ache in the shoulder region, often in the upper trapezius muscle. As the condition becomes established there is the development of increasing pain at rest and at night, the latter becoming quite disturbing and frequently waking the patient in the absence of a history of precipitative movement. Muscle spasm may develop, further limiting shoulder movement, which becomes restricted, with the increase in pain and stiffness at the shoulder. Towards the end of this phase stiffness becomes a major complaint.

O   **What are the characteristics of the adhesive phase?**

Usually after several months the character of pain alters and becomes less severe. There is a reduction in pain at rest and at night but discomfort and a more severe pain at the limits of movement persist. Shoulder movement becomes more restricted during this phase.

O   **What are the characteristics of the resolution phase?**

The pain is less evident and the dominant symptom is restriction of shoulder movement, which often appears less distressing for the patient now that the pain has eased. There is a slow and gradual improvement in range of motion, although this is frequently incomplete. The onset and rate of recovery are variable and unpredictable.

O   **What are the physical findings associated with adhesive capsulitis?**

The physical signs alter to a degree as the condition progresses, with pain, often severe, present in the earlier stages. Differentiation from rotator cuff tendinitis is possible on the basis of there being a global restriction of passive movement rather than simply the loss of abduction and flexion which is often seen with chronic rotator cuff conditions. In the painful phase there is painful restriction of active and passive motion (often mild in the earlier stages). Associated findings are tenderness in the upper trapezius muscle and early scapula hiking in elevation. In the latter phases the important finding is significant restriction of glenohumeral movement with a compensatory increase in scapulothoracic motion during flexion and abduction. Pain may be present but there is less discrepancy between active and passive range. Disuse atrophy of the rotator cuff and deltoid muscles may exist. Joint line tenderness is not a universal finding but is common in the painful phase.

O   **What is the association of diabetes mellitus and adhesive capsulitis?**

Capsulitis is more prevalent in diabetics (prevalence 10–20%), usually occurring at a younger age and often associated with prolonged duration of the diabetes, insulin dependence, the development of limited joint mobility syndrome and widespread microvascular disease. Also bilateral involvement is more common in diabetes. The links between diabetes and capsulitis may revolve around microvascular disease, abnormalities of collagen repair or predisposition to infection.

O   **What is the pathophysiology of adhesive capsulitis?**

Laboratory investigation has revealed little to support the notion that an autoimmune process is involved and there has been no convincing response to immunosuppressive therapy. Histologic studies have failed to demonstrate the presence of inflammatory cell infiltrates granulomas or vasculitis in the joint capsule or synovium. Also, there is nothing to implicate infection, crystal arthropathy or trauma. However, investigators have demonstrated an increase in fibrous tissue, fibroblast numbers and vascularity with no change in the synovial lining and no inflammatory cell infiltrate. To date there has been no association noted between capsulitis and histocompatability antigen carriage in the population and no immunologic disturbance has been demonstrated.

O   **What does clinical diagnostic lab testing reveal in adhesive capsulitis?**

Elevations of erythrocyte sedimentation rate (ESR), acute phase reactants and globulin levels are not usually seen, and calcium metabolism appears normal on testing.

O   **Are there abnormalities on plain radiographs?**

Plain radiographs are not helpful in making the diagnosis except to exclude widespread degenerative changes, calcific tendinitis or neoplasm.

O   **What does arthrography reveal?**

Classical features at arthrography are limitation of joint volume with a loss of the normal dependent axillary fold or pouch and irregularity of the capsular insertion to the anatomical neck of the humerus. Some authors insist that these changes need to be present in order to make a diagnosis of adhesive capsulitis. Ten to thirty percent of patients having arthrography have a demonstrable complete tear of the rotator cuff. However, other studies have suggested that a significant number of patients with a clinical diagnosis of adhesive capsulitis have normal findings at arthrography.

O   What is the role of MRI in the diagnosis of adhesive capsulitis?

The usefulness of magnetic resonance imaging (MRI) in the diagnosis of adhesive capsulitis has also been evaluated. Studies revealed that some changes seen on MRI are specific and sensitive for adhesive capsulitis; however, the decrease in joint fluid is not appreciated. MRI may become a useful, noninvasive way to document capsular thickening, but further studies are needed.

O   What does bone scintography reveal?

Bone scintigraphy may demonstrate increased isotope uptake in the affected shoulder region but this appears to have no predictive value in terms of outcome or response to treatment and is therefore of limited diagnostic value. An average 50% reduction in bone mineral content in the affected humeral head has been demonstrated in bone densitometric studies, although again this is of little diagnostic or therapeutic value.

O   Summarize the therapeutic options for adhesive capsulitis

Technique	Specifics	Outcome	Complications	Comments
Rest, analgesia, ROM	Sling and oral pain medication until patient obtains adequate pain relief When pain subsides enough, begin pendulum and wall crawls to improve ROM; may require continued use of pain medication	Equal to natural history		
Focused active home exercises	Pain control until patient can begin exercises	Lacks good clinical studies	Some believe that too rapid an increase in activity can prolong the disorder	In widespread use
Formal physical therapy	Ultrasound or other physical modalities to ease pain, passive mobilization to increase ROM	Lacks good clinical studies	Some believe that overly aggressive manipulation can prolong the disorder	In widespread use
Oral prednisone	Prednisone dose 10 mg qd for 4 wk, then 5 mg qd for 2 wk	Decrease in pain, no change in ROM	None reported	
Corticosteroid injection	Intra-articular injection; timing and dose varies	Usually decrease in pain, not much change in ROM	Occasional increase in pain	Pain relief is moderate; subacromial injection may be as effective as intra-articular injection
Capsular distention	Intra-articular injection (corticosteroid, anesthetic, or air), 20-30 mL is enough to cause capsular rupture	Can decrease pain significantly, moderate improvement in ROM	Occasional increase in pain after injection	
Manipulation under anesthesia	General anesthesia or interscalene block; manipulation past resistance results in capsular and subcapsular rupture	Marked improvement in ROM	Humerus fracture, neurovascular injury, articular cartilage injury	May require significant pain control and intensive, daily physical therapy after treatment
Surgical capsular release	Open or arthroscopic release of contracted capsular structures	Marked improvement in ROM	Surgical morbidity	May require significant pain control

O   How are AC joint injuries classified?

AC dislocations have been divided into six classifications:

O   How AC joint subluxation/dislocations graded?

Grade I injury involves minor sprain to the joint capsule without ligament disruption. Grade II injury involves subluxation of the joint with downward displacement of the acromion relative to the distal end of the clavicle. There is stretching of the inferior acromioclavicular ligaments, and stretching and possibly a partial tear, but not complete rupture, of the coracoclavicular ligaments. In a Grade III injury complete dislocation of the joint occurs due to rupture of the coracoclavicular ligaments. Grade III injuries can be further classified according to the extent of disruption or perforation of the overlying deltotrapezius fascial or muscle layer by the displaced outer end of the clavicle.

O   **What is the most common mechanism of injury?**

Most AC injuries occur from falling directly on the adducted shoulder. The force of the fall dictates the degree of injury. If the history involves a direct blow to the adducted shoulder, the physical exam is likely to confirm the diagnosis.

O   **What are the key findings on physical examination?**

Pain is well localized to the top of the shoulder in the region of the involved joint, which is tender and often swollen to palpation. Active adduction of the injured shoulder (patient reaches across the chest to grasp the uninjured shoulder) with additional passive adduction by the examiner (crossed-arm adduction test) usually exacerbates the pain. In complete dislocation of the joint a visible step deformity is seen and examination will determine whether or not this dislocation can be reduced. The patient often describes a feeling of their shoulder having dropped due to the downward displacement of the acromion.

O   **What is the rehabilitation treatment plan for grade I, II injuries?**

Grade I joint sprains respond well to ice and NSAIDs, and return to usual sporting activities in 2 days to 2 weeks is common. Grade II sprains may benefit from the use of a sling to diminish strain on the joint until it is asymptomatic, a time period that may range from 1 to 4 weeks. As symptoms abate, gentle passive and active assisted range of motion exercises begin. Strengthening of the trapezius and other shoulder girdle musculature begins isometrically in pain-free positions, and progresses to light isotonic or isokinetic exercises as pain-free range of motion improves. Repetitive shoulder elevation should be kept to a minimum for the first 4 weeks of rehabilitation. The deformity present at the superior aspect of the shoulder, however, will likely persist.

O   **What are the treatment approaches for grade III injuries?**

The rehabilitation of grade III injuries follow a similar protocol as outlined above, but with a longer timeframe. Grade III acromioclavicular separations tend to result in greater limitation of motion and have a higher potential for prolonged disability. In most cases, however, nonsurgical treatment is still the preferred course. The exceptions are types 4, 5, and 6 AC joint injuries. Radiographic findings are the primary method used to diagnose type 4, 5, or 6 fractures. When the injury is diagnosed, an orthopedic surgeon should be consulted for surgical reduction and stabilization. Return to athletic practice and play depends on healing and restoration of near-normal strength and range of motion.

O   **What is the incidence of post injury complications?**

5% to 10% incidence of significant problems with grade III acromioclavicular separations has been reported, regardless of whether or not surgical repair was performed. The most frequent problem is persistent pain, accelerated OA, and osteolysis of the clavicle.

O   **What conservative care approaches are appropriate?**

Conservative care includes use of a sling for comfort and to lessen the chance of further injury in the early post injury stage. Ice and NSAIDs are used to reduce edema and pain. Narcotic analgesia may also be required for a few days. The sling is allowed to be removed for progressively longer periods to perform gentle range of motion exercises. If pain free, isometric exercises may begin early while the limb is in the sling. The sling is discontinued as symptoms allow. If progression to dynamic or sport-specific exercises is hampered by continued symptoms or if the cosmetic deformity is unacceptable to the athlete, then surgical referral for open repair is indicated.

O   **What are the clinical features of AC joint arthropathy?**

Common clinical complaints of those who have AC arthritis are diffuse, lateral shoulder pain and/or local AC joint pain. Nocturnal exacerbation is common. Upper extremity activity and activities of daily living involving the shoulder aggravate the symptoms. The physical exam commonly reveals local tenderness to palpation of the involved joint. Active and passive range of motion of the shoulder may intensify symptoms. Crossed-arm adduction of the involved shoulder with additional passive adduction by the examiner also aggravates pain.

○   **What do imaging studies reveal?**

Degenerative change can be clearly seen on plain radiography and an arthrogram may reveal the presence of a complete tear of the rotator cuff. Traction or weight-bearing views can be taken in order to demonstrate joint instability.

○   **What therapeutic approaches are appropriate for AC joint arthropathy?**

Treatment of osteoarthritis of the AC joint parallels that for other degenerative joints. Common recommendations include activity modification, physical therapy, nonsteroidal anti-inflammatory drugs (NSAIDs) or other analgesics, and corticosteroid injections. Although not widely investigated, corticosteroid injections of the AC joint provide symptom relief for 20 days to 3 months. Injection of the AC joint is performed from a superior approach using a 23- or 25-gauge needle with 1 mL of local anesthetic mixed with 1 mL of an intermediate- or long-acting corticosteroid. Most experts recommend limiting injections to the AC joint to three over 3 to 6 months.

○   **What are the surgical options for AC joint arthropathy?**

Cases resistant to conservative treatment may require surgery, which usually consists of excision arthroplasty of the joint whilst ensuring that instability is minimized. Careful assessment of rotator cuff function is important and in the presence of a significant tear rotator cuff repair or an acromioplasty may be indicated. Excision arthroplasty may also be indicated in the younger patient with chronic symptoms whether due to degenerative change, osteolysis or instability.

○   **What is the incidence of calcific tendinopathy of the RTC tendons?**

Radiologically detectable calcification in the rotator cuff tendons has a reported prevalence of 2.7–7.5%, occurring in symptomatic and asymptomatic shoulders. The calcific deposits are usually composed of hydroxyapatite.

○   **What are the demographics of calcific tendinitis?**

It is most common in the supraspinatus tendon and has been reported as being more common in women, and sedentary individuals. One investigator estimated that 35–45% of individuals with calcification seen on radiography developed symptoms. Frequently bilateral, it usually occurs between the ages of 40 years and 60 years but can present as an acute condition in the younger patient.

○   **What are the symptoms and signs associated with calcific tendinopathy?**

Patients may present with chronic symptoms of pain on movement with a catching sensation probably due to impingement. Acute calcific tendinitis has a quite different presentation with acute severe pain limiting passive or active shoulder movement almost completely, with exquisite point tenderness and occasionally erythema over the involved tendon. The onset of symptoms can be rapid with no history of injury or overuse and this occurs during the resorptive phase of calcification.

○   **How can patients with RTC calcific tendinopathy be classified?**

Patients can be divided into two groups. Firstly, those patients with an acute onset of severe pain and limitation of movement often in the absence of any previous shoulder symptoms. Secondly, patients who have a more chronic catching pain associated with movement presenting as an impingement problem.

○   **What is the pathological basis of RTC calcific tendinopathy?**

There are three stages in the calcification process. In the calcific stage calcium crystals are deposited in matrix vehicles to form large deposits (known as the formative phase). After a variable period of inactivity (resting period) there is spontaneous resorption of the calcium by means of peripheral vascularization and phagocytosis of the deposit (resorptive phase). Following removal of the calcium the space is filled with granulation tissue (post calcific stage).

O **What treatment options are available for this condition?**

Iontophoresis or phonophoresis with acetylsalicylic acid and/or corticosteroids may be beneficial in promoting resorption of the deposit. Some clinicians advocate 'needling' with or without fluoroscopic guidance to disperse and expedite resorption. There is modest evidence to support this intervention. Extracorporeal shock wave therapy has been used in Europe with promising results. The treatments otherwise are analogous to rotator cuff tendinopathy without calcific deposit. For deposits greater than 0.8 cm in size consider arthroscopic debridement.

O **What is the scapulocostal syndrome?**

An adventitious bursa may form on the ventral-medial aspect of the scapula secondary to extrinsic overuse/repetitive injury or intrinsic pathology such as a rib exostosis, or primary benign bone tumor. Alternately a myofascial pain syndrome involving the subscapularis, rhomboid, infraspinatus or rhomboid muscle may be responsible.

O **What types of GHJ dislocation can occur?**

Shoulder dislocations account for almost 50% of all joint dislocations. Most commonly, these dislocations are anterior (90-98%) and occur due to trauma. Most anterior dislocations are subcoracoid in location. Posterior dislocations are less common (2-10%) and are the result of an axial load applied to the adducted and internally rotated arm. Inferior subluxation occurs commonly in hemiplegic shoulders, but true dislocation is rare. Superior migration of the humeral head relative to the glenoid fossa is common in rotator cuff tears, but dislocations are very rare.

O **What is the most common mechanism for anterior GHJ dislocations?**

The usual mechanism of injury is extreme abduction, external rotation, extension, and a posterior directed force against the humerus. The accurate diagnosis of dislocation is not difficult if the humeral head remains in an abnormal position with respect to the glenoid cavity of the scapula, but in cases in which spontaneous relocation occurs prior to the patient's being seen by a physician, the nature of the injury as well as its propensity to recur may be unclear.

O **What recommendations are appropriate for the acute phase of a GHJ dislocation?**

Acute dislocation or chronic laxity in the recreational athlete can often be successfully treated conservatively. Chronic glenohumeral subluxation or dislocation most commonly occurs in the anterior direction (97%). If an acute dislocation has occurred, a period of immobilization aids initial healing of the capsuloligamentous lesion. Application of ice decreases tissue edema and pain. The time period for immobilization must be brief, however, to avoid disuse atrophy, shoulder stiffness, and maladaptive histologic changes in soft tissue and bone. Three to six weeks is adequate.

O **What is the appropriate progression of therapeutic exercise in an anterior shoulder dislocation?**

Gentle isometric strengthening can begin during the period of immobilization. Early motion is important for minimizing adhesions and preserving proprioceptive skills. The caveat is to avoid the combination of abduction, external rotation, and extension, which stresses the already damaged anterior capsule. Strengthening exercises should begin at less than 90 degrees of abduction and anterior to the coronal plane, so as to avoid anterior translation of the humerus. Strengthening exercises should target the dynamic anterior stabilizers, including the subscapularis, pectoralis major, and latissimus dorsi. Later, strengthening of the remaining shoulder muscles is initiated. Once range of motion and strengthening have progressed to the point that the athlete can assume a position of 90 degrees of abduction and external rotation without apprehension, sport-specific exercises may commence. The total period of rehabilitation may vary from 6 weeks to 6 months.

O **What complications can occur with a GHJ dislocation and how are they detected?**

Routine radiographs supplemented with special projections have been advocated in the latter instances to document the presence of osseous and cartilaginous residua of the dislocation, including the Hill-Sachs lesion of the humeral head and the Bankart lesion of the glenoid cavity, which indicate previous anterior dislocation. An osseous Bankart lesion typically is visualized as an elevation of a small sliver of bone and irregularity of the adjacent glenoid rim. A depression along the posterolateral aspect of the humeral head is indicative of a Hill-Sachs lesion. When large and bony, one or both of these lesions will be detected by the conventional studies but when the osseous defect in the humeral head or scapula is small, CT may be required.

○   **What is the risk of recurrent dislocation?**

Nonathletes have a 30% recurrence risk with nonoperative treatment, and athletes have an 82% recurrence risk with nonoperative treatment.

○   **What is the association between the recurrent dislocation risk and age?**

If the dislocation was the patient's first, recurrence rates with nonoperative treatment depend on age, as follows:

Patients aged 1-10 years have a 100% recurrence rate.
Patients aged 11-20 years have a 27-95% recurrence rate.
Patients aged 21-30 years have a 40-79% recurrence rate.
Patients aged 31-40 years have a 40-72% recurrence rate.
Patients aged 41-50 years have a 0-24% recurrence rate

○   **What are SLAP lesions?**

SLAP lesions (superior labrum anterior, posterior) refer to injuries of the superior portion of the glenoid labrum at the insertion of the biceps tendon to the superior labral complex. The biceps tendon reportedly decelerates the arm during throwing, resulting in strenuous forces being placed upon it. SLAP injuries result from excessive stress on the biceps tendon as it inserts into the glenoid labrum. SLAP injuries usually are manifested by pain and clicking and, occasionally, instability after acute pitching or racquet sport activity, catching a heavy falling object, or falling on an outstretched hand. The degree of involvement of the biceps tendon varies, and SLAP lesions can occur in the absence of capsular injuries. SLAP lesions can be evaluated with CT scanning or MR imaging. Often arthroscopic surgery is required for symptomatic lesions.

ELBOW

○   **What is the elbow flexion test?**

A test designed to identify cubital tunnel syndrome. The patient is asked to hold his or her elbow fully flexed for 5 min. The test result is positive if tingling or paresthesias are felt in the ulnar nerve distribution of the forearm and hand.

○   **What is the golfer's elbow test?**

A test designed to identify the presence of inflammation in the area of the medial epicondyle. The patient flexes the elbow and wrist, supinates the forearm, and then extends the elbow. The test result is positive if the patient complains of pain over the medial epicondyle.

○   **What are the ligamentous instability tests?**

Tests designed to assess the integrity of the lateral and medial collateral ligaments of the elbow. The patient's arm is held by the examiner so that the examiner is supporting the elbow and wrist. The examiner tests the lateral collateral ligament by applying an adduction or varus force to the distal forearm with the patient's elbow held in 20° to 30° of flexion. The medial collateral ligament is similarly tested by the application of an abduction or valgus force at the distal forearm. The test result is positive if pain r altered mobility is present.

○   **What are the Tennis elbow tests?**

The following tests are designed to determine he presence of inflammation in the area of the lateral epicondyle:

1) The patient flexes the elbow to approximately 45° and fully supinates the forearm while making a fist. The patient is then asked to pronate the forearm and radially deviate and extend the wrist while the examiner resists these motions. For a positive test result, pain is elicited in the area of the lateral epicondyle. 2) The examiner pronates the patient's forearm, fully extends the elbow, and fully flexes the wrist. For a positive test result, pain is elicited in the area of the lateral epicondyle. 3) The examiner resists extension of the third digit of the hand distal to the proximal interphalangeal (PIP) joint. A positive test is indicated by pain in the area of the lateral epicondyle of the humerus.

O How does olecranon bursitis present clinically?

Pain is usually localized and typically does not occur on passive or resisted movement. It is usually provoked by leaning on the elbow or flexion with a constriction around the elbow such as a coat sleeve. Tenderness should be sought about the tip of the olecranon and will be present, sometimes with palpable thickening of the bursal wall even in the absence of significant effusion and is generally very sensitive to pressure.

O How does septic olecranon bursitis present?

Septic olecranon bursitis occurs less frequently (around 25% of hospital cases) but is important and should not be missed. Usually it occurs following an abrasion or may be associated with an initial cellulitis of the skin. A surface temperature probe, where available, may help distinguish infective from non-infective causes at an early stage. The finding of infection requires appropriate antibiotic therapy and re-aspiration of purulent fluid as necessary. Staphylococcus aureus is the most frequently found organism although S. epidermidis or a streptococcus are less commonly found. Other organisms are rarely implicated. If repeated non-infective bursitis occurs then surgical removal of the bursa should be considered.

O What tests of bursal fluid are recommended?

Aspiration of the bursa both reduces symptoms and allows assessment of the fluid. Along with gross visualization of blood staining, the turbidity of the fluid, white cell count and differential, and Gram stain with culture of the fluid can be undertaken to exclude infection. Comparison of fluid and blood glucose levels may be useful. Polarizing light microscopy can be performed to reveal any crystals. If no infection is suspected local steroid injection may be performed which is effective in speeding recovery. A compressive elastic bandage will help to prevent recurrence of swelling.

O What is radiohumeral bursitis?

Bursitis may also occur between the biceps insertion and the head of the radius. Pain presents at the elbow during wrist rotation. Tenderness is detected over the head of the radius and accentuated during wrist rotation. Response to local anesthetic injection at the site of tenderness aids in diagnosis. Methylprednisolone acetate 20 mg can then be injected.

O What is cubital bursitis?

Cubital bursitis and antecubital cysts may cause swelling and pain at the anteromedial border of the elbow or in the antecubital area. The median nerve may be stretched by the swelling, causing pain radiation into the forearm and hand. Repetitive movement and a roughened surface of the bicipital tuberosity are thought to contribute to the formation of cubital bursitis and antecubital cysts. Rheumatoid arthritis should also be considered. Aspiration and injection with methylprednisolone acetate 20 mg and I mL lidocaine hydrochloride I% is often helpful. Excision may be required.

O What is the epidemiology of lateral epicondylitis?

Around 1-3% in the general population, work-related cases 59 per 10,000 workers per year, 7.4% of industrial workers in the USA at some time are affected by it. It occurs mostly those aged between 40 years and 60 years, the dominant arm being affected most frequently. Some 40–50% of tennis players suffer with it, mainly older players but in clinical practice less than 5% of cases are due to the game. It is found most often in non-athletes and the majority are not manual workers.

O What is the probable pathogenesis of lateral epicondylitis?

The majority of cases are due to a musculotendinous lesion of the common extensor tendon at the attachment to the lateral epicondyle or nearby, especially that portion derived from extensor carpi radialis brevis. Ischemic stress may be important because the tenoperiosteal junction (enthesis) and nearby tendon are relatively avascular, since the blood supply is a watershed of that derived from muscle and bone and working muscle takes up the blood supply at the expense of tendon. This ischemia initiates a partial fibrocartilage transformation of the damaged tissue.

○   **What may precipitate the condition in manual workers?**

In manual workers relative overuse of wrist and finger extensors may precipitate the condition, which most often affects the dominant arm. Sometimes there may be bilateral involvement either due to increased stress placed on the unaffected arm or resulting from a general tendency to soft tissue lesions which occurs in some individuals.

○   **What symptoms and signs are encountered in lateral epicondylitis?**

Pain is localized to the lateral epicondyle but may spread up and down the upper limb. Grip is impaired due to pain, and this may result in restricted daily activities. Tenderness over the epicondyle is usual, although maximum tenderness is sometimes found at nearby sites. The other cardinal sign is increase in pain on resisting wrist dorsiflexion with the elbow in extension. Symptoms may also be precipitated by extending the elbow with the wrist flexed and by resisted middle finger extension. Resisted supination may also be painful. The range of movement of the elbow is usually normal but a few degrees of extension may be lost in some severe and chronic cases.

○   **What clinical condition can mimic aspects of lateral epicondylitis?**

A nerve entrapment around the elbow may produce diagnostic confusion. Radial tunnel syndrome or compression of the posterior interosseous nerve can produce lateral elbow and upper forearm pain. It can be the cause of apparent lateral epicondylitis that is unresponsive to conservative treatment but is believed to be a rare cause of resistant cases.

○   **What is the pathogenesis of radial tunnel syndrome?**

The entrapment of the posterior interosseous nerve has been found to be due to compressive lesions caused by abnormal fibrous bands in front of the radial head, a sharp tendinous origin of extensor carpi radialis brevis, or a radial recurrent fan of vessels. More rarely, a lipoma or ganglion has been found to be the cause. Compression of the posterior interosseous nerve may occur where it passes through supinator muscle just below the elbow joint. A well defined arcade of Frohse is present in 30% of subjects and makes a compression neuropathy more likely. Diffuse pain, sensory signs, symptoms distal to the lateral epicondyle and the presence of muscle weakness may be useful distinguishing features.

○   **What physical modalities may be considered in the management of lateral epicondylitis?**

Ultrasound, by its ability to cross myofascial planes and concentrate near bone, has theoretical advantages. A double blind controlled trial has confirmed an advantage for pulsed therapeutic ultrasound. Sixty-three percent of patients improved and the technique had the merit of being non-painful with a relapse rate lower than that after corticosteroid injection.

○   **What is the role of NSAIDs in managing lateral epicondylitis?**

There is clinical evidence to advocate either topical or oral NSAIDs for shortterm pain management in lateral epicondylitis.

○   **What role does corticosteroid injection therapy play in the management of lateral epicondylitis?**

Local corticosteroid injections are both efficacious and cost effective, with around 90% of subjects responding. But the injection may cause increased pain for up to 72 hours afterwards and a significant number of patients relapse. The injection may be repeated after 2–4 weeks, in the event of either failure to respond or relapse, but should not be repeated more than twice as it is unlikely then to be effective and increases the risk of side effects. In general, it appears that injection improves symptoms in the acute period, but does not enhance outcomes at one year.

○   **What are 4 goals in the rehabilitation of lateral epicondylitis?**

1. Decrease pain and inflammation
2. Identify and correct causal factors

3. Restore strength and flexibility to wrist extensors
4. Return patient to work or sport

O   **What modalities are appropriate in lateral epicondylitis?**

The therapist can augment healing by applying modalities to the lateral epicondylar region. In the acute stage, ice, phonophoresis, or iontophoresis help to lessen inflammation and pain. As the pain subsides, heat, ultrasound, and transverse friction massage can increase local circulation, minimize scar formation, and eliminate metabolic waste products. Other interventions include laser therapy and acupuncture. However, no definitive conclusions can be drawn concerning effectiveness of these modalities for lateral epicondylitis based on literature review.

O   **What is the role for counterforce bracing in lateral epicondylitis?**

Counterforce bracing with a tennis elbow strap diminishes pressure on the injured elbow by creating a "new" origin for the extensor carpi radialis brevis. This "new" muscle origin not only alters the magnitude and direction of the muscle force, but it also effectively bypasses the injured muscle fibers, allowing them to heal. However, no definitive conclusions can be drawn concerning effectiveness of orthotic devices for lateral epicondylitis based on literature review.

O   **What therapeutic exercises may be appropriate for the patient?**

The clinician must determine for each patient the underlying factors that increase the risk of tennis elbow. For many patients, decreased strength or flexibility of the wrist extensors predisposes them to develop tennis elbow. Loss of motion at the elbow joint is not compensated for by shoulder or wrist motions, causing excessive stress to be placed at the elbow. A progressive stretching and strengthening program must be implemented to restore pain free function to the patient. Both concentric and eccentric muscle contractions need to be strengthened and low level endurance needs to be retrained.

O   **If the patient is an avid tennis player what other issues should the clinician address?**

Use of poor technique or improperly fitting equipment contributes to this syndrome when playing tennis. If the racquet grip is too large or too small, both the finger flexors and wrist extensors may be overused. If the strings on the racquet are too taut, the vibration transmitted to the elbow and wrist on ball impact may be too great for the soft tis sue to absorb. Over pronation during the forehand stroke of an overhead serve may cramp the lateral compartment of the elbow joint. In most instances, correction of these causal factors eliminates the need for more invasive treatment.

O   **What rehabilitation issues are addressed subsequent to the acute episode?**

As the symptoms subside, the patient should gradually return to sporting or other functional activities. The above exercise and modification program should be maintained and performed to prevent recurrence. In general, the patient may complain of intermittent symptoms (e.g., painful twinges) when per forming various activities, such as opening a jar or lifting an object. These painful re minders tend to last up to one year from original injury.

O   **How does the efficacy of the different conservative approaches compare?**

Systematic reviews of the efficacy of corticosteroid injection for lateral epicondylitis, compared with physical therapy or NSAIDs, have yielded conflicting results, with comparisons made difficult by different methodologies in various reports.

O   **What prognoses have been reported in lateral epicondylitis?**

Lateral epicondylitis has been considered to be a self-limiting disorder with patients improving with or without treatment within 1 year. This good prognosis contrasts with reported relapse rates of between 18% and 50% 6 months after conservative treatment. In one study 40% of patients had prolonged minor discomfort, which in some persisted for 5 years. Manual workers, especially mechanics, builders and domestic workers are most susceptible to recurrence on resumption of the activity, which induced the initial pain.

○   **What surgical options are available in lateral epicondylitis?**

In most reports surgery aims to lengthen the muscle tendon complex either by the less favored distal tenotomy or by a 'lateral release' procedure involving division of the origin of the common extensor tendon. Subcutaneous division of the tendinous origin of extensor carpi radialis brevis carried out under local anesthetic using a small blade has been used with claimed success in 70% of cases. A more extensive lateral release may be undertaken in conjunction with resection of the proximal third of the annular ligament (a modified Bosworth operation) with a success rate of up to 86%. There is a possibility, however, of this operation resulting in lateral elbow instability.

○   **What surgical intervention has the best success rate?**

The reported success rate of 90% of a simple lateral release without substantial risk is the surgical management of choice. However, no definitive conclusions can be drawn concerning effectiveness of surgical management for lateral epicondylitis based on literature review.

○   **What is medial epicondylitis?**

Medial epicondylitis is a lesion of the common tendon of the wrist flexors (flexor carpi radialis and ulnaris) or the pronator teres tendon where they originate on the medial epicondyle. The incidence of medial epicondylitis is much less than lateral epicondylitis, but the symptoms tend to be more acute. Repetitive wrist flexion from sports or vocational activities tends to cause this condition. **In the US:** Medial epicondylitis accounts for only 10-20% of all epicondylitis diagnoses. Medial epicondylitis is usually found in the dominant elbow of a golfer.

○   **What are the signs and symptoms associated with medial epicondylitis?**

The signs and symptoms associated with medial epicondylitis are:
1. Pain at medial epicondyle, radiating down volar aspect of forearm
2. Pain on active or resisted wrist flexion (with elbow extended)
3. Pain on resisted pronation
4. Pain on passive wrist extension

○   **What are the treatment approaches for medial epicondylitis?**

The treatment approaches are similar to lateral epicondylitis. Oral anti-inflammatories (NSAIDs), rest, and modalities can be used to decrease pain and inflammation. Counterforce bracing can be helpful by creating a "new" muscle origin for the wrist flexors and pronators. (Counterforce bracing will not help if medial epicondylar pain occurs due to valgus instability or ulnar nerve entrapment and can, in fact, worsen these conditions. Determining and correcting the cause of the overuse syndrome remain the key to proper treatment.

○   **What 5 sporting activities tend to increase the risk of medial epicondylitis?**

1. Pitching a baseball: especially throwing a curve ball or screw ball
2. Driving a golf ball using an improper technique
3. Backstroking in swimming using an improper technique
4. Playing excessive racquetball
5. Serving in tennis

Each of the above activities increases the use of the wrist flexors or pronators. Patients may need to seek out a specialized coach or professional athlete to correct the improper technique contributing to the injury.

○   **What are other causes of medial epicondylitis?**

Other causes of medial epicondylitis are decreased strength and flexibility of the wrist flexors.

○   **In these cases what rehabilitation strategies are appropriate?**

A progressive stretching and strengthening program must be implemented. As with lateral epicondylitis, emphasis is on a pain-free program with both concentric and eccentric work occurring. Implementation of the conservative program is imperative, because cortisone injections have not been efficacious in treating this problem.

O **What is little league elbow?**

Little league elbow is the name used to describe a group of elbow problems related to the stress of throwing in young athletes. Throwing can cause medial symptoms as well as lateral and posterior symptoms. The medial symptoms are related to the repetitive valgus distraction forces on the medial elbow.

O **What elbow injury is most common in children?**

The medial epicondyle has the longest exposure to medial distraction forces in the elbow because it is the last ossification center to close. Thus, medial epicondyle apophysitis is the most common elbow injury during childhood (before the appearance of all the secondary ossification centers).

O **What are the findings on examination in medial epicondyle apophysitis?**

Physical examination demonstrates pain to palpation of the medial epicondyle that is exacerbated by resisted wrist flexion and valgus testing of the elbow.

O **What are the treatment approaches in medial epicondyle apophysitis?**

Treatment includes no throwing for four to six weeks, as well as symptomatic treatment with ice and NSAIDs. Correction of throwing mechanics and a progressive throwing program over the subsequent six to eight weeks will help the athlete to return to play. In addition, a position change from pitcher (typically 15 to 30 throws per inning) may help the player to avoid overloading the elbow.

O **What are ulnar collateral ligament (UCL) injuries?**

Ulnar collateral ligament tears occur in the skeletally mature thrower, as well as in wrestlers, gymnasts, or football players who sustain traumatic valgus injury from a fall on an outstretched arm or a tackle while the hand is planted.

O **What are the findings on examination?**

On physical examination valgus stress at 30° of elbow flexion reproduces medial pain and instability.

O **What imaging modalities aid in diagnosis?**

Ulnar collateral ligament tears may be seen on stress radiographs with the application of valgus force. Magnetic resonance imaging (MRI) with contrast arthrography is sensitive for both partial and full thickness ligament injuries.

O **What are the treatment approaches in UCL injuries?**

Treatment includes conservative management for at least six months with no throwing activities. Ice and NSAIDs can be used to control symptoms; the ulnar nerve, which runs behind the medial epicondyle, should be avoided during the application of ice because it can sustain thermal injury from prolonged exposure. The associated strength deficits should be addressed through rehabilitation. An eight-week progressive throwing program after the six-month rest will test the success of conservative management. If symptoms return, surgical intervention may be necessary.

WRIST/HAND

O **What is the Bunnell-Littler test?**

A test designed to identify intrinsic muscle or joint contractures at the PIP joints. The examiner flexes the PIP joint maximally while maintaining the metacarpophalangeal (MCP) joint in slight extension. The test result is positive for a joint capsule contracture d the PIP joint cannot be flexed. The test is positive for intrinsic muscle contracture if the MCP is slightly flexed and the PIP flexes fully.

○   What is Finkelstein test?

A test designed to determine the presence tenosynovitis of the abductor pollicis longus and extensor pollicis brevis tendons. The test is commonly used to determine the presence of de Quervain's disease. The patient makes a fist while holding the thumb inside the fingers. The patient then attempts to deviate ulnarly the first metacarpal and extend the proximal joint of the thumb. If the patient experiences pain, this is recorded ams a positive test result.

○   What is Froment's sign?

A test designed for determining the presence of adductor pollicis weakness from ulnar nerve paralysis. The patient attempts to grasp a piece of paper between the tips of the thumb and the radial side of the index finger. The test result is positive if the terminal phalanx of the patient's thumb flexes or if the MCP joint of the thumb hyperextends (Jeanne's sign) as the examiner attempts to pull the paper from the patient's grasp.

○   What is the Intrinsic-plus test?

A test designed to identify shortening of the intrinsic muscles of the hand. This test is useful and specific when examining the hand of the patient with rheumatoid arthritis, particularly in the early stages prior to any destruction or deformity of the hand. In this test, the MCP joint of the finger being tested is hyperextended. The middle and distal joints flex slightly owing to passive action of tissues. The examiner then further attempts to flex passively the PIP joint of the finger. Any severe restriction to this movement is considered a positive sign.

○   What is Phalen's (wrist flexion) test?

A test designed to determine the presence of carpal tunnel syndrome. The patient's wrists are maximally flexed by the examiner, who maintains this position by holding the patient's wrists together for 1 min. The test result is positive if paresthesias are present in the thumb, index finger, and the middle and lateral half of the ring finger. Note there is also a reverse Phalen's test which is more sensitive for median nerve entrapment at the base of the hand. The maneuver is exactly reversed.

○   What is the tight retinacular ligament test?

A test designed to determine the presence of shortened retinacular ligaments or a tight distal interphalangeal (DIP) joint capsule. The examiner holds the patient's PIP joint in a fully extended position while attempting to flex the DIP joint. If the DIP joint does not flex, the test is positive for either a contracted collateral ligament or joint capsule. The test is positive for tight retinacular (collateral) ligaments and a normal joint capsule if, when the PIP joint is flexed, the DIP joint flexes easily.

○   What is Tinel's sign?

A test designed to detect carpal tunnel syndrome. The examiner taps over the carpal tunnel of the wrist. The test result is positive if the patient reports paresthesia distal to the wrist. Note that originally the Tinel sign was used to elicit neurogenic symptoms of any given sensory nerve in a somatic distribution.

○   What is De Quervain's tenosynovitis?

De Quervain's stenosing tenosynovitis of the abductor pollicis longus and extensor pollicis brevis typically represents an occupation or vocation-related repetitive strain injury due to chronic overuse of the wrist and hand.

○   Which population of patients is most vulnerable?

It is most common in women between 30 and 50 years of age.

O   What is the pathogenesis?

Repetitive activity, involving pinching with the thumb while moving the wrist in radial and ulnar directions, results in frictional inflammation with thickening and stenosis of the fibrous tendon sheath as it passes over the distal radius beneath the flexor retinaculum.

O   What other scenarios can present with this condition?

De Quervain's tenosynovitis may also occur in association with RA, psoriatic arthritis, other inflammatory arthropathies, direct trauma, and pregnancy and during the postpartum period.

O   What symptoms and signs are characteristic?

Most patients report several weeks or months of pain on the radial aspect of the wrist and at the thumb base during pinch grip, grasping, and other thumb and wrist movements. The affected tendon sheath is tender and often swollen. Finkelstein's test is positive and a tendon crepitus may be palpable. Patients may have other forms of pathology such as carpal tunnel syndrome, or trigger finger or thumb.

O   What differential diagnosis is most common?

The diagnosis of de Quervain's tenosynovitis is often confused with osteoarthritis of the first CMC joint and with the intersection syndrome due to tenosynovitis of the second extensor compartment (extensor carpi radialis longus and brevis) at its intersection with the tendons of the first extensor compartment (abductor pollicis longus and extensor pollicis brevis).

O   What treatment recommendations are appropriate?

Treatment of de Quervain's tenosynovitis consists of heat therapy, nonsteroidal anti-inflammatory drugs (NSAIDs), and wrist and thumb immobilization by thermoplastic splinting. A radial gutter light support splint (thumb spica or short opponens) immobilizes the wrist in slight extension and radial deviation and the first MCP joint in slight extension. The IP joint of the thumb is left unrestricted. Alteration of hand activities, avoiding tasks that require repetitive thumb movements or pinch grasping, is important. These measures are usually effective in alleviating symptoms.

O   What other interventions are considered in this condition?

In patients with more severe or persistent pain, one or more local corticosteroid injections can be helpful, giving complete and lasting relief in about 70% of patients. Surgical decompression of the first extensor compartment, with or without tenosynovectomy, is indicated in those with persistent or recurrent symptoms for more than 6 months.

O   What is the intersection syndrome?

In intersection syndrome, pain and swelling occur at the crossing point of the first dorsal compartment muscles (abductor pollicis longus and extensor pollicis brevis) and the radial wrist extensors (extensor carpi radialis longus and brevis). Peritendinitis crepitans may occur with crepitation palpable about 4 to 6 cm proximal to the radial carpal joint on the dorsal surface of the forearm. The condition is seen in those participating in rowing sports or weight training. Treatment includes splinting, NSAIDs, and local corticosteroid injection. Thumb immobilization may be required in severe cases.

O   What is trigger finger?

Trigger finger or thumb, also known, as stenosing digital tenosynovitis or snapping finger or thumb, is the most common repetitive strain injury of the hand. The thumb is the most commonly affected digit, followed by the ring and long fingers. Stenosing tenosynovitis is much more common in women, with a frequency 2-6 times that observed in men. The peak incidence of trigger digit occurred in individuals aged 55-60 years in several series. Increased incidence in the dominant hand is observed.

O   What is the anatomical lesion?

The anatomic lesion is a tenosynovitis of the flexor tendons of the finger or thumb, which results in fibrosis and constriction localized to the first annular pulley that overlies the MCP joint. A tendon nodule often develops at the site of stenosis. The nodule and/or tendon sheath constriction interfere mechanically with normal tendon gliding, resulting in pain over the area of the pulley and snapping or triggering movement of the finger or thumb.

○   **How does trigger finger present?**

Pain along the course of the sheath with resisted flexion (performed isometrically), and pain on stretching the tendon passively in extension, are common. Intermittent locking of the digit in flexion may also develop, particularly upon arising in the morning. Passive extension of the PIP joint of the finger or IP joint of the thumb may produce a crepitus and a popping sensation as the digit is straightened. Examination reveals tenderness over the area of the proximal pulley often associated with linear tenderness and swelling of the flexor tendon sheath, and limitation of digital flexion and extension. A nodule can often be palpated in the palm just proximal to the MCP joint as it moves during finger or thumb flexion and extension.

○   **What is the pathogenesis of trigger finger?**

The most common cause of trigger finger or thumb is overuse trauma of the hands from repetitive gripping activities with increased pull and friction on the flexor tendons. The underlying pathobiologic mechanism for triggering is fibrocartilaginous metaplasia of the pulleys, either due to trauma or disease.

○   **What other systemic conditions can give rise to trigger finger?**

Other causes of flexor digital tenosynovitis include RA, psoriatic arthritis, diabetes mellitus, amyloidosis, hypothyroidism, sarcoidosis, pigmented villonodular tenosynovitis and infections, including tuberculosis and sporotrichosis A.

○   **What management strategies are practiced for this condition?**

Management consists of modification of hand activity, local heat treatment, gentle exercises and NSAIDs as required. One or more corticosteroid injections of the affected flexor tendon sheath are effective and often curative in the majority of patients. A highly satisfactory rate of success can be predicted in female patients and in patients with single digit involvement, a discrete palpable nodule, short duration of symptoms (i.e., <4 mo), or no associated conditions (eg, RA, DM). For those patients who decline injection, consider splinting the involved digit. The MCP joint is splinted in approximately 15° of flexion. Surgical transection of the fibrous annular pulley of the finger or thumb flexor sheath is rarely required for those with chronic symptoms not responding to medical treatment.

○   **What are the outcomes in treatment of trigger finger, intersection syndrome and *De Quervain's tenosynovitis*?**

Whereas splinting, NSAIDs, and other conservative modalities are associated with return to work within 3 to 6 weeks, the addition of treatment by intralesional injection will provide pain relief within 4-7 days, and locking will usually cease within 14 days, saving several weeks of medical leave. Up to 90% of patients have a successful outcome with one to three injections.

○   **How does surgery compare with intralesional injection therapy?**

The cost and time savings of intralesional injection were compared with surgical results in one nonrandomized study, with results favoring injection. Younger patients and patients who refused injection and underwent surgery were compared to those willing to undergo injection. An average of 4 weeks of medical leave was saved by injection, and morbidity and success rates were comparable. In another comparative study, injection of the mixture of corticosteroid and local anesthetic agent had a fourfold greater success rate than that of a local anesthetic alone.

○   **What is a ganglion?**

A ganglion is a cystic swelling overlying a joint or tendon sheath. Ganglia may be unilocular or multilocular, and are thought to result from herniation of synovial tissue from a joint capsule or tendon sheath. The most widely held physiologic explanation attributes cyst formation to mucoid degeneration of collagen and connective tissues. This theory implies that a ganglion represents a degenerative structure that houses the myxoid changes of connective tissue.

O   **What are the demographics of ganglion cysts?**

Ganglion cysts are the most common soft tissue tumors of the hand and wrist. They can occur in patients of any age, including children; approximately 15% of ganglion cysts occur in patients younger than 21 years. Seventy percent of ganglion cysts occur in patients between the second and fourth decades of life. Women are affected 3 times as often as men. No predilection exists for the right or left hand, and occupation does not appear to increase the risk of ganglion formation.

O   **What are the anatomical characteristics of ganglia?**

Ganglions are usually solitary, and they rarely exceed 2 cm in diameter. They can involve almost any joint of the hand and wrist. Dorsal wrist, volar wrist, volar retinacular, and distal interphalangeal ganglion cysts comprise the vast majority of ganglions of the hand and wrist. Dorsal wrist ganglia occurring over the scapholunate ligament of the wrist represent 60-70% of all ganglia. The volar wrist is the next most common site of occurrence; 20% of all ganglia occur in the volar wrist. The flexor tendon sheath of the fingers, particularly at the level of the A1 pulley, is involved in 10-12% of ganglia.

O   **What are indications for treatment?**

Indications for treatment include limitation of motion, pain, weakness, and paresthesias. Treatment is also indicated if malignancy is a concern or if the patient finds the lesion aesthetically displeasing. Cysts that drain externally require attention because of the risk of development of a serious joint or soft tissue infection.

O   **What therapeutic options are appropriate?**

The predominant current nonsurgical method of treatment involves aspiration alone or followed by steroid injection. This is especially successful for tendon sheath ganglions in the hand and digits. Surgical treatment involves total ganglionectomy with removal of a modest portion of the attached capsule.

O   **What is the postoperative rehabilitation for ganglionectomy?**

Postoperative care following excision of wrist ganglion involves placement of a protective dressing, which is left in place for 2-3 days. A bulky dressing or a volar splint is used to reduce pain, bleeding, and swelling. Mobilization is initiated after several days, and range-of-motion exercises are encouraged to restore wrist and finger mobility.

O   **What are the characteristics of Flexor Carpi Radialis and Flexor Carpi Ulnaris Tendinitis?**

Like other tendinopathies about the wrist, irritation of the wrist flexors occurs with stress of the wrist in a particular position. Activities that require forced wrist flexion for prolonged periods, or with repetition, put patients at risk for inflammation about the flexor carpi radialis tendon and the flexor carpi ulnaris tendon. There will be tenderness along the course of the tendon, especially near its insertion. Wrist flexion against resistance with the wrist held in extension reproduces the symptoms.

O   **What is the treatment for Flexor Carpi Radialis and Flexor Carpi Ulnaris Tendinitis?**

Treatment consists of splinting and rest, elimination of the activities that cause pain, and oral nonsteroidal anti-inflammatory medications. Injection of corticosteroid into the flexor carpi radial's or flexor carpi ulnaris sheath may be curative. Sharp pain associated with an intense inflammatory localized reaction is suggestive of calcific tendinitis and is most commonly seen about the flexor carpi ulnaris tendon.

O   **What are the characteristics of hamate fractures?**

A relatively uncommon and under diagnosed cause of palmar pain in young, active individuals is a fracture of the hook of the hamate. These fractures can occur from a fall on an extended wrist, a "dubbed" golf shot, or forcefully striking a ball with a club or bat. Pain in the base of the palm overlying the hamate is the most common presenting symptom. Often, the pain is present only with the activity that caused the fracture, such as driving a golf ball or swinging a bat.

O   **What imaging modality is appropriate?**

Plain radiographs of the wrist are usually read as normal. A carpal tunnel view, obtained with the wrist in a hyperextended position, may demonstrate the fracture. Alternatively, a selective CT scan through the hamate is a more accurate way to confirm the diagnosis

O   **What is the management of hamate fractures?**

If it is diagnosed within 2 to 3 weeks of injury, casting should be attempted to allow the fracture to heal. If this fails, or if it is diagnosed late, surgical treatment is indicated, and most authors favor excision of the hook followed by a gradual return to activities.

O   **What is a carpal boss?**

Often confused with a dorsal ganglion, the carpal boss is a bony, non-mobile prominence on the dorsum of the wrist. It is an osteoarthritic spur that forms at the second or third carpometacarpal joints. The boss is most evident with the wrist in volar flexion. Patients usually present with pain and localized tenderness over the prominence. The condition is twice as common in women as in men, and most patients are in their third or fourth decade of life.

O   **What imaging modality is appropriate?**

Radiographs are best taken with the hand and wrist in 30 to 40 degrees of supination and 20 to 30 degrees of ulnar deviation to put the bony prominence on profile (the "carpal boss view").

O   **What are the treatment options?**

Conservative treatment consists of rest, immobilization, nonsteroidal anti-inflammatory medicines, and occasionally injection with corticosteroids. If it is persistently painful despite these measures, surgical excision of the boss may be necessary but is associated with continued symptoms in a high percentage of patients.

O   **What is Extensor Carpi Ulnaris Tendinitis and Subluxation?**

The extensor carpi ulnaris can become irritated with forced pronation and supination activities, such as putting topspin on a tennis ball. In severe cases, the tendon can begin to sublux about the ulnar head, as its compartment becomes increasingly lax.

O   **What are the presenting symptoms?**

Patients complain of pain with forceful rotation of the forearm, and there will sometimes be an associated snapping of the extensor carpi ulnaris tendon.

O   **What is the recommended treatment?**

Early treatment consists of immobilization of the wrist and often the elbow to prevent pronation and supination. Antiinflammatory medication can help to decrease the inflammation more quickly. If the acute inflammation resolves after an adequate period of rest but the extensor carpi ulnaris tendon continues to be unstable, surgery may be indicated to reconstruct or release the sheath at the wrist.

O   **What other extensor tendinopathies may occur at the wrist?**

The extensor pollicis longus tendon can be irritated as it passes around Lister's tubercle. This condition, unlike other tendinopathies about the wrist, carries a significant risk of tendon rupture. Early diagnosis and sometimes even urgent operative treatment are necessary to prevent this complication. Localized pain, swelling, and tenderness are again the hallmarks of these conditions. Corticosteroid injection are not routinely used in this condition because of a propensity for extensor pollicis longus rupture in chronic cases.

O   **What are the pathological characteristics of scaphoid fractures?**

The scaphoid is more susceptible to injury than any of the other carpal bones because of its unique position bridging the proximal and distal rows of the carpal bones. It is also vulnerable to infarction given the tenuous blood supply it receives.

○   **What clinical evaluation is recommended?**

Any tenderness in the anatomic snuffbox over the dorsal scaphoid should prompt treatment as for a fracture. Treatment involves immobilization in a thumb spica splint or cast and reexamination in 10 to 14 days. If the patient remains symptomatic, radiographs should be repeated. If the radiographs are negative, a bone scan should be obtained. A negative bone scan any time more than 72 hours after injury rules out an occult fracture of the scaphoid.

○   **What clinical treatment approaches are considered?**

Treatment of nondisplaced scaphoid fractures is usually determined by location. Seventy percent of scaphoid fractures are through the waist, 20% are proximal, and 10% are distal. Distal fractures heal rapidly and require 4 to 6 weeks of immobilization in a short arm cast. Proximal and waist fractures require immobilization, first in a long arm thumb spica cast for 6 weeks, then in a short arm thumb spica cast with cast changes every 2 to 3 weeks to prevent loosening of the cast and loss of fixation. Immobilization should continue for 4 to 6 months or until at least 50% bridging or healing is demonstrated by x-ray or, more typically, by computed tomography (CT) scans.

○   **What is scapholunate dissociation?**

The interosseous ligament between the scaphoid and the lunate is a stout structure, especially dorsally, and usually requires a significant force to cause disruption. The typical mechanism of injury is a fall onto the outstretched hand with the wrist extended. Early diagnosis is essential to prevent the late sequelae of carpal collapse.

○   **What imaging modality aids in the diagnosis?**

The key radiographic feature of scapholunate dissociation is (scapholunate interval widening). The anteroposterior rather than the posteroanterior view has been shown to better demonstrate the scapholunate interval.

○   **What treatment is recommended?**

Early surgical intervention is recommended to attempt to maintain carpal alignment and prevent scapholunate advanced collapse.

○   **What is the triangular fibrocartilage complex (TFCC)?**

It comprises the articular disk itself as well as the immediately surrounding ulnocarpal ligaments.

○   **What is the mechanism of injury?**

It can be injured by a variety of mechanisms, both acute and chronic. Hyperpronation and hypersupination of the carpus with loading are the usual causes of acute injuries, whereas repetitive pronation and supination cause more degenerative changes in the TFCC.

○   **What are the clinical characteristics of TFCC injury?**

Tears of the TFCC may present with painful clicking during wrist rotation. Patients generally demonstrate localized tenderness on the midaxial border of the wrist and directly beneath the extensor carpi ulnaris tendon. If forced ulnar deviation of the wrist and gripping reproduce the patient's symptoms, a degenerative tear of the central portion of the TFCC is suspected.

○   **What imaging modalities aid in the diagnosis?**

Plain radiographs are most useful in determining ulnar variance and for ruling out fractures or arthritis as a cause of ulnar wrist pain. Ancillary studies for TFCC tears include 3-compartment arthrography and MRI. Arthroscopy also may aid in the diagnosis as well as surgical management if needed.

○   **What is the initial treatment of TFCC injuries?**

Patients presenting with pain localized to the ulnar side of the wrist often respond to simple splinting and rest. This conservative treatment, as well as nonsteroidal antiinflammatory medications, can be used effectively while the full workup is in progress. A course of rest and splinting followed by a gradual return to activities may completely alleviate their symptoms.

○   **What is a sprain of the pisiform triquetral joint?**

The pisiform-triquetral joint may be sprained; resulting in the pisiform's being displaced distally. This results in pain with wrist flexion or ulnar deviation motions. The pisiform is tender to palpation in the hypothenar aspect of the palm. Reconstructive surgery may be indicated.

○   **What is trapezium first metacarpal joint sprain?**

If trapezium-first metacarpal joint sprain results in subluxation with limitation of pinch grasping, it may suffice to inject the site of tenderness with a steroid-local anesthetic mixture and to prescribe a thumb splint that allows pinch grasping, yet stabilizes the carpometacarpal joint. For persistent symptoms, consider arthroplasty.

○   **What is Dupuytren's contracture?**

This is a relatively common condition characterized by nodular thickening and contraction of the palmar fascia drawing one or more fingers into flexion at the MCP joints. In most patients, Dupuytren's contracture affects the ulnar side of both hands. The fourth finger is usually affected earliest, followed by the fifth, third, and second fingers in decreasing order of frequency.

○   **What is the histopathology reveal?**

Fibrous nodules, resulting from contraction of proliferating fibroblasts in the superficial layers of the palmar fascia, are the earliest abnormality. The dermis is invaded by fibroblastic cells, resulting in puckering, dimpling and tethering of the overlying skin. Dupuytren's disease is initially characterized by marked fibroblastic proliferation and vascular hyperplasia. This is followed by dense, disorderly collagen deposition with thickening of the palmar fascia and nodule formation. Ultrastructurally, contractile, smooth-muscle-like fibroblasts or myofibroblasts, surrounded by bundles of disarrayed collagenous fibrils and completely or partially occluded capillaries are present in the fibrotic nodules and cords.

○   **How does it present clinically?**

There is usually little pain, and if no further progression occurs the hand function is preserved and no treatment is required. However, after a variable period of months or years, the aponeurotic thickening may extend distally to involve the digits. The fingers become flexed at the MCP joints by taut fibrous bands radiating from the palmar fascia, and the hand cannot be placed flat on a table (positive table top test). Although there is no direct involvement of the joints or tendons, progressive flexion deformity of the fingers can lead to severe functional impairment.

○   **What is the etiology?**

The etiology of Dupuytren's contracture is poorly understood.

○   **Who is at risk?**

The disorder is rare in non-Caucasian individuals. Its incidence rises with increasing age, and the sex ratio is predominantly male (5:1). Familial predisposition is frequent, suggesting an autosomal dominant pattern with variable penetrance.

O   What have cytogenetic studies suggested?

Cytogenetic studies of Dupuytren's nodules have shown nonspecific chromosomal abnormalities, including numerical and structural clones and random aberrations, pro phasing and premature centromere separation. A pathogenetic role for local repetitive injury and occupational trauma remains unproven.

O   What other risk factors have been identified?

A relationship to cigarette smoking, producing microvascular occlusion, has been suggested. Dupuytren's contracture has been observed in association with idiopathic epilepsy, alcohol misuse, diabetes mellitus, chronic pulmonary disease and reflex sympathetic dystrophy syndrome.

O   What is the prognosis?

Dupuytren's contracture runs a variable course: some patients show little change or incapacity over a period of many years, while in others fascial contraction progresses rapidly with severe deformity and impairment of hand function within a short period of time.

O   What are the treatment options?

Treatment depends entirely on the rate of progression and severity of the lesions. In patients with mild disease, local heat, stretching exercises, and use of protective padded gloves during heavy manual grasping tasks, are often helpful. Many patients learn the benign nature of the contracture, and adapt to the disorder. In more severe lesions with pain and inability to straighten the fingers, intralesional corticosteroid injections may be beneficial. In those with advanced disease with progressive digital contracture of more than 30°, a positive table top test and functional impairment, surgical intervention (limited or total palmar fasciectomy with or without skin graft replacement), is indicated.

O   What is the risk of recurrence?

The risk of recurrence is increased in young patients with active bilateral disease, and in those with a strong family history and/or other ectopic fibrotic lesions.

O   What is the mallet finger injury?

The so called mallet finger injury to the extensor tendon insertion may also include an avulsion fracture of the dorsal lip of the distal phalanx, but the basic treatment is the same for both types.

O   How is it treated?

Static splinting of the distal interphalangeal joint in full extension is needed until the fracture is healed or the tendon can support the joint against gravity (at least 4–6 weeks). Gentle flexion is allowed thereafter, but full power of the flexor digitorum profundus should not be encouraged for several more weeks. Extension splinting is required at night and during sports for at least 1 month after it has been discontinued for gentle daily activities, and complete function may not be achieved for at least 3 months.

O   What does an avulsion injury of the central extensor tendon slip rehabilitation involve?

Avulsion or tear of the central extensor tendon slip at the base of the middle phalanx requires continuous splinting of the joint in full extension for a minimum of 4 to 6 weeks, with the distal interphalangeal joint usually kept free to allow active flexion and prevent retinacular ligament contractures. Despite this program, a boutonnière deformity may develop, although this condition is seen more often in the untreated or incompletely treated injury. Rehabilitation of such a deformity must include a prolonged period of splinting, at least 6 to 9 months.

○   **How are fracture-subluxations of the proximal interphalangeal joint managed?**

Fracture-subluxation of the proximal interphalangeal joint is sometimes under diagnosed, or dismissed as a rather innocuous injury. However, the long-term disability from its inadequate treatment can seriously affect an athletic career (professional or otherwise). Early concentric reduction of the joint is mandatory and often requires internal fixation or open surgical methods. Prevention of full joint extension is necessary after any type of reduction for this injury, and extension block splinting often is utilized to achieve this goal. Active flexion and extension exercises must be performed for many weeks after injury, and treatment of long-term losses of full extension may require dynamic extension splinting.

○   **What is the Gamekeeper's thumb?**

Tears of the ulnar collateral ligament are the most common sport-related injury to this joint, and are the most common hand injury incurred from skiing.

○   **How is this injury graded and treated?**

Grade I and II sprains have incomplete tears of the ligament, without damage to the adductor tendon aponeurosis; these usually are treated with a thumb spica cast for a minimum of 4 weeks. Grade III injuries are associated with a complete tear of the ligament, which often is displaced superficially to the adductor aponeurosis (the so called Stener lesion). Although the literature reflects some difference of opinion regarding the treatment of grade III tears, most authors advocate open surgical repair of the ligament.

○   **What advice is given regarding return to sport activity?**

Regardless of the degree of collateral ligament sprain, prolonged splinting can protect the healing ligament during resumption of sports activity. Many athletes, especially those who have recurrent injuries, prefer preventive taping of this joint to using rigid splints. High level competitive skiers and other athletes may require concomitant splinting of the interphalangeal joint for adequate protection during sports activity.

HIP

○   **What is Galeazzi's test?**

A test designed to detect unilateral congenital dislocations of the hip in children. The child is positioned supine with the hips flexed to 90° and the knees fully flexed. The test result is positive if one knee is positioned higher than the other.

○   **What is Ober test?**

A test designed to determine the presence of a shortened (tight) iliotibial band. With the patient lying on one side, the lower limb closest to the table is flexed. The other lower limb, which is being tested, is abducted and extended. The knee of the limb is flexed to 90° and is then allowed to drop to the table. If the limb does not, this indicates that the iliotibial band is shortened (tight).

○   **What is Ortolani's test?**

A test designed to identify a congenital hip dislocation in infants. The infant is positioned supine with the hips flexed 90° and the knees fully flexed. The examiner grasps the legs so that the examiner's thumbs are placed on the infant's medial thighs and the examiner's fingers are placed on the infant's lateral thighs. The thighs are gently abducted, and the examiner applies a gentle force to the greater trochanters with the fingers of each hand. Resistance will be felt at about 30° of abduction and, if there is a dislocation, a click will be felt as the dislocation is reduced (see the related Barlow's provocative test).

O **What is Patrick's test?**

A test designed to identify arthritis of the hip. With the patient lying supine, the knee is flexed and the hip is flexed, abducted, and externally rotated until the lateral malleolus rests on the opposite knee just above the patella. In this position the knee on the side being tested is gently forced downward; if pain is produced in the groin, the test result is positive for the presence of hip pathology. If pain is referred to the buttock it suggest SI joint pathology. FABER is an acronym for the combined pattern of movements and is an alternative nomenclature designation.

O **What is the Thomas test?**

A test designed to test for contracture of the hip flexor muscles. In supine position, the patient holds one flexed hip against the chest. The test is positive if the other thigh does not remain against the surface.

O **What is the Trendelenburg test?**

Examines the ability of the hip abductors to stabilize the pelvis on the femur. The patient stands first on the unaffected side, then the affected side. A negative test occurs when the pelvis rises on the opposite side. A positive test occurs when the pelvis on the opposite side drops and indicates a weak or painful gluteus medius, a hip dislocation, or coxa vara.

O **What is one of the most common causes of pain in the hip region?**

Trochanteric bursitis is one of the most common causes of pain about the hip region. The soft tissues that cross the bony posterior portion of the greater trochanter are protected from it by the three trochanteric bursae. The gluteus maximus bursa, which separates the fibers of gluteus maximus from the greater trochanter, is the most important of these bursae. It is not palpable unless it is distended or inflamed.

O **What is the clinical presentation of this condition?**

Patients with trochanteric bursitis present with a deep, aching pain sometimes associated with a burning sensation on the lateral aspect of the hip and thigh. The pain increases with activities such as walking, squatting and climbing stairs, and is associated with a limp in 15% of patients. Typically the pain decreases at rest, although it is frequently worse at night, especially when the patient is lying on the affected side. Tenderness can be elicited on palpation of the area around the greater trochanter which may feel boggy, at least in thin patients. Resisted abduction of the hip when the patient is lying on the opposite side may accentuate the discomfort. The movements of the hip are normal, but in severe cases discomfort can limit motion.

O **Who is at risk for this condition?**

Trochanteric bursitis is more common in women. It can occur as an isolated condition but is more frequently seen in association with damage to the ipsilateral hip joint, mechanical lumbar spine sprain/strain and obesity. Potential precipitating factors include local trauma, leg length inequalities, jogging and other athletic and stressful activities.

O **What comorbid pathology may be encountered in the patient with trochanteric bursitis?**

Trochanteric bursitis is commonly associated with other pathologic conditions. In 1986, Schapira and coworkers described a study of 72 patients with a clinical diagnosis of trochanteric bursitis; 91.6 percent of these patients had associated problems, including osteoarthritis of the same hip (44.5 percent), lumbar spondyloarthrosis (38.8 percent), and rheumatoid arthritis (8.3 percent).

O **Compare trochanteric bursitis with gluteus medius tendinitis?**

Gluteus medius tendinopathy can mimic trochanteric bursitis, but it is distinguished by tenderness on palpation superior to the greater trochanter. Some authors have suggested that a more accurate term is "greater trochanter pain syndrome" to reflect the role that tendinopathy of the gluteus medius and minimus are thought to play. Magnetic resonance imaging (MRI) has documented tendinosis and tears of the gluteus medius; however, the true incidence is unknown because of selection bias in those undergoing MRI.

O   **What muscle imbalances may occur as a result of this condition?**

The alteration in gait secondary to these conditions is often accompanied by a limitation of internal rotation of the hip and reflex tightening of the external rotators. These factors may increase the tension of gluteus maximus on the iliotibial band, and potentiate bursal inflammation.

O   **What imaging abnormalities may be visualized?**

Slight irregularities of the greater trochanter or peritrochanteric calcifications of the bursa are sometimes seen on plain radiographs. Bone scintigraphy may show local increased uptake. The differential diagnosis of increased radio uptake in this region includes stress fractures, local infection and bone and soft tissue tumors. MRI occasionally shows trochanteric bursitis, but these results may not alter clinical recommendations and MRI may not be warranted except to exclude other pathologic conditions.

O   **What is the clinical course of trochanteric bursitis?**

The course of trochanteric bursitis is varied: an acute phase may last several days, followed by the gradual abatement of symptoms. However, in many patients, low grade discomfort may persist for weeks or months.

O   **What treatment options are available for trochanteric bursitis?**

Treatment of both trochanteric bursitis and gluteus medius tendinopathy consists of rest, ice, ITB stretching, strengthening of the hip girdle and trunk musculature (especially gluteus medius), and NSAIDs. Recalcitrant cases usually respond to a local corticosteroid injection. Mechanical precipitants such as leg-length discrepancy, ITB tightness, and pes planus should be addressed. Runners should avoid banked tracks or roads with excessive camber when resuming their running program.

O   **What considerations should be given to recalcitrant trochanteric bursitis?**

Failure of trochanteric bursitis to respond to conservative treatment may be due to tightness of the iliotibial band, as evidenced by a positive Ober's test. Exercises to stretch out the fascia lata in these patients may be worthwhile. In patients with true leg length discrepancy, trochanteric bursitis tends to occur on the longer leg because of the increased stress imposed on the abductors. In these patients, a heel lift may be indicated. Various surgical procedures have been proposed for refractory cases of trochanteric bursitis but these are rarely, if ever, necessary.

O   **Under what circumstances may iliopsoas bursitis manifest clinically?**

The iliopsoas bursa is the largest synovial bursa in the body and is localized anterior to the hip joint between the iliopsoas muscle and the anterior capsule of the hip. Iliopsoas bursitis has been described in association with a variety of hip disorders, including osteoarthritis, rheumatoid arthritis, synovial chondromatosis, pigmented villonodular synovitis, osteonecrosis and septic arthritis. In athletes and workers the cause of pain is thought to be irritation of the iliopsoas tendon over the iliopectineal eminence.

O   **What unusual anatomical feature of the iliopsoas bursa complicates evaluation and management?**

While the bursa communicates with the hip cavity in only 15% of adults, a communication has been documented in most reported cases of bursitis. Several theories may explain this finding: hip synovitis with excessive synovial fluid accumulation may cause enlargement of the iliopsoas bursa via a preexisting communication; a weakened inflamed hip capsule may rupture into the adjacent bursa, creating a new communication; or the bursa itself may be enlarged by the inflammatory process

O   **How does iliopsoas bursitis present?**

The patient will often complain of groin pain or anterior hip region that worsens with passive hip flexion, extension or external rotation.

○ **What imaging studies are considered diagnostically?**

MRI has been proposed as the best diagnostic test to document iliopsoas bursitis, particularly if there is suspected communication with the joint.

○ **What conservative treatment option is recommended?**

The use of deep heating agents, or interferential current combined with gentle stretching of the hip flexors followed by strengthening exercises to the hip musculature. NSAIDs may be beneficial. If there is concomitant RA/OA a cane held contralaterally is indicated. Injection of corticosteroid may also prove beneficial.

○ **What is ischiogluteal bursitis?**

Ischiogluteal bursitis is most commonly seen in patients engaged in jobs, which favor repeated friction of the ischial bursae. In the standing position, the gluteus maximus forms a thick pad over the ischial tuberosity. When the thigh is flexed, as in the sitting position, the distal border of the gluteus maximus moves superiorly, leaving the ischial tuberosity subcutaneous. Weavers repeatedly extend one limb and then the other in the practice of their craft. The repeated friction on the ischial bursa may lead to inflammation of the bursae or 'weaver's bottom' The cause of this bursitis is usually prolonged sitting on a hard surface.

○ **Who is at risk for ischiogluteal bursitis?**

Sedentary people are at risk as well as avid bicyclists. Other common causes include men who keep thick wallets in their back pockets and people with muscle imbalances of the hamstrings and gluteus maximus.

○ **What are the symptoms and signs of ischiogluteal bursitis?**

Patients with ischiogluteal bursitis complain of exquisite pain over the ischium, which is aggravated by sitting and lying. Local tenderness on palpation of the ischium is always found. Enthesitis, such as seen in ankylosing spondylitis and Reiter's syndrome, can give rise to a similar clinical picture. The patient may display an antalgic gait pattern and may have restricted hip flexion.

○ **What therapeutic interventions are recommended?**

Trunk and knee-to-chest stretching exercises while lying on the cushion should be encouraged. The treatment includes removal of the stimulus by padding hard sitting surfaces, removing the wallet from the back pocket, modalities for symptomatic relief, and exercises to restore muscle balance to the hip. A local injection of corticosteroid may be used in refractory cases. Care should be taken not to inject the sciatic nerve, which passes just laterally to the bursa.

○ **What are the clinical presentation and treatment for athletes with ischial bursitis?**

Ischial bursitis may occur as a complication of an injury of the hamstring insertion into the ischial tuberosity. Symptoms include pain while sitting and localized tenderness on examination. Initial treatment consists of rest, ice, NSAIDs, hamstring stretching and strengthening, and protection. Often a doughnut cushion will alleviate the patient's symptoms while he or she is sitting. Aspiration of the bursa and injection of a corticosteroid should be considered for recalcitrant cases. Rarely, surgical excision of the bursa for persistent pain and disability is indicated.

○ **What is adductor tendinitis?**

While the adductor longus, adductor magnus, adductor brevis, and pectineal muscles are all adductors of the hip, of these the adductor longus is most often injured in sports.

○ **What is the mechanism of injury in athletes?**

The mechanisms of injury to the adductor longus include a powerful abduction stress during simultaneous adduction of the leg when performing a cutting movement or overuse, such as repetitive abduction of the free leg in the skating stride. With a sudden change of direction that occurs with sharp cutting movements, a forceful eccentric contraction of the muscle occurs instead of a concentric contraction, causing the strain. While a forceful muscle contraction in an adult may cause a strain in the muscle-tendon unit, the same action in an immature athlete may cause an avulsion fracture.

○   **Who is at risk for Adductor tendinitis?**

Adductor tendinitis tends to occur in patients engaged in sports activities involving straddling, such as horseback riding, gymnastics and dancing, as well as in adepts of aerobic exercise classes, especially in those individuals with an inadequate or insufficient warming up period.

○   **What are the signs and symptoms associated with it?**

The pain is typically felt in the groin and inner aspect of the thigh and is increased by passive abduction of the thighs and active adduction against resistance. Tenderness may also be elicited by local palpation of the adductor muscles, especially near their insertion on the front of the pubis.

○   **What is the differential diagnosis?**

The differential diagnosis of adductor tendinitis include hernias, genitourinary afflictions (prostatitis, epididymitis, urethritis, hydrocele, etc.), osteitis pubis and arthritis of the hip.

○   **What are the treatment recommendations?**

Treatment consists of rest and ice during the acute phase. Nonsteroidal anti-inflammatory drugs, ultrasound and progressive stretching exercises are used in the subacute phase. Local corticosteroid injections are reserved for patients resistant to these conservative modalities.

○   **What is Snapping hip syndrome?**

This syndrome refers to conditions about the hip that cause an audible or palpable "snapping." The cause can be intra-articular or extraarticular. The most common cause involves the snapping of the iliotibial band or the tensor fascia lata over the greater trochanter of the femur (external snapping). Less commonly, the iliopsoas tendon may snap as it slides over the iliopectineal eminence, or the iliofemoral ligament may slide over the femoral head (internal snapping). Other causes may include the long head of biceps femoris gliding over the ischial tuberosity and intraarticular pathology such as subluxation of the hip or the presence of loose bodies.

○   **What are the symptoms and signs associated with the snapping hip syndrome?**

The athlete may describe associated pain, crepitation, and local warmth, but performance is rarely impaired. Physical examination focuses on localizing the source of the click and associated discomfort.

○   **What treatment approach is appropriate?**

Treatment consists of modified activity, correcting muscle imbalance and tightness of the involved structures (eg, the iliotibial band or tensor fascia lata), and correcting biomechanical malalignments using orthoses whenever appropriate, as with a leg-length discrepancy. Corticosteroid injections are appropriate if bursal causes can be identified. Surgery is rarely recommended.

○   **What is Osteitis Pubis?**

Inflammation on each side of the periosteal bone of the symphysis pubis is detectable clinically by local direct point tenderness, and radiographically by erosion, sclerosis, and widening of the symphysis pubis.

○   **What medical pathology may trigger it?**

This disorder may result from regional spread of sepsis following surgery of the prostate gland or bladder, or inguinal herniorrhaphy.

O   **What are the mechanisms operative in athletes who develop osteitis pubis?**

This inflammatory lesion of the bone adjacent to the symphysis pubis is thought to be due to mechanical strain from trauma, excessive twisting and turning in sports such as soccer, or repetitive shear stress from excessive side-to-side motion (as in runners with a crossover arm swing).

O   **Who is at risk?**

It is common in ice hockey, soccer, and distance running. It is also common in exercising pregnant women and women in the postpartum period because of the particular instability of this joint after birth.

O   **How does it present?**

Pain is rarely described by the injured athlete as originating from the symphysis. Instead, pain appears to emanate from the perineal, inguinal, or thigh regions. On examination, however, the pubic symphysis is usually tender to palpation, and the pain can be reproduced by passive abduction and active resisted adduction of the thigh.

O   **What radiographic findings may occur?**

Radiographic changes may not be visible for 2 to 3 weeks. Common bone changes are symmetric resorption of the medial ends of the pubic bones, widening of the symphysis, and rarefaction or sclerosis along the pubic rami. Technetium bone scanning is likely to give positive results. MRI, particularly fat-suppression sequences may document stress around the symphysis but may also detect adjacent areas of pathology or help identify other conditions (e.g., pubic stress fracture). Limited STIR sequences may be economical for the monitoring of changes in the stress reaction with treatment.

O   **What rheumatic conditions are associated with it?**

Osteitis pubis may be secondary to ankylosing spondylitis, chondrocalcinosis, or polymyalgia rheumatica. When the condition is associated with arthritis, pain frequently has no relation to radiographic change. In female patients, subluxation and irregularity of the medial surfaces were found to be correlated with number of children born and not to arthritis.

O   **What is the initial treatment of osteitis pubis??**

The initial focus of treatment is the reduction of inflammation. Rest from the inciting activity is required, with cross training used to maintain aerobic fitness. NSAIDs or even oral corticosteroids may be used. Intraarticular cortisone injection may be of value when other methods are not working.

O   **What is the subsequent rehabilitation approach?**

After the stress has been reduced across the symphysis and the inflammation diminished, a stretching and strengthening program emphasizing abdominal, hip, and short-arc closed chain exercises is instituted. During relative rest, patients maintain fitness with cycling and swimming. Patients typically return to play after 8 to 12 weeks.

O   **What is the course and outcome for osteitis pubis?**

Osteitis pubis can sometimes take as long as 9 months to resolve with conservative care. Reported rates of recurrence and failure to return to previous levels of competition have been as high as 25%, and may be higher in men.

O   **What other modalities are considered?**

Use of a sacral belt to stabilize the pelvis has also provided symptomatic benefit. Obviously, when radiographic progression suggests osteomyelitis, surgical consultation should be obtained. Some surgeons advocate wedge resection of the symphysis pubis for persistent symptoms, but pelvis instability can result in up to one-third of operated patients.

○ **What is Iliotibial band syndrome (ITB)?**

The iliotibial band consists of connective tissue that runs from the ilium to the fibula. In patients with this syndrome, an aching or burning pain is felt at the site where the band courses over the lateral femoral condyle and, occasionally, the pain radiates up the thigh toward the hip. There may also be an abnormal shortened iliotibial tract. The tightness of the iliotibial band can be tested for by having the patient lie on the side with the involved side up. The examiner lowers the straight involved leg forward and downward noting any discomfort, tautness, and tenderness, when compared to the uninvolved leg. Risk factors include a varus alignment of the knee, excessive running mileage, worn shoes, or continuous running on uneven terrain.

○ **What treatment is appropriate?**

The treatment of iliotibial band syndrome includes rest, NSAIDs, stretching, physical therapy, and attention to contributing factors, such as shoes, techniques and running surface. The clinician should address postural dysfunction, muscle imbalance, leg length discrepancies as part of the conservative approach. Local corticosteroid injection into the areas of tenderness can be helpful, but the patient must refrain from running for at least two weeks following the injection.

KNEE

○ **What is the abduction (valgus stress) test?**

A test designed to identify medial instability of the knee. The examiner applies a valgus stress to the patient's knee while the patient's ankle is stabilized in slight lateral rotation. The test is first conducted with the knee fully extended and then repeated with the knee at 20° of flexion. Excessive movement of the tibia away from the femur indicates a positive test result. Positive findings with the knee fully extended indicate a major disruption of the knee ligaments. A positive test result with the knee flexed is indicative of damage to the medial collateral ligament.

○ **What is the adduction (varus stress) test?**

A test designed to identify lateral instability of the knee. The examiner applies a varus stress to the patient's knee while the ankle is stabilized. The test is done with the patient's knee in full extension and then with the knee in 20°-30° of flexion. A positive test result with the knee extended suggests a major disruption of the knee ligaments, whereas a positive test result with the knee flexed is indicative of damage to the lateral collateral ligament.

○ **What is the anterior drawer (sign) test?**

A test designed to detect anterior instability of the knee. The patient lies supine with the knee flexed 90 degrees. The examiner sits across the forefoot of the patient's flexed lower limb. With the patient's foot in neutral rotation, the examiner pulls forward on the proximal part of the calf. Both lower limbs are tested. The test result is positive if there is excessive anterior movement of the tibia with respect to the femur.

○ **What is the Apley grinding test?**

A test designed to detect meniscal lesions. The patient lies prone with the knees flexed 90°. The examiner applies a compressive force through the foot and rotates the tibia back and forth while palpating the joint line with the other hand feeling for crepitation. The test result is positive if the patient reports pain or the examiner feels crepitation. This test is then repeated by applying a distractive force to the leg, and if pain is elicited it is indicative of a ligamentous injury rather than a meniscal injury.

○ **What is the apprehension test?**

A test designed to identify dislocation of the patella. The patient lies supine with the knee resting at 30° flexion. The examiner carefully and slowly displaces the patella laterally. If the patient looks apprehensive and tries to contract the quadriceps muscle to bring the patella back to neutral, the test result is positive.

O **What is the bounce home test?**

A test designed to identify meniscal lesions. The patient lies supine, and the heel of the patient's foot is cupped by the examiner. The patient's knee is completely flexed and then allowed to extend passively If extension is not complete or has a rubbery end-feel ("springy block"), the test result is positive.

O **What is Clarke's sign?**

A test designed to identify the presence of chondromalacia of the patella. The patient ties relaxed with knees extended as the examiner presses down slightly proximal to the base of the patella with the web of the hand. The patient is then asked to contract the quadriceps muscle as the examiner applies more force. The test result is positive if the patient cannot complete the contraction without pain.

O **What is the crossover test?**

A test designed to identify anterolateral instability of the knee. With the patient standing and the uninvolved leg crossed in front of the test leg, the examiner secures the foot of the test leg by carefully stepping on it. The patient rotates the upper torso away from the injured leg approximately 90°. In this position the patient is asked to contract the quadriceps muscles. If this action produces a feeling of "giving way" in the knee, the test result is positive.

O **What is the fluctuation test?**

A test designed to identify significant knee effusion. The knee is placed in a position of 15° flexion. The examiner then places the palm of one hand over the suprapatellar pouch and the other hand anterior to the joint, with the thumb and index finger adjacent to the patellar margins. The examiner tries to feel and assess the shifting or fluctuation of synovial fluid while alternatively pressing down with one hand and then the other.

O **What is the Helfet test?**

A test designed to identify meniscal lesions. The "screw home" mechanism is observed during full extension. With a torn meniscus blocking the joint, the tibial tubercle remains slightly me dial in relation to the midline of the patella, and the final limit of external rotation is prevented.

O **What is the Hughston posterolateral drawer test?**

A test designed to identify the presence of posterolateral rotary knee instability. The procedure is similar to the Hughston posteromedial test except the patient's foot is slightly laterally rotated. The test result is positive if the tibia rotates posteriorly on the lateral side an excessive amount when the examiner pushes the tibia posteriorly.

O **What is the Hughston posteromedial drawer test?**

A test designed to identify posteromedial rotary instability of the knee. The patient lies in a supine position with the knee flexed to 90°. The examiner fixes the foot in slight medial rotation by sitting on the foot. The examiner pushes the tibia posteriorly. The test result is positive if the tibia moves or rotates posteriorly on the medial aspect an excessive amount.

O **What is the Jakob test (reverse pivot shift)?**

It is a test designed to identify posterolateral rotary instability of the knee. This test can be performed with the patient either standing or supine: In the standing position, the patient leans against a wall with the involved extremity toward the examiner. The examiner's hands are placed above and below the test knee, and a valgus stress is applied while the patient flexes the knee. The test result is positive if there is a jerk in the knee or the tibia shifts posteriorly and the knee gives way. The patient lies supine. The examiner supports the patient's knee posteriorly with one hand and the heel with the other hand. The patient's foot is then laterally rotated.

O **What is the Lachman's test?**

A test designed to identify injury to the anterior cruciate ligament. The patient lies supine with the examiner stabilizing the distal femur with one hand and grasping the proximal tibia with the other hand. With the knee held in slight flexion, the tibia is moved forward on the femur. A positive test result is indicated by a soft end-feel and excessive observable movement of the tibia.

○   **What is the Macintosh test (lateral pivot shift)?**

A test designed to identify anterolateral rotational instability (ALRI). The examiner grasps the leg with one hand and places the other hand over the lateral, proximal aspect of the leg. With the knee in extension, a valgus; stress is applied and the leg internally rotated as the knee is flexed. At about 30°-40° of flexion, a sudden jump is noted as the lateral tibial plateau, which has subluxed anteriorly in relation to the femoral condyle, suddenly reduces.

○   **What is the McMurray test?**

A test designed to identify meniscal lesions. The patient lies supine while the examiner grasps the foot with one hand and palpates the joint line with the other. The knee is fully flexed and the tibia rotated back and forth and then held alternately in internal and external rotation as the knee is extended. A click or crepitation may be felt over the joint line with a posterior meniscal lesion, as the knee is extended.

○   **What is the O'Donoghue's test?**

A test designed to detect meniscal injuries or capsular irritation. The patient lies supine, and the examiner flexes the knee to 90°, rotates it medially and laterally twice, and then fully flexes and rotates it again. The test result is positive if pain increases on rotation.

○   **What is the patellar tap test?**

A test designed to identify significant joint effusion. The knee is flexed or extended to discomfort, and the examiner taps the surface of the patella. The test result is positive if a floating of the patella is felt.

○   **What is the posterior drawer test?**

A test designed to identify posterior instability of the knee. The patient lies supine with the knee flexed to 90° as the foot is held in a neutral position by the examiner sitting on it. The examiner's hands grasp the leg around the proximal tibia and attempt to move the tibia backward on the femur. The test result is positive if there is excessive posterior movement of the tibia on the femur.

○   **What is the posterior sag sign (gravity drawer test)?**

A test designed to identify posterior instability of the knee. The patient lies supine with the knees flexed to 90° and the feet supported. The test result is positive if the tibia sags back on the femur.

○   **What is the differential diagnosis for knee pain in childhood?**

Pain in the knee in this age group (2–10 years) is uncommon but is always significant. Intraarticular causes include a torn discoid lateral meniscus and osteochondritis dissecans. Inflammatory causes include pauciarticular juvenile chronic arthritis and septic arthritis. Periarticular causes are osteomyelitis of the lower femur or upper tibia and, at the upper end of the age group, Osgood–Schlatter's disease (traction apophysitis of the tibial tubercle) and Sinding-Larsen–Johansson syndrome i.e. 'Jumper's knee' is due to micro tearing at the inferior patellar pole attachment. Referred pain may come from the hip due to Perthe's disease (Idiopathic osteonecrosis of the femoral head in children aged 3–12 years).

○   **What is the differential diagnosis for knee pain in adolescence?**

Knee pain is common in adolescence (10–18 years). Intraarticular causes are usually related to osteochondritis dissecans or tears involving a discoid lateral meniscus. In girls the anterior knee pain syndrome and patellar maltracking are the most common causes of pain. Inflammatory causes are pauciarticular juvenile chronic arthritis and septic arthritis. Periarticular pain is usually due to Osgood–Schlatter's or Sinding-Larsen–Johansson syndrome. Slipped upper femoral epiphysis in boys frequently presents with knee pain and a limp and is common in this age group. The hip should be carefully examined as loss of internal rotation is an early sign of slipped upper femoral epiphysis.

○ What imaging studies are appropriate initially in adolescent knee pain?

Anteroposterior (AP) and lateral views of the femur and hip, and a bone scan, should be performed in cases of knee pain for which no cause can be found. If slipped upper femoral epiphysis is suspected, AP and lateral radiographs of the hip should be performed.

○ What is prepatellar bursitis?

The prepatellar bursa normally covers the patella and portions of the patellar tendon. With macrotrauma (e.g., a blow) or repetitive microtrauma (e.g., repeated kneeling), the bursa can become inflamed, fill with fluid, and enlarge in volume and area.

○ What are its diagnostic features?

The patient with prepatellar bursitis presents with pain on flexion or direct pressure and reports pain with walking or running. On physical examination, a soft tissue enlargement sometimes warm, tender, and erythematous is found anterior to the patella. Signs of acute inflammation require aspiration and synovial fluid analysis to exclude septic bursitis. Cultures of bursal fluid may need review before corticosteroids are administered.

○ How is it managed?

Treatment usually is nonsurgical, consisting of measures to prevent repetitive trauma, compression, use of oral nonsteroidal anti-inflammatory drugs (NSAIDs), and rest. If this conservative treatment fails, aspiration and corticosteroid injection may be considered. Occasionally, surgical excision is necessary.

○ What is pes anserine bursitis?

The anserine bursa is located medially about 6 cm below the joint line between the attachment of the medial collateral ligament at the medial tibial plateau and the conjoined tendon formed by the gracilis, sartorius, and semitendinosus tendons. Anserine bursitis commonly accompanies medial compartment osteoarthritis of the knee and may be the major source of pain in this condition. Anserine bursitis should be suspected when pain, particularly at night, occurs in the medial knee region over the upper tibia.

○ What alternative presentation may occur in athletes?

The more common site of bursitis in athletes is in the iliotibial band area. Examination reveals tenderness above the lateral joint line and perhaps extending to the joint line itself. The iliotibial band is often tight and may click as it passes over the lateral femoral condyle. Iliotibial bursitis is associated with overuse and with running, bicycling, or other vigorous endurance sports. Treatment for all bursitis is conservative, including stretching, anti-inflammatory medication, or injection of corticosteroids. On rare occasions, bursectomy or partial release of the overlying tendons (e.g., a tight iliotibial band) is necessary.

○ What is jumper's knee?

Patellar tendinitis is a condition which most commonly affects young sportsmen but may also affect older patients. The symptoms are of pain at the inferior pole of the patella, which is brought on by activity, particularly climbing stairs, running and jumping. The condition is due to mucoid degeneration of the patellar tendon at its insertion into the inferior pole of the patella. The majority of cases respond to rest and NSAIDs. For the athlete a graded progressive program in therapeutic exercise is warranted after the acute symptoms have subsided. If the symptoms do not abate injection of a small amount of steroid (0.2 ml) into the tender area is usually helpful. A larger volume should not be injected, since necrosis of the tendon can occur. Occasionally, operative treatment to excise the involved portion of tendon is necessary.

○   **What is popliteus tendinitis?**

This is also an overuse injury which causes pain over the lateral aspect of the joint. It is caused by inflammation of the popliteus tendon and paratenon as it passes beneath the arcuate ligament complex. Popliteus tendinitis has been associated with downhill running or other deceleration activities. Typically, patients are able to run for short distances, but with continued running, posterolateral knee pain develops. Many patients will report pain in the back of the knee, but they will almost always point to the posterolateral area. The main finding is tenderness along the proximal aspect of the popliteus tendon.

○   **What treatment is appropriate?**

A rehabilitation program emphasizing eccentric strengthening of the quadriceps muscle. In addition to strengthening, various treatment modalities that have been recommended include rest, NSAIDs, and localized corticosteroid injection.

○   **What are popliteal cysts?**

Swellings occurring in the popliteal region are common and should be called popliteal cysts regardless of where they originate. They may occur at any age from childhood onwards. They communicate with the knee joint in about two thirds of cases. Approximately 60% arise from bursae and 30% from synovial herniation through the posterior capsule of the joint. Approximately 10% are of indeterminate origin. The bursal cysts most commonly arise from the bursa deep to the semimembranosus on the medial side of the popliteal fossa. The hernial cysts arise most commonly from the medial side.

○   **How do they present clinically?**

The presenting complaint is usually of a swelling at the back of the knee. The swelling may be associated with aching and is more prominent when the knee is extended. The cysts often transilluminate. In children there is usually no other abnormality found on examination of the knee but in adults the cysts are associated with rheumatoid arthritis and osteoarthritis.

○   **How can they be imaged?**

Magnetic resonance imaging (MRI) or ultrasound can aid the diagnosis of Baker's cyst. MRI is advantageous, because it may identify the underlying cause, such as a concomitant meniscal tear. Focus should be in the most common area for Baker's cyst, along the medial aspect of the popliteal fossa beneath the medial head of the gastrocnemius.

○   **What is the differential diagnosis?**

The differential diagnosis includes popliteal artery aneurysm, and solid tumors such as osteochondroma. Occasionally a nerve sheath ganglion or a muscle tumor may cause difficulty with diagnosis. Popliteal cysts may become very large due to a valve effect of the opening into the joint, particularly in rheumatoid arthritis. If they burst they may simulate a deep vein thrombosis. The signs in the calf are similar but differentiation can usually be made due to a history of a swelling in the popliteal fossa and the sudden onset of pain, often with a sensation of water running down the leg.

○   **What is the recommended treatment?**

Treatment in children should be conservative, as the cysts commonly decrease in size spontaneously and those, which are operated on have a high recurrence rate. Treatment in adults should be aimed at the underlying pathology. A large cyst, which is causing pain or interfering with knee movement, should be excised, although marsupialization and drainage into the calf is an alternative. Aspiration and injection of steroid solution may be performed but reaccumulation is frequent.

○   **What is osteochondritis dissecans (OCD)?**

Osteochondritis dissecans occurs most commonly in the knee joint. A fragment of cartilage with its underlying subchondral bone becomes detached and may become loose in the joint. Within the knee, OCD lesions occur at the medial femoral condyle (80% to 85% of cases), the lateral femoral condyle (10% to 15% of cases), and the patella (5% of cases). The reported prevalence of OCD is 30 to 60 cases per 100,000 people. The second decade is the usual time for presentation but it may occur earlier. Bilateral disease is present in 30% to 40% of patients. Males are affected three times more often than females.

○ **What is the etiology of OCD?**

A traumatic origin is supported by multiple studies. Approximately 40% of patients presenting with OCD of the knee have a history of major or repetitive knee trauma, and 60% of patients presenting with OCD participate in a high level of athletic activity; however, it is likely that the etiology of OCD is multifactorial.

○ **What are the pathological changes?**

The pathological changes, which occur, are avascular necrosis of the bone and degenerative changes in the overlying cartilage, with softening, fibrillation and fissuring.

○ **What are the symptoms of OCD?**

Patients with OCD of the knee typically present with poorly localized, aching knee pain and swelling. Symptoms of knee locking or giving way may develop as the disease progresses. The pain is exacerbated by strenuous activity and twisting motions, especially internal rotation of the tibia, which causes the medial tibial spine to strike the lateral aspect of the medial femoral condyle (the site of most OCD lesions). As a result, patients may walk with the affected leg externally rotated. Many patients with lesions of the lateral femoral condyle feel a painful "clunk" with knee flexion and extension.

○ **What are the signs of OCD?**

On physical exam, the affected knee typically maintains full range of motion, unless a loose body causes mechanical locking. Thigh circumference may be diminished on the affected side because of disuse atrophy. A joint effusion may be noted, especially if the patient has been active. With the knee flexed, diffuse tenderness may be elicited over the involved femoral condyle. However, this finding is nonspecific and often seen in patients with patellofemoral disease.

○ **What is Wilson's test?**

Wilson described a useful diagnostic test for OCD of the medial femoral condyle. When the knee is extended, the medial tibial spine rubs against the medial femoral condyle. Patients who have OCD experience pain at approximately 30° of flexion. External rotation of the tibia relieves the discomfort.

○ **What do imaging studies reveal?**

Osteochondritic lesions of the condyles can often be seen on AP and lateral radiographs but are best seen on a tunnel view. The radiographic appearance is diagnostic, showing a well circumscribed fragment of subchondral bone. If the fragment has become detached an irregularity is seen at the site. CT scanning and magnetic resonance imaging (MRI) are useful to confirm the diagnosis and to define the extent of the lesion. In cases of doubt a bone scan may be useful to differentiate osteochondritis dissecans from abnormalities of ossification. A hot spot around the lesion confirms active disease, the uptake decreases with healing of the lesion.

○ **How is it treated initially?**

Nonsurgical management is indicated for a juvenile/young adult patient with a lesion in the medial femoral condyle and no evidence of fragment instability on plain radiographs. The basis of conservative treatment is modification of activity to promote bone healing at the site of fragment separation. An initial 1 to 2 week period of immobilization and minimal weight-bearing is helpful to control pain and initiate healing. However, prolonged immobilization and casting should be avoided because joint motion is important for articular cartilage nutrition and healing.

○ **What is the subsequent treatment for OCD involving the knee?**

Activities should be modified for 6 to 12 weeks Younger patients generally require a shorter period of activity modification than older patients. In general, rapid or strenuous movement of the lower extremities should be avoided, especially high-impact activities such as running, cutting, and jumping. Activities of daily living and upper body exercise are permitted. After the period of activity modification, decisions regarding a patient's return to normal physical activity should be made on an individual basis, based on symptoms. Low-impact exercises such as bicycling or swimming are usually well tolerated and may be recommended initially. This is followed by a gradual return to full activity.

When is surgery indicated?

Surgery may be indicated for juvenile/young adult patients with stable lesions of the medial femoral condyle if conservative therapy fails to relieve symptoms or if there is no radiographic evidence of healing after 12 weeks. Surgical repair is recommended for adult patients regardless of the stability of the lesion. Unstable fragments require surgery regardless of the patient's age.

What factors predispose to patellofemoral pain syndrome (PFS)?

PFS often arises from a combination of intrinsic and extrinsic factors. Factors that predispose individuals to patellofemoral pain include the presence of patella alta, increased Q angle, femoral anteversion, ITB tightness, lateral retinacular tightness, triceps surae tightness, quadriceps and hamstring weakness and excessive pronation. It also may be secondary to fracture or degenerative disease in the knee region. Clinicians should look for all of these factors as well as attempt to mobilize the patella superiorly, inferiorly, medially, and laterally to determine if any soft-tissue restrictions exist.

What symptoms are reported?

Pain in PFS is typically diffuse and poorly localized over the anterior aspect of the knee. Patients will sometimes report that the pain seems to be coming from "behind the kneecap." An early clue to a diagnosis is to ask the patient to point with one finger to the spot of maximal pain. Patients with PFS are often unable to pinpoint pain and instead will rub the front of their knees and complain of diffuse, rather than focal, pain within or over the anterior knee. Buckling or subjective instability in PFS is often noted with stair use and is usually due to pain inhibition of the quadriceps. Bilateral pain is common.

What physical examination findings are evident in standing?

First observe the patient while he or she stands barefoot facing you. Observe the standing Q-angle (i.e., the valgus angle) acting across the knee; angles greater than 25° in females and 20° in males are considered abnormal. Watch for torsional deformities as well as significant hindfoot pronation. Next, observe the patient squat and stand. Note how difficult this is for the patient, as this helps determine the severity of functional deficit.

What physical exam findings are noted in supine/siting?

With the patient sitting on the examining table facing you, observe whether the tibial tubercles are directly below the patellae or are displaced laterally more than 10°, indicating an increased tubercle sulcus angle. Before palpating for tenderness evaluate the patient's patellar mobility and lower-extremity flexibility. With the patient supine on the examination table, perform the patellar tilt test and patella glide test as a first step in evaluating patellar mobility. Next ask the patient to actively flex and extend the knee and observe the dynamic patellar tracking. Palpate and listen for crepitus as the patient moves his or her leg. Compression testing done at differing degrees of flexion assesses pain as the patella moves through the femoral groove.

What other elements of the examination need to be addressed in PFS

Flexibility deficits in the hip external rotators, hamstrings, quadriceps, and gastrocnemius-soleus muscle group may contribute to abnormal patellofemoral biomechanics. Diagnosing asymmetry that results from such deficits is a critical part of managing patellofemoral disorders, because asymmetry should be addressed in a treatment plan that uses stretching exercises to focus on specific muscle groups.

What radiographic studies may be helpful?

Initial evaluation of patients who have patellofemoral complaints usually involves plain radiographic studies. Anteroposterior and lateral views can rule out associated and potentially serious bony conditions such as tumors, infection, or bony loose bodies. Plain radiographic patellar axial views, the sunrise or Merchant view, can demonstrate patellofemoral malalignment, but plain radiographs are less sensitive than computed tomography or magnetic resonance imaging studies in this regard.

❍ What is chondromalacia patellae?

A diagnosis of chondromalacia patellae means softening of the articular cartilage of the patella and can only be made at arthroscopy or arthrotomy. It is a pathological diagnosis and should not be used to describe the clinical syndrome of pain arising from the anterior knee joint. However, patients with anterior knee pain may be found to have chondromalacia patellae. It may be associated with patellar malalignment, in which case it is probably due to impact loading and shearing of the articular cartilage as the patella is compressed against the lateral femoral condyle. Articular cartilage is poor at resisting shear forces, and repetitive impact loading and shear may both be shown to produce cartilage softening.

❍ Summarize the early, intermediate and final phases of PFPS rehabilitation:

Weeks 1 to 2:

1. Use modalities to reduce swelling, inflammation and pain.
2. Use massage, MFR, and patella mobilization to increase flexibility of soft tissues.
3. Begin quadriceps exercises: quad sets, mini squats, wall glides, and modified leg press.
4. Use biofeedback to help recruit the VMO.
5. Stretch the lateral structures if needed: ITB/TFL, hamstrings, and lateral retinaculum.
6. Avoid deep squats, low chairs, and stair climbing.
7. Use patellar tape or brace to decrease pain and increase function.

Weeks 2 to 4

1. Use modalities as needed.
2. Progress quadriceps strengthening in pain-free ROM, avoiding 20' to 50' range.
3. Gently increase knee ROM to full. Continue stretching lateral structures if needed.
4. Begin proprioceptive and balance training in standing.
5. Begin ambulation in all directions.
6. Avoid excessive stair climbing.
7. Begin to wean off patellar tape or brace.

Weeks 4 to 8

1. Progress quadriceps strengthening full range in open and closed chain.
2. Increase resistance and speed of exercise.
3. All transfers should be independent and pain-free.
4. Progress gait training on uneven terrain and for speed.
5. All functional activities should be approaching independent and pain-free.
6. Use of patellar tape or brace should be restricted to high-level activity only

❍ What are the demographics of meniscal injury?

The prevalence of acute meniscal tears is 61 cases per 100,000 persons. The overall male-to-female ratio is approximately 2.5:1. The peak incidence of meniscal injury for males is in men aged 31-40 years. For females, the peak incidence is in those aged 11-20 years. In patients older than 65 years, the rate of degenerative meniscal tears is 60%.

❍ What is the mechanism of injury?

The mechanism of the injury is usually a twisting force applied to the weight-bearing knee, causing entrapment of the meniscus between the tibial and femoral condyles. The resulting tear is usually longitudinal. If the tear is extensive the inner portion may displace into the joint causing the knee to lock (a bucket handle tear). This locking may be intermittent as the torn portion flips in and out of the joint. A tear may extend to the inner margin of the meniscus forming a 'parrot beak' tear. The flap formed can displace into the joint causing intermittent locking. Peripheral meniscal detachment may also occur.

❍ How are meniscal injuries classified?

Classification of meniscal tears provides a description of pathoanatomy. The types of meniscus tears are (1) longitudinal tears that may take the shape of a bucket-handle if displaced, (2) radial tears, (3) parrot-beak or oblique flap tears, (4) horizontal tears, and (5) complex tears that combine variants of the above.

○   **How do meniscal injuries present in older adults?**

In the older age group, where the meniscus is less elastic, degenerative tears can occur. These tears are usually horizontal cleavage tears or radial tears running into the substance of the meniscus.

○   **How do acute meniscal injuries present clinically?**

The history of an acute meniscal tear in a young adult is often characteristic. A twisting injury occurs causing immediate severe pain. The patient is unable to weight bear and may be unable to fully extend the knee if a bucket handle tear has lodged in the joint. The knee swells within several hours. If a cruciate ligament rupture is also present a hemarthrosis will accumulate within an hour. The patient complains of pain well localized to the joint line. Examination reveals a painful knee with tenderness over the joint line adjacent to the tear. An effusion is virtually always present and if the torn portion has displaced into the joint, a springy block to full extension is felt.

○   **How do chronic meniscal injuries present?**

In a chronic tear the patient may complain of pain over the joint line and a feeling of 'catching'. Joint line tenderness is usually present. True locking occurs when the torn portion of the meniscus displaces into the joint causing loss of full extension. Locking due to a meniscal tear always occurs with the knee flexed, although not necessarily weight bearing. Examination of a knee locked due to a meniscal tear reveals a springy block to extension; forced extension is painful. Flexion is usually full or only mildly reduced due to pain. Patients often confuse locking with stiffness and it is important to distinguish between the two. If the knee unlocks with a click or a clunk it is suggestive of a meniscal tear.

○   **What imaging studies/procedures are helpful?**

While the majority of acute and chronic meniscal injuries can be diagnosed on the history and examination, confirmation may be obtained by MRI or arthroscopy. Recently MRI has been found to be accurate, but, if the tear is symptomatic, arthroscopy is preferable as it can be excised at the same time.

○   **What are the MRI criteria for the grading of meniscal injuries?**

This is the criterion standard imaging study for imaging meniscus pathology and all intraarticular disorders. Normal menisci have a homogenous low signal. Abnormal meniscal signals are classified into the following 3 groups:
Grade I - Small area of increased signal within the meniscus
Grade II - Linear area of increased signal that does not extend to an articulating surface
Grade III - Abnormal increased signal that reaches the surface or edge of the meniscus

○   **What is the clinical significance of these grades?**

Grade I and II changes are common in older patients as evidence of the normal aging degenerative process and in young patients as normal perforating vascular channels. Grade I and II changes are not usually seen arthroscopically and do not represent meniscal tears. Grade III changes are meniscal tears.

○   **What is the diagnostic value of aspiration of blood during arthrocentesis in an acute knee injury?**

An aspiration may help identify the underlying cause of the effusion. Blood in the knee is an ominous sign: Since the meniscus itself is avascular, hemarthrosis should not be attributed to a meniscal tear. Rather, the physician should assume that other structures in addition to the meniscus (such as the ACL) may have been injured.

○   **What factors determine if conservative or surgical therapy is warranted??**

Factors that may suggest that conservative therapy is likely to be successful include

Symptoms develop over 24 to 48 hours after injury (as opposed to immediate)
The patient is able to bear weight
There is minimal swelling
There is full range of movement with pain only at the end of range of motion
Pain on McMurray's test is only in the inner range of flexion
Factors that may suggest that surgery will be required include

There was a severe twisting injury and activity could not be continued
The knee is locked or motion is severely restricted
Pain on McMurray's test with minimal knee flexion
Presence of an associated ACL tear
Little improvement in symptoms after three weeks of conservative treatment

○   **What conservative management elements are appropriate?**

A home or outpatient physical therapy program or simple rest with activity modification, ice, and nonsteroidal anti-inflammatory drugs (NSAIDs) is the nonoperative management of possible meniscus tears. The physical therapy program goals are to minimize the effusion, normalize gait, normalize pain-free range of motion, prevent muscular atrophy, maintain proprioception, and maintain cardiovascular fitness. Choosing this course of treatment must include consideration of the patient's age, activity level, duration of symptoms, type of meniscus tear, and associated injuries such as ligamentous pathology.

○   **How is the evaluation and management different in older adults?**

In older patients with degenerative tears an initiating injury may not be remembered. The patient usually complains of acute well localized joint line pain which may wake him from sleep. Examination usually reveals joint line tenderness and a small effusion, although this is not a constant feature. Plain radiographs may reveal mild degenerative change and arthrography or MRI will confirm the diagnosis. Symptoms often settle with conservative treatment but arthroscopic resection of the torn portion of the meniscus may be required.

○   **Compare the disadvantages of treatment options for meniscal tears**

Comparison of Treatment Options for Meniscal Tears

Treatment	Advantages	Disadvantages	Comments
Nonoperative	- Surgery and its risks are avoided - Small peripheral tears may heal on their own - Preferable in patients whose chief complaints are caused by arthritis, rather than a meniscal tear	- May not relieve all symptoms, especially catching and clicking - Potentially repairable tear may become irreparable	- Does not mean no therapy - Requires an exercise program and some physical therapy to prevent quadriceps weakness
Partial meniscectomy	- Often relieves symptoms very well - Rapid return to joint function - Yields poor results if articular cartilage is already damaged	Meniscal tissue is lost, creating some risk for degeneration	Only for patients who are sufficiently bothered by their tear, and for whom meniscal repair is not possible
Meniscal repair	- Provides reliable short-term relief from pain - Helps long-term preservation of joint	- Not all tears are repairable - The risk of complications is higher than for simple meniscectomy - Longer recovery than for meniscectomy	This surgery is not as simple as a meniscectomy and should be performed by a sports medicine specialist
Open meniscectomy	None	Excessive dissection, causing a slower functional recovery	Rare now, but physicians may see patients who had this surgery years ago; arthritis likely

○   **Summarize the postoperative rehabilitation s/p meniscectomy:**

PO week 1
Minimize joint effusion with ice, TENS, and electrical stimulation
Begin knee isometrics, SLR, ankle pumps, and ROM exercises
Ambulate weight bearing as tolerated with assistive device or splint.

Ensure all transfers and bed mobility are independent.
Train basic ADL.
PO Weeks 2 to 4
Minimize joint effusion.
Continue PO Week 1 program for patients with articular cartilage damage.
Progress other patients to: hamstring isometrics, terminal knee extension, hip isotonics, and light stationary bike riding. Emphasize quadriceps strengthening.
Continue ROM stretching and self stretching.
Massage arthroscopic portal sites to prevent adhesions,
Begin gait training without ambulation device for maneuverability.
Train independence in all basic ADL without ambulation device.
PO Weeks 4 to 8
Begin more quadriceps intensive exercise for patients with articular cartilage damage.
Progress other patients to resisted isotonics, isokinetics, and closed chain exercise.
Train balance and proprioception.
Progress stair climbing to step-overstep.
Begin low-level instrumental ADL.
Return to full knee ROM in 6 to 10 weeks.
Return to full function in 3 to 6 months

○   **What is the mechanism of MCL injuries?**

The medial collateral ligament is usually injured as a result of a valgus force, often associated with external rotation of the tibia. The classic example is a skiing injury where the ski moves laterally, causing a valgus external rotation force on the knee. In the acute phase the findings are of swelling and bruising over the course of the ligament with tenderness over the joint line or femoral insertion. Loss of full extension may be present in an incomplete tear due to pain as the ligament comes under tension in the last 20° of extension.

○   **What are the characteristics of medial collateral ligament injuries (MCL)?**

The annual incidence of acute knee injury in the US is estimated to be 300 cases per 100,000 population. Collateral ligament injuries account for 25% of patients presenting to emergency rooms with acute knee injury. Peak incidence of collateral ligament injuries occurs in adults aged 20-34 years. Age patterns are bimodal with highest incidence rates at the ages of 20-34 years and 55-65 years. MCL and LCL injuries can occur at any age.

○   **What concomitant injuries may occur in medial collateral ligament injuries?**

Medial collateral ligament injuries may be associated with meniscal tears or peripheral detachment of the medial meniscus. An associated ACL injury may also be present. If doubt exists about the possibility of coexisting capsular or ACL damage an examination under anesthetic and arthroscopy should be performed.

○   **What initial treatment is most often recommended?**

Conservative management consisting of rest, ice, compression, and elevation (RICE) is the mainstay of care for MCL injuries. Nonsteroidal anti-inflammatory drugs (NSAIDs) are prescribed for pain relief; however, their effect on ligament healing remains controversial. To protect the healing ligament, the knee is placed in a short, hinged knee brace that blocks 20° of terminal extension but allows full flexion. Modalities may be added to provide additional pain relief and to hasten healing; these may include ultrasound, phonophoresis, cold whirlpool, ice, and electrical stimulation.

○   **What weight bearing guidelines are recommended for MCL injury?**

Weight bearing is allowed as tolerated for grade 1 and 2 MCL tears. Pain abates after 3 to 5 days in grade 1 MCL injuries but may continue for up to 2 weeks in grade 2 MCL injuries. For grade 3 tears, initial non-weight-bearing is indicated and the patient advances to partial weight bearing by the second week after injury. By 4 weeks the patient should be fully weight bearing.

○   **What therapeutic exercise program is implemented initially?**

The day after injury the patient begins quadriceps isometric strengthening exercises, straight leg raises, and cocontraction exercises of the hamstrings and quadriceps with the knee flexed 20° and heel pressure directed toward the floor or bed. Closed kinetic chain exercises are implemented and include mini-squats, toe raises, leg presses, cycling, and activities with an exercise band. The bicycle seat is initially raised and gradually lowered as the patient's knee flexion improves. Once the patient achieves 90° knee flexion, passive resistance exercises for the quadriceps and hamstrings can be added.

O **What is an appropriate subsequent rehabilitation program?**

After 4 to 6 weeks of rehabilitation, patients who have grade 1 and 2 MCL injuries may no longer need the brace and may return to sports if they can perform various functional tests: one-legged hopping (both vertical and horizontal), running shuttles, skipping rope, trampoline jumping, using a balance board, and climbing stairs. Grade 3 MCL tears, however, may take as long as 8 to 12 weeks to heal enough to return to activity.

O **What are the characteristics of lateral collateral ligament injuries?**

The lateral collateral ligament is rarely injured in isolation but is usually torn in association with damage to the posterolateral ligament complex (lateral capsule, arcuate ligament and popliteus tendon). The cruciate ligaments may also be damaged. The mechanism of injury is usually a varus force on a flexed knee. The ligament usually ruptures at its fibular insertion or it may avulse the fibular styloid. Peroneal nerve palsy may be associated with a lateral collateral ligament tear and should be looked for at the time of the injury.

O **What is an appropriate rehabilitation treatment approach to an LCL injury?**

Rehabilitation for patients who have LCL tears is similar to the protocol described for MCL injuries: functional activities and closed kinetic chain exercises. Knee brace protection on return to play at approximately 8 weeks is recommended. Grade 3 LCL tears probably are best managed operatively because grade 3 LCL injuries inevitably involve the posterolateral corner of the knee (arcuate complex and popliteus).

O **What are the demographics of Anterior cruciate ligament (ACL) injury?**

Incidence of ACL injury in the United States is estimated to approach 1 case per 3000 individuals. Females are at higher risk of ACL injury when considering sports participation numbers. ACL injuries occur most commonly in individuals aged 14-29 years. Approximately 70% of ACL injuries occur through noncontact mechanisms. The largest proportion of these injuries occur during sports that involve deceleration, twisting, cutting, or jumping. ACL injury can occur as a result of excessive valgus stress, forced external rotation of the femur on a fixed tibia (with the knee in full extension), or forced hyperextension.

O **What are the symptoms of an ACL injury?**

The typical injury involves a noncontact deceleration, cutting movement, or hyperextension, often accompanied by a "pop," with the inability to continue sports participation. The symptoms of an ACL deficient knee are giving way, swelling and pain. The patient experiences symptoms with twisting or jumping maneuvers. The symptoms are due to rotational instability rather than loss of anteroposterior stability. Symptoms of locking may occur, but these are usually due to a coexisting meniscal tear rather than to the ACL rupture itself.

O **What are the clinical findings in an ACL injured knee?**

A hemarthrosis almost always is present because of the plentiful vascular supply to the ACL. There is limited range of motion (ROM), and joint line tenderness. During physical examination, the anterior drawer test is specific for anteromedial band rupture; the Lachman test and pivot shift test are preferential for a disrupted posterolateral band. All three tests are likely to be positive when the ACL is completely torn. A positive Lachman or anterior drawer test with a firm end-point suggests a partial (grade 2) ACL sprain, particularly when the pivot shift is negative.

O **What associated injuries may occur with ACL pathology?**

Associated injury is common. Meniscal tears occur in approximately 50% of cases, with a slightly higher incidence of lateral meniscal tears when compared to medial meniscal injury. Other pathology includes bone bruising in up to 70% of cases (mostly of the lateral femoral condyle), medial collateral ligament injury, and true fractures of the tibial plateaus or femoral condyles.

O   **What do radiographic studies reveal in ACL injuries?**

Radiographs should be taken to look for avulsion injuries of the tibial spines and other associated fractures. A small flake of bone may be seen to be avulsed from the lateral aspect of the tibial condyle just above the fibula. This is called a Segond fracture and if present indicates a 60–70% chance of an ACL injury. If there is doubt about the diagnosis an examination under anesthetic and arthroscopy should be performed.

O   **What treatments may be considered?**

Most cases can be treated conservatively and any subsequent functional instability treated later. In athletes with ACL and associated ligamentous and meniscal damage, acute surgery is indicated. Symptomatic chronic tears of the ACL in young patients, which have not responded to conservative measures, may be treated by intra-articular replacement of the ACL with autogenous tissue, such as patellar or semitendinosus tendon. In older patients extraarticular repair may control the instability.

O   **What consideration should be given to a conservative treatment approach in ACL injury?**

For an isolated ACL injury (a minority of acute weightbearing injuries characterized by hemarthrosis), conservative management with rehabilitation and bracing for six months should be considered, particularly if the athlete is willing to curtail his or her activity.

O   **What are the basic rehabilitation elements of ACL tears treated operatively?**

Although no definitive ACL protocol has been universally agreed on as the most effective, most current protocols stress the following principles:

Initiation of early ROM and weight bearing
Early edema control techniques
Avoidance of excessive stress to the graft (avoiding excessive early open-chain exercises)
Early hamstring strengthening to provide dynamic joint stability and to decrease strain on the graft
Proprioceptive retraining and neuromuscular reeducation
Muscle strengthening and conditioning
Incorporation of closed kinetic chain exercises
Sports-specific agility training
Aerobic cardiovascular training
A bracing algorithm
Criteria-based progression from one level to the next
Criteria-based return to athletic activity

O   **What are the demographics of posterior cruciate ligament injuries (PCL)?**

PCL injuries occur in athletes and multiple-trauma victims. Incidence data are limited. One study estimates that PCL injuries make up as many as 20% of all knee ligament injuries. Another study of all patients admitted to a regional trauma center with severe knee injuries (i.e., dislocations) found that 38% had PCL injuries; 56% of the PCL injuries were unrelated to sports, and 32.9% were sports-related.

O   **What are the mechanisms of PCL injuries?**

Regardless of whether the injury is due to a sports activity or a motor vehicle accident, the mechanism of injury remains fairly consistent: posterior force on the proximal tibia. In motor vehicle accidents this occurs as the proximal tibia strikes the dashboard. In sports, a PCL injury can occur when an athlete falls to the ground on a flexed knee with the foot plantar flexed, so that the proximal tibia strikes the ground first.

O   **What other associated pathology is encountered with PCL injury?**

Isolated PCL injuries do occur, but combined ligamentous injuries are more common. Associated injuries may involve the ACL, medial collateral ligament, lateral collateral ligament, or posterolateral complex. Meniscal and articular cartilage injuries are also commonly seen in association with both acute and chronic PCL injuries, with incidences of 27% and 49%, respectively.

○ **What are the symptoms and signs associated with PCL injury?**

The patient history typically consists of a fall with a blow to the anterior aspect of the proximal tibia. Unlike those with ACL injuries, patients who have PCL injuries usually do not have incapacitating pain, and they report vague symptoms such as unsteadiness or insecurity of the knee. The physical exam usually does not reveal findings typical of a severe ligamentous injury, and often only a mild hemarthrosis will be noted. Most patients with an isolated PCL injury will have nearly full range of motion. Abrasions or lacerations to the anterior proximal tibia should raise the physician's suspicion for a PCL injury.

○ **What is the accuracy of PCL injury selective testing?**

Rubinstein et al assessed the accuracy of PCL injury diagnoses. The posterior drawer was the most sensitive test (90%) and was highly specific (99%). While the quadriceps active test and reverse pivot shift both had high specificity (97% and 95% respectively), they both had low sensitivity (58% and 26% respectively). The authors found an overall clinical exam accuracy of 96%.

○ **What are the outcomes of untreated PCL injury?**

The long-term outcome of patients who have untreated PCL injuries is unclear. As many as 80% to 90% of patients with untreated PCL injuries report occasional pain on follow up. Two studies found that up to 43% of the patients considered walking a problem, and as many as 65% decreased their activity level after the injury.

○ **What conservative rehabilitation program is appropriate in PCL injury?**

Patients who have grade 1 or 2 PCL injuries (less than 1 cm of posterior translation) should first receive nonoperative treatment that includes aggressive quadriceps strengthening and full range of motion maintenance. Patients may return to sports when quadriceps and hamstring strength reaches 90% of the contralateral side. This may take as long as 4 to 6 weeks.

○ **What is a typical postoperative rehabilitation program for a PCL injury?**

The postoperative protocol includes the use of a knee brace in extension with weight bearing as tolerated for 4 weeks, as well as quadriceps strengthening exercises. Later, closed chain exercises are performed at 6 weeks, and proprioceptive training is performed at 12 weeks. Hamstring exercises are delayed for 4 months to decrease the posterior load on the tibia. Patients can begin light jogging at 6 months.

ANKLE/FOOT

○ **What is Achilles tendon rupture and tendinitis?**

Achilles tendon rupture is a complete disruption of the Achilles tendon, observed most commonly in patients aged 30-50 years, usually occurring at a point 4-5 cm proximal to the calcaneus. This area above the calcaneus is the zone of poor blood flow in the tendon. Achilles tendonitis is inflammation of the tendon or paratenon, usually resulting from overuse associated with a change in playing surface, footwear, or intensity of an activity.

○ **What is the pathogenesis of Achilles tendonitis?**

It is usually caused by repetitive trauma and microscopic tears due to excessive use of the calf muscles in ballet dancing, distance running, basketball, jumping and other athletic activities, or from faulty footwear with a rigid shoe counter. The tendon is also a common site for gouty tophi, rheumatoid nodules and xanthomas. Abnormalities of the tendon and peritendinous tissues can be demonstrated by sonography and MRI.

○   **What are the signs and symptoms of Achilles tendonitis?**

Tendinitis of the Achilles tendon is characterized by pain, swelling, tenderness and sometimes crepitus, over the tendon near its insertion. Passive dorsiflexion of the ankle intensifies the pain.

○   **What are the treatment options?**

As with all overuse injuries, the clinician must try to identify and correct the cause of the tendinitis to prevent its recurrence. Patients usually respond well to conservative treatment consisting of:

Oral nonsteroidal anti-inflammatory medication
Ultrasound
Massage
Muscle stretching: maintaining the medial arch during stretch
Strengthening exercises (including eccentric exercise)
Modification of walking surface
Orthotics
Alterations of footwear, such as a heel lift for Achilles tendinitis or a medial wedge for posterior tibialis tendinitis
Proprioceptive retraining on the small balance board

○   **What are other considerations in treatment?**

The Achilles tendon is vulnerable to rupture particularly in elderly individuals. Corticosteroid injections in or near the tendon are of questionable value. They predispose to tendon rupture and should, therefore, be discouraged. Surgical excision of the inflamed peritendinous tissue is rarely required.

○   **What is retrocalcaneal bursitis?**

This is associated with posterior heel pain made worse by passive dorsiflexion of the ankle. Bursal distension produces a tender swelling behind the ankle with bulging on both sides of the tendon. Known causes include rheumatoid arthritis (RA), psoriatic arthritis, ankylosing spondylitis, and Reiter's syndrome. It may also occur in association with Achilles tendinitis as a result of repetitive trauma due to athletic overactivity, particularly in runners. The diagnosis can be confirmed by radiography (showing obliteration of the retrocalcaneal recess), sonography, or MRI.

○   **What treatment is recommended?**

Rest, activity modification, moist heat application, a slight heel elevation using a felt heel pad, and NSAIDs constitute sufficient therapy for most patients. A walking cast and/or a cautious corticosteroid injection into the bursa are sometimes required. Surgical bursectomy and resection of the superior prominence of the calcaneal tuberosity are rarely indicated.

○   **What is retroachilleal or subcutaneous calcaneal bursitis?**

It produces a painful tender subcutaneous swelling overlying the Achilles tendon, usually at the level of the shoe counter. The overlying skin may be hyperkeratotic or reddened. It occurs predominantly in women, and is frequently caused and aggravated by improperly fitting shoes or pumps with a stiff, closely contoured heel counter. Management consists of rest, heat application, NSAIDs, padding, and relief from shoe pressure by wearing a soft, non-restrictive shoe without a counter. Local corticosteroid injections should be avoided. Surgical excision is rarely indicated.

○   **What circumstances may lead to rupture of the Achilles tendon?**

Rupture of the Achilles tendon typically occurs during a burst of unaccustomed physical activity involving forced ankle dorsiflexion. Achilles tendon rupture may result from a sharp blow, a fall or from athletic injuries. It also occurs in elderly patients with pre-existing Achilles tendinitis or retrocalcaneal bursitis, patients with systemic lupus erythematosus or RA receiving corticosteroids, in those on long-term hemodialysis, and following local corticosteroid injections in the vicinity of the tendon.

○ **What signs and symptoms are present?**

The onset is often sudden, with pain in the region of the tendon and difficulty walking or standing on the toes. Swelling, ecchymosis, tenderness and sometimes a palpable gap, are present at the site of the tear. In partial tendon rupture, active plantar flexion of the ankle may be preserved but painful. In those with complete rupture, squeezing the calf muscles with the patient sitting or kneeling on a chair produces little or no passive ankle plantar flexion (positive Thompson calf squeeze test).

○ **What imaging studies are appropriate if surgery is considered?**

The extent and orientation of the rupture can be accurately assessed by MRI or ultrasound.

○ **How do conservative and surgical care compare?**

The outcomes are similar.

○ **What post operative rehabilitation is recommended at 2 weeks?**

At 2 weeks the cast is removed, the wound is inspected, and the staples or sutures are removed. Another short leg cast with the foot in gravity equinus is worn for an additional 2 weeks.

○ **What post operative rehabilitation is recommended at 4 weeks?**

At 4 weeks the cast is changed, and the foot is gradually brought to the plantigrade position over the next 2 weeks. Walking is gradually resumed with partial weight-bearing on crutches during a 2-week period.

○ **What post operative rehabilitation is recommended at 6-8 weeks?**

At 6 to 8 weeks, a short leg walking cast is applied with the foot in the plantigrade position, and full weight-bearing is allowed. Alternatively, a removable brace allowing plantar flexion only may be used. Gentle active range-of-motion exercises for 20 minutes twice a day are begun. Isometric ankle exercises along with a knee and hip strengthening program can be instituted. Toe raises, progressive resistance exercises, and proprioceptive exercises, in combination with a general strengthening program, constitute the third stage of rehabilitation.

○ **What post operative rehabilitation is recommended at 12 weeks?**

At 12 weeks, a reverse-90-degree ankle stop brace or similar device is fitted (if not already in use) and is worn until a nearly full range of motion and strength 80% that of the opposite extremity have been obtained, usually within 6 months. In reliable, well-supervised patients with good tissue repair, this program can be accelerated, with earlier use of dorsiflexion stop orthoses and active range of motion exercises.

○ **What are the characteristics of posterior tibial tendinitis (PTT)?**

Posterior tibialis tendon dysfunction occurs commonly in women between 45 and 65 years old and is associated with pronation or flatfoot deformity and obesity. Predisposing factors to degenerative posterior tibial tendon insufficiency (tearing) include: diabetes mellitus, hypertension, obesity, trauma or surgery to the medial aspect of the ankle and steroid injections. In addition, other inflammatory conditions such as rheumatoid arthritis, seronegative arthropathy and infection may also lead to degeneration of the posterior tibial musculotendinous unit.

○ **What symptoms are characteristic of posterior tibial tendinitis?**

Symptoms begin with the insidious onset of pain and swelling along the medial aspect of the ankle, as well as a sense of fatigue in the foot and arch.

○ **What are the mechanisms of posterior tibial tendon injury?**

The posterior tibial tendon injuries appear to fall into 2 categories: traumatic and degenerative. A traumatic injury usually occurs suddenly, as with a blow to the medial side of the ankle or with a twisting injury that results in a complete or partial tear of the tendon. A chronic tear develops over a period of time and is usually related to a slowly developing degenerative tearing (or stretching) of the tendon.

O   **What are the findings on physical exam?**

The physical exam consists of examination of the ankle for areas of swelling, tenderness, and abnormal positioning of the foot, arch, and medial aspect of the ankle. In addition, attention is paid to the forefoot and to the position of the heel. Palpation of the posterior tibial tendon allows for localization of the pain to the tendon, for identification of localized swelling in and around the tendon, and for palpation of the tendon to determine if a gap in the tendon can be felt.

O   **What is the classic finding associated with PTT?**

One of the classic signs of posterior tibial tendon insufficiency is a "splaying" of the forefoot. This means that the medial aspect of the ankle rolls to the inside causing increased prominence of the medial malleolus. At the same time, as the arch drops, the forefoot moves to the outside (laterally). When this occurs, the abnormality is best seen by viewing the patient's feet while the patient is standing. When viewed from the backside, the affected foot will appear to turn to the outside and "too many toes will be seen".

O   **What are appropriate treatment interventions?**

Treatment is directed at achieving appropriate alignment of the hindfoot with custom-molded orthotics, supportive shoes, physical therapy, rest (sometimes using a short-leg walking cast or boot for 4 to 6 weeks), and nonsteroidal anti-inflammatory medications. Tendon sheath injection are helpful if antiinflammatory agents do not provide adequate relief. Surgical intervention ranges from synovectomy and tendon reconstruction to lateral column lengthening and arthrodeses.

O   **What are the demographics of ankle sprains?**

The number of incident cases have been estimated at 1 per 10,000 persons per day. Ankle sprains are the most commonly seen sports injury, comprising 14-21% of sports injuries. Athletes participating in basketball, volleyball, soccer, and football are especially at high risk for ankle sprains, comprising 25-45% of injuries in these sports. The lateral ankle complex (i.e., the anterior talofibular, calcaneofibular, posterior talofibular ligaments) is the site most commonly injured. Approximately 85% of such injuries are inversion sprains of the lateral ligaments, 5% are eversion sprains of the deltoid or medial ligament, and 10% are syndesmosis injuries.

O   **Which of the lateral ligaments is most frequently injured?**

The anterior talofibular ligament is most often injured.

O   **How are syndesmotic injuries differentiated?**

Injury probably results from an external rotational force. A squeeze test, consisting of compression of the fibula against the tibia at the mid-calf level, will elicit pain near the ankle when the syndesmosis has been injured. These injuries require more prolonged treatment, and they are more likely to result in recurrent ankle sprain and formation of heterotopic ossification.

O   **How do lateral ankle sprain symptoms present?**

A patient with an ankle sprain usually has a history of a twisting injury to the ankle. The patient often recalls stepping on another player's foot, landing wrong, or stepping in a hole. There is usually an immediate onset of pain and some degree of swelling. Weight bearing is painful and difficult. The patient often relates hearing a pop at the time of injury.

O **What role does the anterior drawer test play in assessing ankle stability after a sprain injury?**

An anterior drawer test can assess the stability of the ATFL. Cup the heel in one hand, pull it forward and stabilize the tibia with the other hand. Translation of more than 10 mm or a 3 mm difference between sides suggests ATFL disruption. Comparison of the affected side to the uninjured side is critical since the amount of laxity is highly variable between patients.

O **What role does the talar tilt test play in assessing ankle stability after a sprain injury?**

The talar tilt tests the ATFL and CFL. Invert the ankle and compare the laxity to the uninjured side. A complete rupture of the ATFL and CFL, as evidenced by both talar tilt of at least 20-30° opening and talar tilt of at least 10° greater than the uninjured side, is considered a third-degree ankle sprain.

O **What are the Ottawa ankle rules?**

The decision to obtain postinjury radiographs is based on the Ottawa ankle rules. These guidelines state that an ankle radiographic series (anteroposterior, oblique, and lateral views) should be obtained if bone tenderness is present over the lateral or medial malleolus, or if the patient is unable to bear weight for four steps both immediately postinjury and in the emergency department. Exclusions for use of the Ottawa ankle rules are age younger than 18 years, intoxication, multiple painful injuries, pregnancy, head injury, or diminished sensation due to neurologic deficit.

O **What pathology may be visualized on radiographic imaging of the sprained ankle?**

If radiographs are warranted, they should be examined for fractures of the medial, lateral or posterior malleoli, talar dome, lateral talar process, and anterior calcaneal process. Injuries to the distal syndesmotic ligaments and deltoid ligament will produce widening of the ankle mortise that is manifested by increased medial clear space and lateral talar subluxation.

O **What is the role of stress radiographic imaging in ankle sprains?**

Stress radiographs help document lateral ligamentous ankle injury but are not required to make the diagnosis of an acute ankle sprain. Talar tilt stress radiographs and anterior drawer stress radiographs are primarily used to document mechanical instability as a cause of chronic lateral ankle instability.

O **What is the West Point Ankle Sprain Grading System?**

West Point Ankle Sprain Grading System

Criterion	Grade 1	Grade 2	Grade 3
Location of tenderness	ATFL	ATFL, CFL	ATFL, CFL, PTFL
Edema, ecchymosis	Slight local	Moderate local	Significant diffuse
Weight-bearing ability	Full or partial	Difficult without crutches	Impossible without significant pain
Ligament damage	Stretched	Partial tear	Complete tear
Instability	None	None or slight	Definite

O **How are mild lateral ligament injuries managed?**

Management of type I sprain includes immediate application of cold with compression, elevation, and rest for the first 24 to 48 hours. In mild injury, when the edema subsides, adhesive strapping or elastic support should be applied and continued until symptoms subside. Prevention of further injury includes ankle strapping to limit inversion or eversion, use of elastic ankle supports, and shoes with rigid toe boxes and firm soles. Air or gel stirrup braces, laced supports with malleable metal stays, and lightweight plastic posterior leg splints have been advocated for some ankle problems. The foot should not be held in a plantar flexed position.

O **How does the rehabilitation program progress?**

Following recovery from injury, the athlete may progress from walking to jogging, and then to running in figure-eight's, with gradually tighter circles and broken patterns in order to test the stability of the ankle before competitive activity is resumed.

○   **What therapeutic exercises are appropriate?**

Initial exercises should include foot ankle circles with emphasis on movement toward the area of sprain to strengthen those muscles. Balance retraining and activities to improve kinesthetic awareness of the injured ankle may be necessary. The rehabilitation exercise program should be carried out over several weeks to provide protection against further injury. Incomplete rehabilitation can lead to the problem of recurrent lateral ligament sprain.

○   **What are the demographics of plantar fasciitis?**

Plantar fasciitis is one of the most common overuse injuries, affecting approximately 10% of runners, as well as numerous athletes in basketball, tennis, soccer, gymnastics, and other sports. Overall, it is estimated that more than 2 million Americans receive treatment each year for the condition.

○   **What are the extrinsic and intrinsic risk factors associated with plantar fasciitis?**

Extrinsic factors of plantar fasciitis include training errors, improper footwear, and unyielding surfaces. Intrinsic factors include pes cavus or pes planus, decreased plantar flexion strength, reduced flexibility of the plantar flexor muscles, excess pronation, and torsional malalignments.

○   **What is the pathogenesis of plantar fasciitis?**

It results from repetitive microtrauma causing tearing and stretching of the fibers of the plantar fascia at its narrow proximal calcaneal attachment. Pathologic findings include mucinoid degeneration, necrosis, and metaplasia consistent with a chronic degenerative and reparative inflammatory process and microtears at the fascia-bone junction.

○   **How does it present clinically?**

Pain on the under surface of the heel on weight bearing is the principal complaint. Often, the pain is worse when weight is borne after a period of rest (e.g., in the morning), and eases on walking. Localized tenderness, without swelling, is present over the anteromedial portion of the plantar surface of the calcaneus. Passive dorsiflexion of the toes often accentuates the discomfort.

○   **Who is at risk?**

Plantar fasciitis commonly occurs in obese middle-aged and elderly patients as a result of repetitive trauma from athletic activities, occupations that entail excessive standing and walking, changes in walking surfaces or from changes in shoe wear. It may also occur in young individuals as a result of sport injuries, for example striking the heel with some force, or as an enthesopathy in association with ankylosing spondylitis, Reiter's syndrome or psoriatic arthritis.

○   **What condition may coexist?**

Subcalcaneal (infracalcaneal) bursitis may coexist with plantar fasciitis and distinguishing the two is sometimes difficult. Bursal distention produces a cystic swelling over the plantar aspect of the calcaneus. Unlike plantar fasciitis, dorsiflexion of the MTP joints does not increase the discomfort. It usually occurs in older persons as a result of repetitive trauma from improperly fitting shoes, falls, pounding the heel with some force, prolonged walking, or from recent weight gain.

○   **What is a painful heel fat pad?**

A painful calcaneal fat pad is often confused with plantar fasciitis. The heel pad is normally composed of elastic fibrous tissue septa separating closely packed fat cells. Rupture of the septa in elderly obese patients, under the influence of ordinary weight bearing or suddenly due to a severe impact, results in attrition of the heel pad, poor stress absorption and increased bearing pressure on the calcaneus with reactive bony proliferation.

○   **How does it present clinically?**

Pain is experienced beneath the heel with weight bearing, particularly on standing. The posterior weightbearing portion of the calcaneal tuberosity is tender, in contrast to the more anterior tenderness of plantar fasciitis. Soft tissue radiographs may show decreased density and volume of the calcaneal fat pad, and increased cortical density of the calcaneal tuberosity.

○ What are heel spurs?

Bilateral plantar and calcaneal traction spurs are common in obese, middle-aged, and elderly individuals. They are frequently asymptomatic although heel pain may result from a coincidental plantar fasciitis, Achilles tendinitis or from a painful heel pad.

○ What treatment is considered for plantar fasciitis?

Treatment of plantar fasciitis includes rest, avoidance of running and jumping, stretching, and the use of anti-inflammatory medications. Adding a small heel raise and a soft heel pad can often be helpful. Taping and night splints in the acute phase may provide some symptomatic relief. Orthoses may also be necessary, especially if an athlete has an excessively pronated or cavus foot. If the above modalities do not relieve the symptoms, no more than two cortisone injections into the plantar fascia aponeurosis are of value in some patients. In refractory cases, operative fascial release may be indicated.

○ What therapeutic exercises may be considered for plantar fascitis?

Joint mobilization to the first MTP joint can be used to restore normal mobility to this joint. These modalities must be done in conjunction with an exercise program to strengthen the foot intrinsics, such as towel grasping. It is also imperative to gently stretch out the Achilles tendon. This must be done with the heel in contact with the floor and a small towel roll under the foot to maintain the arch.

○ What is tarsal coalition?

Tarsal coalition is a condition in which 2 or more bones in the midfoot or hindfoot are joined. The most common types of coalitions are those between the calcaneus and either the talus or the navicular bones. Patients with this congenital condition usually present during late childhood or adolescence, but presentations in adulthood have been reported.

○ What are the demographics of tarsal coalition?

The incidence of talocalcaneal coalitions in the general population is thought by most authors in the literature to be approximately 1%. Bilateral coalitions occur in approximately 50% of cases, and they are most often associated with calcaneonavicular coalition. Sex ratios vary, with a male-to-female ratio from 1:1 to 4:1. No statistical difference in racial distributions has been found.

○ How is tarsal coalition classified?

The classification of tarsal coalitions is based on the bones affected. The 2 most common types, calcaneonavicular and talocalcaneal, comprise the majority. Although calcaneocuboid, talonavicular, and cubonavicular tarsal fusions also occur, they are less common.

○ What is the clinical presentation?

Patients with tarsal coalition usually present during the second decade of life, presentations in adulthood have been documented. Complaints include mild pain deep in the subtalar joint and limitation of range of motion. Often, the symptoms are relieved by rest and aggravated by prolonged or heavy activity.

○ What are the distinctive findings on examination?

In cases of calcaneonavicular coalition, pain may be more superficial and originating from the area of the coalition in the sinus tarsi. Palpation may elicit pain at the calcaneonavicular junction laterally. In cases of talonavicular coalitions, the pain is usually more vague, but tenderness may be elicited with palpation of the middle facet region, just anterior to the medial malleolus.

O   **What therapeutic strategies are utilized in the management of tarsal coalition?**

Conservative approaches are generally suboptimal and arthodesis/ostetomy procedures yield superior results.

O   **What are the symptoms suggestive of sinus tarsi syndrome?**

Patients who have sinus tarsi syndrome typically present immediately after the injury with diffuse swelling and pain over the lateral ankle. They have difficulty bearing weight on the affected foot and usually require crutches. At this point the injury is indistinguishable from an acute ankle sprain and should be treated as such. As the swelling decreases over several weeks, patients exhibit less pain with ambulation but will continue to have pain and a feeling of hindfoot instability when they walk down steps or on uneven surfaces. Pain frequently disappears when the foot is at rest or when immobilized with a brace.

O   **What are the findings on physical examination?**

The physical examination will reveal exquisite tenderness over the sinus tarsi. The proximity of the anterior talofibular ligament to the sinus tarsi requires very specific palpation to identify the source of pain. Pain can also be reproduced by testing foot motion in extreme supination and adduction. Pain and instability can be reproduced by having the patient walk down steps or on an uneven surface.

O   **What imaging studies aid in the diagnosis?**

Patients with sinus tarsi syndrome typically have normal radiographs. Magnetic resonance imaging (MRI) is by far the most useful tool in assessing the tarsal canal. Pathologic changes that occur with sinus tarsi syndrome are easily visualized and inflammatory and fibrotic tissue infiltration can be seen by comparing T1and T2 weighted images.

O   **What treatment is beneficial in the management of sinus tarsi syndrome?**

Initial treatment is conservative. In many cases, symptoms can be completely relieved by repeated injections of local anesthetic and corticosteroid into the sinus tarsi. Treatment should also focus on correction of dysfunctional feet with orthoses and physical therapy. Physical therapy should address retraining of the peroneal and calf muscles and include a general strengthening and proprioception program with an exercise band and a tilt board.

O   **What is metatarsalgia?**

Metatarsalgia, or pain and tenderness in and about the metatarsal heads or MTP joints, may either be limited to a single joint or generalized across the ball of the foot.

O   **What are the clinical findings?**

Pain in the forefoot on standing and walking, and tenderness on palpation of the metatarsal heads and sometimes the MTP joints are the main clinical findings. Prominent, dropped central metatarsal heads, plantar calluses and clawed toes are frequently present. Metatarsalgia is a relatively common symptom of diverse causes.

O   **What is the etiology of this condition?**

The condition often follows years of disuse and weakness of the intrinsic muscles due to chronic foot strain from improper foot wear with the toes cramped into tight or pointed shoes. Other causes include attrition of plantar fat pad in elderly individuals, plantar callosities, altered foot biomechanics due to flat, splay, or cavus foot, hallux valgus, hallux rigidus, arthritis of the MTP joints, intermetatarsophalangeal bursitis, trauma, osteochondritis of the second metatarsal head (Freiberg's disease), stress fractures, sesamoiditis, previous forefoot surgery, tarsal tunnel syndrome, interdigital (Morton's) neuroma, hemiplegia, and arterial insufficiency including Buerger's disease

O   **What treatment approaches are considered?**

A properly fitted shoe with a broad toe box a metatarsal pad, or a metatarsal bar placed behind the metatarsal heads is helpful. Rocker soles can relieve and redistribute metatarsal pressure during the push-off phase of gait. Weight reduction is essential in obese patients Calluses can be softened with 20% salicylic acid and collodion; the application is removed after 2 or 3 days with warm soaking. Toe flexion and extension exercises may also be helpful.

○   **What foot orthoses or modified shoe wear are recommended?**

The use of an anterior heel, "earth shoe," running shoe, soft insoles such as Spenco or Plastizote, or comma-shaped inserts are additional methods for relieving weightbearing from the metatarsal region. An extended steel shank inserted between the out sole and mid sole of a shoe can minimize motion at the metatarsophalangeal joints of the first and second toe. Combining soft Plastizote, micropore rubber, cork, and a viscoelastic polymer at pressure points can be utilized.

○   **Where do metatarsal stress fractures most commonly occur?**

Metatarsal stress (or march) fractures, commonly affect the neck or shaft of the second metatarsal.

○   **What is the etiology?**

There is often a history of prolonged use of the foot, such as a strenuous marching in recruits, hiking or distance running (fatigue fractures). Fractures may also occur in patients with RA, osteoporosis, or other metabolic bone disease (insufficiency fractures).

○   **How does it present clinically?**

The patient complains of pain in the metatarsal area on weight bearing in the absence of a clear history of trauma. The dorsum of the foot is edematous, and tenderness is localized to the affected metatarsal.

○   **Can it be imaged radiographically?**

Stress fractures may not be visible on radiographs for 2-6 weeks, and bone scanning or CT are sometimes required for correct diagnosis.

○   **What treatment is recommended?**

Management consists of rest, a stiff-soled shoe, and avoidance of stress-provoking activities until healing occurs. Plantar padding and strapping of the foot, or cast immobilization may occasionally be required.

○   **What or other common sites for stress fracture in the athlete?**

The most common site involved is the junction of the lower third of the medial tibia, followed by the tarsal bones, metatarsals, femur and fibula. In adolescents gymnast's spondylolysis of the pars interarticularis in the lower lumbar vertebrae is notable.

CERVICAL SPINE

○   **What is neck (cervical spine) strain/sprain?**

Neck strain can be defined as nonradiating neck pain associated with a mechanical stress or a prolonged abnormal position of the cervical spine. It is a clinical condition describing a nonradiating discomfort or pain about the neck area associated with a concomitant loss of neck motion (stiffness). One of the most common causes of cervical strain/sprain is termed cervical acceleration-deceleration (CAD) injury. This is frequently called whiplash injury.

○   **What are the demographics of cervical spine strain/sprain?**

Dreyer and Boden showed that, in the general population, the 1-year prevalence rate for neck and shoulder pain is 16-18%. Almost 85% of neck pain results from acute or repetitive neck injuries or chronic stresses and strain. Chronic neck pain, regardless of its cause, is identified in 9.5% of men and 13.5% of women. The average age of patients with a whiplash injury is the late fourth decade.

○   **What is the etiology?**

Consistent with known biologic models, injury to bony, articular (disks and facets), nerve (including root and spinal cord), and soft tissues of the cervical spine (ligament, tendon, muscle) are the most likely sources of dysfunction and pain. Cervical strain is produced by an overload injury to the muscle-tendon unit because of excessive forces on the cervical spine. The cause is thought to be the elongation and tearing of muscles or ligaments. Secondary edema, hemorrhage, and inflammation may occur. The cervical facet capsular ligaments may be injured under whiplash-like loads of combined shear, bending, and compression forces; this mechanism provides a mechanical basis for injury caused by whiplash loading

○   **What injuries can occur as result of whiplash injury?**

Postmortem studies have shown that, after whiplash injuries, ligamentous injuries are extremely common, but disk herniation is a rare event. Strain or tears of the anterior annulus and the alar portions of the posterior longitudinal ligament (when stretched by a bulging disk) are possible causes for discogenic pain after whiplash injury. Injuries of the zygapophysial joint found in clinical and cadaveric studies include fracture, bleeding, rupture or tear of the joint capsule, fracture of the subchondral plate, contusion of the intra-articular meniscus, and fracture of the articular surface.

○   **What structures in the cervical spine are most likely to serve as primary source of nociception in CAD?**

According to Bogduk, the convergence of postmortem studies, biomechanical studies, and clinical studies converge to suggest lesions of the zygapophysial joints as those injured in cases of whiplash.

○   **What is the epidemiology of whiplash injury or cervical acceleration-deceleration (CAD) injury?**

The prevalence of whiplash injury has been measured prospectively. Of those individuals involved in a rear-end MVA, approximately 20% develop neck pain. In data collected by the Quebec Task Force on Whiplash-Associated Disorders, the incidence was 131 whiplash injuries per 100,000 vehicles per year. Barnsley et al estimate that the annual incidence of symptoms due to whiplash injury is 3.8 cases per 1000 population.

○   **How does neck strain/sprain symptoms present?**

Common traumatic events or factors that may lead to cervical strain/sprain injuries include motor vehicle accidents, lifting or pulling heavy objects, awkward sleeping positions, unusual upper-extremity work, and prolonged static positions. Pain is the most common presenting symptom, although the associated complaint of a headache is not unusual. The pain is usually located in the middle to lower part of the posterior aspect of the neck. The area of pain can be limited to a small local point (unilateral) or can cover a diffuse area (bilateral). The pain may not radiate into the arms but may radiate toward the shoulders. The pain associated with a neck sprain is most often a dull, aching pain that is exacerbated by neck motion. The pain is usually abated by rest or immobilization.

○   **Are headaches common after whiplash injury?**

Headaches are the second most common symptom associated with whiplash injury.

○   **Can there be visual symptoms?**

Other symptoms associated with whiplash injuries include visual disturbances manifested by accommodative problems and oculomotor dysfunction mediated through increased sympathetic tone.

○   **Can dizziness occur?**

Dizziness may occur secondary to damage to the vestibular apparatus, with perilymph fistulas causing disequilibrium.

○ **Can cognitive symptoms emerge?**

Cognitive functions, such as concentration, memory, and attention span are decreased in whiplash patients.

○ **Do psychological factors play a role in the symptoms?**

Psychological factors have been suggested as playing a role in the symptom complex and delaying resolution of whiplash injuries. However, recent studies have refuted this notion, demonstrating the lack of correlation between psychological stress and personality traits with the outcome of a whiplash injury. Psychological stress that whiplash patients experience is similar to that associated with chronic pain of any source. The primary reason for psychological dysfunction in association with whiplash injuries is the trauma itself.

○ **What findings occur on examination?**

Physical examination of patients with neck strain usually reveals nothing more than a locally tender area(s) just lateral to the spine. The intensity of pain is variable, and the loss of cervical motion correlates directly with the pain intensity. Muscles most commonly affected include the sternocleidomastoid and the trapezius. Active motion of the cervical spine against any type of resistance causes an increase in pain. Slow passive movement of the neck may allow for a greater arc of motion than determined during the active motion portion of the examination. Other than the preceding abnormalities, the remainder of the physical examination is normal. Specifically the neurologic examination as well as the shoulder examination is normal.

○ **What does radiographic evaluation reveal?**

Radiographic evaluation of patients with neck strain/sprain is normal. On occasion, muscle spasm may be great enough to cause some straightening of the normal lordosis of the cervical spine. This is a nonspecific finding and only indicates that there is significant muscle spasm secondary to pain. The presence of straightening of the cervical spine may be related as frequently to the positioning of the patient as to the presence of acute or chronic neck pain.

○ **What is the presentation of facet arthropathy in the cervical spine?**

Cervical facet pain typically presents as unilateral, dull, aching neck pain with occasional referral into the occiput or interscapular regions, depending on the cervical facet joint injured. Neurologic findings should be normal. Palpation often reveals regional soft tissue changes in response to the underlying injury. Palpation laterally along the facet joints will often reveal an area of focal tenderness and altered mechanics corresponding to the injured facet. Presently clinical suspicion of facet injuries is best confirmed by diagnostic intraarticular facet injections or blockade of the facet nerve supply, that is, medial branch blocks.

○ **What are the typical pain referral patterns for cervical facet arthropathy?**

The C2-C3 facet joint refers pain to the posterior upper cervical region and head, while the C3-C4 facet joint refers pain to the posterolateral cervical region without extension into the head or shoulder. The C4-C5 joint refers pain to the posterolateral middle and lower cervical region, and to the top of the shoulder. The C5-C6 joint refers pain to the posterolateral middle and primarily lower cervical spine and the top and lateral parts of the shoulder and caudally to the spine of the scapula. The C6-C7 joint refers pain to the top and lateral parts of the shoulder and extends caudally to the inferior border of the scapula.

○ **What conservative approaches are considered?**

Treatment of cervical facet joint injuries remains controversial. Intraarticular corticosteroid injections for the treatment of whiplash facet pain are ineffective. Typical conservative care of cervical facet joint injuries without dislocation includes nonsteroidal anti-inflammatory drugs, postural exercises and education, use of a cervical pillow, active and passive stretching, positional releases and manual therapy, specific strengthening, and short term judicious use of modalities to facilitate the above interventions.

○ **What is the role of medial branch blocks in diagnosing cervical facet arthropathy?**

Cervical medial branch blocks are technically easier to perform than intraarticular joint blocks and provide additional diagnostic confirmation of cervical facet arthropathy. The medial branch is located at the waist of the articular pillar and is more readily accessible than the joint, which can be narrowed by degenerative changes. Medial branch blocks also are less risky than joint blocks. The epidural space, intervertebral foramen, and vertebral artery may be entered when attempting a joint block; these structures are not as accessible when performing a medial branch block. However, there are reported adverse effects with medial branch blocks, and transient disequilibrium and presyncope have been noted.

O   **What is the role of radiofrequency neurotomy in cervical facet arthropathy?**

Radiofrequency neurotomy denervates the facet joint by coagulating the medial branch of the dorsal ramus, which denatures the proteins in the nerve. However, the nerve is not destroyed since the medial branch cell bodies in the DRG are not affected. In addition, the nerve may grow back to its target facet joint after 6–9 months depending on the radiofrequency lesion site.

O   **What is the efficacy of radiofrequency neurotomy in cervical facet arthropathy?**

The efficacy of radiofrequency neurotomy was demonstrated in a randomized double-blind trial by Lord et al. Long-term efficacy of radiofrequency neurotomy for chronic cervical pain was verified in patients with neck pain secondary to motor vehicle accidents in an investigation by McDonald et al.

O   **What is the natural course of WAD?**

It was concluded that between 14% and 42% of the patients with whiplash developed chronic complaints (lasting longer than six months), and that 10% of these had constant severe pain.

O   **What treatment approaches are utilized in the acute management of neck strain/sprain?**

The mainstay of treatment of neck strain includes controlled physical activity and brief immobilization in a soft cervical orthosis. The use of a contoured cervical pillow at night may be beneficial. Nonnarcotic analgesics in the form of nonsteroidal anti-inflammatory drugs are helpful in making patients comfortable. These drugs may be continued until the patient's symptoms have resolved. Muscle relaxants may be helpful in the patient who has palpable spasm on physical examination or has difficulty sleeping at night. Physical therapy modalities may take the form of cold (ice) initially or heat (warm bath) subsequently. Intermittent lightweight cervical traction may decrease pain and diminish spasm.

O   **Is there a role for injection therapy?**

Patients with localized pain and severe spasm limiting mobility may benefit from trigger point injection of anesthetic with or without the addition of corticosteroids. The injection relieves pain and blocks reflex spasm. These injections are indicated after 2 to 4 weeks of rest and medication without significant improvement. More recently the role of botulinum toxin injections for paracervical and periscapular myofascial pain syndrome has shown promising efficacy.

O   **What therapeutic exercises are appropriate?**

A course of isometric exercises should begin once the pain is controlled; A/AROM exercises may be initiated. The role of mobilization and manipulation is unclear in acute neck strain/sprain. Modification of the position of the patient while at work may help decrease neck pain.

O   **What is the prognosis?**

Most patients improve within 8-12 weeks. Whiplash injuries may require longer healing and are discussed under facet injuries. If significant pain persists past 4 to 8 weeks, flexion and extension radiographs may be useful to exclude late instability.

O   **What is the evidence supporting a multimodality approach in acute and subacute neck strain/sprain?**

Patients with neck pain as well as people with neck pain plus related headache that lasted at least one month, who received multimodal care that included exercises plus mobilization [movement imposed onto joints and muscles] or manipulation [adjustments] reported greater pain reduction, improved ability to perform everyday activities and an increase in their perceived effects of treatment than those who received no treatment.

O   **Summarize the critical reviews in the therapeutic approaches to the management of neck pain.**

A summary of the evidence on therapy for acute and chronic neck pain after whiplash, without comment on the quality of the studies involved and the magnitude of effect and its duration

Therapy	Acute neck pain	Chronic neck pain
Electromagnetic Therapy	Temporary benefit	No data
Traction	No added benefit	No data
Collars	=Traction and exercise	No data
Rest and analgesia	?=Natural history	No data
TENS or ultrasound	<Rest and analgesia	No data
Multimodal therapy	>TENS or ultrasound	No data
	>Rest and analgesia	No data
Mobilization	>Rest and analgesia	No data
Home exercise	>Rest and analgesia	No data
Tailored physiotherapy	>Rest and analgesia	No data
	=Home exercise	No data

TENS, transcutaneous electrical nerve stimulation.

A summary of the evidence on therapy for acute and chronic neck pain not caused by whiplash, without comment on the quality of the studies involved and the magnitude of effect and its duration.

Therapy	Acute neck pain	Chronic neck pain
Exercise	Effect uncertain	No data
Collars	?=Natural history	No data
TENS	?=Natural history	No data
Neck school	=No treatment	No data
Spray and stretch	=No benefit	No data
Laser	=Placebo	No data
Traction	=Analgesics	No data
Magnets	No data	=Placebo
Acupuncture	No data	=Sham TENS
Physiotherapy	No data	=Acupuncture
Electromagnetic therapy		=Moderate Analgesia
Manipulation	No data	=Drugs
		=Physiotherapy or GP
Mobilization	No data	>/= Salicylates

TENS, transcutaneous electrical nerve stimulation. GP, management by general practitioner.

O   **What is an HNP?**

A herniated disc can be defined as the protrusion of the nucleus pulposus through the fibers of the annulus fibrosus.

O   **How are the HNPs distributed in the cervical spine?**

Cervical intervertebral disc disease accounts for 36% of all spinal intervertebral disc disease, second only to lumbar disc disease, which accounts for 62% of all spinal intervertebral disc disease. Most acute disc herniations occur posterolaterally and in patients around the fourth decade of life when the nucleus is still gelatinous. The most common areas of disc herniation are C6-C7 and C5-C6. The C7 nerve root is affected in 37% to 75.6% of individuals reported in large studies with cervical radiculopathy. The same studies reported frequency of C6 radiculopathy of 15.8% to 48%. C7-TI and C3-C4 disc herniations are infrequent (less than 15%). Disc herniation of C2-C3 is rare.

O   **Succinctly summarize the association of cervical HNP to radiculopathy**

The cervical region accounts for 5-36% of all radiculopathies encountered. Incidence of cervical radiculopathies by nerve root level is as follows: C7 (70%), C6 (19-25%), C8 (4-10%), and C5 (2%).

O   **What are the demographics of cervical radiculopathy?**

Using a combination of clinical symptoms, physical signs, and radiographic, electrodiagnostic and surgical findings, a recent epidemiological study reported the average annual age adjusted incidence of cervical radiculopathy to be 93.2:1000,000. The age specific annual incidence per 100,000 population reached a peak of 202.9 for the age group 50-54 years.

O   **What are the distinctive features of the cervical HNP?**

Unlike the lumbar herniated disc, the cervical herniated disc may cause myelopathy in addition to radicular pain because of the spinal cord in the cervical region. The uncovertebral prominences play a role in the location of ruptured disc material. Pure nerve root compression occurs if extruded disc material enters into the nerve root canal. The uncovertebral joint tends to guide extruded disc material medially where cord compression may also occur.

O   **What patterns of neural impingement and disc herniation occur in the cervical spine?**

The disc herniation usually affects the nerve root numbered most caudally for the given disc level; for example, C3-C4 disc affects the fourth cervical nerve root, C4-C5 the fifth cervical nerve root, C5-C6 the sixth cervical nerve root, C6-C7 the seventh cervical nerve root, and C7-T1 the eighth cervical nerve root. Individual disc herniations do not involve other roots but more commonly present some evidence of upper motor neuron findings secondary to spinal cord compression.

O   **What patterns of symptoms may be observed?**

Not every herniated disc is symptomatic. The presence of symptoms depends on the spinal canal reserve capacity, the presence of inflammation, the size of the herniation, as well as the presence of concomitant disease such as osteophyte formation. In disc rupture, protrusion of nuclear material results in tension on annular fibers and compression of the dura or nerve root causing pain.

O   **What are the two categories of disc herniation?**

Cervical radiculopathies have been divided into two categories according to the hardness of the disc lesion. Individuals usually younger than 45 years of age have soft disc lesions associated with herniation of the nucleus pulposus, resulting in nerve root or cord compression. Hard disc lesions, produced by disc calcifications or osteophytes, occur in individuals older than 45 years of age. Soft disc lesions resolve more frequently than hard disc lesions. Hard discs are more closely associated with cord compression.

O   **What symptoms occur in cervical HNP?**

Clinically, the patient's major complaint is arm pain, not neck pain. The pain is often perceived as starting in the neck area and then radiating from this point down the shoulder, arm, and forearm, and usually into the hand. The onset of the radicular pain is often gradual, although there can be a sudden onset associated with a tearing or snapping sensation. As time passes, the magnitude of the arm pain clearly exceeds that of the neck or shoulder pain. The arm pain may also be variable in intensity, precluding any use of the arm without a range from severe pain to dull, cramping ache in the arm muscles. The pain is usually severe enough to awaken the patient at night.

O   **What other symptoms may occur in cervical HNP?**

Additionally, a patient may complain of associated headaches as well as muscle spasm, which can radiate from the cervical spine to below the scapulae. The pain may also radiate into the chest, mimicking angina (pseudoangina), or the breast. Symptoms including back pain, leg pain, leg weakness, gait disturbance, or incontinence suggest compression of the spinal cord. Paresthesias are poorly localized because a number of nerve roots may result in a similar pain distribution.

O   **What physical findings are evident on examination of the patient with a cervical HNP?**

Physical examination of the neck usually shows some limitation of motion, and on occasion the patient may tilt the head in a cocked robin position (torticollis) toward the side of the herniated cervical disc. Extension of the spine often exacerbates the pain as the intervertebral foramina are narrowed further (Spurling's sign). Axial compression, Valsalva's maneuver, and coughing may also exacerbate or recreate the pain pattern.

O   **What neurological deficits may present?**

A neurologic examination that shows abnormalities is the most helpful aspect of the diagnostic workup, although the examination may remain normal despite a chronic radicular pattern. Even when a deficit exists it may not be related temporarily to the present symptoms but to a prior attack at a different level. To be significant, the examination must show objective signs of reflex diminution, motor weakness, or atrophy. Manual muscle testing has greater specificity than reflex or sensory abnormalities. The presence of atrophy helps document the location of the lesion as well as its chronicity. The presence of subjective sensory changes is often difficult to interpret and requires a coherent and cooperative patient to be of clinical value. The presence of sensory changes alone is usually not enough to confirm the diagnosis.

O   **What are the features of C3 nerve root compression?**

When the third cervical nerve root is compressed, no reflex change or motor weakness can be identified. The pain radiates to the back of the neck and toward the mastoid process and pinna of the ear.

O   **What are the features of C4 nerve root compression?**

Involvement of the fourth cervical nerve root leads to no readily detectable reflex changes or motor weakness. The pain radiate, into the back of the neck and into the superior aspect of the scapula. Occasionally, the pain radiates into the anterior chest wall. The pain is often exacerbated by neck extension.

O   **What are the features of C5 nerve root compression?**

Compression of the fifth cervical nerve root is characterized by weakness of shoulder abduction usually above 90° and weakness of shoulder extension. The biceps reflexes are often depressed and the pain radiates from the side of the neck to the top of the shoulder. Decreased sensation is often noted in the lateral aspect of the deltoid, representing the autonomous innervation area of the axillary nerve.

O   **What are the features of C6 nerve root compression?**

Involvement of the sixth cervical nerve root produces biceps muscle weakness as well as a diminished brachioradialis reflex. The pain again radiates from the neck down the lateral arm and forearm into the radial side of hand (index finger, long finger, and thumb). Numbness occurs occasionally in the tip of the index finger, the autonomous area of the sixth cervical nerve root.

O   **What are the features of C7 nerve root compression?**

Compression of the seventh cervical nerve root produces reflex changes in the triceps jerk with associated loss of strength in the triceps muscles, which extend the elbow. The pain from this lesion radiates from the lateral neck down the middle of the area into the middle finger. Sensory changes occur often in the tip of the middle finger, the autonomous area for the seventh nerve. Patients should also be tested for scapular winging that may occur with C6 or C7 radiculopathy.

O   **What are the features associated with C8 nerve root compression?**

Involvement of the eighth cervical nerve root by a herniated C7-TI disc produces a significant weakness of the intrinsic musculature of the hand. This involvement can lead to a rapid atrophy of the interosseous muscles because of the small size of these muscles. Loss of the interossei leads to significant loss in fine hand motion. No reflexes are easily found, although the flexor carpi ulnaris reflex may be decreased. The radicular pain from the eighth cervical nerve root radiates into the ulnar border of the hand and the ring and little fingers. The tip of the little finger often demonstrates a diminished sensation.

O   **How does the accuracy of electrodiagnosis (EMG/NCS) compare to other diagnostic modalities?**

EMG findings become much more significant in the presence of historical and physical findings consistent with herniation of a disc. EMG and myelography correlate with the level of disc herniation in from 77% to 90% of cases studied. A recent study shows that EMG and MRI findings agree in the majority (60%) of patients with a clinical history compatible with cervical and lumbosacral radiculopathy.

O   **What is the role of EMG/NCS in the diagnosis of cervical radiculopathy?**

The primary use of EMG is to diagnose radiculopathy in cases of questionable neurologic origin. EMG/NCS provides a physiological measure for detecting axonal loss with good sensitivity and high specificity (at least 85%) and can provide information as to which anatomical lesions are truly physiologically significant. Of all the electrodiagnostic methods used to assess patients with suspected radiculopathy, the needle examination is by far the oldest and is still an important and useful procedure.

O   **What are the limitations of EMG/NCS?**

If cervical radiculopathy affects the sensory root only, EMG will be unable to demonstrate an abnormality. An incomplete examination occurs if the patient with acute symptoms is examined early (3 to 21 days from onset of symptoms). Another study should be repeated in 2 to 3 weeks if symptoms persist.

O   **What does a screening EMG/NCS consist of in cervical radiculopathy?**

In general, a screening exam for radiculopathy of at least one marker muscle of each myotome should be assessed. Sampling of appropriate paraspinal muscles may be useful unless there has been a prior laminectomy may be useful.

O   **What EMG findings are characteristic in sampling muscles involved in the cervical radiculopathy myotome?**

Membrane instability, positive sharp waves and fibrillation potentials
other signs of membrane instability and ectopic motor discharge including CRDs, fasciculations, etc.
Large MUAP amplitude
Increased polyphasicity
Decreased MUAP recruitment and interference pattern.

O   **What are radiographic findings in patients with cervical HNP?**

Plain radiographs may be entirely normal in a patient with an acute herniated cervical disc.

O   **What are the problems encountered using plain films in c spine disorders?**

Conversely, 70% of asymptomatic women and 95% of asymptomatic men between the ages of 60 and 65 years have evidence of degenerative disc disease on plain roentgenogram. Views to be obtained include anteroposterior, lateral, flexion, and extension. Oblique views are optional because they increase the cost and radiation exposure without supplying significant additional information. Plain roentgenograms may be used as an initial screening test for those individuals who have failed conservative therapy, who have sustained trauma to the cervical spine, or who are 60 years of age or older with new symptoms of neck pain.

O   **What additional imaging studies may be indicated?**

Additional radiographic studies are indicated for individuals with myelopathic signs, progressive neurologic deficit, treatment failure, and consideration for surgical intervention.

O **What is myelography of the cervical spine?**

Myelography identifies neural compression indirectly by the changes in the contour of structures outlined by water soluble contrast agents, such as iohexol and iopamidol. This invasive procedure requires the introduction of dye through a lateral cisternal puncture at C1-C2. Myelography is able to visualize the entire length of the cervical spine and identify unsuspected abnormalities. Myelography is useful for identifying the exact level of nerve root impingement.

O **What are the limitations of myelography?**

Diagnostic inaccuracies occur secondary to small central disc protrusions and bone spurs. Cervical myelograms have been shown to be abnormal in 21 % of asymptomatic individuals without neck or arm pain.

O **What is the role of CT scanning?**

Computerized tomography (CT) permits direct visualization of compression of neural structures and therefore is more precise than myelography.

O **What are the advantages?**

The advantages of CT over myelography include better visualization of lateral abnormalities such as foraminal stenosis and of abnormalities caudal to the myelographic block, less radiation exposure, and no hospitalization. From the surgical perspective CT is best at distinguishing soft disc compression from hard bony compression.

O **What are the disadvantages?**

Disadvantages of CT include length of time to complete the study and changes in spinal configuration between motion segments.

O **Can CT and myelography be combined?**

Myelographic dye may be injected and CT images obtained. The combination of the two studies gives excellent differentiation of bone and soft tissue lesions and allows direct demonstration of the spinal cord and the spinal canal dimensions. The CT myelogram is accurate in 96% of cervical lesions.

O **What is the role of MRI?**

Magnetic resonance (MR) imaging allows excellent visualization of soft tissues, including a herniated disc in the cervical spine. MR imaging is the radiographic technique of choice for the evaluation of cervical radiculopathy to confirm the presence of anatomic changes that explain clinical findings.

O **What are the limitations of MRI?**

Not all MR imaging disc abnormalities are symptomatic. Exploratory MR imaging has a significant opportunity to find anatomic abnormalities that have no correlation with clinical symptoms. HNP may be observed with MRI in 10% of asymptomatic individuals aged younger than 40 years and 5% of those older than 40 years. Degenerative disc disease (DDD) may be observed with MRI in 25% of asymptomatic individuals aged less than 40 years and 60% of those aged more than 40 years.

O **What is the initial treatment approach to cervical HNPs?**

The initial management of a herniated cervical disc initially is relative rest and brief immobilization in a soft cervical collar. Controlled physical activity should be maintained for at least 2 weeks. After the acute pain begins to abate, the patient should gradually increase activity and decrease the use of the orthosis. Most people are able to return to work in a month in a light duty capacity.

○ **What are the recommendations for drug therapy?**

Drug therapy is an important adjunct to controlled physical activity and immobilization. Anti-inflammatory medications, analgesics, and muscle relaxants have been used in the acute management of these patients. Oral systemic corticosteroids administered in a tapering dosage for 7 days may provide relief in more refractory cases but should not be used routinely. The muscle relaxants and the benzodiazepines have tranquilizing and central nervous system depressant properties. As such, they have at best a limited role in the management of the acute herniated disc patients.

○ **What consideration may be given to injection therapy?**

A trigger point injection may give dramatic relief of referred muscle pain. Epidural corticosteroid injections have shown to improve cervical radicular pain. Cervical epidural injections are most helpful for those individuals with radicular pain in contrast to those with axial pain.

○ **How is traction prescribed in cervical radiculopathy?**

Cervical traction is used to distract the interspace associated with disc herniation. Weights of up to 50 pounds are applied for periods of up to 60 seconds with the head flexed. Traction instruction is usually given by a physical therapist, and the traction may be applied by the patient at home. Traction is used up to 3 times a day for 15-minute sessions for 4 to 6 weeks.

○ **What exercises may be prescribed?**

Cervicothoracic stabilization exercise protocols incorporate the use of helpful rehabilitation principles- ergonomics, posture as well as both regional stretching, strengthening and generalized condition exercises of benefit to the patient. Alternatively, the McKenzie method of mechanical evaluation and treatment of the spine may be utilized. It involves identifying patterns of movements or positions that decrease symptoms and improve the segmental motion.

○ **What is the role of manual medicine techniques in cervical radiculopathy?**

Spinal manipulation and mobilization may restore normal ROM and decrease pain; however, no clear therapeutic mechanism of action is known. Studies document short-term improvement in the acutely injured patient and in those with cervical radiculopathy secondary to disc herniation. No evidence exists that manipulation confers long-term benefit, improves chronic conditions, or alters the natural course of the disorder.

○ **What is the role of epidural steroid injection therapy in cervical radiculopathy?**

Cervical epidural corticosteroid injections may be helpful in alleviating persistent radicular pain and avoiding the need for surgery in patients who have not responded to the above measures. Epidural injections are most effective in patients with radicular pain in whom the clinical examination correlates with findings noted on the imaging study. Symptom relief may last from days to weeks to months. If necessary, a repeat injection can be administered four weeks later and a third injection sometime in the following 6 to 12 months.

○ **Summarize the consensus guidelines for the management of acute and chronic neck pain.**

1. For acute neck pain:
   Simple analgesics or NSAIDs might be used to provide analgesia while patients undergo natural recovery, but in the knowledge that the efficacy of these agents may be no greater than that of a placebo;
   There is no evidence to justify the use of major tranquilizers or tricyclic antidepressants.
2. In the first 8 weeks after onset:
   Patients could be treated with rest and analgesia, but a more rapid resolution of pain might be achieved by the use of ice, and passive mobilization; although a home exercise program offers just as much chance of rapid resolution and a greater chance of being pain free at 2 years.
   Instruction to resume normal activities is as efficacious as other measures.
3. In the face of refuting data, and given the availability of a proven alternative: traction, electromagnetic therapy, collars, TENS, ultrasound, neck school, spray and stretch, laser therapy and traction are not justified.
4. For chronic neck pain:
   There is to date insufficient scientific evidence on which to judge the role of physical therapy;
   The use of analgesics might be justified on humanitarian grounds but not on the basis of evidence of efficacy;
   If NSAIDs are used, their efficacy should be determined and patients carefully monitored for side effects;
   Intraarticular injections of corticosteroids into the cervical zygapophyseal joints are not indicated;

Disc excision and fusion for neck pain without neurological signs might be entertained on the basis of uncontrolled clinical trials of this procedure, but this form of therapy is best reserved for the context of clinical trials approved by an ethics committee and designed to determine its efficacy and safety.
Radiofrequency neurotomy can be used to provide a complete relief of pain in patients rigorously diagnosed as suffering from cervical zygapophyseal joint pain.

O   **What problems may arise during the conservative treatment course?**

Despite appropriate conservative care, approximately a small percentage of patients presenting with acute cervical radiculopathy will continue to have significant and debilitating arm pain and possibly persistent neurologic deficits. These patients should be referred for surgical consultation after a minimum of 6 weeks to 3 months of conservative care. Patients without neurologic deficit or significant arm pain do not benefit from surgical intervention over the long run.

O   **What is cervical spondylosis?**

Cervical spondylosis describes a nonspecific degenerative process of the spine, which may result in varying degrees of stenosis of both the central spinal canal and root canals. Factors contributing to this narrowing include degenerate disc, osteophyte, and hypertrophy of lamina, articular facets, ligamentum flavum and posterior longitudinal ligament. Other relevant pathological processes include loss of the cervical lordosis and vertebral body subluxation. A congenitally narrow canal will precipitate the early development of symptoms.

O   **What is cervical myeloradiculopathy?**

When the secondary bony changes of cervical spondylosis encroach on the spinal cord, a pathologic process called myelopathy develops. When this involves both the spinal cord and nerve roots, it is called myeloradiculopathy.

O   **Which patient population is affected?**

Myelopathy is the most serious and difficult sequelae of cervical spondylosis to treat effectively. Less than 5% of patients with cervical spondylosis develop myelopathy, and they usually range from 40 to 60 years of age. However, cervical spondylotic myelopathy (CSM) is the most common cause of spinal cord dysfunction in individuals older than 55 years of age.

O   **What is the anatomical definition of stenosis?**

Cervical stenosis is associated with an anteroposterior (AP) diameter of less than 10 mm, while diameters of 10-13 mm are relatively stenotic in the upper cervical region. Space-occupying bodies such as the foreshortened and thickened ligamentum flavum and posterior longitudinal ligament, bulging of disc material, and loss of cervical lordosis add to the risk of static stenosis. Dynamic stenosis may occur secondary to segment instability causing compression of different portions of the spinal cord with flexion or extension.

O   **What is the typical pattern on spinal cord involvement?**

The pathologic course of cervical spondylotic myelopathy is characterized by early involvement of the corticospinal tracts and later destruction of anterior horn cells, demyelination of lateral and dorsolateral tracts, and relative preservation of anterior columns. Static and mechanical factors and ischemia are critical to the development of cervical spondylotic myelopathy. Free radical- and cation-mediated cell injury, glutamatergic toxicity, and apoptosis may be of relevance to the pathophysiology of cervical spondylotic myelopathy.

O   **How does it present?**

Cervical pain is uncommon. The typical presentation in the upper limbs is numb, clumsy hands with difficulties with buttons, coins, and fine manipulation. Patients will typically complain of tingling in the hands and feet. Weakness of the small muscles of the hands is commonly seen. Legs are often unsteady with a tendency to "jump" at night. Patients can have a surprisingly good exercise tolerance, and spastic weakness tends to occur in more advanced cases. Bladder disturbance is generally seen with more advanced disease. Sensory signs are less common than might be expected from the frequency of symptoms.

O   **What are the 5 syndromes of CSM?**

Five distinct syndromes exist that are characterized by degenerative radiographic and clinical signs of spinal cord compression: (1) lateral nerve root compression with radicular pain, weakness, or paresthesia; (2) myelopathy with long tract signs and symptoms; (3) myeloradiculopathy combined with both root and long tract signs and symptoms, which is the most common form; (4) spinal cord tissue vascular ischemia from anterior spinal artery compression with nonspecific motor and sensory deficits; and (5) anterior syndrome secondary to a posterior disc bulge during neck flexion impinging on the anterior horn of the cord with painless upper extremity weakness and normal lower extremities.

O   **What are the characteristics of upper extremity neurological findings?**

The upper extremity findings may start out unilaterally and include hyperreflexia, brisk Hoffmann's sign, and muscle atrophy (especially hand muscles).

O   **How does pyramidal tract pathology manifest?**

Pyramidal tract weakness and atrophy are more commonly seen in the lower extremities and are the most common abnormal physical signs. The usual clinical findings in the lower extremities are spasticity and weakness. Weakness and wasting of the upper extremities and hands along with fasciculations may also be the result of combined CSM syndrome including myelopathy and radiculopathy.

O   **How do sensory deficits manifest?**

Sensory deficits in spinothalamic (pain and temperature) and posterior column (vibration and proprioception) function should be documented. Alterations of sensation may include numbness, loss of temperature on the contralateral side, loss of proprioception, or decreased dermatomal sensation. Usually there is no gross impairment of sensation; rather, a patchy decrease in light touch and pinprick is seen.

O   **How are DTRs affected?**

Hyperreflexia, clonus, and positive Babinski's sign are seen in the lower extremities. Hoffmann's sign and hyperreflexia may be observed in the upper extremities.

O   **What radiographic features are detected?**

Roentgenographic evaluation may include anteroposterior, lateral, flexion-extension, atlanto-occipital, and oblique views. Roentgenograms of the cervical spine in these patients often reveal advanced degenerative disease, including spinal canal narrowing with prominent posterior osteophytosis, variable foraminal narrowing, disc space narrowing, facet joint arthrosis, and instability. These findings are usually more prominent in the lower cervical spine.

O   **What is the Pavlov ratio?**

The Pavlov ratio is determined by dividing the anteroposterior diameter of the canal by the anteroposterior diameter of the corresponding vertebral body. The ratio is usually 1.0.

O   **What does myelography reveal?**

Myelography is a diagnostic technique that introduces dye into the spinal canal to exhibit the presence of posterior or anterior defects compressing neural elements. Posterior defects are secondary to facet arthrosis and buckling of the ligamentum flavum. Anterior defects are secondary to changes in the posterior longitudinal ligaments and intervertebral discs.

○ **What is the role of MRI?**

MR imaging is the noninvasive examination of choice for the evaluation of CSM. The spinal cord is visualized in sagittal and axial planes. MR imaging is able to detect the extent of spinal cord compression and alterations of the spinal cord proper.

○ **What role does CT imaging play?**

CT is superior to MR imaging for the identification of osteophytes. CT/myelography is useful for distinguishing disc tissue from osteophytes.

○ **What conservative treatment options are there for the patient with CSM?**

Evaluating the efficacy of any particular treatment strategy for CSM is difficult because reports show that as many as 18 percent of patients with CSM will improve spontaneously, 40 percent will stabilize and approximately 40 percent will deteriorate if no treatment is given. Conservative therapy should be attempted in those individuals without severe neurologic compromise or those who are poor surgical risks. Conservative therapy includes immobilization with a firm cervicothoracic orthosis, if there is evidence of degenerative cervical spine instability; nonsteroidal anti-inflammatory drugs, muscle relaxants, epidural corticosteroid injections, and physical therapy to address weakness, limb muscle and truncal imbalances and gait disturbance.

○ **What is the rationale for surgical intervention?**

There are data from a single prospective randomized study indicating that patients with mild to moderate cervical spondylotic myelopathy do not benefit more from surgery than from conservative measures. Whether patients with more severe forms of cervical spondylotic myelopathy would benefit from surgery remains an unanswered question. The longer the duration of preoperative symptoms and the worse the severity of these preoperative symptoms, the less the benefit from surgery. The goal of surgery in the myelopathic patient is to decompress the spinal canal to prevent further spinal cord compression and vascular compromise.

○ **What are the surgical options?**

Literature review regarding spondylotic myelopathy does not clearly demonstrate the superiority of either the anterior or posterior approach. No randomized prospective clinical trials have been performed. Options include (1) single or multiple level ACDFs, (2) single or multiple level anterior corpectomy with fusion, (3) laminectomy with or without fusion, and (4) laminoplasty. Choice of the approach is based on the location of pathology, risks and benefits of each procedure, and geometry of the spinal canal.

○ **What complication can occur in patients with congenital stenosis?**

Patients with congenital narrowing of the spinal canal are at risk of developing transient neuropraxia in the absence of spondylosis. These patients may develop transient quadriplegia with hyperflexion or hyperextension of the neck. These people are usually athletes who undergo direct pressure on the head. These patients should be evaluated for the presence of spinal stenosis, which would preclude participation in contact sports.

○ **What is the Klippel-Feil syndrome (KFS)?**

The term Klippel-Feil syndrome is used to identify all patients with congenital fusion of the cervical vertebrae that involve two segments, block vertebrae, or the entire cervical spine.

○ **How does this syndrome present?**

The condition is detected throughout life, often as an incidental finding. Patients with upper cervical spine involvement tend to present at an earlier age than those whose involvement is lower in the cervical spine. Most patients present with a short neck, decreased cervical ROM, and a low hairline, which occurs in 40-50% of patients. Decreased ROM is the most frequent clinical finding. Rotational loss usually is more pronounced than is the loss of flexion and extension.

○   **What is the likelihood of neurological manifestations in KFS?**

Neurological problems may develop in 20% of patients. Occipitocervical abnormalities were the most common cause of neurological problems. Hearing loss is common with Klippel-Feil syndrome. The hearing loss can be sensorineural, conductive (one third of cases), or mixed.

○   **What is the likelihood of torticollis in KFS?**

Torticollis and facial asymmetry occur in 21-50% of patients with Klippel-Feil syndrome.

○   **What is Torticollis?**

Torticollis is the common term for various conditions of head and neck dystonia, which display specific variations in head movements characterized by the direction of movement.

○   **How often is cervical dystonia posttraumatic?**

Posttraumatic cases account for 10-20% of cases; the others are idiopathic.

○   **What is the age and gender distribution?**

Onset of idiopathic cervical dystonia typically occurs when patients are aged 30-50 years. Onset of posttraumatic cervical dystonia is within days of injury for the acute form and 3-12 months after injury for the delayed form.

○   **What are the characteristics of posttraumatic cervical dystonia?**

Posttraumatic cervical dystonia is divided into 2 subtypes, acute onset (initiated immediately to a few days after head and neck trauma) and delayed onset (3-12 mo after head and neck trauma).

○   **What are the characteristics of the acute type?**

Characteristics of acute posttraumatic cervical dystonia include local pain immediately following trauma such as concussion or whiplash injury, followed within days by a marked limitation in range of motion of the neck and an abnormal posture of the head without phasic components, elevation of the shoulder, and eventual hypertrophy of the trapezius. Two characteristics distinguish acute posttraumatic from idiopathic and delayed posttraumatic cervical dystonia: (1) no increase in symptoms with effort and (2) no inhibitory response to sensory tricks.

○   **What are the characteristics of the delayed type?**

Delayed-onset posttraumatic cervical dystonia is nearly identical to idiopathic cervical dystonia and includes activation by effort and the ability to minimize symptoms by the use of sensory tricks.

○   **What therapies are available for patients with cervical dystonia?**

Therapy of cervical dystonia includes local trigger point injections (lidocaine and corticosteroids), cooling spray and stretching, range-of-motion exercises, or drug therapy (benztropine, amantadine, and selective dopamine antagonists). Botulinum toxin injection is often selected option particularly if drug therapy is not tolerated or efficacious. Surgical denervation is indicated in patients resistant to all medical therapy. In patients with cervical dystonia who respond to botulinum toxin therapy, selective peripheral denervation of the posterior branches of the cervical roots may be helpful.

○   **What is the role of botulinum toxin in the management of cervical dystonia?**

Identifying the specific muscles involved in cervical dystonia prior to the injection is important. The sternocleidomastoid, trapezius, splenius capitis, and levator scapulae muscles are injected most commonly. An EMG study of 100 patients found that 2 or 3 muscles commonly are abnormal. Eighty-nine percent of patients with rotating torticollis had involvement of the ipsilateral splenius capitis and contralateral sternocleidomastoid with or without the additional involvement of the contralateral splenius capitis. Patients with lateral torticollis had ipsilateral sternocleidomastoid, splenius capitis, and trapezius involvement, while retrocollis was produced by bilateral splenius capitis activity.

O   **What is the therapeutic time window for botulinum toxin injection therapy?**

Beneficial effect from toxin injection usually is apparent in 7-10 days. Maximum response from the toxin is reached in approximately 4-6 weeks and lasts for an average of 12 weeks. Injections usually are repeated every 3-4 months.

O   **What is the most common side effect?**

Dysphagia

LUMBAR SPINE

O   **What are the demographics of lumbar spine sprain/strain*?**

Surveys suggest that the lifetime incidence of LBP ranges from 60-90% with a 5% annual incidence. For persons younger than 45 years, mechanical LBP represents the most common cause of disability, and it is the third most common cause of disability in persons aged older than 45 years. Of all cases of mechanical LBP, 70% are due to lumbar strain or sprain, 10% of cases are due to age-related degenerative changes in discs and facets, 4% of cases are due to herniated discs, 4% are due to osteoporotic compression fractures, and 3% are due to spinal stenosis. All other causes account for less than 1% of cases. *
Alternatively designated as mechanical low back pain in some nomenclature systems and clinical publications.

O   **What are other significant demographic factors associated with lumbar spine sprain/strain?**

The people most affected tend to be those in their fourth, fifth, and sixth decades. It has essentially the same rates in women as in men. It is not clear whether low back pain is more prevalent in certain races. In the United States, there are demographic differences in rates of low back pain. Rural areas tend to have higher rates than urban areas, and the South, the West, and the Midwest have higher rates than the Northeast.

O   **What is the etiology?**

The etiology of lumbar spine sprain/strain is not always clear but may be related to ligamentous, arthrogenic or muscular strain secondary to either a specific traumatic episode or continuous mechanical stress. Low back pain that is associated with lumbar spine sprain/strain may be related to anatomic structures that are tonically contracted in the resting position. Low back pain may also occur during motion if the stress is greater than the supporting structures can sustain or if the components of the lumbosacral spine are structurally abnormal.

O   **What are examples of specialized provocative tests for the LS spine/pelvis?**

Clinical Test	Affected System	Indication
Gaenslen's sign	MSK	Sacroiliac joint disease
Schober Test	MSK	Estimate lumbar flexion
Straight leg raise	NS	Spinal nerve root disorders
Lasègue test	NS	Spinal nerve root disorders
Femoral nerve stretch	NS	Spinal nerve root disorders
Crossed straight leg raise	NS	Spinal nerve root disorders
Valsalva maneuver	NS	Spinal nerve root disorders

O   **Provide a plausible pathophysiologic model to describe the pathogenesis of mechanical low back pain (LBP)**

The concept of a biomechanical degenerative spiral has an appealing quality and is gaining wider acceptance. This concept postulates the breakdown of the annular fibers and allows PLA2 and glutamate, cytokines, interleukins, alpha TNF, to leak into the epidural space and diffuse to the DRG. The weakened vertebra and disc segment become more susceptible to vibration and physical overload resulting in the compression of the dorsal root ganglion stimulating release of Substance P. Substance P, in turn, stimulates histamine and leukotriene release, leading to an altering of nerve impulse transmission. The neurons become sensitized further to mechanical stimulation, possibly causing ischemia, which attracts polymorphonuclear cells and monocytes to areas that facilitate further disc degeneration and produce more pain.

❍   To what degree do skeletal muscle groups acting on the spine contribute to mechanical LBP?

Recent studies have demonstrated significant abnormalities in paraspinal muscle function. Dynamometry and postural endurance testing has demonstrated paraspinal weakness and excess fatigability in patients with low back pain. Muscle wasting and weakness can arise rapidly because of reduced motor unit recruitment owing to fear of pain or reflex inhibition. Muscle imbalance predisposes to mechanical disruption that perpetuates mechanical disadvantage. The endurance of back muscles related to a task is a more useful predictor of incidence of back pain than is the absolute strength of these muscles.

❍   Can deconditioning of the paraspinal muscles contribute to mechanical LBP?

Radiographic evaluation of cross-sectional views of patients with back pain demonstrate decreased muscle mass in paraspinous and psoas muscles. Decreased muscle mass results in decreased muscle power that puts individuals at risk for persistent muscle injury.

❍   How do patients with mechanical LBP present?

Patients with muscle strain have back pain as their main complaint. The pain can be limited to a small local area or can cover a diffuse area of the lumbosacral spine but does not radiate to the lower extremities. At times, there may be a referral of pain to the buttocks or posterior thigh. Such referral of pain does not necessarily connote any mechanical compression of the neural elements and should not be called sciatica.

❍   How does injury relate to the onset of symptoms in mechanical LBP?

The patient may experience pain simultaneously with an injury. Subsequently, the pain increases in intensity and grows larger in its distribution after a few hours. The change in pain is associated with increasing edema in the injured structure along with the reflex contraction of surrounding muscles that limit motion. The patient may be able to continue to be active for a few hours. However, marked pain and stiffness occur the next day after sleeping. Flexion or extension of the spine may cause pain. Pain occurs with the motion that contracts the injured muscle. Certain motions may be painless, while others cause incapacitating pain. In general, muscle strain will be increased with activity and relieved with rest.

❍   What exam findings may be encountered if the injury is mostly muscular?

On physical examination, any active motion of the involved muscle against resistance will cause pain. If a patient stands and is asked to bend laterally against resistance, resulting in muscle contraction without motion, he will complain of discomfort in the damaged muscle. The damaged muscle is tender on palpation. Passive stretching of the muscle will also cause pain.

❍   If the injury is ligamentous how does this present on exam?

Patients with ligamentous sprains (disruption of the attachment of ligaments to bone) also develop localized back pain. Patients with supraspinous ligament sprains do not develop pain with active or passive extension but experience pain when the damaged ligament and its attachment to bone are stressed with flexion. Diagnosis of other ligamentous sprains is more difficult, since these structures are deep inside the back. Passive movements that put stress on the involved ligament will cause back pain, but identifying the specific location of injury is difficult.

❍   What is the multifidus triangle?

Not infrequently, patients with muscle or ligamentous strain will develop pain in the low back in an area lateral to the fourth and fifth lumbar vertebrae and medial to the posterior iliac crest. This area of pain also spreads down so the sacrum. This area, referred to as the multifidus triangle, contains a number of tissues, including facet joints, transversus ligament, quadratus lumborum and multifidus muscle, iliolumbar ligament, and dorsolumbar fascia, which may be sources of low back pain. The greatest portion of stress placed upon the lumbosacral spine is concentrated in this area, making it a common location for tissue injury.

O **What congenital abnormalities may appear on LS spine radiographs?**

The most common congenital abnormality is spina bifida occulta, which is found most frequently at the first sacral vertebra. Another abnormality is sacralization or incorporation of the transverse process of the fifth lumbar vertebra into the sacrum. A sixth lumbar vertebra in addition to the normal number of five also is occasionally seen with lumbarization of the spine. Most congenital abnormalities are asymptomatic.

O **What treatment strategies are appropriate for acute mechanical LBP?**

The therapy of lumbar spine sprain/strain includes controlled physical activity, nonsteroidal anti-inflammatory drugs, muscle relaxants, and physical therapy. Lumbar spine sprain/strain is generally improved with controlled activity.

O **What role does bed rest play in therapy?**

A period as short as 2 days has been shown to be effective at relieving back pain. Continuing bed rest to 7 days did not appreciably decrease pain or hasten return to work. Convincing the patient to limit activities is a primary goal of therapy. Controlled physical activity allows the injured tissues to rest, permitting a greater opportunity for healing without re injury. Bed rest is kept to a minimum.

O **Is there evidence to support the role of increased activity in acute mechanical LBP?***

Increasing evidence supports the use of active exercise relatively early in the course of lumbar spine sprain/strain to maximize function. As soon as the very acute pain is diminished, patients should be encouraged to increase physical activity. A physical therapist may be used if the patients require encouragement to remain mobile.* *Note that in the most recent Cochrane systematic database review this consensus opinion has come into question.*

O **What pharmacotherapy is appropriate?**

Nonnarcotic analgesics in the form of nonsteroidal, antiinflammatory drugs, tramadol and mild opioids are helpful in making patients comfortable while their injury heals. Nonsteroidal drugs with a rapid onset of action are most helpful in patients with acute pain. These drugs may be continued until the patients' symptoms have resolved. Muscle relaxants may be helpful in the patient who has palpable spasms on physical examination or has difficulty sleeping at night because of muscle pain. The combination of nonsteroidal, anti-inflammatory drug with a muscle relaxant is better than a nonsteroidal alone in improving pain relief in low back pain patients with muscle spasm on physical examination.

O **What is the role of injection therapy?**

Patients with very localized pain and severe spasm limiting mobility may benefit from a soft tissue (trigger point) injection of local anesthetic with or without the addition of corticosteroid preparation. The injection relieves pain and blocks reflex spasm. These injections should be given to compliant patients who will limit their activity during the natural course of healing. Increased activity may cause additional damage to musculoligamentous structures, which may not be recognized by the patient in whom the protective mechanism of pain has been blocked by injection.

O **What role is there for orthoses?**

Braces are reserved for patients who must remain active while healing continues. Braces may be recommended for subacute or chronic low back pain. Rigid LSOs are not well tolerated. Semirigid and nonrigid LSOs are better tolerated, but, their efficacy is ambiguous.

O **Summarize the efficacy data for therapeutic interventions in mechanical LBP from systematic reviews**

Results from Systematic Reviews

Intervention	Reviews	Trials	Patients	Summary of Reviewers Conclusions
Drugs				
Analgesics	1	1	29	Negative
Antidepressants	6	10	408	Conflicting
Injections(epidural, facet)	4	15	898	Conflicting
Muscle relaxants	1	1	50	Positive
NSAIDs	2	9	1126	Conflicting
Opioids	1	2	38	Positive
Education/behavior				
Back schools	7	17	2575	Conflicting
Bed rest	1	2	203	Uncertain
EMG biofeedback	1	5	176	Negative
Cognitive/behavior	3	15	999	Conflicting
Couple therapy	1	1	56	Negative
Multidisciplinary teams	3	8	561	Positive
Physical treatments				
Acupuncture	6	20	645	Conflicting
Exercises	6	21	1980	Conflicting
Laser	2	1	20	Negative
Orthoses	3	5	806	Conflicting
Spinal manipulation	9*	27	3050	Conflicting
TENS	4	8	397	Conflicting
Traction	3	16	108	Conflicting

O   **What is the prognosis for acute mechanical LBP?**

The prognosis is good for recovery from mechanical LBP. At one month, 35% of patients can be expected to recover; at 3 months, 85% have recovered; and at 6 months, 95% have recovered.

O   **What is the risk of recurrence?**

Recurrence at one year is 62%, and at 2 years 80% of patients have had one or more recurrences.

O   **What therapeutic options are considered for subacute LBP?**

Regaining flexibility in tight structures are key adjunct treatments to flexion, extension, and lumbar stabilization exercising. Resisted strength training as well as aerobic conditioning have all been effective in reducing pain and improving function. Modalities, such as moist heat and ultrasound, are commonly used in the treatment of LBP. In addition, flexion, extension, and lumbar stabilization exercises can be performed in the therapeutic pool. Exercise and physical agents cannot always correct a mechanical problem in the back. Manual therapy consisting of joint mobilization, muscle energy, massage, strain-counterstrain, and MFR can be used safely on elderly patients by skilled clinicians

O   **What does the return to work curve reveal about mechanical LBP?**

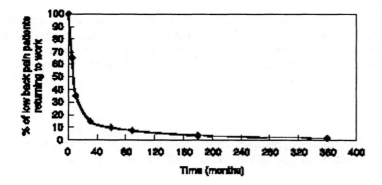

O   **What are the risk factors for chronicity?**

Risk factors for occurrence and chronicity.		
	Occurrence	Chronicity
Individual factors	Age	Obesity
	Physical fitness	Low educational level
	Strength of back	High levels of pain and disability
	and abdominal muscles	
	Smoking	
Psychosocial factors	Stress	Distress
	Anxiety	Depressive mood
	Mood/emotions	Somatization
	Cognitive functioning	
	Pain behaviour	
Occupational factors	Manual handling of materials	Job dissatisfaction
	Bending and twisting	Unavailability of light duty on
	Whole-body vibration	return to work
	Job dissatisfaction	Job requirement of lifting for 3/4
	Monotonous tasks	of the day
	Work relations/	
	social support	
	Control	

O **Compare and summarize consensus guidelines for therapy of acute and chronic mechanical LBP**

Evidence of treatments for acute and chronic low back pain.		
	Acute low back pain	Chronic low back pain
Beneficial	Advice to stay active	Exercise therapy
	NSAIDs	Behavioural therapy
	Muscle relaxants	Multidisciplinary treatment
		programmes
Likely to be beneficial	Analgesics	Analgesics
	Spinal manipulation	Back schools in occupational
		settings
		Massage
		NSAIDs
Unknown effectiveness	Acupuncture	Acupuncture
	Back schools	Anti-depressants
	Epidural steroid injections	Epidural steroid injections
	Lumbar supports	Lumbar supports
	Massage	Muscle relaxants
	TENS	Spinal manipulation
	Traction	TENS
	Trigger point injections	Trigger point injections
	Thermal therapy	Thermal therapy
	Ultrasound	Ultrasound
Unlikely to be beneficial	Specific exercises	Bed rest
		EMG biofeedback
Ineffective or harmful	Bed rest	Facet joint injections
		Traction

NSAIDs, non-steroidal anti-inflammatory drugs; TENS, transcutaneous electrical nerve stimulation; EMG, electromyogram.

O **What are the epidemiological characteristic features of acute lumbar HNP?**

Lumbosacral radiculopathy occurs in 2% of the population. Of these cases, 10-25% develop symptoms that persist for more than 6 weeks. Most disc ruptures occur during the third and fourth decade of life while the nucleus pulposus is still gelatinous. The time of the day a herniation occurs may relate to diurnal alterations in spinal anatomy. The most likely time of the day associated with increased forces on the disc is in the morning.

O **What anatomical levels are most likely to be involved?**

The perforations usually arise through a defect just lateral to the posterior midline where the posterior longitudinal ligament is weakest. The two most common levels for disc herniation are L4-5 and L5-S1, accounting for 98% of lesions; pathology at the L2-3 and L3-4 can occur but is relatively uncommon. Overall, 90% of disc herniations are at the L4-L5 and L5-S1 levels. Less than 10% of herniations occur at higher lumbar levels.

O   **What pattern of neural compression occurs with lumbar HNPs?**

Disc herniations at L5-S1 will usually compromise the first sacral nerve root; a lesion at the L4-5 level will most often compress the fifth lumbar root, while a herniation at L3-4 more frequently involves the fourth lumbar root.

O   **What are the presenting symptoms?**

Clinically, the patients' major complaint is a sharp, lancinating pain. In many cases, there may be a prior history of intermittent episodes of localized low back pain. The pain not only is present in the back but also radiates down the leg in the anatomic distribution of the affected nerve root. It will usually be described as deep and sharp, progressing from above downward in the involved leg. Its onset may be insidious or sudden and associated with a tearing or snapping sensation in the spine. Occasionally when sciatica develops the back pain may resolve since once the annulus has ruptured, it may no longer be under tension.

O   **What other symptoms occur?**

Finally, the sciatica may vary in intensity; it may be so severe that patients will be unable to ambulate and they will feel that their back is "locked." On the other hand, the pain may be limited to a dull ache, which increases in intensity with ambulation. Pain is worsened in the flexed position and relieved in extension of the lumbar spine. Characteristically, patients with herniated discs have increased pain with sitting, driving, walking, coughing, sneezing, or straining.

O   **What findings may be encountered on physical exam?**

The physical examination will demonstrate a decrease in the range of motion of the lumbosacral spine, and patients may list to one side as they try to bend forward. On ambulation, patients walk with an antalgic gait, holding the involved leg flexed so as to put as little weight as possible on the extremity.

O   **What exam findings occur in an S1 lesion?**

When the first sacral root is compressed, the patient may have triceps surae weakness and be unable to repeatedly rise up on the toes of that foot. Atrophy of the calf may be apparent, and the ankle (Achilles) reflex is often diminished or absent. Sensory loss, if present, is usually confined to the posterior aspect of the calf and lateral side of the foot.

O   **What exam findings occur in an L5 lesion?**

Involvement of the fifth lumbar nerve root can lead to weakness in extension of the great toe, and in a few cases to weakness of the evertors and dorsiflexors of the foot. A sensory deficit can appear over the anterior leg and the dorsomedial aspect of the foot down to the great toe. There are usually no primary reflex changes, but on occasion, a diminution in the posterior tibial reflex can be elicited. There must be asymmetry in obtaining this reflex for it to have any clinical significance.

O   **What exam findings occur in an L4 lesion?**

With compression of the fourth lumbar nerve root, the quadriceps muscle is affected; the patient may note weakness in knee extension, which is often associated with instability. Atrophy of the thigh musculature can be marked. A sensory loss may be apparent over the anteromedial aspect of the thigh, and the patellar tendon reflex can be diminished.

O   **What is the straight leg raising test (SLR)?**

The straight leg raising test detects irritation of the sciatic nerve.

O   **What is its pathological significance?**

The passive raising of the leg by the foot with the knee extended stretches the sciatic nerve, its nerve roots, and dural attachment. When the dura is inflamed and stretched, the patient will experience pain along its anatomic course to the lower leg, ankle, and foot. Dural movement starts at 30° of elevation. Pain of dural origin should not be felt below that degree of elevation. Pain is maximum between 30° to 70° of elevation. Symptoms at greater degrees of elevation may be of nerve root origin, but may also be related to mechanical low back pain secondary to muscle strain or joint disease.

O   **What effect does dorsiflexion of the foot have?**

Dorsiflexion of the foot will exacerbate the radicular pain. Pain may also be experienced in the leg below the knee when the contralateral normal leg is raised.

O   **What does the presence of contralateral pain reflect?**

The presence of contralateral pain suggests a large central lesion in the spinal canal causing traction on the opposite nerve root when the normal leg is raised.

O   **What is the femoral stretch test?**

Dural irritation of nerve roots from L2 to L4 are tested by the femoral stretch test in the prone position. With the knee bent, the thigh is elevated from the examining table. The test is positive if pain is reproduced in the front of the thigh (L2 and L3) or the medial aspect of the leg (L4).

O   **Under what circumstances should plain radiographs be considered in 'sciatica'?**

Plain radiographs may be recommended for patients who have a systemic medical illness such as an inflammatory arthropathy, infection, tumors, or significant fractures. Numerous guidelines have suggested that criteria for obtaining plain films include older age, systemic illness, previous malignancy, neurologic deficits, drug or alcohol abuse, and significant trauma.

O   **When should bone scans be considered in 'sciatica'?**

Bone scan is best reserved for the patient with one of the following:

Constitutional symptoms of fever and/or weight loss
Pain with recumbency
Failure to respond to conservative therapy
Abnormal laboratory tests including elevated sedimentation rate or anemia.

O   **What are the Waddell signs?**

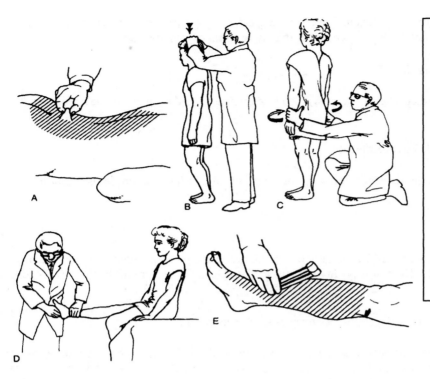

Waddell tests:

A) Superficial sensitivity to light pinch.

B) Axial loading causing low back pain.

C) Passive rotation of the shoulders and pelvis in the same plane causing back pain.

D) Straight leg raising test in the seated position. Stroking the skin on the bottom of the foot distracts the patient.

E) Stocking distribution of sensory deficit.

O   **What is a limitation of CT scanning lumbar spine disorders?**

CT will not visualize intradural lesions unless radiographic contrast media is present intrathecally.

O   **What is an indication to consider CT-myelogram in lumbar spine disorders?**

CT enhanced with contrast (CT-myelogram) is especially helpful in patients with multiple disc abnormalities, multilevel radiculopathies, extruded free disc fragments, a disc fragment in the lateral recess, stenosis of the spinal canal or lateral recess.

O   **Is MRI or CT imaging superior for vertebral osteomyelitis?**

MRI is more sensitive in the detection of vertebral osteomyelitis than plain radiographs or CT.

O   **What is a limitation of MRI in lumbar spine disorders?**

As with CT and myelography, MRI findings are only significant in patients with correlating clinical symptoms and signs. Herniated discs are noted in 10% of asymptomatic young women and bulging discs in up to 45%.

O   **Which imaging modality is preferred for the diagnosis of HNP or stenosis?**

A consensus is growing that MRI is the most useful technique for lumbar spine imaging. In the diagnosis of herniated discs and spinal stenosis, MRI has sensitivity equal to or greater than CT or myelography.

O   **How does EMG compare with other modalities in diagnosing nerve root pathology?**

Electrodiagnostic examination has a degree of accuracy in identifying patients with nerve root compression similar to that of MRI and clinical examination. A recent study shows that EMG and MRI findings agree in the majority (60%) of patients with a clinical history compatible with cervical and lumbosacral radiculopathy. Overall sensitivity varies from 30-90% for EMG (needle examination) to 50-80% for H-reflexes. EMG provides a physiological measure for detecting axonal loss with good sensitivity and high specificity (at least 85%) and can provide information as to which anatomical lesions are truly physiologically significant. Needle examination is thus critical in maintaining high diagnostic specificity in eliminating unnecessary and sometimes risky or costly interventions.

O **What are 6 relative indications for EMG/NCS in 'sciatica'?**

1. When added information will alter treatment plans.
2. Imaging studies show an abnormality that does not correlate with symptoms.
3. Imaging findings are normal despite clinical suspicion.
4. There is a suspicion of polyneuropathy, myopathy, or entrapment neuropathy.
5. It is clinically important to determine the age of the lesion.
6. It is clinically important to demonstrate which of numerous anatomic lesions in the spine is causing radicular symptoms.

O **What are the treatment approaches of radiculopathy?**

Physical therapy for acute radiculopathy should emphasize analgesia through passive modalities, stretching activities, and soft tissue mobilization initially and then advance to McKenzie-type activities to regain segmental motion. Once segmental activity has been normalized or improved and the patient's pain has reduced, then the patient may begin a walking program and a progressive lumbar stabilization program. The stabilization program should be steadily advanced and the patient should have a generalized conditioning program initiated as well.

O **What is the prognosis of acute lumbar HNPs?**

Recovery in 3 months is typical of 75% of patients.

O **What are indications for surgery?**

The choice of surgical treatment and its timing is controversial. The indications for surgery other than cauda equina syndrome are progressive neurological deficit and pain that cannot be controlled by other means.

O **What are the surgical outcomes?**

The outcome of neurologic dysfunction is the same in patients treated aggressively or without invasive measures, although recovery is quicker with surgery.

O **What is the role for epidural steroid injections (ESI)?**

Recent studies have demonstrated positive efficacy of lumbar ESIs when proper placement is confirmed by using fluoroscopic guidance and radiographic confirmation through the use of contrast. Approximately 60-75% of patients receive some relief after ESIs. Benefits include relief of radicular pain and LBP (generally relieving leg pain more than back pain), improvement of quality of life, reduction of analgesic consumption, improved maintenance of work status, and obviating the need for hospitalization and surgery in many patients. Although numerous articles support the benefit of ESIs for LBP, other studies dispute the efficacy of these procedures.

O **What factors influence the likelihood of beneficial outcome from lumbar ESI?**

In general, patients who have had symptoms fewer than 3 months have response rates of 90%. When patients have radiculopathy symptoms for fewer than 6 months, response decreases to approximately 70%. Response decreases to 50% in patients who have had symptoms for over 1 year. Patients with shorter duration of symptoms also have more sustained relief than those with chronic pain. Patients with chronic back pain have better response if they develop an acute radiculopathy.

O **What are the goals of back school?**

Back schools may be used to prevent initial episodes of back pain or as part of a treatment program to prevent recurrent attacks; most schools deal primarily with prevention of recurrences. The goals of the back school in the short run are to reduce pain, encourage appropriate rest, and emphasize the good prognosis of most back pain problems. Teaching patients proper body mechanics, to develop coping skills for episodes of pain, to accept shared responsibility for their recovery, and to improve their general physical condition to help prevent recurrent back pain are the long range goals.

○   What are the methods used in back school?

The methods used by back schools to teach patients may be cognitive (classroom instruction of basic facts), physical (demonstrations of appropriate exercises Ad work habits), and motivational (encouragement to be an active participant in their own care). A number of back schools have been developed that utilize a combination of these methods.

○   What is a type I spondylolisthesis?

Type I, dysplastic spondylolisthesis, is secondary to a congenital defect of either the superior sacral or inferior L5 facets or both with gradual slipping of the L5 vertebra. The female-to-male predominance is 2:1. This type accounts for approximately 15-20% of cases of spondylolisthesis. Symptoms usually develop during the adolescent growth period.

○   What is a type II spondylolisthesis?

Type II, isthmic or spondylolytic, in which the lesion is in the isthmus or pars interarticularis, has the greatest clinical importance in persons under the age of 50. The spondylolytic (isthmic) type is the most common cause of spondylolisthesis. Approximately 82% of cases of isthmic spondylolisthesis occur at L5-S1. Another 11.3% occur at L4-L5. If a defect in the pars interarticularis can be identified but no slipping has occurred, the condition is termed spondylolysis. If one vertebra has slipped forward on the other (horizontal translation), it is referred to as spondylolisthesis. Type II spondylolisthesis occurs secondary to a lytic process (fatigue fracture of the pars interarticularis), elongation (attenuated) of an intact pars, or acute fracture.

○   What is a type III spondylolisthesis?

Type III, or degenerative spondylolisthesis, occurs secondary to degeneration of the lumbar facet joints with alteration in the joint plane allowing forward or backward displacement. Degenerative spondylolisthesis is most common in an older age population. The L4-L5 vertebral space is affected 6-10 times more commonly than at other levels. Black women are affected 3 times more commonly than white women. There is no pars defect and the vertebral body slippage is never greater than 30%.

○   What is a type IV spondylolisthesis?

Type IV traumatic spondylolisthesis, is associated with acute fracture of a posterior element (pedicle, lamina, or facets) other than the pars interarticularis.

○   What is a type V spondylolisthesis?

Type V, pathologic spondylolisthesis, occurs because of a structural weakness of the bone secondary to a disease process such as a tumor.

○   What are the demographics of spondylolysis?

The affected population shows a 2:1 male-to-female predominance. White men are affected more commonly than black men, and white women are affected more often than black women. A family history of spondylolysis and/or spondylolisthesis is commonly found. High-risk activities include gymnastics, rowing, tennis, wrestling, weightlifting, and football; all of these create mechanical stresses that play an important role in development of spondylolysis. A 4.4% incidence of spondylolysis and a 2.6% incidence of spondylolisthesis at age 6 years and a 5.4% and 4.0% prevalence, respectively, has been reported in adulthood.

○   What symptoms occur in spondylolisthesis?

The most common clinical manifestation of spondylolisthesis is low back pain. The pain is improved with extension of the spine and exacerbated with flexion. The degree of slippage does not necessarily correlate with the degree of pain experienced by the patient. Besides back pain, these patients can also complain of leg pain. This occurs because there is frequently a buildup of a fibrocartilaginous mass at the site of the defect, which can cause pain by irritating the nerve root as it exits the neural foramen. Once the symptoms begin, the patient usually has constant low-grade back discomfort that is aggravated by activity and relieved by rest.

O   **What are the physical findings in spondylolisthesis?**

The physical findings of spondylolisthesis are fairly characteristic. In the absence of any radicular pain, the patient exhibits no postural scoliosis, but there is usually an exaggeration of the lumbar curve and a palpable "step off." Hamstring tightness is commonly found in the symptomatic patient with spondylolysis or spondylolisthesis.

O   **What are the radiographic findings in spondylolisthesis?**

Forward subluxation of the body (spondylolisthesis) is best visualized on the lateral roentgenogram. The amount of slippage is graded by the system of Meyerding. The top of the sacrum is divided into four parallel quarters, posterior to anterior. A slip of 25% or less of the sacrum is Grade 1, while movement of 75% or more of the sacrum is Grade IV.

O   **How much dynamic AP translation occurs normally in the lumbar spine with extension-flexion?**

Normal lumbar vertebral levels should have less than 3.0 mm of dynamic AP translation on extension and flexion views of the spine.

O   **What other imaging study is helpful in spondylolysis?**

Advances in bone scintigraphy in the form of single photon emission computed tomography (SPECT) allows for the identification of lesions not imaged by planar bone scan. SPECT is able to detect fractures in the pars interarticularis, transverse process, and vertebral body not detected by plain bone scan.

O   **What is retrolisthesis?**

In extreme degeneration of intervertebral discs, a retrolisthesis may occur. With decreased disc height, excess motion occurs in adjacent vertebral bodies, allowing posterior motion. L1 and L2 vertebrae seem more commonly affected by this process.

O   **What conservative therapy is appropriate?**

When the symptoms are acute, rest is indicated. If leg pain is a significant problem, antiinflammatory medication can be quite beneficial. Stabilization exercises should be started once the patient is in a remission, and the patient is usually advised to wear a corset during occasional strenuous activity. Brace therapy with semirigid LSOs may be helpful in decreasing symptoms in patients with spondylolisthesis. Flexion exercises are more effective than extension exercises for the treatment of spondylolisthesis.

O   **What are the risk factors for progression of slippage?**

For the younger population, the following factors are known to correlate with higher risk of slip progression:

Younger age (<15 y)
High-grade listhesis (>30%)
Female sex
Ligamentous laxity
Type 1 (dysplastic) slip
Lumbosacral hypermobility

O   **What are the surgical indications in spondylolisthesis?**

Neurologic signs - Radiculopathy (unresponsive to conservative measures), myelopathy, neurogenic claudication
Any high-grade slip (>50%)
Type 1 and type 2 slips, with evidence of instability, progression of listhesis, or lack of response to conservative measures
Traumatic spondylolisthesis
Iatrogenic spondylolisthesis
Type 3 (degenerative) listhesis with gross instability and incapacitating pain
Postural deformity and gait abnormality

O   **What guidelines should patients receive regarding activity?**

Once patients experience symptoms secondary to spondylolisthesis, it is unreasonable to expect them to perform heavy work or participate in high-performance athletics. These individuals should be restricted in regard to activities generally involving heavy lifting or repetitive bending.

O   **What are the anatomical criteria for lumbar spinal stenosis (LSS)?**

Interpedicular distance, considered subnormal if less than 18 mm, commonly increases from upper to lower lumbar segments. Some sources define pure absolute central canal stenosis as a midsagittal canal diameter of less than or equal to 10 mm, pure relative at 10-12 mm, and mixed as a combination thereof. Mid-sagittal canal diameter less than 15 mm and transverse diameter less than 20 mm usually are considered abnormal. Posterior disc height of 4 mm or less and foraminal height of 15 mm or less may suggest foraminal stenosis; nevertheless, clinical correlation is required.

O   **Is there a strong correlation between clinical findings and imaging criteria definition?**

No convincing correlation has been found between clinical symptoms and radiologic findings in a study of 100 symptomatic patients with LSS. Similarly, no correlation has been shown between physical function and radiologic findings.

O   **What are the pathological changes are associated with lumbar spinal stenosis?**

Pathologic studies of the lumbar nerve root canal show that lumbar spondylosis is associated with reduction in the vertical dimension due to disc space narrowing, posterior bulging of the intervertebral discs, retropulsion of annulus fibrosus remnants, and the formation of sclerotic ridges around the vertebral endplates. There are also osteoarthritic changes involving the facet joints and thickening of the ligamentum flavum.

O   **What is central canal stenosis?**

Central canal stenosis, commonly occurring at an intervertebral disc level, defines midline sagittal spinal canal diameter narrowing that may elicit neurogenic claudication (NC) or pain in the buttock, thigh, or leg. Such stenosis results from ligamentum flavum hypertrophy, inferior articulating process (IAP), facet hypertrophy of the cephalad vertebra, vertebral body osteophytosis, and herniated nucleus pulposus (HNP).

O   **What is lateral canal stenosis?**

Lateral recess stenosis (i.e., lateral gutter stenosis, subarticular stenosis, subpedicular stenosis, foraminal canal stenosis, intervertebral foramen stenosis) is defined as narrowing (less than 3-4 mm) between the facet superior articulating process (SAP) and posterior vertebral margin. Such narrowing may impinge the nerve root and subsequently elicit radicular pain. This lateral region is compartmentalized into entrance zone, mid zone, exit zone, and far-out stenosis.

O   **What are the demographics of LSS?**

Approximately 250,000-500,000 US residents have symptoms of spinal stenosis. This represents about 5 of every 1000 Americans older than 50 years. Lumbar spinal stenosis occurs more commonly in males. This may be a combination of a congenitally narrow canal linked with occupational risk. LSS remains the leading preoperative diagnosis for adults older than

65 years who undergo spine surgery. The incidence of lateral nerve entrapment is reportedly 8-11%. Some studies implicate lateral recess stenosis as the pain generator for 60% of patients with symptomatology of failed back surgery syndrome.

O   **What lumbar nerve roots are most commonly involved?**

Incidence of foraminal stenosis increases in lower lumbar levels because of increased dorsal root ganglion (DRG) diameter with resulting decreased foramen (i.e., nerve root area ratio). Jenis and An cite commonly involved roots as L5 (75%), L4 (15%), L3 (5.3%), and L2 (4%).

O   **What is the most often reported symptom in lumbar spinal stenosis?**

The most characteristic symptom is pseudoclaudication, defined as any discomfort that occurs in the buttock, thigh or leg on standing or walking, which is relieved by rest and is not produced by peripheral vascular insufficiency. At times, similar symptoms can occur while lying down and are relieved only by walking around. Such discomfort is generally described as pain but occasionally is appreciated as numbness or weakness, with many patients experiencing various combinations of these symptoms. Katz and colleagues report that the historical findings most strongly associated with LSS include advanced age, severe lower extremity pain, and absence of pain when the patient is in a flexed position.

O   **How is pseudoclaudication relieved?**

Pseudoclaudication is generally relieved by lying down or sitting and adopting a posture of flexion at the waist.

O   **How often are the symptoms bilateral?**

Forty percent of cases have bilateral symptoms.

O   **What neurological findings are encountered in lumbar spinal stenosis?**

Restriction of straight leg raising (Lasègue's sign) is present in only 10% of cases of sciatica due to lumbar spinal stenosis. Ankle jerks are absent in 40%, knee jerks are absent in 10%, and a small percentage have sensory loss or weakness. Katz and colleagues report physical examination findings most strongly associated with LSS include wide-based gait, abnormal Romberg test, thigh pain following 30 seconds of lumbar extension, and neuromuscular abnormalities;

O   **What is the role of CT scanning in the diagnosis of LSS?**

CT scan provides excellent central canal, lateral recess, and neuroforaminal visualization. Additionally, CT scan offers contrasts between intervertebral disc, ligamentum flavum, and thecal sac. Unfortunately, CT scan, like MRI, yields a high false-positive rate (35.4% when correlated with surgically proven LSS).

O   **What is the role of MRI in the diagnosis of LSS?**

MRI remains the imaging modality of choice for LSS. The advantages include nonionizing radiation and superior multiplanar soft tissue visualization without osseous artifact. A trefoil shaped central spinal canal may provoke more symptoms than a round or oval canal by depressing the lateral recess. Unfortunately, MRI abnormalities have been documented in 20% of asymptomatic subjects.

O   **How does myelography compare to CT and MRI?**

Myelography is less sensitive and specific than CT scan or MRI.

O   **What do electrodiagnostic studies reveal in lumbar spinal stenosis?**

Wilbourn and Aminoff report variable EMG/NCS findings, including multiple, bilateral lumbosacral radiculopathies in 50% of LSS patients, with prominent chronic motor unit action potential (MUAP) changes, and fibrillations solely in distal musculature. The remaining 50% of patients demonstrate other varied abnormalities. Diagnostically, EMG complements MRI in assessing radiculopathy. Specifically, EMG rarely presents false-positive results and carries high specificity (85%).

○   **What is the role of dermatomal somatosensory evoked potentials (DSEPs) in the diagnosis of LSS?**

Using CT scan and MRI comparison standards, Kraft and colleagues demonstrated 78% sensitivity and 93% predictive value with DSEPs for an anatomical study positive for LSS when using multiple root disease (MRD) criteria. When criteria of multiple root disease and single root disease (SRD) were added, the sensitivity rose to 93%, with a positive predictive value of 94%.

○   **Summarize nonoperative Treatment for Degenerative Lumbar Spinal Stenosis**

Nonoperative Treatment for Degenerative Lumbar Spinal Stenosis

Method	Comments
Medications	Decrease inflammation, provide pain relief
NSAIDs	Provides pain relief
Acetaminophen	Decrease inflammation; diminish radicular symptoms and pain
Oral corticosteroids	Decrease paravertebral muscle spasm
Muscle relaxants	Not routinely used, but may help in acute flares
Narcotics	Decrease radicular symptoms
Tricyclic antidepressants	Decrease radicular symptoms
(eg, nortriptyline hydrochloride)	Decrease pain; increase ambulatory capacity in some patients
Anticonvulsants (eg, gabapentin)	
Calcitonin injections	
Physical Therapy	
Conditioning	Encourages weight loss; improves aerobic conditioning
Stretching	Promotes muscle relaxation and limberness, improves lumbosacral motion, and decreases muscle spasm
Strengthening	Improves muscle tone in back and abdominal muscles
Modalities	May benefit some patients, but results are inconsistent
(eg, heat, ice, ultrasound, electrical stimulation)	
Activity Modification	
Riding stationary bicycle or leaning forward on a treadmill	Promotes lumbosacral flexion; is usually well-tolerated
Bracing	
Lumbosacral corset (soft)	Supports weak musculature; provides minimal immobilization
Lumbosacral orthosis (rigid)	Decreases symptoms by immobilization; should be prescribed in slight flexion

○   **What physical rehabilitation interventions may be considered?**

The therapist can use modalities (e.g., hot packs, ultrasound, massage) to decrease paravertebral muscle guarding. Because lumbar extension exacerbates the symptoms, the therapist should prescribe a program of (Williams') flexion exercises to increase both flexibility and strength. These exercises also open up the intervertebral foramen, decreasing nerve root compression. In addition, lumbar stabilization exercises, performed with a reduced lumbar lordosis (i.e., a posterior pelvic tilt), are beneficial for this condition. However, a lumbar stabilization program can be difficult for some patients to learn. The therapist should also prescribe an appropriate conditioning program, such as stationary bike riding, for this patient population.

○   **What are surgical indications?**

Indications for surgery vary according to the patient characteristics but include sphincter and sexual dysfunction due to compression of conus medullaris or cauda equina, severe radicular symptoms, particularly if there are progressive neurologic motor deficits, and radicular symptoms failing to respond to conservative management.

○   **What is the most common surgical procedure for LSS?**

In the lumbar spine, the mainstay of decompressive surgery is single or multilevel laminectomy for canal decompression and foraminotomy for nerve root decompression. The need for fusion with or without fixation in stable spinal stenosis is controversial. The method employed by most is posterolateral intertransverse fusion bilaterally through a midline approach with autologous hip graft, local autograft (bone harvested during decompression), or allograft (i.e., cadaveric). The use of internal fixation is also controversial. Pedicle screw fixation has become the most widely accepted device for spinal stabilization, but they have associated morbidity and increased operative time. Interbody fusion is another method of further stabilizing the lumbar spine.

○ **What are the surgical outcomes?**

Johnsson and colleagues document improvement in 60% of surgically treated patients with 25% worsened, compared with improvement in 30% of conservatively treated patients and no change in 60%.

○ **What is the role of ESI in LSS?**

Epidural steroid injection (ESI) provides aggressive-conservative treatment for LSS patients who demonstrate limited response to oral medication, physical therapy, and other noninvasive measures. Studies of ESI for LSS treatment demonstrate mixed results due to varying injection and guidance techniques, patient populations, follow-up periods and protocols, ancillary treatments (eg, physical therapy, oral medication), and outcome measures. This lack of consistency limits the ability to assess ESI efficacy for LSS. Studies report that 50% of patients with LSS or HNP-provoked radicular pain received temporary relief and that such results were close to those associated with the placebo effect. ESI may do little to relieve chronic lateral recess stenosis-related radicular pain.

○ **What other invasive procedures may be utilized in the treatment approach to lumbar spinal stenosis?**

Medial branch /dorsal ramus blocks and RF denervation procedures, spinal cord stimulators.

○ **What is the natural clinical course of LSS?**

Johnsson and colleagues' single study of the natural course of LSS reports unchanged symptoms in 70% of patients, improvement in 15%, and worsening in 15% after a 49-month observation period. Walking capacity improved in 37% of patients, remained unchanged in 33%, and worsened in 30%.

○ **Summarize a plausible differential diagnosis with treatment options for low back pain**

Diagnosis and Workup for Different Causes of Low Back Pain						
	Mechanical LBP	**Herniated Disk**	**Spinal Stenosis**	**Metastases**	**Ankylosing Spondylitis**	**Epidural Abscess**
Age (yr.)	30-60	35-45	50-70	>50	20-40	40-60
Pain description and location	Dull, low back and buttocks	Electric, knifelike, radiates to foot	Aching and burning in buttocks and thighs	Insidious, unrelenting, severe lumbar pain	Insidious, unrelenting back and buttock pain	Sharp and severe, bilateral buttock and leg pain
Comorbidities	None	None	DJD of spine	Primary cancer	Uveitis, arthritis, aortic insufficiency	Immunocompromised state
Physical examination findings	Normal	Altered dermatomal sensation, pain on SLR, possibly altered reflexes	Pain with spinal extension	Variable	Decreased axial mobility, decreased chest expansion	Leg weakness, gait disturbance, +/- altered rectal tone, +/- altered reflexes
Laboratory results	Normal	Normal	Normal	Electrolyte abnormalities, especially calcium and phosphate	Often elevated ESR	Elevated ESR, often positive blood cultures, +/- leukocytosis
X-ray studies	None needed	MRI if prolonged pain, progressive pain, progressive neurologic deficits	CT-myelogram MRI	Plain films, often MRI or CT to better delineate lesions	Plain films show sacroiliitis	MRI indicated
Treatment	Analgesics, spasmolytics, Manual therapy Therapeutic exercise	Conservative for 3 months (including ESI), then consider surgery if necessary	Conservative (including ESI) versus laminectomy with noninstrumented arthrodesis	Combination of steroids, radiation, Bracing and possibly surgical stabilization	Physical therapy, nonsteriodals, DMARDs, Biological agents	Surgical decompression and intravenous antibiotics

O   **What is scoliosis?**

Scoliosis is lateral curvature of the spine. The term is usually applied to curves in excess of 10°. Scoliotic curves may be either structural (fixed), characterized by fixed rotation on forward bending, or compensatory, tending to maintain body alignment of the head over the pelvis and normal position on forward bending.

O   **What are the demographics of idiopathic scoliosis?**

Studies of adults have recognized scoliosis between 3.9% to 6% individuals. Other studies using the 10° definition of scoliosis have placed the overall prevalence in the 1.9-3.0% range. The incidence is only slightly greater in girls than in boys, but scoliosis is more likely to progress and require treatment in girls than in boys. The daughters of affected mothers are more likely than other children to have scoliosis, but identical twins are not uniformly affected.

O   **What is lumbar scoliosis?**

When the apex of the curve is from L2 to L4, the curve is termed lumbar. When the apex is at L5 or the sacrum, the curve is termed lumbosacral.

O   **What is kyphoscoliosis?**

Kyphoscoliosis is lateral curvature of the spine associated with either increased posterior or decreased anterior angulation in the sagittal plane in excess of the accepted normal curve for that area. Kyphoscoliosis affects both the thoracic and lumbar spine. It can be acquired or congenital. Congenital kyphosis and kyphoscoliosis are much less common than congenital scoliosis. Although congenital kyphosis and kyphoscoliosis are uncommon but potentially dangerous spinal deformities that, in contrast to congenital scoliosis, can occasionally result in paraplegia.

O   **What is the outline of the scoliosis research society classification of scoliosis?**

The major categories include idiopathic, neuromuscular, congenital, neurofibromatosis, mesenchymal disorders, rheumatoid disease, trauma, extraspinal contractures, osteochondrodystrophies, and infection of bone, metabolic disorders, disorders related to the lumbosacral joint, and tumors.

O   **What is the classification of Idiopathic scoliosis?**

Idiopathic scoliosis can be divided into three groups on the basis of age at onset: infantile (birth–3 yr.), juvenile (4–10 yr.), and adolescent (11 yr. and older). Adolescent idiopathic scoliosis is much more common than juvenile-onset scoliosis; infantile idiopathic scoliosis is extraordinarily rare.

O   **What are the characteristics of infantile scoliosis?**

Occurs between birth and 3 years of age. Usually noticed in the first year of life. More common in boys particularly from Europe. Left thoracic curve occurs more common, and often resolves spontaneously. Few patients will have progressive curves which can be quite severe requiring early bracing and even surgery.

O   **What are the characteristics of Juvenile scoliosis?**

Occurs between 4-10 years of age. Incidence is equal for boys and girls. Most curves are right thoracic. Curves are progressive in nature and need close follow up.

O   **What are the characteristics of Adolescent scoliosis?**

Usually diagnosed at the age of 10. Most curves are right thoracic and thoracolumbar. Curves have a strong tendency to progress during adolescent growth spurt. Extremely active, athletic teenage girls with delayed menses are most of risk for curve progression.

O   **What are the typical curve patterns seen in idiopathic scoliosis?**

Right thoracic curves are most common. They can develop rapidly and must be treated early or severe cosmetic deformity. Cardiopulmonary compromise will ensue when curves reach 60 degree.
Thoracolumbar curves are also common. They are usually not as deforming.
Lumbar major curves are less common. Most (65%) are left lumbar curves. They are not deforming but can lead to disabling back pain in later life and during pregnancy.

O   **What are the nonstructural forms of scoliosis?**

Nonstructural (compensatory) forms of scoliosis include those related to postural, hysterical, nerve root, inflammatory, leg length, and hip abnormalities.

O   **What is the pattern of skeletal maturation in the spine?**

Growth plate of the vertebra form a solid union at full maturation. At 6-8 years of age in girls (7-9 years old in boys), a calcific ring develops at the superior and inferior aspect of the vertebra. This ring gradually fuses with the vertebral body at the age of 14-15. Complete fusion occurs at age 21-25.

O   **What history is obtained in adolescent patients with scoliosis?**

In taking the history of adolescents, the physician should inquire about family history and connective tissue, neuromuscular and traumatic disorders. Positive responses to these inquiries help identify those individuals who have specific reasons for developing scoliosis (neurofibromatosis, Marfan syndrome, muscular dystrophy) and do not belong in the idiopathic group. Include the following items specifically:

Chronological age
Age at recognition of deformity. The longer the muscle imbalance, the more the distortion.
Impression of the rate of progression
Associated symptoms: pain, fatigue, cardiopulmonary symptoms. History of night pain resolved with ASA is concerning for osteoid osteoma. Back pain in young children can be due to spondylosis or spondylolisthesis and disc herniation.
Developmental factors: rate of growth, appearance of 2nd sexual characteristics (menarche). Rapid scoliotic curve changes occurs during rapid spine growth period. Progression usually halts or is much slower at skeletal maturity.
Genetic factors: racial origin. Infantile idiopathic scoliosis is more common in Britain and Europe.

O   **Is there an association between scoliosis and spine pain?**

Systematic surveys have documented that musculoskeletal back pain occurs more commonly among patients with scoliosis than among matched controls. No correlation is consistently associated with degree of curvature

O   **What is the origin of motion related pain in scoliosis?**

Patients may complain of pain with certain motions of the spine. Patients with scoliosis do not have parallel facet joints. The planes of the facets are at an angle. The soft tissues on the concave side of the curve tend to shorten, resulting in a mechanical restriction of motion. With spinal flexion past a certain degree, ligamentous and capsular tissues are stretched, resulting in pain. In addition, extension of the spine may cause impingement of the asymmetric facet joints, resulting in low back pain.

O   **What is the basic physical examination for idiopathic scoliosis?**

Specific examination should be done to identify scapular asymmetry and unilateral prominence, waist asymmetry, shoulder level, and asymmetry in the distance between the arms and the torso. As the patient bends over, prominence of one side of the rib cage is noted. From the rear, a measurement of the distance right or left from the gluteal cleft to a line drawn from C7 to the ground is a measurement of spinal imbalance. Inability to bend side to side may be secondary to intraspinal lesions such as a tumor, herniated disc, or osteoid osteoma, as well as scoliosis.

O   **What is Cobb's angle?**

Cobb's method is used to measure spine curvature. The vertebrae forming the ends of the curve are those that are most severely tilted toward its concavity. Lines are drawn along the upper border of the superior end-vertebra and along the lower border of the inferior end-vertebra. Perpendiculars are erected from each of these lines and are extended to intersect. Cobb's angle is the angle formed by the intersection of these two perpendicular lines.

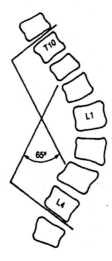

O   **How is radiographic progression of scoliosis defined?**

In general, young patients with mild scoliosis can be safely seen in follow up and X-ray done every 6-9 months. For faster progressive curves, X-ray every 3 months is recommended. In adolescents, a progression of 1 degree/month is normal, where as a significant progression is 3-5 degree/month.
Thus to diagnose a progression of scoliosis, a definite increase of a curvature of greater than 5° must be seen on roentgenographic evaluation.

O   **What are risk factors for clinically significant progression?**

In general, the following rules apply:

Thoracic curves causes more deformity and disability.
The earlier the age of onset, the greater the deformity and disability later in life.
Some prognostic signs of x-ray for active progression of scoliosis are: osteopenia of the vertebra near the apex of the curve, narrowed intervertebral disc space, and wedging of the apical vertebra.

O   **How is scoliosis managed in the young adult?**

Treatment in the young adult is directed toward the prevention of future problems. If the curve is less than 40° in the lumbar spine and the pain is not severe, nonoperative treatment can be employed. This includes analgesics and anti-inflammatory medication, local facet injections, physical therapy, and braces. The Milwaukee brace is (CTLSO) a mainstay of nonoperative therapy in young individuals and is used to prevent progression of spinal curvature. For the most part this form of bracing is rarely effective in the adult population.

O   **How is the severity of rotatory scoliosis measured?**

The severity of rotation of the vertebrae associated with scoliosis may be determined by the method of Nash and Moe, which is graded by the location of the pedicle on the concave side of the scoliosis. With Grades 1 and 2 the convex pedicle is visible on AP view. With Grades 3 and 4, the convex pedicle has twisted out of view.

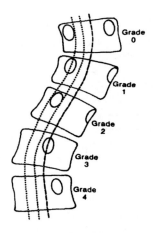

Grade 0
Grade 1
Grade 2
Grade 3
Grade 4

○ **How is scoliosis managed in the young adult?**

Treatment in the young adult is directed toward the prevention of future problems. If the curve is less than 40° in the lumbar spine and the pain is not severe, nonoperative treatment can be employed. This includes analgesics and antiinflammatory medication, local facet injections, physical therapy, and braces. The Milwaukee brace is (CTLSO) a mainstay of nonoperative therapy in young individuals and is used to prevent progression of spinal curvature. For the most part this form of bracing is rarely effective in the adult population.

○ **What are indications for surgery?**

If the curve is > 40° or if discomfort cannot be controlled or the curve is progressive, surgery is indicated. The aim of surgery is to straighten the spine as much as is safely possible and to stabilize it in a corrected position. A number of instrumentation devices have been developed and utilized for scoliosis.

○ **What is the prognosis of untreated idiopathic scoliosis?**

Untreated scoliosis is associated with major disability and death. In the adult, pain may become progressive and severe as increasing degenerative changes occur in facet joints and intervertebral discs. Respiratory insufficiency may limit stamina and work potential in those with double curvature (thoracolumbar scoliosis). Premature death may also be a complication of severe scoliosis. Nachemson reported a mortality twice that of the normal population at age 40 from cardiorespiratory causes in nontreated scoliosis patients of all types.

○ **Summarize the clinical evidence supporting the role of bracing in idiopathic scoliosis**

Three studies that set the standards of bracing for this high risk group:

Lonstein and Winter: 1020 patients treated with Milwaukee brace. Those patients with thoracic curves of 20-29 degrees and Risser 0-1, only 40% showed progression at the end of bracing (vs. 68% if not braced).
Durand: 477 patients. At 2-5 year follow up, only 21% of patients had progressed.
Bassett: 71 patients with curves 20-29 degrees and Risser 0-1. Only 36% of those with thoracic curves progressed.

○ **Summarize the clinical monitoring and conservative treatment of scoliosis**

Milwaukee brace for thoracic curves and TLSO for lumbar or thoracolumbar curves.
No bracing needed for curves less than 20 degrees.
Curves of 20-29 degrees need bracing when 2 or more years of growth remain or if there is evidence of progression.
Curves or 30-39 degrees should be braced at the first visit if growth remain.
No bracing needed for patients with Risser 4 or 5.
Brace should be worn 20-22 hours per day and taken off for hygiene and strengthening exercises.
Patients should be seen on a monthly basis for brace adjustment with X-ray taken every 6 months.
Weaning off brace: When the child is more mature and the curve holds its position, the child is allow more time out of the brace. The weaning period takes about 2-3 years until the age of 15 in girls and 16 ½ in boys.

○   **Summarize the indications for surgical intervention**

Severe cosmetic changes in the shoulder and trunk.
Adolescents with curve more than 45 degrees.
Relentless curve progression
Major curve progression in spite of bracing
Inability to wean the patient from the brace
Significant thoracic and lumbar pain
Progressive loss of pulmonary function.
Emotional or psychological inability to accept the brace.

○   **What general surgical procedure principles are considered?**

The primary goal of scoliosis surgery is to achieve a solid bony fusion. The surgical technique used to achieve such an arthrodesis is vastly more important than the instrumentation system that the surgeon needs to use, if any. Modern instrumentation systems have been shown to allow for adequate curve correction but with little or no ability to diminish associated rib humps.

○   **What are the considerations for postoperative bracing?**

With the advent of large-rod multiple-hook constructs, such as the Cotrel-Dubousset system and its direct decendents, bracing has been de-emphasized. It is almost as likely that a patient will not receive a postoperative brace as receive one, whereas previously, bracing was much more widespread. In certain specific circumstances, postoperative bracing is still almost always used, such as anterior thoracic or thoracolumbar instrumentation procedures or surprisingly weak bone stock.

○   **What are the postoperative bracing guidelines?**

When a brace is used, it is typically to be worn full-time for at least 6 weeks, followed by a period in which the brace may be off for bathing with subsequent progressive weaning. As a rule of thumb, patients may also miss up to 6 weeks of school (if their procedure is done at such time of the year), and up to 6 months may be required before they resume most of their normal activities. Vigorous sports may be restricted for at least a year, in some instances permanently (based on risk versus benefit discussions between patients, families, and their surgeons).

COMPLEX REGIONAL PAIN SYNDROME

○   **Compare and contrast Complex regional pain syndrome type 1 (reflex sympathetic dystrophy) and Complex regional pain syndrome type 2 (causalgia)**

Complex regional pain syndrome type 1 (reflex sympathetic dystrophy)
1. The presence of an initiating noxious event or a cause of immobilization.
2. Continuing pain, allodynia, or hyperalgesia with which the pain is disproportionate to the inciting event.
3. Evidence at some time of edema, changes in skin blood flow, or abnormal sudomotor (sweat gland) activity in the painful region.
4. The diagnosis is excluded by the existence of conditions that would otherwise account for the degree of pain and dysfunction.
Note: criteria 2, 3, and 4 are necessary for a diagnosis of complex regional pain syndrome (1 is not always present).
Complex regional pain syndrome type 2 (causalgia)
1. The presence of continuing pain, allodynia, or hyperalgesia after a nerve injury, not necessarily limited to the distribution of the injured nerve.
2. Evidence at some time of edema, changes in skin blood flow, or abnormal sudomotor activity in the region of the pain.
3. The diagnosis is excluded by the existence of conditions that would otherwise account for the degree of pain and dysfunction. Note: all 3 criteria must be satisfied.

○   **Provide a differential diagnosis for a patient to exclude CRPS.**

Musculoskeletal	Bursitis Myofascial pain syndrome Rotator cuff tear Undiagnosed local pathology (fracture or sprain)
Neurologic	Poststroke pain syndrome Peripheral neuropathy Postherpetic neuralgia Radiculopathy
Infectious	Cellulitis Infectious arthritis
Vascular	Raynaud's disease Thromboangiitis obliterans (Buerger's disease) Thrombosis Traumatic vasospasm
Rheumatic	Rheumatoid arthritis Systemic lupus
Psychiatric	Factitious disorder Hysterical conversion reaction

○   What recent clinical research findings have elucidated the pathogenesis of CRPS?

1) The Sudeck concept of an exaggerated regional inflammatory response is supported by new data indicating that, in patients with acute RSD, immunoglobulin G labeled with 111 Indium is concentrated in the affected extremity.
2) A study with 31P (phosphorus) nuclear magnetic resonance (NMR) spectroscopy showed an impairment of high-energy phosphate metabolism, which explains why these patients are unable, rather than unwilling, to exercise.
3) Electron microscope studies of skeletal muscle biopsies showed reduced mitochondrial enzyme activity, vesiculation of mitochondria, disintegration of myofibrils, abnormal depositions of lipofuscin, swelling of endothelial layers, and thickening of the basal membrane, which are all signs of oxidative stress. Oxygen consumption is reduced in limbs affected by RSD, and reduction of pain following treatment with oral vasodilators has been described.
4) After a partial nerve lesion, excessive antidromic activation of undamaged afferent C fibers and neuropeptide release, leading to acute vasodilation within the innervation territory of the affected nerve, were demonstrated.
5) The frequency of the presence of human lymphocyte antigen-DQ1 (HLA-DQ1) was increased significantly in RSD compared with control frequencies. This association provides an indication of an organic basis.
6) Positron emission tomography (PET) in patients with chronic post-traumatic neuropathic pain or neuralgia revealed significantly decreased level of thalamic activity contralateral to the symptomatic side compared to normal controls.

○   What potential sites and mechanisms of interaction between sensory and sympathetic systems?

Coupling between postganglionic sympathetic efferent neurons and the sensory afferent neurons can occur at different sites. Site 1— at the periphery in cutaneous or deeper tissues; site 2—within the peripheral nerve by ephaptic mechanisms; and site 3—in the dorsal root ganglion, where sprouting of noradrenergic neurons has been observed after peripheral nerve lesions.

○   What possible mechanisms of interaction between sympathetic postganglionic fibers and nociceptors in the periphery?

Chemical coupling between norepinephrine (and possibly other transmitters) released from sympathetic terminals and afferent neurons via an adrenoceptor mechanism. Even though an excitatory effect of norepinephrine on postsynaptic a-receptors is suspected, actions on postsynaptic inhibitory alpha-2 receptors cannot be ruled out. Indirect chemical coupling may occur via activation by norepinephrine of a-adrenoceptor on secondary cells such as mast cells, leukocytes, or platelets. These cells in turn may release chemical mediators that activate nociceptive afferents. Indirect coupling may also result from alterations in the microvascular milieu of the sensory terminals, resulting in altered excitability of the afferents.

○   What morphologic evidence for an interaction between sensory and sympathetic systems after nerve injury?

Catecholamine-fluorescent axons in an L5 dorsal root ganglion (DRG) of normal rats, and 50 days after sciatic nerve ligation have been studied. In normal rats, the fluorescent axons are perivascular in the DRG. In contrast, in the DRG of animals with lesions, fluorescent axons run between profiles of neurons or form basket-like rings around large diameter sensory neurons.

○   What is a plausible model for CRPS?

According to experimental data, small-diameter polymodal C and Aδ afferent neurons are sensitized after noxious stimuli, this could suggest a rationale for hyperalgesia to heat and algesic agents. Central spinal mechanisms may also play a role, including the sensitization of central neurons following either intense mechanical stimuli or continuous nociceptive input. Alterations in non-nociceptive neurons may also be a source of noxious stimuli. Experimental evidence in humans or non-human primates tends to implicate alpha 1-adrenorecptors in sympathetic efferent, afferent aberrant coupling, whereas data from the majority of animal studies have identified the alpha 2-adrenoreceptor as being responsible for excitation, sensitization of nociceptive afferents, in some cases via prostaglandin E$_2$.

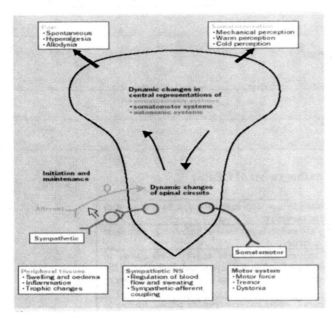

O   Does it occur in children?

RSD is less frequent in children than in adults. In the former group of patients, RSD is more common in girls than in boys; more often involves the lower extremity, has unique radionuclide features, generally follows a physical injury, and is self-limited and benign, with no clinical residua.

O   What is the incidence of CRPS?

The mean age of CRPS patients ranges from 36 to 42 years with women predominating (60% to 81%). The upper extremity is involved in 44% to 61% of cases, and the lower extremity in 39% to 51%. The etiology of CRPS is typically an injury (often minor): 16% after a fracture, 10% to 29% after a strain or sprain, 3% to 24% postsurgery, 8% after contusion or crush injury, and 6% are spontaneous, 2% to 17% other causes, or of unknown etiology.

O   In what clinical conditions can CRPS emerge?

Any neurally related visceral, musculoskeletal, neurologic, or vascular condition is a potential source for RSD, although an incipient cause frequently is not identifiable.

Trauma (often minor) ranks as the leading provocative event
Ischemic heart disease and myocardial infarction
Cervical spine or spinal cord disorders
Cerebral lesions
Infections
Surgery
Repetitive motion disorder or cumulative trauma, causing conditions such as carpal tunnel

O **What is the prognosis and recurrence rate of CRPS?**

The prognosis for the chronic CRPS patient is poor, with less than 10% reporting resolution 4 to 18 years after onset. CRPS may also recur in the same or a different limb after it has resolved, with a 1.8% annual incidence of recurrence.

O **What are the stages of CRPS/RSD?**

STAGE I	STAGE II	STAGE III
Onset of severe, pain limited to the site of injury	Pain becomes even more severe and more diffuse	Marked wasting of tissue (atrophic) eventually become irreversible.
Increased sensitivity of skin to touch and light pressure (allodynia).	Swelling tends to spread and it may change from a soft to hard (brawny) type	For many patients the pain becomes intractable and may involve the entire limb.
Localized swelling	Hair may become coarse then scant, nails may grow faster then grow slower and become brittle, cracked and heavily grooved	A small percentage of patients have developed generalized RSD affecting the entire body
Muscle cramps	Spotty wasting of bone (osteoporosis) occurs early but may become severe and diffuse	
Stiffness and limited mobility	Muscle wasting begins	
At onset, skin is usually warm, red and dry and then it may change to a blue (cyanotic) in appearance and become cold and sweaty.		
Increased sweating (hyperhydrosis).		
In mild cases this stage lasts a few weeks, then subsides spontaneously or responds rapidly to treatment.		

O **What signs and symptoms are reported in CRPS patients?**

Frequency of signs and symptoms among CRPS patients[a]

[a] NA, not applicable. Items were assessed as objective sign or subjective symptoms only.

Variables	Signs (%)	Symptoms (%)
"Burning" pain	NA	81.1
Hyperesthesia	NA	65.1
Temperature asymmetry	56.3	78.7
Color changes	66.4	86.9
Sweating changes	24.2	52.9
Edema	56.1	79.7
Nail changes	9.3	21.1
Hair changes	8.5	18.7
Skin changes	19.5	24.4
Weakness	56.1	74.6
Tremor	8.8	23.7
Dystonia	14.0	20.2
Decreased range of motion	70.3	80.3
Hyperalgesia	63.2	NA

Frequency of signs and symptoms among CRPS patients*
Allodynia					74.0			NA

○   **What is the myofascial pain association with RSD?**

The majority of cases (56% to 61%) have a myofascial component associated with CRPS. Myofascial dysfunction is more prevalent in the affected upper extremity (69% to 70%) than the lower extremity (42% to 47%).

○   **What skeletal changes can occur?**

Patchy bone demineralization is observed in 50% of chronically affected patients, especially in a periarticular distribution. All these clinical features of CRPS may also be observed in patients with no history of pain however.

○   **What do plain radiographs reveal in CRPS?**

X-rays may show patchy periarticular demineralization within 3-6 weeks. The extent of osteoporosis is more than expected from disuse alone, and it is a common abnormality revealed on radiographs.

○   **What role does three-phase bone scan play in the diagnosis of CRPS?**

A 3-phase bone scan may be helpful both in revealing findings typical for the diagnosis of RSD and also in excluding other conditions that could cause the patient's symptoms. A false negative bone scan is fairly common. The 3-phase bone scan often is considered sensitive and specific, particularly in the early phase (less than 20 weeks) of the syndrome, but a study by Warner reports that the 3-phase bone scan has shown a diagnostic sensitivity of only 44%. Abnormal increased activity must be diffuse, not focal. The most suggestive and sensitive findings on bone scan include diffuse increased activity with juxta-articular accentuation uptake on the delayed images (Phase 3).Phases 1 and 2 are less sensitive and specific for RSD.

○   **What does thermography reveal in CRPS?**

This test (Infrared not liquid crystal) demonstrates limb temperature differences quantitatively, but it is nonspecific. Bruehl noted that thermography may be useful in situations where sensitivity and specificity are equally important; an asymmetry cutoff of 0.6°C appears optimal. If specificity is more important, a cutoff of 0.8°C or 1.0°C may be considered.

○   **What does sudomotor function testing reveal in CRPS?**

Sudomotor function testing: Chelimsky found that autonomic testing in 396 patients with pain demonstrated abnormalities in resting sweat output, resting skin temperature, and quantitative sudomotor axon reflex test predicted the diagnosis of CRPS I with 98% specificity.

○   **What do sweat tests reveal in CRPS?**

The sympathetic skin response (SSR) provides useful information on sudomotor dysfunction in patients with RSD; however, it is not possible yet to determine the final value of SSR for the diagnosis of RSD. Quantitative sudomotor axon reflex test (QSART): In QSART, the stimulated sweat output is greater and is prolonged when sympathetic hyperfunction is present.

○   **What do electrodiagnostic studies reveal in CRPS?**

Results of electromyography (EMG) and nerve conduction studies (NCS) typically are within the reference range in RSD. In fact, if the EMG and nerve studies identify a nerve lesion, by definition, the condition is not CRPS type I but still may be CRPS type II instead. Single fiber EMG examination also shows no definite abnormalities. The electrodiagnostic studies may be normal because C-fiber abnormalities cannot be well detected. Patients with allodynia (eg, extreme pain even when clothing touches the involved limb or when a breeze blows across it) may have a difficult time tolerating EMG and NCS.

○   **What does Quantitative sensory testing reveal in CRPS?**

The purpose of quantitative sensory testing (QST) is to quantify perception thresholds objectively. QST uses very precise reproducible stimuli, allowing comparison of symptomatic to asymptomatic areas, comparison to age-matched and sex-matched controls, and changes with time or treatment. This provides the physician with information about the severity and progression of the sensory dysfunction. The standard QST involves determination of vibrotactile detection thresholds, an Ab-fiber mediated sensation, cool detection thresholds, an A delta fiber–mediated sensation, and warm thermal thresholds, a C-fiber mediated sensation, in appropriate areas. Heat and cold pain thresholds also are obtained with the patient's permission and with the patient controlling the amount of stimulus applied.

O **What does Laser Doppler imaging reveal in CRPS?**

Laser Doppler imaging, with appropriate stressors, provides a simple, fast, noninvasive, and painless method for the study of segmental autonomic function. This type of imaging study provides excellent spatial information, eliminates many sources of artifact, and can be used to test skin autonomic reflexes bilaterally, both rapidly and repeatedly. Along with baseline images, mild stressors (inspiratory gasp, cold pressor positional dependency) are used to quantify skin vasoconstrictor reflexes. The first author has found these methods to be especially useful in helping to distinguish between sympathetically mediated and sympathetically independent pain conditions.

O **What role does diagnostic sympathetic ganglion block have in assessing CRPS?**

The IASP consensus group did not recognize response to sympathetic ganglion block as part of the diagnostic criteria for CRPS, since such responses, while often dramatic and impressive, are not universal. Further, response to such blocks is more indicative of sympathetically maintained pain, which includes other etiologies in addition to CRPS.

O **What is the primary goal of physical (PT) and occupational therapy (OT)**

The primary objective of physiotherapeutic modalities is goal-oriented functional restoration. The algorithm for physical and occupational therapy can be divided into four general steps that should be customized to individual needs: (1) desensitization of the affected region; (2) mobilization, edema control, and isometric strengthening; (3) stress loading, isotonic strengthening, range of motion, postural normalization, and aerobic conditioning; and (4) vocational and functional rehabilitation as well as ergonomic reconditioning. In general, progression through PT and OT will require concurrent application of psychological and pharmacological modalities. Despite the widespread conviction that physiotherapeutic modalities are beneficial for patients with CRPS, the effect of physiotherapy on the natural course of disease is unknown. To date, only the short-term efficacy of physical therapy compared with placebo therapy has been shown for patients with CRPS.

O **What is the role of behavioral medicine in CRPS rehabilitation?**

The recent International Association for the Study of Pain consensus report recommends that patients with pain less than 2 months in duration generally do not require formal psychological intervention. The panel of experts recommended that after 2 months, patients with CRPS should receive psychological evaluation, including psychometric testing, to identify and treat psychological disease, such as anxiety, depression, or personality disorder. All factors that contribute to patient disability should be determined. Counseling, behavioral modification, biofeedback, relaxation therapy, group therapy, and self-hypnosis should be considered. Therapies aimed at improving patient motivation and coping skills are necessary. For patients with pain longer than 6 months in duration, additional psychological testing maybe warranted. Despite the fact that principles derived from cognitive behavioral theory are effective for treatment of chronic pain in general, the value of cognitive–behavioral psychotherapy and psychometric testing specifically for patients with CRPS has not been fully determined.

O **Provide paradigms for the global treatment hierarchy for CRPS.**

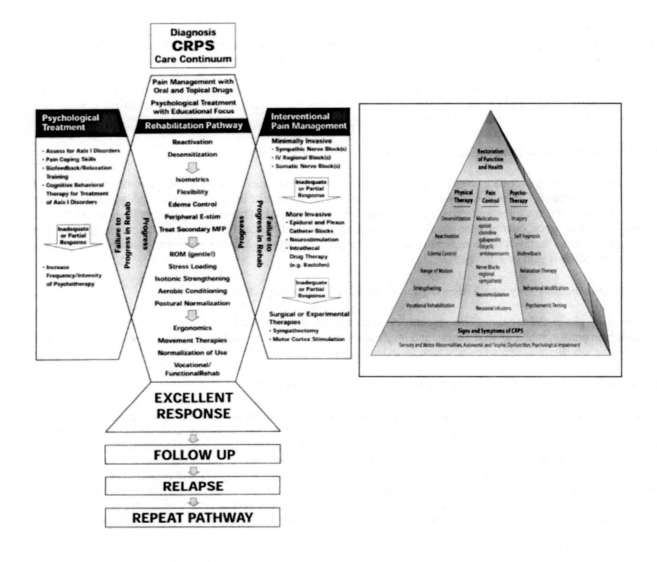

○ **What is the role of stellate ganglion and lumbar ganglion block in CRPS?**

Nerve blocks are recommended primarily to reduce pain and facilitate physiotherapy and functional rehabilitation Nevertheless, a retrospective study showed that the prophylactic use of stellate ganglion blocks in patients with a previous history of CRPS decreased recurrence rate of disease from 72% to 10% after reoperation on the affected extremity.

○ **What invasive therapies are available for CRPS?**

Implantable devices, such as spinal cord stimulators, are being increasingly used in intractable CRPS to produce symptomatic relief. Neuromodulatory modalities include peripheral nerve, spinal cord, and thalamic stimulation. The efficacy of most of these therapies has not been shown by placebo-controlled trials in CRPS patients. In a recent prospective, randomized, controlled study, patients with CRPS who received spinal cord stimulation combined with physiotherapy obtained greater pain relief and improvement in health-related quality of life compared with patients who received physiotherapy alone. Spinal cord stimulation produced analgesia in patients with CRPS who had undergone previous sympathectomy. The role of epidural or intrathecal opioid/clonidine/baclofen pump delivery may also ne considered in refractory cases before surgical interventions are selected.

○ **What surgical interventions may be considered?**

Surgical or chemical sympathectomy and radiofrequency ablation of sympathetic ganglia are options when conservative therapies have failed. The diagnosis of SMP should be confirmed with placebo controlled tests before considering sympathectomy as a therapeutic option. However, a potential risk of sympathectomy is the development of postsympathectomy neuralgia, which may represent denervation supersensitivity of adrenoceptors. Amputations of the affected limb have been performed for pain refractory to medical therapy, for limbs with recurrent infections, and to improve residual function. Unfortunately, relief of pain is achieved only in a minority of patients after amputation.

○   **What pharmacotherapies have had promising results?**

Oral corticosteroids (30- 40 mg of prednisone) in the first 4–6 weeks for two weeks may be useful to reduce the high turnover metabolic state. At present, however, calcitonin 100–160 IU daily for 4–8 weeks, followed by one injection every second day for 3–6 weeks is preferred to oral corticosteroids in the early stage, particular when urinary hydroxyproline excretion is increased and/or hyperdynamic blood flow is demonstrated.

○   **What other pharmacotherapies are available?**

Drug Category	Example of Drugs Used
Analgesics	Nonsteroidal anti-inflammatory drugs, corticosteroids (prednisone), tramadol (*Ultram*), opioids
Antidepressants	Amitriptyline (*Elavil*), doxepin (*Sinequan*), nortriptyline (*Pamelor*), trazodone (*Desyrel*)
Anticonvulsants	Carbamazepine (*Tegretol*), gabapentin (*Neurontin*), phenytoin (*Dilantin*), topiramate Topamax), lamotrigine (Lamictal), Levetiracetam (Keppra®), Zonisamide (Zonegran ®).
Antiarrhythmics	Mexiletine (*Mexitil*)
Calcitonin	Calcitonin injections (*Calcimar*)
Oral opioids (controversial)	Hydromorphone (*Dilaudid*), morphine, oxycodone (*Percocet*)
Sympathomimetics	Clonidine patch (*Catapres-TTS*), phentolamine IV (*Regitine*), epidural blocks, guanethidine (not available in the United States), bretylium (*Bretylol*), calcium channel blockers, beta-blockers, alpha-blockers
Muscle relaxants	Clonazepam (*Klonopin*), baclofen (*Lioresal*)
Topical analgesics	Capsaicin cream (*Zostrix*), lidocaine transdermal (*Lidoderm*)5% patches

OSTEOPOROSIS

○   **What is osteopenia?**

Osteopenia occurs when bone resorption exceeds bone formation no matter what the specific pathogenesis. Diffuse osteopenia is found in osteoporosis, osteomalacia, hyperparathyroidism, neoplasm, and a variety of other conditions.

○   **What is osteoporosis?**

Osteoporosis is established when the decrease in bone mass is greater than that expected for a person of a given age, sex, and race, and when it results in structural bone failure manifested by fractures.

○   **What are the current bone mineral density (BMD) definitions of osteoporosis?**

Condition	Definition
Normal	BMD is within 1 SD of a "young normal" adult (T score above -1)
Osteopenia	BMD is between 1 and 2.5 SD below that of a "young normal" adult (T score between -1 and -2.5)
Osteoporosis	BMD is 2.5 SD or more below that of a "young normal" adult (T score at or below -2.5)

○   **What risk factors are associated with osteoporosis?**

Advanced age
Female gender
Asian, white, or Hispanic ethnicity
Small body size/weight (<127 lb [57.7 kg])
Positive family history in first-degree relative(s)
Premature natural or surgical menopause
History of prolonged amenorrhea
Low calcium intake
Low vitamin D intake or exposure
Immobilization/sedentary lifestyle
Smoking
Alcoholism
Eating disorders (especially anorexia nervosa)

○   **Compare and contrast demographics for gender and osteoporosis and hip fracture**

**Osteoporosis and Risk of Hip Fracture in Men
and Women: A Comparison**

Factor	Men	Women
Peak bone mass	10 to 12% greater than in women	
Lifetime risk of hip fracture at age 50	6%	17.5%
Sex distribution of hip fractures worldwide	30%	70.0%
U.S. incidence of hip fracture at age 65	4 to 5 per 1,000	8 to 10 per 1,000
Mortality from hip fracture	31%	17.0%

○   **Where do osteoporotic fractures most frequently occur?**

These fractures are most typical in the spine, proximal portion of the femur, and distal portion of the radius; they are produced by trabecular or cortical bone loss, or both, depending on the site of involvement.

○   **What are the most frequent causes of generalized osteoporosis?**

Senescent osteoporosis and postmenopausal osteoporosis constitute the most common causes of generalized osteoporosis.

○   **How does bone mass change with age?**

The peak bone mass is approximately 20 per cent greater in men than in women and is greater in black than in white persons. In general, a gradual loss of skeletal mass occurs beginning in the fifth or sixth decade of life in men and in the fourth decade in women. After the age of about 50 years, bone loss takes place at a rate of 0.4 per cent each year in men; after the age of approximately 35 years, women lose bone at a yearly rate of 0.75 to 1 per cent, which increases to a rate of 2 to 3 per cent after the menopause. Up to the age of 80 years, women appear to be affected four times more frequently than men. After this age, there is no sex difference in the frequency of osteoporosis.

○   **What changes happen in trabecular and compact bone with age?**

Although loss of both compact and trabecular bone occurs in older men and women, the magnitude of the loss of compact bone in women after the menopause is much greater than that in men. Concomitant reduction of trabecular bone is evident, and the resulting diminution of bone mass produces a decrease in strength and a propensity to fracture.

○   **Is there an association between axial and appendicular osteoporosis?**

Generally it is reported that patients with osteoporosis in the vertebral column have a high frequency of femoral fracture, particularly in the transcervical and subtrochanteric regions of the femoral neck. The rate of occurrence of osteoporosis in older patients with such fractures has been estimated at 75 to 85 per cent. These fractures occur spontaneously or after minor trauma and may be accompanied by fractures of the ribs, humerus, or radius.

○   **What mechanisms may be responsible for involutional and postmenopausal osteoporosis?**

Microradiographic analysis has shown a striking increase in the resorptive surface, suggesting that excessive bone resorption is the fundamental abnormality in postmenopausal and senile osteoporosis. Even more recently, morphometric methods based on tetracycline-estimated rates of apposition have revealed impaired bone formation in many patients with osteoporosis.

○   **What deficiency may be responsible for postmenopausal osteoporosis?**

Estrogen deficiency resulting from menopause (or oophorectomy) has been implicated in the pathogenesis of such osteoporosis. The negative calcium balance relates principally to an increase in bone resorption and a reduction in the efficiency of calcium absorption.

○   **What clinical diseases and conditions contribute to secondary osteoporosis?**

Endocrine	Marrow Disorders	Gastrointestinal Disorders	Connective Tissue Disorders	Miscellaneous
Hypogonadism	Lymphoma	Gastrectomy	Marfan's syndrome	Immobilization
Hypercortisolism	Multiple myeloma	Malabsorption	Ehlers-Danlos syndrome	Chronic obstructive pulmonary disease
Hyperthyroidism	Disseminated carcinoma	Primary biliary cirrhosis or other	Kümmell's Disease	Radiation treatment
Hyperprolactinemia	Chronic alcoholism	Gastrectomy		Chronic renal disease/renal failure
Hyperparathyroidism		Anorexia nervosa		Rheumatoid arthritis
Diabetes mellitus		Severe malnutrition		Osteogenesis imperfecta

○   **What medications have been associated with secondary osteoporosis?**

Glucocorticoids
Excess thyroid hormone
Anticonvulsants (phenytoin, carbamazepine, phenobarbital)
Heparin
Cyclosporin A
Gonadotropin-releasing hormone analogues e.g. leuprolide
Highly active antiretroviral therapy for human immunodeficiency virus (HIV)
Chemotherapeutic agents causing Hypogonadism e.g. aromatase inhibitors
Excess vitamin A or D
Methotrexate
Loop diuretics e.g. furosemide
Neuroleptics, metoclopramide, and other drugs that raise prolactin

○   **What diagnostic work up is indicated for male patient with osteoporosis?**

Laboratory Evaluation for Osteoporosis in Men

Initial screening*	Additional tests†
Complete blood cell count	Serum protein electrophoresis to

Calcium	screen for multiple myeloma 24-hour
Phosphorus	urine collection to rule out
Alkaline phosphatase	hypocalciuria or hypercalciuria
Kidney and liver function tests	Estradiol level‡
Vitamin D (25-hydroxyvitamin D)	Parathyroid hormone to screen for
Thyroid-stimulating hormone level	hyperparathyroidism
Total testosterone	

O   **What is the mechanism for steroid induced osteoporosis?**

Histologic studies have revealed decreased bone formation and increased bone resorption, the latter being manifested as increased osteoclastic cell numbers, activity, and resorption sites. The decrease in rate of bone formation has been attributed to direct corticosteroid inhibition of osteoblast formation. Moderate doses of steroids decrease the synthesis of bone collagen by preexisting osteoblasts and the conversion of precursor cells to functioning osteoblasts. Laboratory analysis reveals negative calcium balance and hypercalciuria.

O   **Compare the overall demographics of gender associated osteoporosis as it relates to age**

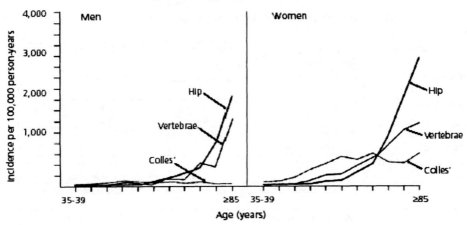

O   **How do vertebral fractures manifest clinically?**

Vertebral fractures typically present with acute back pain after sudden bending, lifting or coughing but fractures may be asymptomatic and just present with progressive kyphosis. Most vertebral fractures occur in the middle and lower thoracic and upper lumbar spine; most commonly the twelfth thoracic and first lumbar vertebrae. The pain associated with fracture is variable in quality and may be sharp, dull or nagging and is often aggravated by movements. The pain tends to be localized to the fracture site but may radiate anteriorly into the abdomen. However, radiation down into the legs is uncommon. Acute episodes of pain usually settle after 4–6 weeks; severe back pain which persists for many weeks is unusual and the diagnosis of uncomplicated vertebral fracture should be questioned when this occurs.

O   **Are all vertebral compression fractures symptomatic?**

In some cases vertebral fracture is painless and discovered as an incidental finding; loss of height may be a more objective measure of fracture in these patients.

O   **What chronic problems may arise a result of vertebral compression fractures?**

Further or multiple fractures may occur at variable intervals ranging from months to years in some patients (crush fracture syndrome) leading to continuous dull back pain often in association with progressive dorsal kyphosis.. Back pain in this situation usually arises from the apophyseal joints.

O   **What factors predispose to proximal radius and femur fractures?**

Fractures of the distal forearm and proximal femur usually follow falls. Factors, which increase the likelihood of falling include: poor vision, impaired coordination, abnormal gait, associated neurologic and rheumatic diseases, and use of sedatives and other drugs. Approximately 30% of subjects aged 65 years or older will fall once or more per year but only 3% will sustain a fracture.

○ **Does the direction of a fall influence the type of fracture sustained?**

Falls forward are more likely to result in Colles' fractures and falls backwards are more likely to result in hip fractures.

○ **What other fractures may occur in osteoporosis?**

Rib fractures, pubic rami and sacral fractures occur in osteoporosis.

○ **How do compression fractures of the vertebrae affect height?**

Each complete compression fracture causes about one centimeter loss in height and in severe cases with multiple fractures height loss of between 10–20 cm may occur.

○ **What features may be encountered in the vertebral radiographic assessment of osteoporosis?**

In the spine radiographic evidence of reduced bone mass, evident as increased radiolucency and sometimes referred to as osteopenia, may be apparent before fracture, but as up to 30% of bone mineral may be lost before this is apparent radiographically, this sign is not always present. Other radiologic features include accentuation of vertebral endplates and prominence of vertical trabeculae due to relative loss of horizontal trabeculae. Changes in the shape of vertebral bodies usually suggest fracture and may consist of anterior wedging (loss of anterior height with normal posterior height), biconcave or 'codfish' vertebrae (loss of mid vertebral height) or crush/compression fracture (overall loss of vertebral height).

○ **What is the most sensitive finding on X-ray of a thoracic vertebral compression fracture?**

Diagnosis of fracture based upon a reduction in anterior, posterior or mid vertebral height of 15–20% appear most sensitive. Wedging, biconcavity and compression may all be apparent in the same patient. Herniation of the intervertebral disc into the vertebral body (Schmorl's nodes) can also occur in osteoporosis.

○ **What radiographic features may be encountered in the long bones of patients with osteoporosis?**

Long bones may show cortical thinning due to endosteal resorption. In the pelvis and ribs, osteoporosis is manifest by increased radiolucency, abnormal trabecular structure and cortical thinning.

○ **Compare the diagnostic modalities used to assess BMD**

Method	Utility	Versatility	Ease	Availability	Cost	Radiation Dose
RA	+	-	+	-	+	+
SXA	+	-	++	-	+	+
pDXA	+	-	++	+	+	+
DXA	+	++	+	+	-	+
QCT	++	-	-	-	-	-
pQCT	+	-	+	-	-	+
QUS	+	-	++	+	+	++

Abbreviations: DXA, full-table dual X-ray absorptiometry; QCT, quantitative computed tomography; QUS, quantitative ultrasonography; pDXA, peripheral dual X-ray absorptiometry; RA, radiographic absorptiometry; SXA, single X-ray absorptiometry; +, good; ++, excellent; -, poor.

○　**What do data of racial differences in BMD measurement reveal?**

Available data suggest a descending scale of bone density according to race as follows: Blacks > Polynesians > Hispanics > Caucasians > Asians.

○　**What are useful indications for the measurement of osteoporosis?**

The most useful indications for bone density studies involve prediction of fracture risk. As bone density declines, fracture risk increases. A decrease in bone mass of 1 standard deviation is associated with a 50% to 100% increase in fracture incidence. Bone mass measurement is clinically useful in identifying estrogen-deficient women with low bone mass so that appropriate decisions can be made with regard to medication such as anti-resorptive therapy. If bone mineral density is 1 standard deviation below the mean as compared to the density in premenopausal women, treatment can be recommended to decrease fracture risk. No intervention for fracture prevention is necessary if density is more than 1 standard deviation above the mean.

○　**What is the most often selected treatment for postmenopausal women with osteoporosis?**

Medications used to prevent and treat osteoporosis fall into two categories: drugs that inhibit bone resorption (antiresorptive agents) and drugs that stimulate bone formation (anabolic agents). Five antiresorptive agents have Federal Drug Administration (FDA) approved labeling for use in the prevention or treatment of osteoporosis: the bisphosphonates, alendronate and Risedronate; the selective estrogen-receptor modulator (SERM), raloxifene; calcitonin, and estrogen. The only anabolic agent with FDA approval is teriparatide

○　**What are the bisphosphonates?**

Bisphosphonates are a class of synthetic compounds that are analogues of pyrophosphate, a physiologic inhibitor of bone mineralization. These compounds adhere to the hydroxyapatite content of bone and are important inhibitors of osteoclastic bone resorption.

○　**How do the bisphosphonates impact osteoporosis?**

Bisphosphonates increase the bone density in women with postmenopausal osteoporosis by about 5% to 10% over 1 year, after which bone density plateaus.

○　**What other agents are used in managing osteoporosis?**

Calcitonin- injectable/nasal spray, raloxifene, calcium, vitamin D

○　**What are the recommendations regarding calcium supplementation?**

The National Osteoporosis Foundation recommends 1500 mg of elemental calcium daily for post-menopausal women who are not taking estrogen.

○　**What are the recommendations regarding vitamin D therapy in osteoporosis?**

The primary function of vitamin D is to increase active intestinal calcium absorption. The current United States Dietary Reference Intake (DRI) from the National Academy of Sciences recommendation for vitamin D intake in persons aged 51 to 70 years is 10 µg per day (400 IU/day). Higher doses of vitamin D (800–1000 IU/day) in elderly persons (age ≥ 65y) may be required for optimal bone health.

○　**Summarize the pharmacotherapeutic options for osteoporosis.**

Clinical Presentation	Drug regimen	Comments
History of fragility fractures, osteoporosis by BMD criteria	Calcium, 1,500 mg/d; vitamin D, 800 units/d	All patients with osteoporosis should be given adequate calcium and vitamin D
	Alendronate (Fosamax) 5-10 mg/d (or 70 mg once weekly); risedronate (Actonel), 5 mg/d or 35 mg/week	Potent bisphosphonates are associated with ~50% reductions in vertebral and non-vertebral fractures
	Raloxifene (Evista), 60 mg/d	50% reduction in vertebral fracture was observed
	Calcitonin nasal spray (Miacalcin), 200 IU/d	Calcitonin led to ~50% reduction in vertebral fracture; no apparent effect on non-vertebral fracture was observed
	Parathyroid hormone: hPTH (1-34), 20 mcg/d for 18 months	Substantial improvement in BMD and 60% reduction in vertebral and non-vertebral fractures in recent clinical trials were observed.
Fragility fractures but normal to high BMD	No indicated therapy	Fractures may be unrelated to osteoporosis
No fracture history but low BMD	Same drugs as above	Those with BMD T-scores >(-)2 may be managed with calcium and vitamin D alone
Low BMD, no fractures, but at risk for bone loss in near future (early menopause, starting glucocorticoids)	Alendronate, 5mg/d; 35mg/week; risedronate, 5mg/d or 35mg/week; raloxifene 60 mg/d	Depending on the circumstances, all these agents are indicated for prevention of bone loss leading to osteoporosis.
Disorders requiring more than brief administration of glucocorticosteroids, (also cyclosporines and tacrolimus) including patients undergoing organ transplantation	Alendronate (Fosamax), 5-10 mg/d 35-70mg/week; risedronate, 5 mg/d or 35 mg/week	Potent bisphosphonates conserve BMD and protect against fractures in glucocorticoid related osteoporosis

Abbreviations: BMD, bone mineral density; d, day; hPTH, human parathyroid hormone; IU, International Units; mg, milligrams; mcg, micrograms.

O   **What are the physiological benefits of therapeutic exercise in osteoporosis?**

Weight bearing exercises promote bone growth by increasing mechanical load and stress on bone. Walking decreases bone loss in the trabecular bone of the spine. Strength training results in preservation of bone mineral density and increases muscle mass, strength, and balance.

O   **What are the appropriate elements of a therapeutic exercise program for osteoporosis patients?**

A recommended exercise program should include trunk extension and isometric exercises, upper and lower body resistance training and postural and flexibility education. Stretching of the pectoral and intercostal muscles is helpful for improving chest expansion. Exercises should be performed at least two or three times per week. Walking, biking, and calisthenics are effective and often advised. Dancing, performed several times weekly, leads to increased spinal bone density and can also be considered.

O   **What is Percutaneous vertebroplasty (PV)?**

Percutaneous vertebroplasty (PV) involves the percutaneous injection of polymethylmethacrylate (PMMA) into the site of the vertebral fracture. The cement hardens, stabilizing the fracture.

O   **What is Percutaneous kyphoplasty (PK)?**

Percutaneous kyphoplasty (PK) involves a similar technique. However, the collapse and wedging of the compression fracture is initially "reduced" by the placement of an inflatable balloon catheter into the vertebral body. The balloon is inflated, restoring vertebral height and diminishing anterior wedging of the vertebral body. Inflation of the balloon also creates a cavity within the vertebral body that can then be filled with injected PMMA.

○   What is the efficacy for PV and PK?

These procedures stabilize the fracture, and provide nearly immediate pain relief in 90% to 100% of patients. In addition, kyphoplasty restores vertebral height by almost 50% in approximately 70% of patients.

○   What are the complications associated with these procedures?

The complication rates associated with PV and PK are 1% to 3% for treatment of osteoporotic fractures.

Hemorrhage
Rib or vertebral posterior element fracture
Transient fever
Worsening of pain for several hours after the procedure caused by heat generated cement polymerization
Nerve root irritation
Cement embolization to the lungs via the paravertebral venous plexus;
Pneumothorax for thoracic lesions
Infection

○   What is the role of spinal orthosis in the management of osteoporotic fractures of the vertebral column?

Spinal orthoses may be used in two stages of management of osteoporosis patients. The principle of bracing during the acute stage is to provide spine immobilization in extension posturing through necessary trunk contact. The main objective of bracing during the chronic stage is to assist or substitute for the compromised postural muscles and ligaments of the spine. Bracing also may be considered when bone loss is severe and when further compression fractures may develop during conventional daily activities.

○   What is the postural training support?

Spinal orthoses, such as the postural training support (PTS) can be helpful by decreasing kyphotic posture through counteracting the anterior compressive forces that are exerted on the vertebral bodies. Improvement of body mechanics, which includes proper static and dynamic posturing and prevention of kyphosis, is a major component of treatment. A PTS of minimal weight (1 to 2 pounds) applied below the scapulae and above the waistline biomechanically shifts the upper trunk from a forward position to a more neutral position. This will reduce the exaggerated compressive forces on the lower thoracic spine that are induced through the weight of the head and upper trunk structures.

○   What strategies may compensate for impaired balance in the patient with osteoporosis?

Osteoporotic patients, especially those with kyphosis, have unique difficulties in maintaining balance. Dynamic and standing balance can often be improved with instruction in particular balance strategies, as well as the use of ambulatory devices. Tai Chi has proven effective in this regard. Home modifications such as improved lighting, removal of throw rugs, and installment of grab bars may improve safety. Visual impairment, if present, should be corrected. Because poor depth perception and reduced ability to perceive contrast appear to pose more of a risk than poor acuity, environmental adjustments may be most beneficial. Modification of the risk of falling should remain an essential component of treatment in the osteoporotic patient.

○   Summarize the treatment of osteoporosis in men

Treatment of Osteoporosis in Men
Medications and supplements
Calcium, 1,000 to 1,500 mg per day

Vitamin D, 400 to 800 IU per day
Bisphosphonates
Alendronate (Fosamax), 10 mg per day or 70 mg per week,
at a cost of $62 to $66.50 per month*
Risedronate (Actonel), 5 mg per day, at a cost of $67 per month*
Teriparatide (Forteo), 20 mcg per day, at a cost of $560 per month*
Other
Physical therapy evaluation and instruction for cane or walker use
Regular exercise to increase muscle tone, improve balance
Occupational therapy to assess home fall risk
Avoidance of tobacco and excess alcohol
Decrease fall risk—review of medications, especially antihypertensive
agents

TOTAL JOINT ARTHROPLASTY

O   **What are indications for total hip prostheses?**

Total joint replacement arthroplasty is indicated in individuals with a painful, disabling arthritic joint that is no longer responsive to conservative treatment.

O   **What does the total hip prosthesis consist of?**

The total hip prosthesis commonly consists of a metal femoral stem component articulating with an ultra-high-molecular-weight polyethylene (UHMWPE) acetabular cup. The stem may be fixed to the head or, in the modular designs, stems and heads of different sizes may be interchanged.

O   **What structural elements are used in designing weight bearing articulating surface components?**

Weight bearing articular surfaces are most often fabricated of cobalt-chromium-molybdenum alloy because of its greater wear resistance, whereas implant components such as the femoral stem of hip implants are sometimes made of titanium alloy because its modulus of elasticity is nearer that of bone, thereby potentially causing less stress shielding of the adjacent bone. Also, titanium alloys may form a more intimate bond with bone. The use of ceramic (aluminum oxide or zirconium oxide) femoral heads articulating with polyethylene acetabular components is gaining proponents because these ceramics have excellent frictional and wear characteristics with polyethylene.

O   **What is PMMA (Polymethylmethacrylate)?**

It is a space filling, load-transferring material, technically described as a grout or lute. It does not bond chemically to bone, nor to the surface of metal components, nor to UHMWPE under operative conditions. PMMA can withstand considerable compression but fails more readily under tension or shear forces, since it is about three times stronger in compression than in tension. In a sense, it has the qualities (and the orthopaedic uses and limitations) of the mortar between the bricks of a building. If the cement is not tightly packed between the bone and the implant components, and if gaps or spaces are left between the surfaces, the cement may break because it will be partly subjected to shear and tension rather than pure compression.

O   **How is PMMA secured?**

Mechanical bonding is then accomplished by applying pressure to the PMMA to force it into the textured spaces or pores on the implant surface. Similarly, PMMA bonds securely to cancellous bone if, while it is in the low viscosity (semi-liquid or creamy) state, it is forced into the interstices of the bone. A secure mechanical bond is extremely important because it prevents motion at the bone-cement interface.

O   **What are the consequences of motion at the cement interface?**

Motion results in poor load transfer and also can generate and distribute wear debris. These phenomena can result in bone absorption, component loosening, and even bone or component fracture.

○   How do PMMA fixation and non PMMA fixation compare?

In total joint arthroplasty PMMA bone cement is used to fix the components securely in bone and to distribute loads evenly from the surface of the components to the bone surface, thereby reducing stress (force per unit area) in the supporting bone. Without cement, in a press fit situation, it is more likely that load will be transferred at a few small points of contact, resulting in higher bone stresses at these locations.

○   What features of porous coating of arthroplasty components are clinical significant?

Bone ingrowth occurs most readily if three criteria are met: the pores are greater than 40 mm in diameter, micro motion is absent, and the porous surface is in intimate contact with bone. Bone ingrowth will provide stability; fibrous tissue ingrowth may provide some stability, but it is less ideal for a three-dimensional interlock. Macro motion may cause the development of a smooth membrane that will encapsulate the component without ingrowth and progressively result in loosening.

○   What is the advantage of porous coated components?

In revision and post mortem, histological sections from coated implants consistently demonstrated direct bone-implant contact without an intervening fibrous membrane over most of the implant surface. The two most widely evaluated materials are hydroxyapatite (HA) and tricalcium phosphate (TCP). hydroxyapatite ceramic or tricalcium phosphate.

○   What is a limitation of porous coated implants?

With porous coated hip implants, weight bearing may be restricted for 6 weeks and progression to full weight bearing begins only at 8-12 weeks to allow for enough bony interdigitation to avoid micro motion. The components are initially held rigidly to bone by being "press fit" or by the use of screws. More recent follow up studies suggest that immediate weight bearing as tolerated is not associated with accelerated loosening over time.

○   What are implant related complications?

The current view is that the predominant, long-term cause of failure of hip or knee replacement appears to be particulate wear debris, which stimulates macrophages to produce substances eliciting osteoclastic bone resorption. Wear debris also may contribute to loosening of total knee and other joint arthroplasty components in a similar fashion.

○   Why is infection at the implant site problematic?

Another implant-related complication is infection. Implant surfaces and metallic wear debris and corrosion products may lower the local resistance to infection. Also, if bacteria adhere to implant surfaces, they are more difficult to treat with antibiotics than the same entities present in intercellular space or body fluids.

○   What are the issues impacting the risk of infection in arthroplasty surgery?

With respect to infections in general, the use of prophylactic antibiotics, laminar flow operating enclosures, body exhaust suits for the surgical team, and other measures currently keep the early infection rate of total joint implants to less than 1%. However, when a total joint arthroplasty becomes infected, it is a catastrophic complication that usually requires one or more major surgical procedures, prolonged hospitalization, and high cost in patient morbidity and economic outlay.

○   What is the role of antibiotic prophylaxis?

A number of surgeons have reported a significant decrease in the infection rate when prophylactic antibiotics are used. Wilson, Aglietti, and Salvati reported a decrease from about 11% to 1%. Lidwell et al. found the incidence of joint sepsis to be 0.1% when clean air systems and body exhaust suits were combined with prophylactic antibiotics. The antibiotics most often prescribed are the cephalosporins and the synthetic penicillins. Antibiotics are continued intraoperatively for lengthy procedures and for 24 to 48 hours postoperatively.

O **What is the preferred surgery in younger active patients with hip disease?**

Arthrodesis is often the preferred operative choice for young, vigorous patients with unilateral hip disease and especially for young, active boys or men with avascular necrosis or degenerative arthritis secondary to femoral neck fracture or a slipped capital femoral epiphysis. The patient often can lead an active life after the hip has been fused in the proper position. Techniques of arthrodesis with internal fixation that do not require spica cast immobilization make arthrodesis more acceptable to many patients. If necessary at a later age, the arthrodesis can be converted to a total hip arthroplasty.

O **What weight bearing guidelines are commonly used after THA?**

The consensus is to begin active physical rehabilitation on the first postoperative day with the patient being helped to sit up. Bed mobility and transfer training, if tolerated, are initiated. With cemented prostheses, weight bearing as tolerated is generally started immediately unless the quality of the bone stock was poor. With uncemented porous coated femoral components, controversy still exists as to the initiation of weight bearing immediately after surgery.

O **When can patients progress to full weight bearing (FWB)?**

The patient should be fully weight bearing by 8-12 weeks. The extent of weight bearing must be determined by communication with the orthopedic surgeon.

O **How does the use of bone grafts influence the timing of weight bearing in THA?**

Longer, limited weight-bearing periods are required if bone grafts were used. The mean consolidation time is 4 months for morselized cancellous grafts and 11 months for allografts that are larger than 3 cm.

O **What requirement regarding ambulation must be met before the patient with THA is discharged?**

Safe walking with a walker or crutches outside the parallel bars is essential before the patient may be discharged home.

O **How do standard and rolling walkers compare for the THA patient?**

A rolling walker allows a reciprocal gait pattern in patients who are allowed full weight bearing. It also obviates the need to lift the device to advance it, which may be painful in patients with upper extremity impairments. Also, a rolling walker requires 50% less energy than a standard walker to walk the same distance. However, a rolling walker is more difficult to use on carpet, particularly if the wheels are small. A standard walker is better for patients who 1) are not allowed full weight bearing, 2) cannot tolerate full weight bearing, or 3) tend to fall forward.

O **Which exercise may be ill advised for the THA patient?**

Straight-leg raising should be avoided after use of the uncemented technique because it increases stress on the hip.

O **What precautions are necessary in a posterolateral surgical approach for THA?**

Patients in whom a posterolateral approach was used must be carefully taught not to internally rotate, adduct, or flex their hips to more than 70 to 90 degrees. These motions force the head of the femur toward the weakened area of surgical exposure and capsulotomy and dislocation will more likely occur.

O **What are the precautions in an anterior or lateral approach?**

Patients in whom an anterior or lateral approach with an anterior capsulotomy was used must avoid hyperextension as well as external rotation and adduction, especially when getting out of bed on the surgical side.

O **What is multidirectional instability?**

Multidirectional instability, that is, the potential to dislocate in any direction, may be present when there is insufficient tension or strength in the surrounding soft tissues to keep the femoral head in the acetabular component. This may be seen following revision surgery where the exposure is wide, or when prosthesis with a relatively short neck has been used. A lower extremity that is internally rotated and with a shortened femoral neck may lead to a posteriorly dislocating hip; a leg that is extremely externally rotated with the hip extended may lead to an anterior dislocation.

O   **What radiographs should be obtained to assess for dislocation?**

If there is any question of a dislocation having occurred, an x-ray study of the hip, including an anteroposterior view and a crossed-leg lateral view (which does not require moving the affected limb between views), is mandatory.

O   **What precautions are taken for a trochanteric osteotomy?**

The use of a direct lateral (Hardinge) or trans-trochanter incision with osteotomy of the greater trochanter requires that no active abduction exercises performed.

O   **What preoperative exercises and education are appropriate?**

Preoperatively, instruct the patient in respiratory exercises, isometric gluteal and quadriceps sets, ankle pumps, and total hip precautions (THPs).

O   **What rehabilitation occurs in the acute phase?**

During the acute recovery phase (PO Days 0 to 5)

1. Maintain strict THPs
2. Begin isometrics and straight-plane isotonic exercises
3. Begin reconditioning exercises to unaffected extremities
4. Begin transfers to the unaffected side
5. Begin assisted ambulation on level surfaces
6. Use appropriate dressing and toileting equipment.

O   **What rehabilitation occurs in the 1st week post operative phase?**

From day 1-7 postoperatively
1. Maintain strict THPs
2. Add light resistance to the exercise program
3. Begin working on speed as well as control
4. Begin isotonic exercise in standing posture if FWB
5. Begin prone-lying to stretch out hip flexors
6. Emphasize independence in bed mobility and transfers
7. Ambulate in all directions with appropriate device
8. Emphasize independence in basic ADL (with device).

O   **What rehabilitation occurs in the period of 2-4 weeks postoperatively?**

From 2 to 4 weeks postoperatively
1. Maintain strict THPs
2. Progress resistive exercise when appropriate
3. Customize the program to the patient's interests
4. Stretch out hip flexors and Achilles tendon
5. Teach car transfers
6. Advance patients with uncemented THAs to FWB on physician's orders
7. Ambulate for progressive distance and speed
8. Emphasize independence in basic ADL (with device)

O   **What rehabilitation occurs in the 4-12 week phase?**

From 4 to 12 weeks postoperatively

1. Maintain THPs, but less strictly
2. Return to driving, sexual activity, part-time work
3. Continue progressive resistive exercise
4. Begin developmental sequence with THPs
5. Begin high-level gait activities
6. Begin proprioceptive and balance activities
7. Normalize gait pattern on all surfaces
8. Work on ambulation velocity and maneuvering ability
9. Begin instrumental ADL, wean off assistive devices.

○   **What is the incidence of dislocation and its risk factors?**

Although dislocations are uncommon, an incidence of approximately 3%, they usually occur early in the postoperative period. Dislocation precautions should however be observed for *at least* 8 to 12 weeks. Several factors may contribute to this risk, including (1) a history of previous hip surgery or revision total hip replacement, (2) a posterior surgical approach, (3) faulty positioning of one or both components, (4) impingement of the femur on the pelvis or residual osteophytes, (5) impingement of the neck of the femoral component on the margin of the socket, (6) inadequate soft tissue tension, (7) insufficient or weak abductor muscles, (8) avulsion or nonunion of the greater trochanter, and (9) noncompliance or extremes of positioning in the perioperative period. Age, height, weight, and preoperative diagnosis do not appear to be causative factors. However, in many series, dislocation occurred in women more often than in men.

○   **When should a THA patient return to driving?**

Arthroplasty patients require a minimum of 3 weeks following surgery to recover normal reaction time on the left side of the operation. The patient with right THA should be allowed to resume driving at 8 weeks postoperatively. However, many surgeons, as a matter of personal preference, suggest waiting for the period of dislocation precautions (i.e., 8–12 weeks) before allowing their patients to drive.

○   **What impairments of strength occur after THA?**

Gait analysis and force-plate data suggest that recovery of strength in the musculature about the hip is a prolonged process. Between 3 and 6 months after surgery, muscle strength is still only 50% of normal. Long et al. reported persistent weakness in all patients at 2 years, supporting the need for a prolonged, supervised exercise regimen.

○   **What occupational guidelines may be used with THA patients?**

Many patients with sedentary occupations can return to work after 4 to 8 weeks. At 3 months they can return to occupations requiring limited lifting and bending. It is precarious to encourage patients to return to manual labor after total hip arthroplasty.

○   **What guidelines are given for patients with athletic inclinations?**

Limited athletic activity is permitted. Swimming, cycling, and golfing are acceptable. Jogging, racquet sports, and other activities requiring repetitive impact loading or extremes of positioning of the hip are unwise, and patients should be warned that such activities increase the risk of failure of the arthroplasty.

○   **What nerve injuries may occur in association with THA?**

The sciatic, femoral, obturator and peroneal nerves may be injured by direct surgical trauma, traction, pressure from retractors, extremity positioning, limb lengthening or thermal or pressure injury from cement. The incidence of nerve injury has been reported to be 0.7% to 3.5% in primary arthroplasties. Amstutz et al. reported a 7.5% incidence of nerve palsies after revision procedures.

○   **Why is sciatic nerve injury more common in revision arthroplasty?**

The surgical exposure for a revision procedure usually is technically difficult. The sciatic nerve may be bound within scar tissue posteriorly and is susceptible to direct injury during the exposure. Injudicious retraction of firm, noncompliant soft tissues along the posterior edge of the acetabulum may cause a stretch injury or direct contusion of the nerve.

O   What pattern of nerve injury is most common?

Based on clinical and electromyographic studies, investigators concluded that subclinical nerve injury is the rule rather than the exception and in most instances is caused by surgical trauma. More recently, another group of investigators used somatosensory evoked potential (SSEP) to monitor the sciatic nerve during revision procedures. Neurological compromise was noted in 32% of patients, primarily caused by excessive retraction during exposure of the posterior aspect of the acetabulum or by extremes of positioning of the extremity for femoral cement removal. No patient had clinically apparent nerve palsy after surgery.

O   What complication should be considered in the presence of a complete sciatic neuropathy?

Subgluteal hematoma should be suspected in patients with pain, tense swelling, and tenderness in the buttock and thigh and with evidence of a sciatic nerve deficit.

O   What may account for isolated peroneal nerve injuries?

Postoperative positioning may cause isolated peroneal nerve palsy. Triangular abduction pillows usually are secured to the extremity with straps, which, if applied tightly over the region of the fibular neck, may cause peroneal nerve compression.

O   Are vascular injuries common in THA?

Vascular injuries as a result of total hip arthroplasty are rare (0.2% to 0.3%).

O   How should hematomas be managed in THA?

The main object of treatment is to prevent a secondary infection of the hematoma; bacterial contamination must be prevented, and prophylactic antibiotics are indicated until the hematoma has resolved. Usually observation is the only other treatment required. Hematomas should not be drained in the patient's room by aspiration or by removing several sutures. In the rare instances in which a hematoma must be evacuated because of marked stretching of the skin, excessive pain, sciatic neuropathy, or the need to ligate a bleeding vessel, the procedure must be carried out in the operating room under sterile conditions. If the skin over the hematoma becomes necrotic, the potential for infection is greater. Local debridement and repeat wound closure are indicated to reduce the risk of infection.

O   What is the incidence of bladder infections after THA?

Bladder infection is the most common complication involving the urinary tract, and its reported incidence is 7% to 14% after total hip arthroplasty.

O   What problems may be of concern with leg length discrepancy?

A correlation between leg length discrepancy and the onset of lower back symptoms has not been documented. Likewise, increased joint reaction force and premature mechanical failure have not been linked to leg length discrepancy. However, leg lengthening in excess of approximately 1 cm frequently is a source of significant patient dissatisfaction despite an otherwise technically satisfactory operation, and the degree of dissatisfaction is vastly underestimated by the commonly used hip rating systems. In such cases a heel or shoe lift may partially correct discomfort and gait disturbance.

O   Once a dislocation occurs what conservative management may be pursued?

If the components are in satisfactory position, closed reduction is followed by a period of brief bed rest in abduction. Subsequently a prefabricated abduction orthosis that maintains the hip in 15 degrees of abduction and prevents flexion past 60 degrees, although removable devices are not practical in noncompliant patients. Immobilization for 6 weeks to 3 months is recommended.

O   **What is the incidence of HO after THA?**

The incidence of this complication averages about 13% but varies from about 3%, as reported by Collis and Johnson, to 50% as reported by Riegler and Harris. It usually is painless but may restrict motion to a varying extent; usually it has little clinical significance. It is higher in patients with seronegative spondyloarthropathies.

O   **Does it adversely affect functional outcome in THA?**

Marked limitation of motion or bony ankylosis is uncommon, and significant loss of function has been reported in only 2% to 7%. Loss of motion is the predominant functional limitation resulting from heterotopic ossification. It does not cause limp or loss of strength. An operation to remove the heterotopic bone rarely is indicated because pain usually is not severe, and excision of established heterotopic bone is a difficult procedure.

O   **What is the morbidity and mortality of venous thromboembolic disease in THA?**

Thromboembolic disease is the most common serious complication arising from total hip arthroplasty. It is the most common cause of death occurring within 3 months of surgery and is responsible for more than 50% of the postoperative mortality after total hip arthroplasty. Deep vein thrombosis also can lead to postphlebitic syndrome in the lower extremities. The mortality rate for emboli in total hip arthroplasty patients who do not receive prophylactic medication is reported to be five times greater than that for abdominal and thoracic surgery in patients in the same age group. On the basis of objective criteria and with no prophylactic medication, the incidence of deep vein thrombosis is more than twice that observed after general abdominal surgery.

O   **What is the incidence of VTE disease associated with THA?**

Without prophylaxis, venous thrombosis occurs after total hip replacement in as many as 40% to 70% of patients, and fatal pulmonary emboli occur in approximately 2%. This data includes both asymptomatic and symptomatic VTE.

O   **Where does thromboembolism manifest?**

Thromboembolism may occur in vessels in the pelvis, thigh, and calf. Most thrombi probably develop in the deep veins in the calf and subsequently extend into the thigh, but isolated thrombi in the pelvis or deep femoral veins may develop. Eighty percent to 90% of thromboses occur in the operated limb. Thrombi in the calf alone previously were thought to be unlikely to cause pulmonary emboli. However, proximal propagation of calf thromboses occurs in as many as 30% of patients, and investigators found that 31% of patients with untreated calf thrombosis developed clinically significant pulmonary emboli 3 to 8 weeks after surgery.

O   **What are the temporal features of thromboembolic disease in THA?**

The temporal relationship of deep vein thrombosis and pulmonary embolism to surgery remains controversial. The first diagram represents the temporal rate of DVT. The second diagram represents the temporal rate of pulmonary embolism.

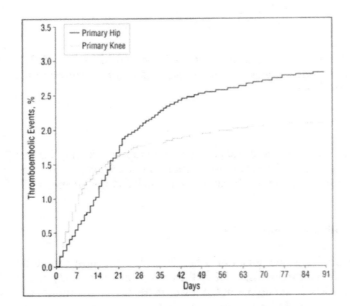

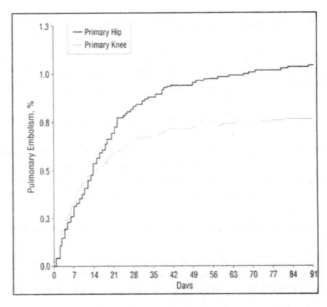

○   **What are the 7ᵗʰ ACCP guidelines for VTE prophylaxis in THA and TKA?**

In summary for patients undergoing elective THA the seventh ACCP conference proposes the following recommendations regarding anticoagulants: (1) LMWH (at a usual high-risk dose, started 12 h before surgery or 12 to 24 h after surgery, or 4 to 6 h after surgery at half the usual high-risk dose and then increasing to the usual high-risk dose the following day); (2) fondaparinux (2.5 mg started 6 to 8 h after surgery); or (3) adjusted-dose vitamin K antagonists (VKA) started preoperatively or the evening after surgery (INR target, 2.5; INR range, 2.0 to 3.0). The use of aspirin as a thromboprophylaxis agent is controversial. The seventh ACCP Consensus Conference statement does not recommend aspirin as sole prophylaxis for any surgical procedure.

○   **What other complications can occur in THA?**

Periprosthetic fractures, early and late infection, loosening and stem failure.

○   **How many TKA designs are used?**

There are three basic types of total knee arthroplasty: totally constrained, semi constrained, and totally unconstrained. The amount of constraint built into an artificial joint reflects the amount of stability that the hardware itself provides. As such, a totally constrained joint has the femoral portion physically attached to the tibial component and requires no ligamentous or soft tissue support. The semi constrained total knee arthroplasty has two separate components that glide on each other, but the physical characteristics of the tibial component prevent excessive femoral glide. The totally unconstrained device relies completely on the body's ligaments and soft tissues to maintain the stability of the joint.

○   **Which are used most frequently?**

Although three designs are available, the semi-constrained knee implants and the totally unconstrained knee implants are most often utilized. In general, the totally unconstrained implants afford the most normal range of motion and gait.

○   **What is unicompartmental TKA?**

Unicompartmental knee arthroplasty replaces the joint surfaces on one side of the knee only (usually the medial compartment). Unicompartmental knee arthroplasty provides better relief than tibial osteotomy and greater range of motion than does a total knee arthroplasty as well as improved ambulation velocity.

○   **What are key epidemiological factors associated with TKA?**

The most frequent principal diagnoses associated with total knee replacement procedures are osteoarthrosis and allied disorders (90.9%) followed by rheumatoid arthritis and other inflammatory poly arthropathies (3.4%). The knee is the joint most often replaced in arthroplasty procedures. The most common age group for total knee replacements is 65 to 84. Women in this age range are more likely to undergo total knee arthroplasty than their male counterparts.

O   **What preoperative rehabilitation should be considered?**

Preoperatively, instruct the patient in respiratory exercises, isometric knee exercises, transfers, and crutch-walking.

O   **What does the rehabilitation consist of during days 1-3 postoperatively?**

1. Check wound for drainage and check skin for areas of breakdown
2. Apply ice, compression, and elevation to the knee before and after treatment
3. Begin isometric knee exercise
4. Begin active -assistive SLR with splint and terminal knee extension
5. Use CPM 5 hours daily, progressing motion 5' to 10' per day or use "drop and dangle" technique to regain knee flexion
6. Begin total body reconditioning
7. Begin bed-to-chair transfers and toilet transfers with a raised toilet seat
8. Begin gait training with an ambulation device and a splint.

O   **What does the rehabilitation consist of during day 4-14 postoperatively?**

1. Check skin integrity
2. Continue anti-inflammatory modalities
3. Progress exercise to resistive with tubing or light weights
4. Emphasize quadriceps exercises
5. Improve knee ROM by using PNF, MFR, patella mobilization, passive stretch, and bicycle riding
6. Teach independence in all transfers
7. Continue gait training without a splint
8. Begin stair climbing with railing
9. Train independence in basic ADLs.

O   **What does the rehabilitation consist of during days 4-14 postoperatively?**

1. Emphasize quadriceps strengthening
2. Increase knee motion (5' to 105')
3. Train one-legged standing balance (5 to 10 seconds)
4. Begin proprioception training
5. Gait-train on all surfaces, including stairs
6. Train independence in basic ADL.

O   **What are the outcomes associated with the use of CPM in TKA?**

Continuous passive motion is a commonly used device post knee arthroplasty. A systematic review found significant improvements in active knee flexion and analgesic use two weeks postoperatively with the use of continuous passive motion and physiotherapy compared to physiotherapy alone. In addition, length of hospital stay and need for knee manipulations were significantly decreased in the continuous passive motion group. Continuous passive motion combined with physiotherapy may offer beneficial results for patients post knee arthroplasty. However, the potential benefits will need to be carefully weighed against the inconvenience and expense of CPM.

O   **What impairments occur after TKA?**

After reintegration into the community, patients require up to one year to achieve 80% of normal muscle strength, walking speeds remain at 10-20% below age matched controls; stair climbing time is 40-50% slower than age matched controls (even at 1 year). Most patients who participated in sports prior to surgery are able to return to low impact sport activities and exercise regimens. Patients are able to return to sedentary, light, and medium work categories. Patients who are on sick leave greater than 180 days preoperatively are less likely to return to work.

○   **What is the risk of thrombolic events associated with TKA?**

The overall incidence of DVT after TKA without any form of mechanical or pharmaceutical prophylaxis has been reported to range from 40% to 88%. The risk of asymptomatic PE may be as high as 10% to 20%, with symptomatic PE reported in 0.5% to 3% of patients and a mortality rate of up to 2%. Proximal thrombi, in the popliteal vein and above, occur in 3% to 20% of patients and have been thought to pose a greater risk of PE than thrombi in calf veins, which have been reported in 40% to 60% of patients.

○   **What is the risk of infection using prophylactic antibiotics in TKA?**

With prophylactic antibiotics, the rate of TKA infection was 1.6% in a follow-up study of 4171 knee arthroplasties by Wilson, Kelley, and Thornhill, with most infections occurring late and presumably due to hematogenous origins.

○   **What patellar complications occur in patients with TKA?**

Patellofemoral complications, including patellofemoral instability, patellar fracture, patellar component failure, patellar component loosening, patellar clunk syndrome, and extensor mechanism tendon rupture, have been cited as the most common reasons for re operation. This has led many authors to advocate TKA without patellar resurfacing for patients with osteoarthritis and adequate patellar cartilage.

○   **What nerve injuries can occur in TKA?**

Peroneal nerve palsy is the only commonly reported nerve palsy after TKA. It occurs primarily with correction of combined fixed valgus and flexion deformities, as are common in patients with rheumatoid arthritis. The incidence of peroneal nerve palsy in the Swedish Knee Arthroplasty project was 1.8% in 2273 rheumatoid patients. The true incidence may be somewhat higher because mild palsies may recover spontaneously and not be reported.

○   **What is the risk of supracondylar fractures in TKA?**

Supracondylar fractures of the femur occur infrequently after TKA (0.2% to 1%).

○   **What are the indications for TSA?**

The primary indication for shoulder arthroplasty is pain from glenohumeral arthritis with resultant loss of function that is unresponsive to conservative treatment. Stiffness, in the absence of pain, rarely is an indication for shoulder arthroplasty. Other indications include rotator cuff tear arthropathy, osteonecrosis, and previous failed surgery.

○   **What are the contraindications for TSA?**

There are no specific age limits for total shoulder arthroplasty, but the patient should be well motivated and a reasonable surgical risk. Contraindications to shoulder arthroplasty include active or recent infection or a neuropathic joint. Paralysis with complete loss of function of both the deltoid and the rotator cuff also is a contraindication. However, loss of function of either the deltoid or the rotator cuff is not a contraindication to shoulder arthroplasty because this can be treated with muscle transfers and soft tissue procedures. Debilitating medical status and uncorrectable glenohumeral instability also are contraindications to shoulder arthroplasty.

○   **What components are most often used for TSA?**

Total shoulder arthroplasty, that is, replacement of the humeral head and the glenoid articulating surface with prosthetic components, is a well-established procedure. When performed properly and when rehabilitation is proper, results can be just as good as after the more common arthroplasties of the knee and the hip. Three types of total shoulder replacement components are available: (1) unconstrained, (2) semiconstrained, and (3) constrained. By far the greatest experience and most success have been achieved with the unconstrained types, most notably as reported by Neer et al. in 1982. Numerous other reports of long-term success using the Neer unconstrained components have appeared during the last 20 years.

○   **What are the rehabilitation interventions for the first 4 days after TSA?**

1. Begin active elbow, wrist, and hand exercises
2. Begin active-assistive shoulder elevation (scaption) and rotations in supine position
3. Begin passive pendulum exercises
4. With doctors orders, begin assisted abduction (depends on rotator cuff repair)

○   **What are the rehabilitation interventions for 4-14 days after TSA?**

1. Add assisted IR and extension exercises in standing
2. Progress intensity of stretch in assisted elevation and ER
3. Begin strengthening: active supine elevation with emphasis on eccentric lowering

○   **What are the rehabilitation interventions for 2-4 weeks after TSA?**

1. Progress stretches of elevation and rotations, add posterior capsule stretch
2. Progress strengthening to active standing elevation with emphasis on eccentric lowering
3. Progress rotator cuff and deltoid strengthening to isometrics and resisted isotonics with Thera-Band
4. Begin light ADL only

○   **What are the rehabilitation interventions 2 months after TSA?**

1. Begin strengthening of large scapular muscles
2. Ensure coordination of scapulohumeral muscles
3. Continue program twice daily for 2 years for optimal results

○   **What are complications associated with TSA?**

Complications are, for the most part, caused by biomechanical factors. As would be expected, complications occur more frequently after total shoulder arthroplasty than after hemiarthroplasty. Complications include glenoid loosening, tuberosity nonunion or malunion, glenohumeral instability, rotator cuff tears, periprosthetic fracture, infection, nerve injury, deltoid rupture, humeral loosening, impingement, heterotopic bone formation, mechanical failure of components, and loss of motion.

FIBROMYALGIA AND MYOFASCIAL PAIN SYNDROME

○   **What are the ACR criteria for fibromyalgia?**

1. History of widespread pain.
Pain is considered widespread when all of the following are present: pain in the left side of the body, pain in the right side of the body, pain above the waist, pain below the waist. In addition, axial skeletal pain (cervical spine or anterior chest or thoracic spine or low back) must be present. In this definition, shoulder and buttock pain are considered as pain for each involved side. "Low back" pain is considered lower segment pain. Thus, pain at three widespread sites (e.g., right arm, low back and left leg) will satisfy the criterion of widespread pain.
2. Pain in 11 of 18 tender point sites on digital palpation.
Pain (mild or greater) on digital palpation must be present in at least 11 of the following 18 tender point sites: Occiput: bilateral, at the suboccipital muscle insertions. *Low cervical:* bilateral, at the anterior aspects of the intertransverse spaces at C5-7. *Trapezius:* bilateral, at the midpoint of the upper border. *Supraspinatus:* bilateral, at origins above the scapula spine near the medial border. *Second rib:* bilateral, at the second costochondral junctions, just lateral to the junctions on upper surfaces. *Lateral epicondyle:* bilateral, 2 cm distal to the epicondyles. *Gluteal:* bilateral, in upper outer quadrants of buttocks in anterior fold of muscle. *Greater trochanter:* bilateral, posterior to the trochanteric prominence. *Knee:* bilateral, at the medial fat pad proximal to the joint line.

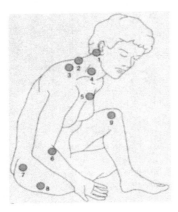

O   **What is the objective criteria for palpating tender points?**

Digital palpation should be performed with an approximate force of 4 kg. For a tender point to be considered "positive" the subject must state that the palpation was painful. "Tender" is not to be considered "painful."

O   **What were the sensitivity and specificity of the ACR fibromyalgia criteria?**

The combination of widespread pain, defined as bilateral, above and below the waist, and axial, and at least 11 of 18 specified tender points, yielded a sensitivity of 88.4% and a specificity of 81.1%.

O   **What is the prevalence of fibromyalgia in the US?**

At any given point in time, conservative estimates suggest that 3-6% of the general population, including children, meet the criteria for diagnosis of fibromyalgia. This assumption makes fibromyalgia over twice as common as rheumatoid arthritis. Physicians may find that approximately 8% of their patients have fibromyalgia. In a rheumatology and physiatry practice, however, as many as 15% of evaluated patients have fibromyalgia. This incidence implies that 1 in every 10 patients evaluated in a medical practice has fibromyalgia.

O   **Who is at risk for fibromyalgia?**

Seventy-three to eighty-eight percent of patients have been female, and the mean patient age has varied from 34 to 57 years, depending on the patient populations.

O   **What is the cardinal symptom in fibromyalgia?**

The cardinal symptom of fibromyalgia is diffuse, chronic pain. The pain often begins in one location, particularly the neck and shoulders, but then becomes more generalized. Generally patients state that 'it hurts all over' and they have difficulty locating the site of pain arising from articular or non-articular tissues. Patients describe the muscle pain often as burning, radiating or gnawing and the intensity of the pain as modest or severe but varying greatly.

O   **Is sleep dysfunction a prominent symptom in fibromyalgia?**

Sleep dysfunction is considered an integral feature of fibromyalgia syndrome. Seventy percent of patients with fibromyalgia recognize a connection with poor sleep and an increased pain, along with feeling unrefreshed, fatigued, and emotionally distressed. Several studies have linked abnormal sleep with these symptoms.

O   **What is the most reliable finding on physical exam in patients with fibromyalgia?**

Thus, the only reliable finding on examination is the presence of multiple tender points. Although various sets of 'best' tender point discriminators in fibromyalgia have been proposed, the current nine pairs of tender points should be routinely examined since they were chosen for classification criteria.

O   **What is the differential diagnosis of fibromyalgia?**

Distinguishing Features of Conditions That May Otherwise Mimic Fibromyalgia

Condition	Distinguishing Features
Diabetes mellitus	Elevated serum glucose or glucosuria
Early collagen vascular disease	Elevated erythrocyte sedimentation rate; elevated C-reactive protein
Electrolyte imbalance	Elevated or diminished serum electrolytes
Hypothyroidism	Hoarseness, bradycardia, abnormal deep-tendon reflexes
Inflammatory/metabolic myopathies	Elevated creatine phosphokinase
Myofascial pain syndrome	Equal sex distribution; unilateral muscle pain not associated with stiffness or fatigue; often responds to local injection
Multiple sclerosis	Abnormal brain imaging; abnormal cerebrospinal fluid
Neuropathy	Abnormal electromyography
Polymyalgia rheumatica	Patients usually elderly; high erythrocyte sedimentation rate; shoulder and hip girdle pain
Psychogenic rheumatism	Diffuse body wide pain, including control points, with normal workup
Seronegative spondyloarthropathy	Occurs mainly in young men; axial pain and stiffness with sacroiliac tenderness
Somatoform pain disorder	Pain not localizing to fibromyalgia tender points; clinically inexplicable pain with back movement, rectum function, intercourse, urination

O   **What is the association of fibromyalgia and depression?**

Approximately 25% of fibromyalgia patients have current major depression and 50% have a lifetime history of major depression.

O   **What other symptoms do fibromyalgia patients experience?**

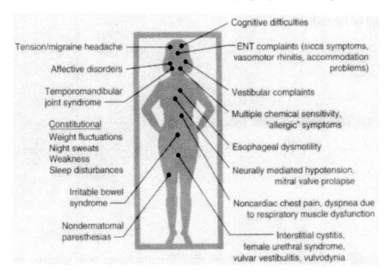

O   **What is the current evidence of the pathogenesis of fibromyalgia?**

Evidence has not been convincing or consistent that fibromyalgia is a disorder of muscle energy metabolism, an inflammatory disease of muscle, an immunopathologic disease of muscle, a generalized disorder of pain perception , a depressive equivalent, a neuroendocrine disturbance, a disorder of serotonin or somatomedin-C metabolism, a mere sleep disturbance, a perturbation of central nervous system/caudate pain perception , or a result of prior domestic violence or sexual abuse.

O   **What is the possible pathogenesis of nociceptive dysfunction in fibromyalgia?**

Fibromyalgia represents a disorder of generalized heightened pain sensitivity. Primary or secondary alterations in substances such as serotonin, endorphins or substance P may integrate the changes in sleep, pain and mood. For example, the level of substance P in the cerebrospinal fluid was three fold higher in fibromyalgia patients than in normal controls. Substance P release is influenced by serotonin, and serotonin deficiency, in either the peripheral or central nervous system, could cause an exaggerated perception of normal sensory stimuli. Fibromyalgia patients have reduced pain tolerance to pressure, heat and electrical pulse, both at classic tender points and control points. The regional cerebral blood flow, as detected by single photon emission computed tomography, was reduced in the left and right hemi thalamus and the right heads of the caudate nuclei in fibromyalgia compared to controls. These areas of the brain are important in pain perception.

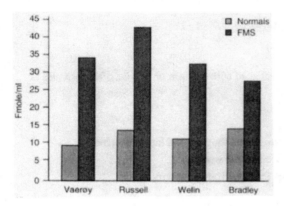

Levels of substance P in fibromyalgia patients compared with controls summary of studies

O   **What is the evidence of neurohormonal disorders in fibromyalgia?**

There is also evidence to suggest neurohormonal abnormalities in fibromyalgia. Two studies have demonstrated reduced levels of growth hormone in some patients with fibromyalgia. Growth hormone is important in muscle homeostasis and excreted primarily during stage 4 sleep. Fibromyalgia patients were noted to have low urinary free cortisol and a decreased cortisol response to corticotropin releasing hormone (CRH). Plasma neuropeptide Y levels were also low in fibromyalgia. These studies all suggest a relative adrenal hyporesponsiveness, which could be the result of a chronic stress reaction.

O   **What have been the models of the pathophysiology of fibromyalgia?**

Investigations of the pathophysiology of fibromyalgia

Sleep

Nociception

Substance P

Neurohormonal (somatomedin C/growth hormone, prolactin, ACTH, arginine/vasopressin, neuropeptide Y)

Muscle (energy) metabolism

Immunologic

Psychologic/depressive equivalent

Stress/trauma-related

Viruses

O   **Are NSAID effective in fibromyalgia?**

'Therapeutic doses of naproxen and ibuprofen and 20 mg daily of prednisone were not significantly better than placebo in clinical trials. Nonsteroidal anti-inflammatory drugs (NSAIDs) may have a synergistic effect when combined with central nervous system (CNS) active medications, but they may be no more effective than simple analgesics.

O   **What CNS active medications are effective in FM?**

In contrast, certain CNS active medications, most notably the tricyclics amitriptyline and cyclobenzaprine, have been consistently found to be better than placebo in controlled trials. The doses of amitriptyline studied have been 25-50 mg, usually given as a single dose at bedtime. In one report, amitriptyline was associated with significant improvement compared with placebo or naproxen in pain, sleep, fatigue, patient and physician global assessment and the manual tender point score. Cyclobenzaprine, 10-40 mg in divided dose, also improved pain, fatigue, sleep and tender point count. However, clinically meaningful improvement with the tricyclic medications has occurred in only 25-45% of patients and the efficacy of these medications may level-off over time.

O   **Summarize drug therapy results of controlled clinical trials showing benefits for fibromyalgia symptoms**

Drug therapy: results of controlled clinical trials showing benefits for fibromyalgia symptoms

Class/Drug	Dose	Study results	Study
Antidepressants			
Amitriptyline (Elavil®)	10–50 mg hs	Improved pain rating	Carette (1994); Scudds (1989)
Fluoxetine (Prozac®)	20 mg qd	Improved pain rating, global well-being	Wolfe (1994); Goldenberg (1996)
Citalopram (Celexa®)	20–40 mg qd	Improved FIQ, pain	Anderberg (2000)
Cyclobenzaprine (Flexeril®)	10–40 mg qd	Improved depression, FIQ, pain	Bennett (1988); Quimby (1989);
NMDA Receptor Antagonists			
Ketamine (Ketalar®)	0.3 mg/kg IV	Improved FIQ, tender points	Sorensen (1997); Graven-Nielsen
Combination therapy			
Alprazolam (Xanax®) + Ibuprofen	3 mg qd +600 mg qid	Improved tender points, pain	Russell (1991)
5HT3 antagonists			
Ondansetron (Zofran®)	4 mg qd	Improved pain, tender points, headaches	Hrycaj (1996)
Hormones			
Growth hormone	Different dosing sq	Improved FIQ, tender points, global well-being	Bennett (1998)

O   **What non-pharmacological treatments are appropriate in fibromyalgia?**

Although widely utilized in the treatment of fibromyalgia, non medicinal therapy has been rarely studied in a controlled fashion. Those few treatments evaluated in controlled studies include cardiovascular fitness training (CFT), EMG biofeedback, hypnotherapy and cognitive behavioral therapy.

O   **What other treatment options may be considered?**

Other less well studied non-medical treatments include transcutaneous electrical nerve stimulation (TENS), acupuncture, laser treatment and tender point injections.

O   **What is the efficacy of therapeutic exercise in fibromyalgia?**

Aerobic exercise should be regarded as a legitimate and useful treatment component in the management of FMS. Improvement can be expected in aerobic performance, tender points, and global well being. Pain intensity, fatigue and sleep may or may not improve; psychological function can not be expected to improve. Evidence therefore supports improvement of only limited symptoms of this disorder. There is some evidence that strength training may be beneficial for FMS (improved pain, musculoskeletal performance and psychological function).

O   **What is the efficacy of Mind body medicine modalities in the treatment of FM?**

Various mind/body therapies that attempt to follow the biopsychosocial model appear to be strong in specific health domains pertinent to FM, such as pain, insomnia, and psychological functioning. Mind/body treatment components can include autogenic training, relaxation exercises, meditation, cognitive-behavioral training, and education. It has been reported that there is wide use of mind/body treatments among FM patients with a corresponding high degree of satisfaction. When compared, nonpharmacological treatment appears to be more efficacious in improving self-report of FMS symptoms than pharmacological treatment alone. A similar trend was suggested for functional measures.

O   **What is an optimal program for fibromyalgia?**

Thus, the optimal intervention for FMS would include nonpharmacological treatments, specifically exercise and cognitive-behavioral therapy, in addition to appropriate medication management as needed for sleep and pain symptoms.

O   **What is myofascial pain syndrome (MPS)?**

Simons et al have defined regional MPS as a condition in which the patient has "hyperirritable spots" or "trigger points" within taut bands of skeletal muscle or fascia that are painful on compression and can give rise to characteristic referred pain, tenderness, and autonomic nervous system symptoms. Pain from MPS can be described as deep and achy, and it is occasionally accompanied by a sensation of burning or stinging. Patients may also report restricted range of motion in the area affected. MPS is limited to one area or quadrant of the body.

O   **What is the relationship of trigger and tender points?**

Differentiation of Myofascial Pain Syndrome From Fibromyalgia

Feature	Trigger Points of Myofascial Pain Syndrome	Tender Points of Fibromyalgia
Tender points	Localized	Multiple, generalized
Musculoskeletal pain	Localized	Generalized
Taut band	No variation from normal	No variation from normal
Twitch response	No variation from normal	Probably normal
Referred pain	More frequent	Less frequent
Fatigue	Less frequent	More frequent
Poor sleep	Less frequent	More frequent
Paresthesia	Less frequent	More frequent
Headaches	Less frequent	More frequent
Irritable bowel	Less frequent	More frequent
Sensation of swelling	Less frequent	More frequent

O   **What are the diagnostic criteria for MPS?**

Recommended Criteria for Identifying Latent and Active Trigger Points

Essential Criteria
Taut band palpable (if muscle is accessible)
Exquisite spot tenderness of a nodule in a taut band
Patient's recognition of current pain complaint by pressure on the tender nodule (identifies active trigger point)
Painful limit to full passive stretch range of motion

Confirmatory Observations
Visual or tactile identification of local twitch response
Observation of a local twitch response induced by needle penetration of a tender nodule
Pain or altered sensation (in the distribution expected from a trigger point in that muscle) on compression of a tender nodule
Electromyographic demonstration of spontaneous electrical activity characteristic of active loci in the tender nodule of a taut band

O   **What is the prevalence of MPS?**

Because of the heterogeneity of nomenclature and patient populations the prevalence is quite variable, 12.5- 55% has been reported in the literature.

O   **What is the pathogenesis of MPS?**

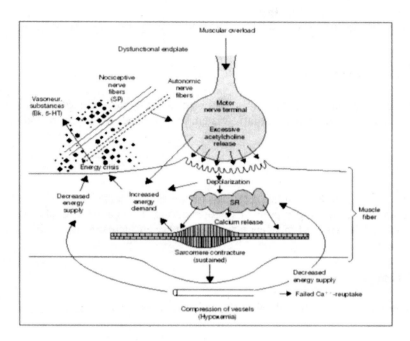

O   How are active TPs classified?

Trigger points are generally classified as either active or latent, and range from 2 to 5 mm in diameter. Active trigger points are hypersensitive and can be associated with two types of pain which may occur spontaneously with muscle use, or with palpation on examination. Most commonly a sharp localized pain, which is well demarcated, can be elicited, as can a radiating pain, described as a subcutaneous ache, with slightly blurred edges that project well beyond the originating trigger point.

O   What is the zone of reference?

The radiating pain, which is quite stereotypic for the individual muscle, displays continuous pain in the zone of reference. These pain reference zones may or may not mimic more traditionally recognized dermatomal, myotomal, or sclerotomal referred pain patterns.

O   What physical findings are evident?

Active trigger points cause restricted motion of the muscle in which they abide. Palpation of the active trigger point with sustained deep pressure will elicit an alteration of the pain in the zone of reference which may occur immediately or be delayed a few seconds. This pattern of referred pain is both reproducible and consistent with patterns observed in other patients with similar trigger points. The zone of reference can therefore serve as a guide for the clinician in locating irritable trigger points for the purpose of treatment. In contrast, the tender points of fibromyalgia display only hypersensitivity.

O   What is the relationship between active and latent trigger points?

Active trigger points that cause referred pain are commonly produced by an acute strain, due to sudden overload of' the muscle, or chronic repetitive strain of the muscle. Referred pain may spontaneously subside within a few days or weeks if the demands on the muscle are reduced and if it is not immobilized. Without perpetuating factors, an active trigger point tends to revert to and persist as a latent trigger point. When latent, the trigger points are quiescent and result primarily in muscle tightness and dysfunction without the presence of persistent or spontaneous pain except when palpated.

O   What are perpetuating factors in MPS?

Perpetuating factors may be mechanical i.e. postural, structural, periarticular pathology; They may be systemic sleep disorders, nutritional deficiencies, metabolic derangements; they may be psychogenic- depression, anxiety, malingering. In the presence of one or more perpetuating factors, trigger points usually persist and become chronic. They may then propagate to other muscles as secondary and satellite trigger points. While one stress activates acute myofascial pain, other factors generally perpetuate it.

○   **Is there a relationship between acupuncture and trigger points?**

The relationship between trigger points and acupuncture points is frequently questioned. Investigators compared the congruence of trigger point locations with the locations of acupuncture points related to pain and found an overall correspondence of 71%.

○   **What is the local twitch response?**

The elicitation of a "local twitch response" produces a reproducible visible shortening of the muscle band and has been associated with electromyographic changes. In locating an active trigger point, palpation during the examination should produce replication or alteration of the patient's complaint. The affected muscles may also display an increased fatigability, stiffness, subjective weakness, and restricted range of motion.

○   **How reliable are trigger point examination techniques?**

Studies have yielded conflicting results regarding interrater and intrarater reliability for the myofascial pain examination for trigger points.

○   **What are some common sites and symptoms of MPS?**

Reference Zones and Symptoms Associated With Common Muscle Trigger Points

Muscle pain	Location symptoms	Associated Structure	of referred
Head and Neck Splenius			
Splenius cervicis, semispinalis cervicis, rotatores, multifidi	Occiput	Headache behind eyes	
Upper trapezius	Back of neck, temporal region	--	
Sternocleidomastoid	see below	Ataxia Dizziness otalgia increased lacrimation, coryza, scleral congestion	
Clavicular	Across forehead, in and behind ear		
Sternal	Occiput, cheek, periorbital area, down toward sternum	Can mimic sinus pain	
Splenius capitis	Retro-orbital or temporo-orbital region	Vertex headache	
Temporalis, masseter, medial and lateral pterygoid	Teeth, jaw	--	
Shoulder, Thorax, and Arm			
Anterior serratus	Side of chest to border of scapula	Decreased maximum chest expansion, shortness of breath	

Pectoralis major and minor	Breast, ulnar aspect of arm	--
Levator scapulae	Base of neck	Neck stiffness; Sequelae of cervical whiplash injury seen with depression and anxiety
Infraspinatus	Glenohumeral joint, down upper arm	Can mimic cervical radiculopathies
Supraspinatus	Middle deltoid, elbow	Can mimic cervical radiculopathies
Back and Buttock		
Quadratus lumborum	Low back	--
Iliocostalis	Lower quadrant abdomen to buttocks	--
Gluteus maximus	Sacrum, inferior surface of buttock	--
Thigh, Leg, and Foot		
Quadriceps femoris		--
Rectus femoris	Knee cap, distal half of anterior thigh	
Vastus intermedius	Upper part of thigh	
Vastus medialis	Medial aspect of knee	
Biceps femoris	Calf	--
Gastrocnemius	Over calf to instep of foot	--
Soleus	Heel, ipsilateral sacroiliac joint	--

O What treatment approaches may be considered in MFPS?

Recognition and correction of perpetuating factors
Spray and stretch therapy
Topical and deep heat modalities
Ice massage
Muscle relaxants
NSAID
Dry needling
Accupressure
Local anesthetic injections
Botulinum toxin injections
Post isometric relaxation exercises
MFR techniques/soft tissue mobilization
Interferential current stimulation
Relaxation exercises

FRACTURE REHABILITATION

Fracture Treatment Protocols

Fracture	Initial Physical Therapy Program	Advanced Physical Therapy**
Scapula scapular body acromion process coracoid process glenoid neck glenoid fossa	**Days 1-5:** shoulder pendulum exercises elbow, forearm; wrist, hand AROM; grip strengthening **Weeks 2-3:** gentle PROM-AAROM shoulder; deltoid, rotator cuff isometrics **If stable fracture pattern-** shoulder PROM-AAROM initiated 1 week post injury, ROM, strengthening progressed to tolerance	**Stable:** PROM/strengthening as tolerated **Unstable:** strengthening at 3 months; progress to isometrics, surgical tubing, and free weights
Clavicle displaced nondisplaced	**Stable** **Day 1 post-stabilization:** early shoulder AROM-AAROM to tolerance; shoulder isometrics; elbow, forearm, wrist, hand AROM; grip strengthening **Unstable:** limit ROM as fracture pattern dictates	**Stable:** PROM/strengthening as tolerated **Unstable:** strengthening at 6-8 weeks; return to activity in 10-12 weeks
Humerus		
1. Proximal fractures greater tuberosity lesser tuberosity surgical neck anatomic neck	**Day 1 post-stabilization:** elbow, forearm, wrist, hand AROM; grip strengthening **Days 2-5:** pendulum shoulder exercises Weeks 1-3: early gentle AAROM shoulder joint within mobility limitations; deltoid, biceps, triceps, isometrics Weeks 3-6: AROM, gentle PROM shoulder	**Week 12:** begin strengthening; progress to isometrics, surgical tubing, free weights, isokinetics; scapular stabilization exercises are important
2. Humeral shaft	**Day 1 post-stabilization:** elbow, forearm, wrist, hand AROM grip strengthening **Days 2-5:** Pendulum shoulder exercises **Weeks 1-3:** Early gentle AAROM shoulder joint within mobility limitations: deltoid, biceps, triceps, isometrics **Weeks 3-6:** AROM, gentle PROM shoulder	**Weeks 10-12:** strengthening **Week 12:** progression the same as for the proximal humerus
3. Distal humerus	Day 1 post-stabilization: shoulder AAROM-AROM; wrist, hand active range of motion-CPM (elbow) as M.D. indicates **Days 2-5:** gentle elbow, forearm AROM; deltoid isometrics; grip strengthening **Weeks 8-10:** gentle PROM-AAROM elbow, forearm	**Weeks 10-12:** strengthening Week 12: isokinetics
Radius & Ulna		
3. Olecranon	**Days 1-7 post-stabilization:** early gentle AAROM-AROM forearm, elbow (initiated after 2-3 days); shoulder, wrist, hand AROM; grip strengthening	**Weeks 10-12:** PROM; strengthening
4. Radial head	**Days 1-7 post-stabilization:** early elbow AROM shoulder, wrist, hand AROM; grip strengthening	**Weeks 10-12:** PROM; strengthening
3. Forearm isolated radius, ulna - both bones Monteggia/Galeazzi	**Days 1-5 post-stabilization:** immediate shoulder, hand AROM; early, gentle AAROM forearm, elbow, wrist as fracture stability allows; grip strengthening	**Weeks 10-12:** PROM **Week 12:**
4. Distal radius	**Days 1-5 post-stabilization:** immediate AROM shoulder, elbow, fingers; initiation of gentle wrist AROM as immobilization allows (after cast removal than splint); grip strengthening	**Weeks 8-10:** PROM; light activity **Weeks 10-12:** strengthening
Wrist & Hand		
Carpal MC Phalanx	**Days 1-5 post stabilization:** early AROM-AAROM fingers, wrist, forearm as fracture and stabilization allow; elbow, shoulder AROM; fine motor control, desensitization; techniques as indicated	**Weeks 8-10:** PROM; light activity **Weeks 10-12:** strengthening

Table 2. Lower Extremity: Acetabulum to Femur

Fracture	X-Rays Needed	Immobilization	Fixation	Mobility Precautions
Acetabulum Posterior wall; posterior	AP Pelvis Judet Views	Distal Femoral Traction	Lag screws reconstruction	**Kocher-Langenbeck** **approach:** (posterior), avoid

columns; anterior wall; anterior column; transverse; T-shaped; posterior column/posterior wall; transverse/posterior wall; both column; anterior column with posterior hemitransverse (Letournel classification)	CT San (3mmCuts)		plates	active hip extension rotation Ilioinguinal approach: (anterior), avoid active hip flexion, vigorous trunk and abdominal flexion **Extended iliofemoral approach:** (posterolateral), no active hip abduction 6-8 weeks; weight-bearing; NWB 8-12 weeks; positioning ROM; posterior wall involvement - no hip flexion greater than 70 degrees for 6 weeks
Pelvis 1. Anterior ring public symphysis rami	AP, inlet & outlet Pelvis, CT scan	See pelvic fracture disruption protocol	plating external fixation lag screws	TDWB-WBAT 10-12 weeks post injury (depends on associated, posterior ring involvement)
2. Posterior Ring Sacrum SI fracture/dislocation iliac wing Femur			screws plating	TDWB-WOLWB 10-12 weeks
1. Femoral head	AP PelvisAP/Lat hip	Distal Femoral Traction	Screw fixation hemiarthroplasty THA (in elderly patient as fracture dictates)	Toe-touch weight-bearing 8-12 weeks no straight leg raises (SLR)TTWB, WBAT dependent on prosthesis fixation (see femoral neck fracture)
2. Femoral neck	AP PelvisAP/Lat both hips (uninjured side with templates)	Buck's Traction	screws dynamic hip screw endoprosthesis (elderly)	WB as necessary for balance for ambulation WB as necessary for balance for ambulation WBAT **ROM precautions:** avoid simultaneous/combination movements of the operative hip. Allow flexion, extension, abduction, adduction or rotation in cardinal planes of motion with no restriction; no SLR 6 weeks **Posterior surgical approach:** no hip flexion greater than 60 degrees, avoid hip adduction, internal rotation past neutral; no SLR 6-8 weeks WB as necessary for balance for ambulation
3. Intertrochanteric femur	AP PelvisAP/Lat hip	Buck's Traction	DHS IM nail	TTWB; no SLR; no active hip abduction with blade-plate fixation
4. Subtrochanteric femur	AP PelvisAP/Lat Femur	Distal Femoral Traction	DHS Blade plate IM nail	Interlocked nail/plate TTWB 6-8 weeks
5. Femoral shaft	AP/Lat Femur AP/Lat KneeAP Pelvis If severely comminuted get scanogram opposite femur	Distal Femoral or proximal tibial traction	IM nail DCP, LC, DCP	Note: Knee immobilizer, external support may be needed To allow early crutch training if quad control slowly achieved; DCP fixation same as IM nail protocol
6. Supracondylar, intracondylar femur	AP/Lat Femur AP/Lat KneeAP Pelvis	Knee Immobilizer	condylar blade plate; condylar buttress plate; screws	TDWB 10-12 weeks

Table 3. Lower Extremity: Patella to Foot				
Fracture	**X-Rays Needed**	**Immobilization**	**Fixation**	**Mobility Precautions**
Patella	AP/Lat Knee	knee immobilizer	cylinder cast,	**Stable: WBAT**

Fracture				
Nondisplaced; displaced			lag screw (s) tension-band wiring	**Unstable:** TTWB 4-8 weeks
Tibia				
1. Tibial plateau	AP/Lat Knee CT Scan	knee immobilizer	buttress T-plate DCP screws	TDWB 8-12 weeks NO TKE exercise (avoid excessive end-range anterior tibial glide)
2. Tibial Shaft	AP/Lat tibia	Cadillac Splint	IM nail reamed and unreamed; plates and screws; external fixator	PWB 6-8 weeks TDWB 8-12 weeks PWB 6-8 weeks
Ankle				
1. Pilon	AP/Lat Ankle Mortise View AP/Lat Tibia	Cadillac Splint Calcaneal Traction	screws and plates	NWB 12 weeks
2. Medial malleolus, posterior malleolus, lateral malleolus (Weber A, B, C)	AP/Lat Ankle Mortise View	Cadillac Splint	screws, plates, and tension-band wiring	PWB 8-12 weeks
Foot				
1. Calcaneus extraarticular intraarticular	Lat Foot Oblique Foot Harris Heel View CT Scan (3mmCuts)	Cadillac Splint Use a lot of Padding to protect from Inevitable swelling.	Reconstruction plate H-plate; lag screw K-wires	NWB 12 weeks
2. Talus	Lat Foot Oblique Foot	Cadillac Splint With toe plate	lag screws K-wires (rare)	NWB 12 weeks
3. Metatarsals and phalanx	AP/Lat & oblique Foot	Cadillac Splint With toe plate	screws, wires, and pins	closed reduction immobilization

Table 3. Lower Extremity: Patella to Foot (Continued)

Fracture	Initial Physical Therapy Program	Advanced Physical Therapy**
Patella Nondisplaced; displaced	Days 1: bilateral UE strengthening; ankle AROM; knee CPM post-op if indicated Days 2 to discharge: quad hamstring isometrics***; knee/AROM as fracture pattern allows***; SLR***	Weeks 4-8: strengthening; progress knee A/AAROM; begin quad Isometrics and SLR if there was quad mechanism involvement Week 8: WBAT, wean from crutches; concentrate on short arc/end range; quadriceps strengthening; closed kinetic chain activities (i.e., cycling, partial squats, leg press); balance proprioceptive training
Tibia 1. Tibial plateau	**Day 1-discharge:** bilateral UE & contralateral LE strengthening; AAROM, isometrics, AP involved LE; bed mobilization/transfer and ambulation training **Weeks 6-8:** TKE initiated; A/AAROM operative LE; hip girdle, quad & hamstring strengthening; balance/proprioception training	Weeks 12-14: WBAT, wean from crutches, gait retraining; strengthen quads, hamstrings, abductors, flexors, extensors, and lower trunk muscles; initiate balance/proprioceptive awareness training; aerobic/fitness & functional training
2. Tibial Shaft	**Day 1-discharge:** bilateral UE & contralateral LE strengthening; AAROM, isometrics, AP involved LE; bed mobilization/transfer and ambulation training **Weeks 6-8:** TKE initiated; A/AAROM operative LE; hip girdle, quad & hamstring strengthening; balance/proprioception training	Weeks 12-14: WBAT, wean from crutches, gait retraining; strengthen quads, hamstrings, abductors, flexors, extensors, and lower trunk muscles; initiate balance/proprioceptive awareness training; aerobic/fitness & functional training
Ankle 1. Pilon	**Immediate post-stabilization:** bilateral UE strengthening; gluteal, quad, hamstring isometrics **Day 2 to discharge:** hip, knee toe AROM; SLR, TKE **Week 2:** ankle subtalar AROM; progressive hip and knee strengthening	Week 12: PROM initiated; strengthening; balance/proprioceptive awareness training; WBAT, wean from crutches; closed kinetic chain program
2. Medial malleolus, posterior malleolus, lateral malleolus (Weber A, B, C)	same as pilon fracture	Weeks 8-10: gait progression after fracture healing; AROM/PROM ankle and subtalar joints; balance/proprioceptive awareness training
Foot 1. Calcaneus extraarticular intraarticular	**Preoperative:** UE strengthening; uninvolved extremity strengthening Involved extremity hip, knee isometrics; crutch training for short distance	Month 3: gradually increase weight-bearing starting at 20 lbs to FWB over 1 mo; gradually wean from assistive devise as patient tolerates; pool therapy if

	(primary elevation of extremity) **Day 1:** UE strengthening; uninvolved extremity AROM strengthening involved extremity hip- knee isometrics; AROM, Toe AROM to tolerance **Days 2-3:** crutch training, NWB involved extremity (limited time in dependent position) **Days 4-7:** early ankle, subtalar AROM when surgical incision is sealed **Week 1 to month 3:** continue early AROM ankle, subtalar, toes; gentle PROM toe dorsiflexion and plantar flexion; progress involved extremity; hip-knee conditioning Same as calcaneus	available; gait training, re-education; desensitization techniques as needed; ankle subtalar AAROMisometrics; low impact endurance training **Months 4-6:** gait progression, advanced balance and proprioceptive activities; ankle, subtalar isometric, isotonic strengthening with tubing/theraband; no free weights; soft-tissue immobilization **Month 6:** ankle, subtalar PROM; joint mobilization; isokinetic assessment, strength-endurance training; advanced balance, gait training as indicated
2. Talus	**Day 1 post-stabilization:** bilateral UE strengthening; hip, knee AROM, isometrics; ankle, subtalar, toe AROM as fracture Pattern allows	
3. Metatarsals and phalanx		Same as calcaneus **Weeks 8-12:** WBAT; wean from crutches; proprioceptive/balance training; closed kinetic chain activities

Terminology:
1. (NWB) Nonweight-bearing - patient may not use extremity for any weight-bearing activity
2. (TDWB) Touch-down weight-bearing - extremity may touch the ground just during rest, not during ambulation
3. (TTWB) Toe-touch weight bearing - toe may touch ground just for balance
4. (WOLWB) Weight-of-leg weight-bearing - approximately 20-30 lbs
5. (PWB) Partial weight-bearing - weight limit specified by M.D.
6. (WBAT) Weight-bearing as tolerated - patient may bear weight through extremity as tolerated
7. (TKE) Terminal knee extension - short-arc quadriceps strengthening exercise
8. (SLR) Straight leg raises - isometric strengthening exercises with hip flexion
9. (UE) Upper extremity
10. (LE) Lower extremity
*Post-stabilization to healing
**After fracture healing
***Note: No active quads if quadriceps mechanisms involved or disrupted

LIMB AMPUTATION

○   **What are the etiologies of limb amputation?**

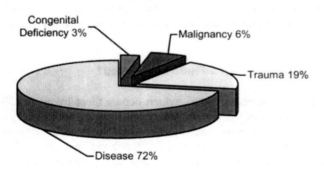

Congenital Deficiency 3%
Malignancy 6%
Trauma 19%
Disease 72%

Amputation of the lower limb is performed significantly more frequently than amputation of the upper limb. Amputation of the distal segment of the limb is more common than that of the proximal segment. Amputations can occur at any age, but for lower extremities, the elderly are most commonly affected, with men more frequently affected than women. Upper limb amputation affects men between the second and fourth decades most frequently, and the right upper extremity is more likely to be amputated than the left. The most common reasons for lower limb amputation are infection, arterial occlusive disease, and complications of diabetes mellitus. Less frequent but important causes are trauma, malignancy, and peripheral neuropathies. For the upper limb, trauma followed by malignancies and acute arterial insufficiency is the most common causes.

O   **What are the concomitant factors in characterizing the etiology of traumatic limb amputation?**

Traumatic loss of a limb, the second most common cause of amputation, occurs most frequently in vehicle- or work related accidents, as a result of violence such as gunshots, or after severe burns and electrocution. Trauma related amputation occurs most commonly in young adult men but can happen at any age to men or to women. Because the mechanism of injury in traumatic amputation is quite variable, this type of amputation is usually classified or categorized according to the severity of tissue damage. The extent of injury to the musculoskeletal system depends on several factors: (1) movement of the object that causes the injury; (2) direction, magnitude, and speed of the energy vector; and (3) the particular body tissue involved.

O   **What are the two types of traumatic amputation?**

In partial traumatic amputations, at least one-half the diameter of the injured extremity is severed or significantly damaged. This kind of injury can incur extensive bleeding, because all of the blood vessels involved may not vasoconstrict. A second type of traumatic amputation occurs when the limb becomes completely detached from the body. As much as 1 liter of blood may be lost before the arteries spasm and vasoconstrict.

O   **What time frame is optimal for initial surgical intervention?**

For optimal outcome, surgical intervention is usually necessary within the first 12 hours after the accident for revascularization or for treatment of the amputated site.

O   **What are the optimal circumstances for limb replantation?**

When replantation is considered, the window of opportunity is much narrower. The decision to replant is a difficult one and is influenced by the patient's age and overall health status, the level of extremity injury, and the condition of the amputated part. Replantation has been most successful in the distal upper extremity. The goal of upper extremity replantation is to provide a mechanism for functional grasp rather than cosmetic restoration of the limb. The period of recovery and rehabilitation after replantation is often significantly longer than that after amputation.

O   **Are there substantial psychological ramifications as well as physical ramifications in traumatic limb amputation?**

Persons with trauma-related amputation undergo extreme physiologic changes as well as psychological trauma. With the sudden loss of a body part, the patient may experience an extended period of grieving. Addressing the patient's psychological needs as well as physical needs is equally important for optimal outcome. An interdisciplinary team approach to rehabilitation is the most effective means to address the comprehensive needs of the patient who has unexpectedly lost a limb to trauma.

O   **What are the current epidemiologic and etiologic factors in cancer related limb amputation?**

Amputation due to cancer is generally a result of osteogenic sarcoma (osteosarcoma), which occurs most frequently in the adolescent and young adult years. Since the early 1990s, advances in early detection, improved imaging techniques, more effective chemotherapy regimens, and better limb resectioning and salvage procedures have reduced the need for amputation in osteosarcoma. Tumor resection followed by limb reconstruction frequently provides a functional extremity. Weight bearing is limited, and the limb is protected by an orthosis, early in rehabilitation. Once satisfactory healing occurs, full weight bearing and near normal activity can be resumed. With new techniques, 5-year survival rates for individuals with osteosarcoma. Increased from approximately 20 % in the 1970s to 80 % in the 1990s.

O   **What are the epidemiologic and etiologic factors with regard to congenital limb deficiency?**

The actual incidence of congenital limb deficiencies is difficult to assess secondary to incomplete or limited databases and terminology inconsistencies. Some estimates suggest an incidence of 1 per 2,000 births; other studies indicate a slightly higher ratio of 1 per 1,692 live births.

O   **How many categories of congenital limb deficiency are recognized?**

Six categories of limb deficiencies have been recognized:

1. Failure of formation of parts, indicating a partial or complete arrest in limb development.
2. Failure of differentiation or separation of parts, where the basic structures have developed but the final form is not completed.
3. Duplication of parts, such as polydactyly.
4. Overgrowth, also called gigantism, and generally caused by skeletal overgrowth.
5. Congenital constriction band syndrome, characterized by constriction bands, which may compromise circulation to the distal part.
6. Generalized skeletal abnormalities.

O   **During what time period in development is the embryo/fetus most likely to develop a congenital limb deficiency?**

Embryologic differentiation of the upper limbs occurs most rapidly at 5-8 weeks after gestation, often before pregnancy has been recognized or confirmed. During this period the upper limbs are particularly vulnerable to mal-formation.

O   **What are the characteristics of upper congenital limb deficiencies?**

Upper limb deficiencies in children vary from minor abnormalities of the fingers to major limb absence.

O   **What is the etiology of congenital limb deficiency?**

The etiology of limb malformation is unclear potential contributing factors cited in the research literature include:

Exposure to chemical agents or drugs.
Fetal position or constriction.
Endocrine disorders.
Exposure to radiation.
Immune reactions.
Occult infections and other diseases.
Single gene disorders.
Chromosomal disorders.
Other syndromes with unknown causes.

For many children, an upper limb deficiency is their only anomaly. However, as many as 12% of these children have coexisting nonlimb malformations.

O   **How are limb deficiencies classified at birth?**

Limb deficiencies that are present at birth are classified according to an international standard based on skeletal features. These deficiencies are referred to as transverse or longitudinal. Transverse deficiencies are described by the level at which the limb terminates. In longitudinal deficiencies, a reduction or absence occurs within the long axis of the limb, but normal skeletal components are present distal to the affected bones.

O   **What role do prosthetics play in the child with congenital limb deficiency?**

The use of prosthetics is a common intervention for children with congenital limb deficiencies. Sometimes surgery is necessary to prepare the existing limb for the most effective use of prosthesis, especially after periods of rapid growth. The goal of prosthetics training for the child should be to enhance the function of the limb and to provide a cosmetic replacement for a missing limb. Rehabilitation strategies are designed with the child's cognitive, motor, and psychological development in mind.

O   **What are the etiologies of upper extremity amputation?**

Almost 90% of upper limb amputations are the result of traumatic injury. Only a small number of upper extremity amputations are the consequence of peripheral vascular disease, tumor, infection, and congenital limb deficiencies. The distribution of these etiologies is vastly different from that of the lower limb. Traumatic amputation occurs primarily in young men between the ages of 20 and 40; the ratio of men to women with new upper limb loss is approximately 4:1. Although as many as 12,000 new upper limb amputations occur each year, nine times as many lower limb amputation surgeries are performed.

○ **What are the circumstances that give rise to traumatic upper extremity amputations?**

Many traumatic amputations of the upper extremity are a result of carelessness when using machinery or equipment or of tampering with safety features that have been installed on equipment to prevent such injuries. Farming accidents in the midwestern states account for most new traumatic upper limb amputations in the United States. Many of these accidents occur when an individual attempts to clear a chute without turning the equipment off or tries to force vegetation through the chute manually, such that clothing becomes entangled and draws the limb into the machine. Other accidental amputations may result from being caught in industrial presses, from frostbite, or from electrical burns. The latter frequently require high proximal debridement and bilateral amputation because of the pattern of electrical injury in the human body.

○ **What are the demographics of the dysvascular amputee?**

75% percent of lower extremity amputations are in individuals who are in the later years of life, with largest group falling in the 55-65 age bracket. Ischemic disease is implicated in 80% of these patients, and more one-half have diabetes mellitus.

○ **What is the mortality associated with dysvascular amputees?**

The 3-year survival for patients with diabetes who have undergone an extremity amputation is approximately 50%. Of those who have had any part of the foot or leg amputated, 20% are likely to die within 2 years.

○ **What comorbidities are associated with the dysvascular amputee?**

In older patients, foot and lower extremity symptoms and compromise are most often a result of a more proximal cause. Individuals with peripheral vascular disease who are at risk of lower extremity amputation usually have evidence of concurrent cardiac and cerebral atherosclerotic disease. In a study of patients who were undergoing cardiac catheterization at the Cleveland Clinic, a 31% coexistence of abdominal aneurysm, 26% coexistence of cerebrovascular disease, and 21 % coexistence of lower extremity ischemia were seen.

○ **Do patients with coexisting diabetes mellitus (DM) have higher rates of morbidity and mortality?**

Patients with diabetes mellitus present an even higher risk of complications related to extensive atherosclerotic disease. Cerebral and coronary artery disease manifest their effects earlier in the diabetic versus the nondiabetic population. Coronary artery disease has the greatest mortality for persons with type 2 diabetes.

○ **What are the characteristics of PVD in patients with diabetes mellitus type 2?**

The prevalence of PVD among persons with diabetes, whether men or women, is significantly greater than in those without diabetes. The Framingham Heart Study found a four to five times greater relative risk of intermittent claudication in persons with diabetes, even when controlling for blood pressure, cholesterol, and smoking. The age adjusted rate of lower extremity amputation among people with diabetes in the United States is approximately 15 times that of the nondiabetic population. More than 50 % of the lower limb amputations in the United States are diabetes related, although persons diagnosed with diabetes represent only 3 % of the population.

○ **Have advances in medical and surgical diagnosis and treatment of DM and PVD eliminated the need for amputation?**

Although major improvements have been made in noninvasive diagnosis, surgical revascularization procedures, and wound-healing techniques, between 2% and 5% of individuals with PVD and without diabetes and between 6% and 25% of those with diabetes eventually undergo an amputation.

○ **What are the most common factors directly responsible for the necessity of amputation of a lower lib segment in**

patients with DM type 2?

Nonhealing or infected neuropathic ulcer precedes approximately 85% of nontraumatic lower extremity amputations in individuals with diabetes. The most frequently cited criteria for amputation among persons with diabetes include gangrene, infection, non healing neuropathic ulcer, severe ischemic pain, absent or decreased pulses, local necrosis, osteomyelitis, systemic toxicity, acute embolic disease, or severe venous thrombosis.

○   **What topics are covered in pre-amputation counseling?**

To fill these information gaps, the patient and family benefit from pre amputation counseling from members of the rehabilitation team and from a prosthetic user who can provide firsthand information

1.   Pain will certainly be present following surgery and its duration and intensity may not be predictable. The patient seeking pain relief as a result of amputation may not be satisfied, as the RL or phantom limb may also be painful.
2.   Phantom sensation (and possibly pain) will likely be present following surgery.
3.   Exercise and proper positioning in the early postoperative period will be very important to future rehabilitation.
4.   A general time frame for acute hospitalization, wound healing, preprosthetic rehabilitation, and prosthetic use is very helpful to the patient.
5.   A discussion of this information with an amputee as closely matched demographically as possible will provide the patient with a more credible view of the future.
6.   Early contact with the patient also allows members of the rehabilitation team to evaluate the patient's premorbid status and current problems so that appropriate goals and plans can be made.

○   **What does the amputee clinical examination consist of?**

A general physical examination that documents body weight, height, peripheral circulation, skin integrity, limb dominance, overall health, comorbidities, and mental status is necessary. The examination of the residual limb (RL) should include the soft-tissue length and shape, bone length and shape, and skin integrity, pliability, and mobility. Scar tissue is assessed, as is the RLE's tolerance to pressure, traction, and weight bearing. Sensation is also evaluated as well as the presence of neuroma or areas of hypersensitivity. The clinician should document the range of motion (ROM) and strength of the proximal joints. The status of the contralateral limb and the ROM, strength, and sensation of the other limbs are critical data in the planning of the rehabilitation program. Balance and coordination are also essential and should be tested. Patients with peripheral neuropathy or skin grafts use vision as a compensatory mechanism for the lack of sensation in the prosthesis and the other limbs. Eye examination should be encouraged, as many patients need updated prescription eyeglasses and vision care.

○   **What specific findings should be addressed in the assessment of a patient with transtibial amputation?**

Assessment of the transtibial RL involves similar considerations. The length is categorized as short, mid, or long. Strength and ROM of the hip and knee are evaluated. Assessment of hip and knee extension is particularly important. As with the transfemoral RL, location of scars, presence of skin or vascular grafts, and the nature of the surgical technique (myodesis or myoplasty) are also noted. The configuration of the distal end and its ability to bear weight are also important factors.

○   **For the amputee with dysvascular disease what clinical indicators contribute to the readiness of lower limb prosthetic training?**

Simple clinical indicators such as the ability to ambulate with a walker or crutches for 30 to 40 ft, while blood pressure and pulse rate are monitored, are adequate to determine whether the patient will be able to achieve the goal of limited household ambulation. Patients with a documented ejection fraction of 15% should be able to ambulate very short distances with an artificial limb. The cardiac risk in this population does not appear to be significantly increased when using a prosthesis or walking short distances.

○   **Given the multifactorial influences on clinical outcomes for amputees, what other patient data should be obtained?**

Cognition
Psychological status

Comorbid medical conditions of the musculoskeletal, peripheral neurological, visual, integumentary and cardiovascular systems

○   **What vocational and recreational interest should be addressed?**

Other areas of importance that should be evaluated include the vocational and recreational activities that the patient performed in the past and wants to pursue in the future. Certain vocational or avocational activities may require alternative specialized prosthetic devices, training, or use of no prosthesis. Devices that may be exposed to extreme weather, water, or other elements that may be corrosive or destructive to the prosthesis should be made of special materials to protect the RL and the prosthesis.

○   **What social support issues should be considered?**

Social support systems play an important role in the amputee's rehabilitation. The rehabilitation program for a person living with an able-bodied spouse in an elevator-accessible single floor apartment is different from that of a person living alone in a third-story walk-up apartment.

○   **What specific findings should be addressed in the assessment of a patient with transfemoral amputation?**

For the transfemoral level of amputation, assessing the length (short, mid, long) of the RL, ROM of the hip (particularly extension), and strength of the hip (particularly abduction, extension) is important.

Knowledge of the type of surgical technique used for amputation is important; in particular, surgical reattachment of the adductor group (myodesis) has a significant impact on future function.

The configuration of the distal end of the femur and the presence of heterotopic ossification or bone growth at the tip should be noted.

Other characteristics of the RL that should be noted include location of surgical scars, position and type of grafts (skin or vascular), and ability to bear weight distally. These factors should be considered when the prosthetic socket is fabricated.

Surgical revision should be considered when heterotopic bone, scars, grafts, or other features of the RL prevent adequate prosthetic fabrication.

○   **What specific findings should be addressed in the assessment of a patient with transradial amputation?**

For the transradial level of amputation (short, mid, long), evaluation of the ROM and strength of the elbow, shoulder, and scapula and the quantification of pronation and supination are necessary. The position of surgical scars, configuration of the distal end, and type of surgical closure carried out (myodesis or myoplastic), and the ability of the RL to receive distal pressure and weight bearing are assessed. Contractility of the underlying muscle is of particular importance if a myoelectric device is to be considered.

○   **What issues should be addressed when carrying out an assessment of a bilateral upper extremity amputee?**

For the bilateral upper-limb amputee, the ROM and strength of shoulder and neck and trunk flexibility are important factors. One should assess the ability to use lower limbs for functional activities such as opening doors, stabilizing objects, feeding, and other essential functions.

The ideal length of the limbs is determined by using a ratio of height; for very-proximal-level amputations, the forearm section is made shorter to improve elbow lift power by reducing the lever arm length. It is necessary to determine the optimal prosthetic control systems to be used (body power versus external power or both).

For externally powered devices, myoelectric or switch control can be used. Externally powered devices require more maintenance than body-powered devices.

○   **What elements of the clinical assessment of a bilateral lower extremity amputee are to be emphasized?**

For patients who have had bilateral lower-limb amputation, the evaluation should focus on the strength, dexterity, and ROM of the upper limbs and the ability to use the upper limbs for support during walking. Assessment of the cardiopulmonary systems is essential in view of the expected increase in metabolic cost during walking. Limb lengths should be determined based on the ability to transfer from sitting to standing (18 inches to the knee may be sufficient) while keeping a lower center of mass for improved balance and more efficient energy utilization during standing and walking.

O   **What issues need to be addressed in prosthetic selection and utilization?**

Choosing prosthetic components based on needs, desires, and available funding sources, as well as accessibility to maintenance, is critical. Projecting the patient's dependency on the prosthetic devices will permit determining the need for a wheelchair or a second set of artificial legs (maybe waterproof ones to be used also during showers).

O   **What interventions are recommended for the post operative care of the residual limb?**

Care of the RL focuses on several areas including wound healing, volume containment, optimization of strength and ROM, and desensitization.

O   **What are the available methods for volume containment of the residual limb?**

Volume containment can be achieved through several approaches. Ideally, the immediate postoperative rigid dressing, applied in the operating room, provides edema control as well as mechanical protection for the limb. As an alternative, the removable rigid dressing can be used, allowing the patient greater participation. The Unna boot also prevents swelling but requires no particular skill in its application. Ace bandages, tubular compression dressings, or stump shrinkers provide elastic compression and may be favored for their simplicity and neatness.

O   **What is the progression of gait training for the patient with a lower extremity amputation?**

Gait training begins with weight bearing and weight shifting, using the parallel bars for upper limb support. The patient gradually progresses to ambulation in the parallel bars. The therapist may find it difficult to focus the patient on proper technique including equal step length and appropriate weight shifting. Gait deviations frequently develop owing to the patient's eagerness to begin walking. As the patient establishes a consistent gait pattern and can maintain good form, he or she advances to use of a walker, crutches, and unilateral support devices. Once the patient is comfortable with level surfaces; he or she progresses to walking on stairs, curbs, and ramps, as well as uneven terrain. The patient also learns safe techniques for transfers, including to and from the floor.

O   **What monitoring is considered during this period?**

Frequent monitoring of the skin allows for prompt corrections of socket fit problems and avoids skin break down. Skin checks are done more frequently for the new prosthetic user and for the patient with delicate skin. Initially, checking the skin every 10 to 15 minutes or after every one or two walks may be necessary. Once the patient and therapist are comfortable with the socket fit, skin monitoring can occur less frequently. Prosthetic wearing tolerance gradually increases over the first few weeks. Some patients can only wear the pros-thesis for 2 to 3 hr/day during the first week of gait training.

O   **What is the pattern of wear and monitoring during the terminal phase of training?**

This gradually increases until it is worn all day (12–16 hours). Throughout the rehabilitation process, the patient should become well versed in skin care. The patient learns to monitor the skin of the RL, noting signs of appropriate weight bearing and watching for evidence of skin irritation or breakdown. When the prosthesis is not worn, the patient wears a stump shrinker or an Ace bandage to prevent edema and provide volume containment.

O   **What are the key elements of the occupational therapy treatment plan?**

As the amputee progresses with ambulation and management of the prosthesis, ambulatory self care activities and homemaking activities can be addressed. Occupational therapy works with the patient to learn safe techniques for bathing, dressing, and toileting using the prosthesis. Many patients need to perform homemaking tasks as well. The therapist should include meal preparation, laundry, shopping, and other household chores in the training routine of these individuals, using the prosthesis if possible.

O   **What concerns regarding the socket for the lower extremity amputee need to be considered for the provision of the definitive prosthesis in the transtibial amputee?**

Concerning the socket, it is vital to allow the patient's RL to mature before fabrication of the permanent socket. The soft-tissue bulk of the RL decreases significantly, owing to resolution of edema as well as disuse atrophy of muscles and adipose tissue. These changes occur primarily during the first 2 to 5 months following the amputation. The definitive prosthesis frequently uses a suction suspension mechanism that is not usually recommended for a preparatory pylon because of fluctuations in RL girth. Patients often will require new instruction on donning techniques for the suction socket.

O   **What concerns regarding the socket for the lower extremity amputee need to be considered for the provision of the definitive prosthesis in the transfemoral amputee?**

Transfemoral level amputees will have significant changes in their abilities depending on the knee unit prescribed, and instruction in mobility and gait should vary based on the type of mechanism used in the permanent prosthetic device. For example, patients ambulating with a cadence responsive knee with swing and stance control will require a different gait pattern compared to patients using a weight activated knee unit. They will also have different mechanisms for transferring from sitting to standing and ascending and descending stairs and inclines.

O   **What are the major concerns in the transition of an upper extremity amputee from a preparatory to definitive prosthesis?**

For the upper limb amputee, early prosthetic fitting is vital to the acceptance of the prosthesis. Generally, the first prosthesis uses conventional or body powered componentry. Myoelectric or externally powered prostheses are not usually recommended at this stage because of the fluctuation in girth as the RL matures. This fluctuation will make it difficult to achieve the intimate fit between the skin and socket needed for the myoelectric system to work properly. Additionally, one should verify that the patient would be a prosthetic user before incurring the higher cost of an externally powered prosthesis. Upper limb amputees who are progressing from conventional to myoelectric prosthetics require a period of retraining, to instruct them in the proper use and care of the new prosthesis.

O   **What are reasonable expectations and requirements for a transtibial amputee to engage in running activities?**

A commonly stated desire for athletic ability is to be able to run again. This goal should be considered for all active amputees, even if it is to run just a short distance for a bus or to get out of danger. A good socket fit is crucial for running for both transtibial level and transfemoral level amputees. A good fit allows the patient to tolerate the tremendous amount of pressure and reaction forces translated to the limb without too much discomfort.

O   **What are the elements of a training program for potential runners with a transtibial amputation?**

For the healthy, active transtibial-level amputee, running is fairly easy to achieve. When the patient is ambulating independently without an assistive device, he or she is ready to begin training. Hopping and jumping activities will assist with building the patient's tolerance for increased force transmitted to the limb. A gradual progression from fast walking, to a trot and then a run is usually successful. The treadmill can be useful to progress the patient to higher speeds.

O   **What are the clinical considerations for ambulation in a patient with bilateral transfemoral amputation?**

Ambulation should be attempted only when adequate cardiac function, strength, balance, and endurance exist; the use of multi axis ankle feet systems with lower height and weight activated knee locking mechanisms should facilitate the patient's ability to ambulate. The clinician can avoid unnecessary expenditures of resources in the geriatric population by careful selection of potentially functional ambulation candidates who have had bilateral transfemoral amputations.

O   **What prosthetic device is appropriate for a transfemoral amputee to engage in running activities?**

The transfemoral level amputee requires increased training to achieve running. Thus the appropriate components such as cadence responsive knees are vital to achieve a step over step running pattern. Without a cadence responsive knee unit, the patient has to wait for the shank of the prosthesis to come forward, resulting in an extra hop on the sound limb.

O   **What are the elements of the training program for a transfemoral amputee to engage in running?**

Training techniques for the transfemoral running gait often begin with weight-bearing activities, balance activities, and exercise to improve pelvic and hip control. Initially there is an emphasis on hopping and jumping, to increase tolerance to increased forces translated to the residual limb. Fast walking and ambulating with an exaggerated step length and then a progression to jogging or running can occur.

O   **How does the energy expenditure of the lower extremity amputee compare with the energy expenditure of normal healthy individuals?**

In normal healthy individuals of the energy cost of walking for helping individuals with a mean the speed of 83 m/min as 0.063 kilocalories per minute per kilogram and 0.000764 kilocalories per meter per kilogram of body weight. Individuals with transtibial amputation walk 36 % more slowly, expending 2 % more kilocalories per minute and 41% more kilocalories per meter to cover a similar distance. For individuals with transfemoral amputation, gait speed is 43% slower, whereas energy cost is reflected as 5 % less kilocalories per minute and 89% more kilocalories per meter.

O   **What factor is critical in determining the degree of energy expended in gait in a lower extremity amputee?**

Preservation of the anatomic knee joint appears to be especially important. A classic study by Waters et al demonstrated that, for young adults with traumatic transtibial amputation, gait speed, oxygen rate, and oxygen cost were quite close to normal values reported by Perry. For those with traumatic transfemoral or dysvascular amputation, diminishing gait speeds kept oxygen consumption close to that of normal adult gait. However, oxygen cost increased well beyond the normal value of 0.15 mg/kg/m. Although gait speeds reported in a more recent study by Torburn et al are much higher, the difference in performance between traumatic and dysvascular groups was consistent. Other studies report oxygen costs of prosthetic gait at between 28% and 33% above normal for individuals with transtibial amputation and between 60% and 110% above normal for individuals with transfemoral amputation.

O   **What is the relationship between gait speed and O_2 rate consumption in a lower extremity amputee?**

Although the relationship between gait speed and oxygen rate (consumption) in prosthetic gait is linear, just as it is in unimpaired gait, the slope is significantly steeper. The clinical implication of this relationship is that the rate of energy consumption and of cardiac work, at any gait speed, is higher for those with amputation and that the threshold for transition from aerobic to anaerobic metabolism is reached at lower gait speeds.

O   **What are practical ramifications of the energy expenditure studies?**

Because of this high energy cost, many older individuals with amputation related to vascular disease may be limited in their ability to become functional community ambulators, instead walking slowly with the assistance a walker or cane. Individuals with bilateral transfemoral amputation are rarely able to become community ambulators with prostheses, instead choosing a wheelchair for long distance mobility. It is important to recognize that the most individuals with unilateral transtibial and transfemoral amputation, regardless of age or etiology dedication, the energy cost of walking with a prosthesis is less than that expended when walking without using crutches or walker.

O   **What are some relative contraindications to ambulatory activity with lower extremity prostheses?**

Several factors are relative contraindications to prescribing prostheses for the bilateral lower-limb amputee. These include lack of motivation, significant cognitive impairment, severe cardiac disease, severe contractures, and severe neurologic impairment. The degree of cardiac compromise a patient can tolerate while walking with bilateral prostheses is unclear. An ejection fraction of 20% may be chosen as an arbitrary cutoff, but no hard data exist to substantiate this. Prosthetic ambulation is possible in the setting of significant cardiac compromise because amputees adjust their walking speed to keep relative energy demands at a manageable level.

REHABILITATION OF THE BOWEL AND BLADDER

○ **What is the incidence of neurogenic bladder?**

Incidence of neurogenic bladder dysfunction depends on the primary cause. Etiology and level of central or peripheral nervous system injury correlate with different causes and classifications of bladder dysfunction. Bladder disorders are reported in 40-90% of patients with MS. Estimates of incidence of urologic symptoms in patients who have sustained a CVA vary, ranging from 33-60% in the acute setting and persisting in 15% at 6 months to 1 year. Incidence of urologic dysfunction in patients with Parkinson disease has been reported to be 37-72%. Incidence of urinary incontinence is higher in patients with dementia and other types of cognitive impairment (eg, TBI, CVA, Parkinson disease) than in the general population. Incidence of bladder disorders is nearly universal in children with myelomeningocele and in patients with SCI.

○ **Summarize the differential diagnosis for patients with established incontinence.**

Lower Urinary Tract Causes of Established Incontinence

Urodynamic Diagnosis	Some Neurogenic Causes	Some Nonneurogenic Causes
Detrusor overactivity	Multiple sclerosis	Urethral obstruction/incompetence
	Stroke	Cystitis
	Parkinson's disease	Bladder carcinoma
	Alzheimer's disease	Bladder stone
Detrusor underactivity	Disk compression	Idiopathic (common in women)
	Plexopathy	Chronic outlet obstruction
	Surgical damage (e.g., abdominoperineal resection)	
	Autonomic neuropathy (e.g., diabetes mellitus, alcoholism, B_{12} deficiency)	
Outlet incompetence	Surgical lesion (rare)	Urethral hypermobility (type 1 and 2 SUI)
	Lower motor neuron lesion (rare)	Intrinsic sphincter deficiency (type 3 SUI)
		Postprostatectomy
Outlet obstruction	Spinal cord lesion with detrusor-sphincter dyssynergia (rare)	Prostatic enlargement
		Prostate carcinoma
		Prolapsing cystourethrocele
		After bladder neck suspension

SUI, stress urinary incontinence.

○ **Summarize medications that can contribute to urinary incontinence.**

Medications That May Affect Continence

Type of Medication	Examples	Potential Effects on Continence
Sedatives/hypnotics	Long-acting benzodiazepines (e.g., diazepam, flurazepam)	Sedation, delirium, immobility
Alcohol	Polyuria, frequency, urgency, sedation, delirium, immobility	
Anticholinergics	Dicyclomine, disopyramide, antihistamines	Urinary retention, overflow incontinence, delirium, impaction
Antipsychotics	Thioridazine, haloperidol	Anticholinergic actions, sedation, rigidity, immobility
Antidepressants	Amitriptyline, desipramine	Anticholinergic actions, sedation

Medications That May Affect Continence

Type of Medication	Examples	Potential Effects on Continence
Antiparkinsonian medications	Trihexyphenidyl, benztropine mesylate (not L-dopa/selegiline)	Anticholinergic actions, sedation
Narcotic analgesics	Opiates	Urinary retention, fecal impaction, sedation, delirium
α-Adrenergic antagonists	Prazosin, terazosin, doxazosin	Urethral relaxation may precipitate stress incontinence in women
α-Adrenergic agonists	Nasal decongestants	Urinary retention in men
Calcium channel blockers	All	Urinary retention; nocturnal diuresis from fluid retention
Potent diuretics	Furosemide, bumetanide	Polyuria, frequency, urgency
Angiotensin-converting enzyme inhibitors	Captopril, enalapril, lisinopril	Drug-induced cough can precipitate stress incontinence in women and in some men with previous prostatectomy
Vincristine	Urinary retention	

○ **What are the characteristics of urinary tract infections (UTI) with a neurogenic bladder?**

Urinary tract infections are a frequent cause of morbidity in patients with neurogenic bladder. Patients with neurogenic bladder who lack sensation do not experience dysuria. Instead, symptoms may include fever, tachycardia, a feeling of uneasiness, signs and symptoms of autonomic dysreflexia, malodorous urine, increase in spasticity in patients with upper motor neuron lesions, and lethargy. The main morbid feature of urinary tract infection is that, if left untreated, it may lead to urosepsis and/or pyelonephritis.

○ **Are patients with neurogenic bladder prone to bladder stone formation?**

Predisposition to bladder stone formation is noted at 4 weeks in patients with SCI as a result of hypercalcemia and hypercalciuria and may persist 12-15 months or even longer. Incidence of kidney stone formation is highest in patients with indwelling catheters, up to 8%. Kidney stones are the leading cause of renal dysfunction in SCI.

○ **Are patients with neurogenic bladder at a higher risk for bladder cancer?**

Incidence of bladder cancer is higher in SCI patients who have had an indwelling Foley catheter for 10 years or more than in other patients with SCI. Squamous cell carcinoma and transitional cell carcinomas are the types of bladder cancer commonly diagnosed in SCI patients.

○ **What physical findings are assessed in the patient with neurogenic bladder?**

1.	Determine the motor level of the lesion, including completeness of lesion in SCI patients. Ascertain the extent of the patient's hand function and ability to perform transfers and activities of daily living (ADL). Hand function is especially important in SCI patients who are to perform self-catheterization.
2.	Conduct sensory testing to determine sensory level, especially in SCI patients. Include testing with light touch, pinprick, proprioception, and sacral sensation.
3.	Test reflexes and include normally tested muscle stretch reflexes, the bulbocavernosus reflex, cremasteric, and anal reflexes. Use the bulbocavernosus reflex to test integrity of the pudendal nerve and the S2-S4 segments.
4.	Determine the condition of the skin in the perianal area. In patients with chronic neurogenic bladder, the skin typically shows areas of chronic irritation manifested by areas of excoriation and redness, usually superseded by fungal infection.
5.	Establish the state of vaginal and bladder supports, particularly in patients with suspected stress incontinence. Relaxation of the bladder neck and weakness of the sphincter mechanism are common in these patients.
6.	Evaluate the status of the prostate, especially in men aged 60 years or more. Prostatic enlargement, which can cause secondary urologic symptoms, usually manifests as urinary retention.
7.	Note the presence of cognitive impairment or dementia. Such patients are at risk for incontinence due to disinhibited bladder contractions.

○　**What pathophysiological findings of suprapontine lesions are associated with neurogenic bladder?**

Suprapontine lesions (eg, due to CVA, MS, dementia, brain tumors, TBI) lead to uninhibited bladder contractions possibly secondary to loss of cerebral cortex inhibition at the sacral micturition center. Facilitation of the spin bulbospinal reflex also is affected.

○　**What pathophysiological findings of supra sacral lesions are associated with neurogenic bladder?**

Supra sacral lesions are associated with the group of neurogenic bladder problems caused by spinal cord lesion from trauma, tumors, or spina bifida. These lesions cause interruption of the spin bulbospinal reflex, which leads acutely to areflexia, then usually to detrusor hyperreflexia and uncoordinated micturition with detrusor sphincter dyssynergia.

○　**What pathophysiological findings of sacral lesions are associated with neurogenic bladder?**

Sacral lesions include lesions affecting the conus medullaris, the cauda equina, and S2-S4 peripheral nerves. Common causes of sacral lesions are trauma, stenosis, tumors, peripheral neuropathy, and infection. In general, lesions of this type lead to variable loss of parasympathetic and somatic nerve function. Detrusor areflexia, bladder neck incompetence, and/or loss of external sphincter function may occur.

○　**What laboratory studies are indicated in the patient with neurogenic bladder?**

1.　Urinalysis and urine culture with sensitivity to rule out infection
2.　24-hour creatinine clearance
3.　Residual urine volume: Usually determined by bladder scanning after void; it may be measured directly by catheterization if bladder scan is not available It reflects bladder and outlet activity during the emptying phase of micturition. An acceptable quantity of up to 150 mL of postvoid residual urine with voiding frequency greater than every 2 hours, if the patient is not experiencing frequent urinary tract infections.

○　**What radiologic studies are indicated for the patient with neurogenic bladder?**

Plain film of the urinary tract, bladder, and kidneys is indicated to determine presence of radiopaque calculi in conjunction with ultrasonography. Excretory urography or intravenous pyelography can be used for visualization of the collecting system. Isotope studies (eg, technetium 99 m dimercaptosuccinic acids [DMSA]) are used for evaluation of function of renal cortex. Ultrasonography is used for routine evaluation of the upper urinary tract to Evaluate for presence of ureteral obstruction, scarring, masses, and either renal or bladder calculi

○　**What does cystometry consist of?**

It evaluates filling and storage phases of detrusor function by measuring changes in intravesical pressure with increases in bladder volume Normal adult bladder capacity is around 400-750 mL, with bladder pressures normally not exceeding 15 cm H_2O during filling phase. Bladder volumes determined and recorded during first sensation of filling, voiding urgency, and maximal filling Assesses voluntary voiding phase after filling and efficacy of emptying It Assesses the leak point (i.e., the pressure at which voiding occurs) .

○　**What abnormal findings may occur in cystometric study of the neurogenic bladder?**

Abnormal findings include decreased bladder compliance with intravesical pressures exceeding 15 cm H_2O with steep rising curve in the cystometrogram, possibly due to bladder inflammation, bladder fibrosis, or detrusor hypertrophy. Involuntary detrusor contraction (i.e., phasic increase in intravesical pressures during filling phase) reflects presence of detrusor hyperreflexia in patients with suprapontine lesions (eg, from CVA, Parkinson disease). This phenomenon also is seen in patients with supra sacral spinal cord disease (eg, SCI, MS, spina bifida). A noncompliant bladder with a reduced capacity demonstrates a steep curve which is associated with neurogenic lesions, inflammation, or severe outlet obstruction. Absence of contractions in attempting to void, as seen in areflexic bladders, may be seen in patients with sacral lesions or peripheral neuropathy.

○　**What is the role of EMG in neurogenic bladder evaluation?**

Electromyography (EMG) is used to measure electrical potentials generated by depolarization of the detrusor muscle and urethral sphincter. Anticipated normal findings include incremental increase in EMG activity in the external sphincter during filling phase secondary to increased recruitment of motor units. Prior to voiding, diminished EMG activity in the external sphincter is expected. Relaxation of the external sphincter is followed by bladder contraction.

O **What abnormal findings may occur in neurogenic bladder EMG?**

Abnormal EMG patterns include absence of recruitment and low levels of EMG activity as in patients with complete SCI. Inappropriate increase may be observed in EMG activity of the sphincter, leading to detrusor contraction against a closed sphincter or detrusor sphincter dyssynergia.

O **How does Video urodynamics assist neurogenic bladder investigation?**

Evaluation of complex lower urinary tract pathology is performed using video urodynamics. This technique involves EMG studies during 3 phases in conjunction with periodic screening of synchronous cystourethrographic studies of the bladder and outlet. Video urodynamics is particularly useful in detection of sites of bladder outlet obstruction and detrusor-sphincter dyssynergia.

O **What is the Valsalva or Credé maneuver?**

The Credé maneuver is manual compression of the bladder, used in patients with decreased bladder tone or areflexia and low outlet resistance. Facilitation of the Credé maneuver by an attendant is useful, particularly in individuals who are quadriplegic. Increasing intravesical pressure also may be achieved through the Valsalva maneuver (i.e., abdominal straining).

O **How can a patient accomplish initiation of reflex bladder contraction?**

Pinching or stimulating the lumbar and sacral dermatomal levels is used to provoke reflex bladder contraction. Patients with SCI may use this technique if there is no outlet obstruction or detrusor sphincter dyssynergia.

O **What is timed voiding?**

A program of timed voiding is useful in patients with weak sphincters or in patients with hyperreflexic bladders. These patients are put on a schedule of frequent bladder emptying before actual bladder contraction. Timed voiding should be scheduled every 2-4 hours.

O **What is the role of clean intermittent catheterization in neurogenic bladder management?**

The practice of clean intermittent catheterization (CIC) is used primarily in patients with neurogenic bladder disease such as in cases of SCI. Prerequisites for use include sufficient outflow resistance to maintain continence between catheterizations, bladder with low pressure, and adequate bladder capacity, ideally more than 300 mL. Encourage fluid restriction to limit bladder volumes to less than 400 mL. Schedule catheterization 3-6 times per day. Problems with this technique include urethral trauma and predisposition to bacteriuria and/or urinary tract infections. Usually SCI patients with lesions at C7 and below can manage self-catheterization. To avoid development of latex allergy, use non latex catheters for chronic use. Lubrication with 2% lidocaine helps to limit pain and trauma. At times, use of a curved tip (coudé) catheter may be necessary if there is difficulty introducing a standard catheter.

O **When can External condom catheters be used to manage the neurogenic bladder**

Men with spinal cord lesions higher than C7 who are unable to perform self-catheterization are the most likely to benefit from the use of external condom catheters. If outlet obstruction is present, a sphincterotomy is needed. The patient must have reflex bladder contractions. Skin breakdown can occur, especially in patients with poor hygiene. Urinary tract infections can occur.

O **What is the role for indwelling catheters in neurogenic bladder management?**

Indwelling catheters are either suprapubic or urethral. Patients frequently choose this option for convenience and as a last resort when all other measures have failed. It is also an option for persons who are unable to catheterize themselves and who prefer not to have the caregiver do CIC. Catheter care includes monthly catheter changes, sterilization of collection bags, and irrigation. Urinary colonization and infections are common. Long term users should have routine cystoscopy to rule out bladder cancer. The pediatric and geriatric populations with adequate bladder emptying use diapers or incontinence pads.

○ **When is transurethral resection of the bladder neck indicated?**

Transurethral resection of the bladder neck is indicated in patients with obstruction at the bladder neck when medical therapy has failed to produce satisfactory results.

○ **When is external sphincterotomy indicated?**

External sphincterotomy is indicated in patients with supra sacral lesions causing failure to empty when other therapeutic modalities have not been successful. Candidates for this procedure should have adequate detrusor contractions.

○ **When is stenting indicated?**

Stenting makes use of removable stents inserted into the urethra via cystoscopy. Indications are similar to those for sphincterectomy.

○ **When is urethral overdilation indicated?**

Urethral over dilation is performed only in females and has the same objective as sphincterotomy.

○ **What is an external compressive procedure?**

External compressive procedure involves creation of a fascial sling around the bladder neck, using a fascial strip from either the abdominal rectus muscle or tensor fascia lata.

○ **When is implantation of an artificial internal sphincter considered?**

Implantation of an artificial sphincter is used most commonly in children with myelomeningocele who have an incompetent sphincter mechanism.

○ **When is bladder augmentation utilized in the management of the neurogenic bladder?**

Bladder augmentation is used primarily in patients with refractory hyperreflexic bladders when medical treatment has failed to alleviate symptoms. In this procedure, the bladder is opened and patched using a reconfigured segment of bowel. Augmentation also is used to achieve a normal bladder capacity in children and adolescents, often in conjunction with the artificial sphincter.

○ **What is the Mitrofanoff procedure?**

The Mitrofanoff procedure uses the appendix to create a channel between the abdominal wall and the bladder. This procedure is particularly useful in patients who are unable to reach the urethra for CIC or in patients with limited hand function due to SCI. In general, it is easier to manipulate clothing and pass the catheter through the umbilicus than to transfer, remove lower extremity garments, and perform urethral CIC.

○ **What is the role for intravesical administration of capsaicin?**

Several studies have investigated the efficacy of intravesical administration of capsaicin, a neurotoxin for C-afferent fibers, for treatment of detrusor hyperreflexia. The results of one study showed improvement in manifestations of bladder disorders, including decreased voiding frequency, fewer leakages, and increased cystometric capacity.

○ **What is the role of electrical stimulation in the management of the neurogenic bladder?**

Electrical stimulation involves use of electrodes driven by an implanted receiver to stimulate detrusor contractions. Electrodes usually are placed in the anterior sacral roots. Bilateral S2-S4 rhizotomies are usually a prerequisite to prevent spontaneous hyperreflexic contractions. This technique may be useful for patients who can transfer independently but who have incontinence between catheterizations.

O **Profile bladder active medications that may be used in the management of urinary incontinence.**

Pharmacological agents used in the treatment of urinary incontinence

Type of Incontinence	Drug	Dose Range	Common Side Effects	Contraindications
Urge	Oxybutynin (Ditropan®)	2.5-5 mg TID-QID	Anticholinergic effects[b]	Untreated angle-closure glaucoma, GI tract obstruction urinary retention
	Oxybutynin XL (Ditropan XL®)	5-30 mg QD	Anticholinergic effects[b]	Same as for Ditropan
	Tolterodine (Detrol®)	1-2 mg BID	Anticholinergic effects[b]	Urinary retention, gastric retention, uncontrolled narrow-angle glaucoma
	Propantheline (Pro-Banthine®)	7.5-30 mg TID-QID	Nausea, insomnia, weakness, postural hypotension	Myasthenia gravis, acute hemorrhage
	Imipramine (Tofranil®)	25 mg QD[a]	Anticholinergic effects[b]	Untreated narrow angle-closure glaucoma, GI obstruction, urinary retention
	Dicyclomine (Bentyl®)	10-20 mg TID	Anticholinergic effects[b]	Concurrent use of monoamine oxidase inhibitors
	Flavoxate (Urispas®)	100-200 mg TID-QID	Nausea, vomiting, dry mouth, headache, blurred vision	Pyloric or duodenal obstruction, GI hemorrhage
Stress	Pseudoephedrine (Sudafed®)	15-60 mg TID	CNS stimulant effects[d]	Severe hypertension, severe coronary artery disease Use of monoamine oxidase inhibitors
	Imipramine (Tofranil®)	25 mg QD[a]	Nausea, insomnia, weakness, postural hypotension	Use of monoamine oxidase inhibitors
	Conjugated estrogen (Premarin®)	0.3-1.25 mg PO QD[c] 2 grams or fraction topical QD[c]	Headache, breast tenderness	Known or suspected breast or uterus cancer
Overflow Outlet obstruction:	Terazosin (Hytrin®)	1-10 mg QD	Dizziness, hypotension, headache drowsiness	Known sensitivity
	Doxazosin (Cardura®)	1-8 mg QD	Dizziness, hypotension, headache drowsiness	Known sensitivity
	Prazosin (Minipres®)	1-9 mg QD	Dizziness, hypotension, headache drowsiness	Known sensitivity
	Tamsulosin (Flomax®)	0.4 mg QD	Headache, dizziness, malaise	Known sensitivity
Atonic bladder:	Bethanecol (Urecholine®)	10-50 mg BID-QID[e] 50-100 mg QID[f]	Rare with oral administration	IM or IV. Hyperthyroidism, peptic ulcer, bronchial asthma, cardiac diseases

a. Starting dose 25 mg/day. Increased by increments by 25 mg/week until clinical response or anticholinergic effects is observed.
b. Dry mouth, blurred vision, dry skin, constipation, urinary retention
c. If uterus intact, add Provera 2.5-5 mg QD
d. Nervousness, restlessness, insomnia, dizziness
e. Per manufacturer's recommendations
f. Believed to be more effective.

O **What clinical follow up is needed fore patients with neurogenic bladder?**

Patients with indwelling catheters must undergo annual cystoscopy for detection of bladder tumors since they have increased risk for squamous cell and transitional cell carcinoma if they have had indwelling catheters for more than 10 years. Recommend cystoscopy more frequently if patient has increased risk factors (eg, smoking, history of recurrent urinary tract infections). Annual renal and bladder ultrasounds are recommended. Perform voiding cystourethrogram as needed. Schedule DMSA as indicated. Determine glomerular filtration rate as needed. Order urinalysis and urine culture with sensitivity at least once a year and as needed.

○ **Summarize the appropriate treatment strategies for neurogenic bladder disorders**

FUNCTIONAL CLASSIFICATION	TREATMENT OPTIONS
INCONTINENCE (failure to store) Due to bladder hyperreflexia (e.g., suprapontine lesions such as stroke, TBI, MS, neoplasm, hydrocephalus, PD)	1. Behavioral: timed voids, fluid restrictions 2. Collecting devices: diaper, catheter (condom or indwelling) 3. Clean intermittent catheterization 4. Drugs: anticholinergics, musculotropics, tricyclic antidepressant, intrathecal baclofen, prostaglandin inhibitors 5. Surgery: augmentation, continent diversion, denervation procedures, neurostimulation procedures
INCONTINENCE (failure to store) Due to the outlet or sphincter incompetence (e.g., children with myelodysplasia; stress incontinence in women with infra-sacral lesion and denervated pelvic floor; or rarely, men with complete denervation)	1. Behavioral: timed voids, pelvic floor exercises, biofeedback, fluid restrictions 2. Collecting devices: diaper, catheter (condom or indwelling) 3. Drugs: a-adrenergic agonists, imipramine, estrogen cream 4. Surgery: collagen injection, fascial sling, artificial sphincter, Teflon injection, neurostimulation
Retention (failure to empty) Due to bladder areflexia (e.g., spinal shock in SCI; MS; peripheral neuropathies; Sacral lesions such as spinal trauma, herniated lumbar disc, spinal tumors, myelodysplasia, A V malformation, lumbar stenosis, arachnoiditis)	I. Behavioral: timed voids, bladder stimulation (suprapubic jabbing, transurethral electrical bladder stimulation), Valsalva's and Credé's maneuvers 2. Collecting devices: indwelling catheter 3. Clean intermittent catheterization 4. Drugs: cholinergic agonists, intravesical prostaglandins, narcotic antagonists 5. Surgery: neurostimulation
Due to outlet or sphincter dyssynergia (e.g., supra sacral traumatic SCI)	I. Behavioral: anal stretch void, suprapubic tapping, biofeedback 2. Collecting devices: indwelling catheters 3. Clean intermittent catheterization 4. Drugs: (X-adrenergic blockers, oral striated muscle relaxant (baclofen, diazepam, dantrolene), intrathecal baclofen 5. Surgery: sphincterotomy incision, bladder neck incision, prostate resection, pudendal neurectomy, stent, sphincterotomy

○ **Provide a definition of constipation**

Straining at stool at least 25% of the time
Presence of lumpy or hard (pellet-like) stools at least 25% of the time
Feeling of incomplete evacuation at least 25% of the time
Fewer than three bowel movements in a week
*For the diagnosis of chronic constipation, the patient must have had two or more of the listed complaints for at least 12 months and not be taking laxatives.

○ **What is the differential diagnosis for chronic constipation?**

CAUSES OF CONSTIPATION
Dietary factors
Dehydration
Low residue
Malnutrition
Endocrine/metabolic disorders
Addison's disease
Diabetes mellitus
Glucagonoma
Hypercalcemia
Hypokalemia
Hyponatremia
Hypothyroidism
Hypomagnesemia
Panhypopituitarism
Pheochromocytoma
Porphyria
Pregnancy
Uremia
Environmental factors
Change in bathroom habits (eg, use of bedpan)
Excess heat leading to dehydration
Inability to get to bathroom without assistance
Strange or hurried environment
Medications (see Table 3)
Metals
Bismuth
Heavy metals (especially lead)
Iron
Myopathies
Amyloidosis
Myotonic dystrophy
Scleroderma
Neurogenic disorders
Autonomic neuropathy
Cerebrovascular events
Chagas' disease
Dementia
Ganglioneuromatosis
Hirschsprung's disease
Hypoganglionosis
Multiple sclerosis
Neurofibromatosis
Paraplegia
Parkinson's disease
Spinal cord injury or tumor
Trauma
Psychogenic
Cognitive impairment
Depression
Eating disorders
Sedentary living/immobility
Other conditions
Anorectal disorders (eg, fissures, thrombosed hemorrhoids, rectocele)
Cardiac disease
Degenerative joint disease
Diverticulosis
Ignoring the urge to defecate
Megacolon
Motility disturbances (eg, colonic inertia or spasm, irritable bowel syndrome)
Postsurgical abnormalities
Prolonged immobility
Radiation
Strictures
Tumors
Volvulus

Weak abdominal muscles

O **What drugs are associated with constipation?**

DRUGS ASSOCIATED WITH CONSTIPATION

Analgesics
Opioids
Anticholinergics
Antihistamines
Antiparkinsonians
Antipsychotics
Antispasmodics
Anticonvulsants
Antidepressants
Lithium
Tricyclic antidepressants
Antidiarrheals
Antihypertensives
Calcium channel blockers
Clonidine hydrochloride
Antitussives
Codeine and derivatives
Cholesterol-lowering agents
Bile acid sequestrants
Diuretics
Minerals
Aluminum-containing antacids
Calcium supplements
Iron supplements
Neurogenic agents

O **Classify the bowel active medications**

CLASSIFICATION OF LAXATIVES
Luminally-active agents
        Hydrophilic colloids; bulk-forming agents (psyllium, bran, etc.)
        Osmotic agents (nonabsorbable inorganic salts or sugars)
        – sugars and alcohols: lactulose, mannitol, sorbitol, glycerin
        – polyethylene glycol
        Saline laxatives: magnesium sulfate, magnesium hydroxide, etc.
        Stool softeners (docusate)
        Lubricants (mineral oil)
Nonspecific stimulants or irritants
        Diphenylmethane derivative (bisacodyl)
        Anthraquinones (senna, cascara sagrada)
        Castor oil

O **Summarize the medication profiles available for administration in chronic constipation**

Laxatives	Adult dosage	Onset of action (hr)
First line agents		
Bulk formers		
- Psyllium (eg, Metamucil)	7 g PO qd-tid	12-72
- Methylcellulose* (eg, Citrucel)	2 g PO qd-tid	12-72
Second-line agents		
Hyperosmotics		
- Lactulose (eg, Cephulac)	15-60 mL PO qd-tid	24-48
- Polyethylene glycol (eg, CoLyte)	200-2,000 mL PO qd-tid	0.5-1

- Glycerin (eg, Sani-Supp)	3 g PR qd-bid	0.25-0.5
- Sorbitol solution (70%)	15-60 mL PO qd-bid	
Salines**		
- Magnesium hydroxide (eg, Milk of Magnesia)	5-15 mL PO tid	0.5-3
- Magnesium citrate (eg, Citro-Nesia)	4 mL/kg-300 mL PO qd	0.5-3
- Sodium phosphate (eg, Fleet Phospho-soda)	20-30 mL PO qd-bid with 12 oz of water	0.5-3
Third-line agents		
Anthraquinones		
- Cascara sagrada	325 mg (or 5 mL) PO qhs	6-12
- Senna (eg, Senokot)	Two 187-mg tablets PO qid	6-12
Emollients (stool softeners)		
- Docusates (eg, Colace)	100 mg PO qd-bid	24-72
- Mineral oil	5-45 mL PO qhs	6-8
Stimulants		
- Phenolphthalein (eg, Ex-Lax)	90 mg PO qhs	6-12
- Castor oil (eg, Purge)	15-60 mL PO qhs	2-6
- Bisacodyl (eg, Dulcolax)	10-30 mg PO or 10 mg PR qhs	6-12

*Aspiration risk in the elderly. **Use with caution in patients with dehydration or cardiac or renal disease.

○   **Provide an algorithm to treat fecal loading**

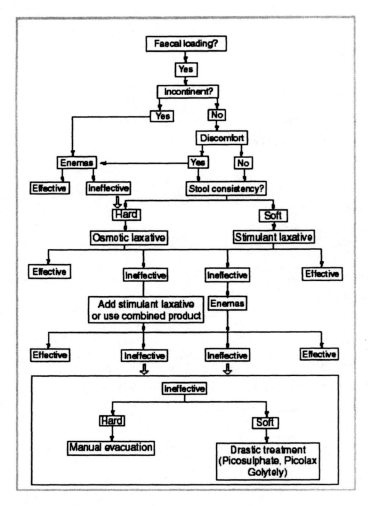

○   **Provide a differential diagnosis for fecal incontinence**

Anal sphincter/pelvic floor incompetence
Obstetric injury to the anal sphincter
Age-associated decrease in anal sphincter squeeze pressure
Pudendal neuropathy (following pregnancy)
Traction neuropathy (associated with chronic constipation)
Denervation atrophy following pudendal nerve injury
Post surgery (e.g. following anal stretch for recurrent anal fissure
or low anterior resection for rectal carcinoma)
Diarrhea
"Overflow" incontinence in patients with fecal impaction
Infection
Medication (e.g. antimicrobials, excessive laxatives)
Post radiation therapy
Colonic disorders (inflammatory bowel disease, diverticulosis,
colorectal carcinoma)
Neurological diseases
Communication and/or mobility problems (e.g. dementia,
post CVA)
Spinal cord injury
Cauda equina injury
Multiple sclerosis
Parkinson's disease
Absent or decreased sensation of rectal filling (e.g. diabetic
neuropathy)
Others
Reduced rectal compliance

Rectal prolapse

O   **Provide an algorithm for a patient with fecal incontinence.**

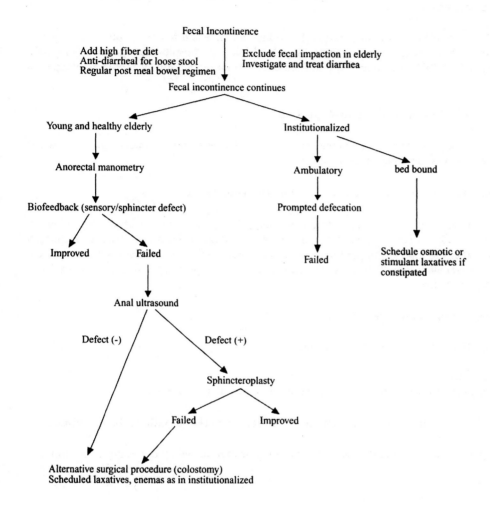

Fecal Incontinence

Add high fiber diet
Anti-diarrheal for loose stool   Exclude fecal impaction in elderly
Regular post meal bowel regimen   Investigate and treat diarrhea

Fecal incontinence continues

Young and healthy elderly   Institutionalized

Anorectal manometry   Ambulatory   bed bound

Biofeedback (sensory/sphincter defect)   Prompted defecation

Improved   Failed   Failed   Schedule osmotic or
                                                                stimulant laxatives if
                                                                constipated

Anal ultrasound

Defect (-)   Defect (+)

Sphincteroplasty

Failed   Improved

Alternative surgical procedure (colostomy)
Scheduled laxatives, enemas as in institutionalized

O   **What is the uninhibited bowel?**

Dysfunction is caused by neurologic lesions interfering with the cortical interrelationships with the pontine defecation center. Patients with stroke, brain injury, or other supra-conal lesions, when stimulated by anorectal filling, can maintain fecal continence owing to the intact pontine defecation center.

O   **What are the features of upper motor neuron bowel dysfunction?**

When neurologic lesions interrupt the pontine defecation center, such as in spinal cord injury above the conus medullaris, there is evidence that with rectal filling, not only the internal but also the external anal sphincter relax. Defecation occurs by mass contraction mediated through the myenteric plexus of the colon. By mechanical and chemical stimulation of the rectal mucosa, similar results are seen, probably by stimulating the myenteric plexus and spinal reflex. UMN colon has been described as spastic.

O   **What are the features of lower motor neuron bowel dysfunction?**

When lesions of the conus destroy either the sacral defecation center or the related nerve supply to the rectum and anus, there is denervation of the external sphincter, which results in a patulous external anal sphincter, and with rectal filling, the internal sphincter relaxes. With distention of the colon and rectum, stimulation of the myenteric plexus of the colon does occur, which leads to mass action peristalsis and internal sphincter relaxation. Lower motor neuron lesions result in both rectal stasis, drier stool because of the prolonged transit time, and at times incontinence of feces.

○   **What is the incidence of bowel dysfunction?**

An estimated 4.4 million individuals in the US suffer from constipation. Fecal incontinence and fecal impaction occur in 0.3-5% of the general population. Difficulty with evacuation of feces may be higher in hospitalized patients and older individuals, estimated to be in the range of 10-50%. No good study of incidence of neurogenic bowel problems by specific cause has been conducted.

○   **What endoscopic studies are indicated in neurogenic bowel function?**

Endoscopic studies include rectosigmoidoscopy, anoscopy, and colonoscopy to visualize anatomical abnormalities or lesions. Endoscopy has the limitation that it cannot assess the function of the GI tract.

○   **What historical information is needed to evaluate the patient with neurogenic bowel?**

Establish history of premorbid bowel function and patterns, including frequency, timing, consistency of stools, eating and dietary habits, use of bowel medications and/or digital stimulation, and presence of gastrointestinal disease. Determine history of prior neurologic insult and whether the injury is upper motor or lower motor neuron to anticipate symptomatology and clinical findings. Assess impact of bowel symptoms that affect the patient's ability to perform activities of daily living (ADL) and continue social and work responsibilities.

○   **What symptoms may occur in neurogenic bowel disorders?**

1. Loss of voluntary control over defecation, known as fecal incontinence
2. Difficulty with evacuation
3. Associated neurologic bladder symptoms
4. Associated symptoms of autonomic dysreflexia in patients with spinal cord lesions at T6 and above.

○   **What are the physical characteristics of the external anal sphincter under normal and pathological conditions?**

The external anal sphincter is normally puckered. Lower motor neuron impairment is manifested by flattening or scalloping.

○   **What is the anocutaneous reflex?**

Stimulation with pinprick in the perianal region leads to visible reflexive anal contraction. Anocutaneous reflex is normally present if S2, S3, S4 reflex arc is intact. This reflex does not correlate with internal sphincter function. Sensory examination tests the integrity of sacral dermatomes to light touch and pinprick.

○   **What findings are assessed on rectal examination?**

Assess the tone of the external sphincter by digital examination. Use this examination to assess the bulbocavernosus reflex. Lower motor neuron impairment is manifested by reduced or absent tone. Rectal sensation usually is absent in lesions above L3.

○   **What is the bulbocavernosus reflex?**

Squeezing the glans penis or clitoris (or applying traction on an indwelling catheter) results in palpable rectal contraction. This reflex is normally present in most patients. The reflex is brisk with upper motor neuron lesions and is absent in lower motor neuron lesions or spinal shock.

○   **What Imaging Studies are indicated in the assessment of the patient with neurogenic bowel disorders?**

Appropriate studies include flat plate, both supine and upright, barium enema, and defecography. These tests all provide visualization of structural defects, identification of abnormal air patterns, and kinetics of defecation. Use serial radiographic studies for evaluation of colonic transit time after the patient has ingested radiopaque beads with food.

○ **What other tests may be indicated in the patient with neurogenic bowel disorders?**

Manometry by kymography and/or catheter use measures pressure and volume changes by intraluminal balloons and catheter, respectively. These tests help determine anorectal pressures and colonic migratory contractions. The saline infusion continence test quantitatively determines continence to liquid after rectal saline infusion. Electromyography determines the state of innervation of the rectal muscles by their respective motor nerves.

○ **What medical emergencies may occur in patients with neurogenic bowel disorders?**

Bowel perforation is a surgical emergency resulting from fecal impaction with eventual distention, then perforation. Refer the patient immediately for surgical intervention if clinical and radiologic findings suggest bowel rupture.

○ **What surgical procedure is often utilized to manage neurogenic fecal incontinence?**

The surgeon may consider muscle transposition with innervated adductor longus, gluteus maximus, or other free muscle grafts to replace the puborectalis sling. A surgeon may use this technique in patients with incomplete motor lesions with some sensation. This technique can lead to some degree of restoration of fecal continence.

○ **What procedure is appropriate for patients with rectal dyssynergia?**

In patients with rectal dyssynergia, consider myotomy since incomplete relaxation of the internal anal sphincter leads to functional outlet obstruction and may cause dysreflexia in susceptible patients.

○ **When should colostomy be considered?**

Colostomy/ileostomy may be considered in highly refractory cases or when stool incontinence complicates other problems such as pressure sore management.

○ **What is Appendicocecostomy (antegrade continence enema [ACE] procedure)?**

The appendix is used as a conduit between the skin and cecum. Enema fluid can be introduced using a catheter. This procedure is used in chronic refractory neurogenic bowel when there is insufficient rectal tone to allow use of rectal enemas. Appendicocecostomy is used most often in children with spina bifida.

○ **What is the role of biofeedback and behavioral training in neurogenic bowel disorders?**

Biofeedback and behavioral training are of benefit to improve sensory and motor awareness in patients with incomplete neurogenic bowel lesions, especially in children.

○ **What other treatment options are available?**

Other options to relieve symptoms include a pulse irrigation evacuation system using intermittent rapid pulses of warm water to break up stool impactions and stimulate peristalsis. Some clinicians also advocate use of a bowel management tube with attached balloon and subsequent administration of saline enema for fecal evacuation in children with neurogenic bowel dysfunction. The balloon helps to provide anal occlusion to retain the enema fluid in persons with weak or absent anal sphincter function.

○ **What bowel training program is used for patients with upper motor neuron disorders?**

The bowel training program (BTP) is essential to begin as early as possible, as soon as the acute ileus stage has resolved. Patients should ideally start on an everyday program, in the evening or in the morning. It is useful to perform the BTP shortly after a meal (breakfast or dinner) so that the natural peristalsis may assist somewhat in the program. The regular BTP, at least initially, should consist of a suppository and digital stimulation with a gloved finger. If there is stool in the vault, this should be cleaned out, then the suppository inserted with a gloved, lubricated finger. Digital stimulation refers to a circular movement and gentle stretching of the anus to stimulate the defecation reflex. After 10 minutes, the digital stimulation can be repeated. It normally takes 20 to 30 minutes for evacuation from the suppository. If at all possible, the patient should be transferred to a commode during the program to allow gravity to assist. Eventually, the BTP can be changed to an every other day program; some patients need to maintain an everyday program to avoid accidents during daily activities.

O   **What bowel training program is used for patients with lower motor neuron disorders?**

Since lower motor neuron (LMN) lesions result in atonic bowels, manual evacuation is frequently necessary. Firmer stools often help with manual evacuation so fluid restriction and avoidance of too many stool softeners are necessary. As with the upper-motor-neuron program, rectal suppositories, digital stimulation, and upright posture are useful. Maintenance of a regular schedule (e.g., every day between 8 and 9 AM) for the BTP helps promote success in avoiding accidents. Patients should be taught to avoid Valsalva forces during transfers to prevent expulsion of stool. During bowel case procedure for LMN patients, bowel care should be started with patients in the seated position and digital stimulation initiated. Intermittent Valsalva force and abdominal wall contraction along with transabdominal massage of the colon in a clockwise manner helps advance the stool. Digital removal is repeated with digital stimulation until there is no further palpable stool.

NEUROLOGIC DISORDERS

STROKE

○ **Provide an operative definition of stroke syndrome**

Stroke is the clinical term for acute loss of circulation to an area of the brain, resulting in ischemia and a corresponding loss of neurologic function. Classified as either hemorrhagic or ischemic, strokes typically manifest with the sudden onset of focal neurologic deficits, such as weakness, sensory deficit, or difficulties with language. Ischemic strokes have a heterogeneous group of causes, including thrombosis, embolism, and hypoperfusion, whereas hemorrhagic strokes can be either intraparenchymal or subarachnoid.

○ **What is the incidence of stroke?**

The average age-adjusted incidence of first stroke has been reported to be 114 cases per 100,000 population, but ranges from 81 to 150 per 100,000 populations in various studies depending on whether completed strokes as well as transient ischemic attacks (TIAs) are included. The incidence of stroke rises sharply with age and doubles with each decade after age 55. Men have a 30% to 80% higher rate than women. African-Americans have higher incidence rates than whites.

○ **What is the prevalence of stroke?**

Stroke prevalence (the number of people who have had a stroke in a given population at a point in time) has been reported to be 500 to 800 cases per 100,000 populations from Rochester, Minnesota. Stroke prevalence in the United States has increased by 20% in recent years, owing to the increased survival of stroke patients, although the incidence of stroke has decreased. Similar figures have been reported from other countries as well.

○ **What is the mortality related to stroke?**

Stroke is a major public health problem, ranking among the top three causes of death in most countries. It affects the brains of almost a half million people every year, causing 150,000 deaths, and there are now approximately 3 million stroke survivors in the United States. The average age-adjusted mortality rate is 50 to 100 per 100,000 population per year in the United States.

○ **What is the temporal pattern of stroke mortality?**

Mortality from stroke is highest for the first 30 days after stroke. The average 30-day mortality ranges from 17% to 34%. Stroke mortality decreases over the next 18 months, and at this point approaches that of the general population matched for age and gender. Fifty percent of 30-day survivors will live at least another 5 years.

○ **Compare key demographics for stroke in the United States**

Population Group	Prevalence	Incidence New and Recurrent Attacks	Mortality	Hospital Discharges	Cost
2001	2001	2001	2001	2001	2004
Total population	4,800,000 (2.0%)	700,000	163,538	931,000	$53.6 billion
Total males	2,100,000 (2.3%)	327,000 (47%)*	63,177 (38.6%)*	391,000	—
Total females	2,700,000 (1.7%)	373,000 (53%)*	100,361 (61.4%)*	539,000	—

White males	2.2%	277,000	53,428	—	—
White females	1.5%	312,000	87,037	—	—
Black males	2.5%	50,000	7,907	—	—
Black females	3.2%	61,000	11,095	—	—
Mexican-American males	2.3%	—	—	—	—
Mexican-American females	1.3%	—	—	—	—

○ **Is the mortality rate different for intracerebral hemorrhage?**

The 30-day mortality rate for hemorrhagic stroke is 40-80%. Approximately 50% of all deaths occur within the first 48 hours.

○ **What are the most common causes for mortality among stroke patients?**

The most frequent cause of death was transtentorial herniation, followed in frequency by pneumonia, cardiac causes, and pulmonary embolism. Cardiovascular disease is the most common comorbidity associated with stroke and has a negative impact on outcome.

○ **What is the rate of recurrence for stroke?**

Recurrent strokes account for 25% of all acute stroke events. The recurrence rate is 4% to 10% per year and is highest in the first year (approximately 13%). The risk thereafter is 4% per year.

○ **What is the categorical distribution of the basic stroke syndromes?**

Ischemic stroke accounts for more than 80 percent of all strokes. ICH usually accounts for 10 to 30 percent of cases depending on the origin of the patient, with greater relative frequencies reported in Asians and blacks. Frequency of SAH is usually a third to a half that of ICH. Among patients with brain ischemia, cardioembolism accounts for 20 to 30 percent of cases, atherothrombotic infarction accounts for 14 to 40 percent, and small deep infarcts due to penetrating artery disease (lacunes) account for 15 to 30 percent of cases.

○ **Summarize stroke syndromes by anatomy**

Stroke Syndromes by anatomy	
Cortical strokes	
Middle cerebral artery	contralateral hemiparesis and sensory loss, face and upper extremity more involved contralateral hemianopsia aphasia/aprosodia gaze abnormalities extinction on simultaneous touching, apraxia
Anterior cerebral artery	contralateral hemiparesis and sensory loss, lower extremity more involved disconnection syndrome abulia, akinetic mutism
Posterior cerebral artery	contralateral hemianopsia with macular sparing disconnection syndrome
Lacunar syndromes of cerebral hemisphere (no diplopia)	
Ventral posterior thalamus	pure sensory loss without weakness
Post limb Internal Capsule	pure motor weakness without sensory loss, confusion or visual field defect (may also be caused by cerebral peduncle infarct)
Genu of internal capsule	Dysarthria clumsy hand syndrome

Subthalamic nucleus	Contralateral Hemiballismus
Midbrain syndromes (Clue: III nerve palsy or vertical gaze problem)	
Tegmentum, red nucleus, III n	Claude's syndrome: Ipsilateral III palsy & contralateral ataxia
above plus cerebral peduncle	Benedikt's syndrome: above plus contralateral weakness
III nerve + cerebral peduncle (red nucleus spared)	Weber's syndrome: ipsilateral III palsy + contralateral weakness
Dorsal midbrain	Parinaud's syndrome: paralysis of up gaze, convergence- retraction nystagmus, lid retraction
Above + paramedian midbrain	Nothnagel's syndrome: III palsy, vertical gaze paralysis, ipsilateral ataxia
Pontine syndromes (VI nerve, horizontal gaze problem or VII nerve palsy)	
Middle cerebellar peduncle + corticospinal tract	Raymond-Cestan syndrome: ipsilateral ataxia + contralateral weakness
Paramedian pons	One-and-a-half syndrome: ipsilateral horizontal gaze palsy plus contralateral INO
Ventral pons	Millard-Gubler syndrome: VI & VII palsy, contralateral hemiparesis
Medulla syndromes (clue: facial sensory loss or Horner's syndrome, ipsilateral tongue, palate, SCM paralysis.)	
Dorsolateral medulla	Wallenberg's syndrome: ipsilateral ataxia, Horner's syndrome, facial sensory loss, contralateral loss of pain & temperature
Lateral medulla	Ipsilateral ataxia, Horner's syndrome, facial sensory loss, ipsilateral paralysis of soft palate, vocal cords or sternocleidomastoid

❍ Classify stroke by etiology

Classification of stroke by etiology

Large artery atherosclerotic disease	Vertebrobasilar system: bilateral or shifting symptoms, visual field defect, brainstem symptoms such as diplopia, ataxia Carotid or anterior system: hemiparesis, visual field defect, aphasia, confusion
Small vessel or penetrating artery disease (Lacunar)	Hypertrophy of the media and deposition of fibrinoid material into vessel wall Small infarcts of deep regions of brain or brainstem 15% of all strokes
Cardiogenic embolism	Common source of cardiac emboli Acute Myocardial infarct Left ventricular aneurysm Dilated cardiomyopathy Cardiac arrhythmia: especially atrial fibrillation Valvular disease: rheumatic mitral valve disease, calcific aortic stenosis, Mitral valve prolapse, endocarditis, prosthetic heart valves Intracardiac tumors: atrial myxoma Intracardiac defects with paradoxical embolism: ASD, patent foramen ovale, atrial septal aneurysm
Hemodynamic changes (low flow)	Cardiac pump failure, decreased systemic perfusion pressure, systemic hypotension Resulted in border zone or watershed infarcts 5% of all strokes, more common in young patients
Nonatherosclerotic vasculopathies	Cervicocephalic arterial dissection Moyamoya Fibromuscular dysplasia Cerebral vasculitis 1% of all strokes
Hypercoagulable disorders	Deficiencies in anticoagulant proteins: Antithrombin III, Protein C, Protein S, Heparin cofactor II, disorders of fibrinogen Secondary hypercoagulable states: nephrotic syndrome, polycythemia vera, sickle cell disease, TTP, paroxysmal hemoglobinuria

O   **What are the risk factors for stroke?**

Nonmodifiable risk factors for stroke

Age: Exponential increase in risk with age
Gender: men has greater stroke incidence, but woman lives longer, therefore outnumber men in total strokes
Family history: first degree relative
Race: Stroke mortality of African American is double that of White Americans.
Modifiable risk factors

Hypertension:
Isolated systolic hypertension increases stroke risk by 2 to 4 times
treatment of hypertension substantially reduces the risk of stroke by about 36% - 42%
68% of persons are estimated to be aware of their hypertension, less than 30% are controlled
Cardiac diseases:
Nonvalvular atrial fibrillation (NVAF)
36% of strokes in those between 80 and 89 years of age are attributed to NVAF
Valvular heart disease, myocardial infarction, coronary artery disease, congestive heart failure, ECG evidence of left ventricular hypertrophy
Diabetes mellitus
Hyperlipidemia: degree and progression of carotid atherosclerosis are directly related to cholesterol and LDL, inversely proportional to HDL. Treatment recommendation
Asymptomatic carotid stenosis:
<75% stenosis, risk is 1.5%/year
>75% stenosis, risk is 3.3%/year
Smoking:
> 40 cigarette/day, stroke risk increases 2X
cessation of cigarette smoking reduces the risk of stroke substantially within 2-5 years
Heavy alcohol consumption increase risk, light alcohol consumption may reduce stroke risk.
Transient ischemic attacks: average annual risk for stroke, MI, or death 7.5%/year.
Physical Inactivity: see lifestyle modification

O   **What are appropriate treatment recommendations for stroke prevention?**

Risk Factor	Treatment Goal	Recommendations
Hypertension	SBP <140 mm Hg and DBP <90 mm Hg; SBP <135 mm Hg and DBP <85 mm Hg if target organ damage is present	Lifestyle modification and antihypertensive medications
Smoking	Cessation	Provide counseling, nicotine replacement, and formal programs
Diabetes mellitus	Glucose <126 mg/dL (6.99 mmol/L)	Diet, oral hypoglycemics, insulin
Lipids	LDL <100 mg/dL (2.59 mmol/L) HDL >35 mg/dL (0.91 mmol/L) TC <200 mg/dL (5.18 mmol/L) TG <200 mg/dL (2.26 mmol/L)	AHA Step II diet: ≤30% fat, <7% saturated fat, <200 mg/d cholesterol. If target goal not achieved, add drug therapy (eg, statin agent) if LDL >130 mg/dL (3.37 mmol/L) and consider drug therapy if LDL 100–130 mg/dL (2.59–3.37 mmol/L)
Alcohol	Moderate consumption (< or = 2 drinks/d)	
Physical activity	30–60 minutes of activity at least 3–4 times/wk	Moderate exercise (eg, brisk walking, jogging, cycling, or other aerobic activity) Medically supervised programs for high-risk patients (eg, cardiac disease)
Weight	< 120% of ideal body weight for height. Check ideal weight.	Diet and exercise

SBP indicates systolic blood pressure; DBP, diastolic blood pressure; AHA, American Heart Association; HDL, high-density lipoproteins; TC, total cholesterol; and TG, triglycerides

O   **What are the treatment considerations according to ischemic stroke subtypes?**

Ischemic Stroke Subtype	Recommendations
Atherosclerotic carotid disease	

>70% stenosis	Carotid endarterectomy of definite benefit if done with acceptable morbidity and mortality. Antiplatelet agents
50–69% stenosis	Carotid endarterectomy of potential benefit depending on risk factors Antiplatelet agents
<50% stenosis	Carotid endarterectomy of no benefit. Use Antiplatelet agents
Intracranial artery stenosis	
50 to 99% stenosis of an intracranial artery (carotid; anterior, middle, or posterior cerebral; vertebral; or basilar)	Patients with TIA or stroke in the territory of the stenotic artery qualified for inclusion in the study. 88 treated with warfarin and 63 treated with aspirin. The rates of major vascular events were 18.1 per 100 patient-years of follow-up in the aspirin group compared with 8.4 per 100 patient-years of follow-up in the warfarin group. (The Warfarin Aspirin Symptomatic Intracranial Disease Study. Neurology. 1995 Aug;45(8):1488-93.)
Cardiac embolism	
Definite source:	Oral anticoagulation (unless contraindicated):
Nonvalvular atrial fibrillation	INR 2–3 (target 2.5) lifelong therapy
Left ventricular thrombus, recent Myocardial infarction	INR 2–3 (target 2.5) 6-month therapy
Prosthetic Valvular heart disease	INR 3–4 (target 3.5) lifelong therapy
Possible cardiac source	Antiplatelet agents (oral anticoagulation undergoing evaluation)
Other infarct subtypes including small-vessel lacunar disease and cryptogenic stroke	Antiplatelet agents

○   What neurological deficits occur with occlusion of the posterior cerebral artery?

Cardioembolism is the most common cause of PCA stroke. Approximately 5% of ischemic strokes involve the PCA or its branches. Death from PCA stroke is uncommon. Rate of morbidity from PCA stroke is high. Recovery of visual field deficits is very limited. Patients may be unable to drive or read, resulting in major limitations in their quality of life, despite normal motor function. Posterior cerebral artery occlusions affect vision and thought, producing homonymous hemianopsia, cortical blindness, visual agnosia, altered mental status, and impaired memory.

○   What are the neurological manifestations of occlusion of the middle cerebral artery (MCA)?

The middle cerebral artery (MCA) is by far the largest of the cerebral arteries and is the vessel most commonly affected by cerebrovascular accident (CVA). Of MCA territory infarcts, 33% involve the deep MCA territory, 10% involve superficial and deep MCA territories, and over 50% involve the superficial MCA territory. Middle cerebral artery (MCA) occlusions commonly produce contralateral hemiparesis, contralateral hypesthesia, ipsilateral hemianopsia (blindness in one half of the visual field), and gaze preference toward the side of the lesion. Agnosia is common, and receptive or expressive aphasia may result if the lesion occurs in the dominant hemisphere. Since the MCA supplies the upper extremity motor strip, weakness of the arm and face is usually worse than that of the lower limb.

○   What is the distinction between the superior division and inferior division of the MCA territory?

Superior division infarcts lead to contralateral deficits with significant involvement of the upper extremity and face and partial sparing of contralateral leg and foot. Inferior division infarcts of the dominant hemisphere lead to Wernicke aphasia. Such infarcts on either side yield a superior quadrantanopsia or homonymous hemianopsia, depending on the extent of infarction. Right inferior branch infarcts also may lead to a left visual neglect. Finally, resultant temporal lobe damage can lead to an agitated and confused state.

○   What is the major mechanism responsible for MCA infarcts?

Most of the sources in the literature support embolism as the primary etiology of MCA strokes. Primary atherosclerosis of the MCA and branches accounts for only 7-8% of symptomatic MCA disease.

240 PHYSICAL MEDICINE AND REHABILITATION REVIEW

O What are the neurological manifestations of ACA occlusion?

Occlusion of the ACA is uncommon, occurring in only 2% of cases, often through atheromatous deposits in the proximal segment of the ACA. The anterior choroidal artery supplies the lateral thalamus and posterior limb of the internal capsule. Occlusion of the anterior choroidal artery occurs in less than 1% of anterior circulation strokes. Anterior cerebral artery occlusions primarily affect frontal lobe function, producing altered mental status, impaired judgment, contralateral lower extremity weakness and hypesthesia, and gait apraxia.

O What are the neurological manifestations of vertebrobasilar artery occlusions?

Studies show that embolic phenomena cause infarction in vertebrobasilar territory in 9-40% of reported cases. The vertebrobasilar bed appears less susceptible than carotid circulation to embolic occlusion. Approximately one fourth of strokes and TIAs occur in the vertebrobasilar distribution. Vertebrobasilar artery occlusions are notoriously difficult to detect because they cause a wide variety of cranial nerve, cerebellar, and brainstem deficits. These include vertigo, nystagmus, diplopia, visual field deficits, dysphagia, dysarthria, facial hypesthesia, syncope, and ataxia. Loss of pain and temperature sensation occurs on the ipsilateral face and contralateral body. In contrast, anterior strokes produce findings on one side of the body only.

O What is a lacunar infarction?

These are infarctions that measure less than 1.5cm in diameter and associated with small penetrating branches of the cerebral arteries.

O Summarize the clinical profile of Intracerebral Hemorrhage (ICH)

Intracerebral Hemorrhage (ICH)

Overview

10% of strokes is caused by ICH.
Main Causes:
Less than 40 years old: vascular malformations and illicit drug use.
40 to 69 years old: hypertension predominates.
Elderly: cause is often unknown, possible amyloid angiopathy.
Other causes:
Use of anticoagulants, thrombolytics, and probably aspirin.
Carotid endarterectomy (especially in the setting of recent ipsilateral infarct or severe postoperative hypertension)
Head trauma.
Prognosis

Mortality: varies between 20% and 56%.
Depends on several variables:
Age
Level of consciousness
Hematoma volume
Ventricular extension of the hemorrhage
30 days after onset: 12% normal or with minor handicap.
Surgical vs. Nonsurgical Treatment

No data from randomized clinical trials
Hematomas of putaminal, thalamic, and lobar location.
Data from many nonrandomized clinical studies with multiple types of biases seems to indicate:
Small supratentorial hematomas (volume < 20 $_{cm2}$) do well without surgical treatment
Large hematomas (volume > 60 cm2) do poorly regardless of whether they are treated surgically or nonsurgically.
Cerebellar Hemorrhage:
Small hemorrhage < 3 cm in diameter in a cerebellar hemisphere and that is without hydrocephalus by CT scan, tend to do well without requiring surgical treatment.
Hemorrhages > 3 cm in diameter and are associated with hydrocephalus and effacement of the quadrigeminal cistern on CT scan have a notorious tendency to progress to brainstem compression and poor outcome unless they are treated surgically.
In addition, the presence of clinical signs of lateral pontine tegmental involvement (ipsilateral horizontal gaze palsy, facial palsy, facial hypesthesia) are an indication for surgical drainage, since further progression of symptoms is likely to result in respiratory arrest and death.

Presence of these clinical or CT signs are indications for emergency surgical treatment, which, if hydrocephalus is present, should include immediate ventriculostomy while preparations are being made for posterior fossa craniotomy for drainage of the hematoma.

Lobar Hemorrhage

Intermediate size: volume of 20-60 $_{cm2}$ are often considered candidates for surgical treatment, especially in instances when progressive deterioration in the level of consciousness occurs in association with CT evidence of enlargement of the hematoma.

This approach is favored by the superficial location of the hematoma, which makes surgical trauma less likely.

An additional reason to consider surgical treatment is the documentation of a vascular lesion with potential for rebleeding, such as an arteriovenous malformation or cavernous angioma.

Thalamic and Caudate Hemorrhage

Deeply located paraventricular hemorrhages often cause ventricular hemorrhage and hydrocephalus.

Emergent ventriculostomy can result in a dramatic reversal of obtundation and neurologic deficits.

O **What is the incidence of subarachnoid hemorrhage (SAH)?**

Spontaneous subarachnoid hemorrhage (SAH) occurs at a rate of 10 to 20 per 100,000 population, at a mean age of 50 years. A ruptured aneurysm is the cause in 70% to 90% of patients

O **Where does SAH most commonly arise from?**

Aneurysms are most commonly located at the circle of Willis involving the anterior communicating artery complex, MCA trifurcation, carotid artery, and posterior communicating artery. Arteriovenous malformations and "unidentified" sources make up the remainder. SAH accounts for 5% to 10% of all strokes.

O **What is the prognosis for patients with SAH?**

In North America, approximately 30,000 individuals are affected each year, of which 40% to 45% die within the first month, most from the initial bleed. Studies using global measures of outcome report that 45% to 75% of SAH survivors experience a "good outcome," having minimal to no neurologic deficit and becoming independent in basic activities of daily living (ADLs). However, recent studies indicated that a high percentage of these patients continue to experience cognitive, behavioral, and social difficulties.

O **What complication can occur with both SAH and intraventricular hemorrhage?**

Both SAH and intraventricular hemorrhage are risk factors for hydrocephalus, which occurs in 15% to 20% of patients with SAH. Patients with SAH should be monitored closely for the development of hydrocephalus, which in addition to occurring acutely, can present many months after SAH as a decline in function, gait, or cognition or simply as a failure to reach expected goals.

O **Summarize the clinical profile of Subarachnoid Hemorrhage (SAH)**

Subarachnoid Hemorrhage (SAH)

Overview

6-16 per 100,000 / year
Risk of SAH increases with age and peaks at 50 years
Risk factors for SAH:
Smoking
Putative factors: increasing age, female gender, black race, alcohol abuse, and binge drinking.
There appears to be an inverse relationship between body-mass index and the incidence of SAH.
Spontaneous intracranial hemorrhages: 77% caused by aneurysms.
Types: saccular, mycotic & fusiform
Other causes of SAH
Trauma
Vascular malformations of brain & spinal cord
Blood dyscrasias
Less common causes: tumors, infection, and vasculopathies.
Autopsy prevalence of aneurysm: 1%
10% died and never reached the hospital
Signs & Symptoms

Headache: sudden onset and very severe
Meningeal signs
A warning leak may occur in up to 50% of the patients several days or weeks prior to the hemorrhage.
Diagnosis

CT head without contrast detects 80-90% of the SAH in first 24 hours.
The longer the interval between onset of symptom and scan, less likely CT will show the bleed.
At 3 weeks after bleed, almost 0%.
If the history is right, CT head negative, consider LP.
MRI may be more sensitive in detecting SAH for onset > 4 days ago.
20% of patient may have multiple aneurysms.
20-25% of cases, Angiogram negative, recommended that a repeat study be performed in 2 weeks.

Recurrent Bleed

4% chance of recurrent hemorrhage within the first 24 hours
1.2% chance each day during the first 2 weeks.
Total 20% risk for rebleeding within 14 days.

Prognosis

For those that reach the hospital:
1/3 comatose
1/3 develop neurologic deterioration
1/3 good recovery possible

O   **Do SAH survivors more closely resemble stroke or TBI patients clinically?**

SAH survivors tend to resemble more closely traumatic brain injury (TBI) patients rather than patients with cerebral infarction in terms of their cognitive, behavioral, and functional deficits. The general pattern of recovery following SAH is also similar to that of TBI, but in general, given the same deficit and same time after the event, the prognosis for SAH is not as good as for TBI, but better than for cerebral infarction.

O   **What is the typical pattern of motor recovery for the stroke patient?**

There is general agreement that the greatest neurologic recovery occurs during the first 3 months after the stroke, and remains statistically significant up to 6 months. Slow recovery may continue up to 1 year but does not reach statistical significance. Some investigators even reported functional recovery up to 2 years. The reasons for this are not entirely clear.

O   **What is the prevalence of hemiparesis in the post stroke population?**

When seen within the first week after onset, 73% to 88% of stroke survivors have some degree of hemiparesis. Hemiparesis is present in 50% of stroke survivors at 6 months and in 30% at 1 year. The degree of neurologic recovery varies depending on the type of stroke.

O   **What classical pattern of motor recovery was described by Twitchell?**

In 1951, Twitchell described a classic pattern for motor recovery and prognostic signs for improvement. In the initial stages, the paretic limb is flaccid, followed by a return of reflexes and development of spasticity. Return of voluntary movement follows in a sequential proximal to distal pattern. Movements are initially in a synergistic pattern (flexor synergies in the upper limb and extension synergies in the lower limb) followed by increased volitional control of individual movements and a decrease in spasticity. Motor recovery may plateau at any point, but usually by 8 to 12 weeks. The lower limb usually shows more recovery than the upper limb, owing to both greater involvement of the arm in the most common middle cerebral territory infarct, and the need for the recovery of more complex fine motor control for functional use of the arm.

O   **What is the prognosis for proprioception in the stroke patient population?**

Proprioception is a key factor in executing and relearning motor function. One study by Smith et al found that 1 week after stroke onset, approximately 44% of the patients had decreased proprioception. Proprioception recovered in 87% of the survivors by 8 weeks. Twelve percent to 49% of the patients with right-sided CVA experience a neglect syndrome. Gross neglect appears to resolve to a large extent in a majority of patients by 8 to 12 weeks, but subtle deficits impacting on function in a busy or distracting environment often remain.

O   **What is the prognosis of visuospatial deficits in stroke patients?**

Stroke patients who initially experience severe visuoperceptual deficits may continue to have the deficits for more than 1 year. Visual field defects are reported in 17% of stroke survivors, but recovery has not been studied extensively. Complete hemianopsia is a bad prognostic sign, and in one study 49% of the patients with complete field defects did not survive to 28 days. Of the remaining survivors, persistent full field defects were seen in 39%, 27% improved to a partial visual field defect, and 34% made full recovery. Those who recovered completely did so within 2 to 10 days after stroke onset.

O   **What is the prognosis of language dysfunction?**

Approximately 24% to 33% of stroke survivors have language dysfunction. Wade et al performed a population-based study of 545 stroke patients and found that 24% were aphasic when seen within 1 week of onset. At 6 months, 12% of the survivors still had evidence of significant aphasia, but 44% of the patients and 54% of the caregivers thought that the speech was abnormal, probably representing mild impairment. The period of greatest language recovery is during the first 3 months, but the different types of aphasia have different recovery pat-terns. Global aphasia tends to show more functional recovery between 6 months and 1 year rather than during the first 6 months (i.e., improved ability to communicate, but not necessarily improved language). The presence of aphasia has been variably associated with increased disability.

O   **What is the prognosis for bladder recovery among stroke patients?**

Bladder incontinence is commonly seen following stroke. It has been noted in approximately 30% to 70% of stroke survivors when seen at 1 week. Many patients will recover bladder function within 1 month. One study by Barer reported results of 362 stroke patients with bladder dysfunction; more than half were incontinent when first seen in the 24 hours after onset. 29% were still incontinent at 1 month. This percentage improved to 14% at 6 months. Bladder continence is a reliable positive prognostic indicator. 97% of stroke patients who were continent on day 1 survived. The majority of patients who were continent at 1 month were home within 6 months.

O   **What is the incidence and prognosis for post stroke dysphagia?**

Dysphagia is present shortly after stroke onset in approximately 50% of stroke survivors, but the rate decreases to 4% by 1 year. Gordon et al studied 91 stroke patients: 41 (45%) had dysphagia at onset, and 35 (86%) of these regained swallowing function within 14 days. Barer assessed 357 patients within 48 hours. 29% had difficulty with swallowing water and 58% showed improvement within 1 week. At 1 and 6 months, swallowing dysfunction was associated with other complications that hamper functional recovery.

O   **What is the incidence of post stroke depression?**

Post stroke depression is common, occurring in 25% to 60% of survivors, and often persists for at least 1 year. Post stroke depression is often under diagnosed and is frequently thought to be reactive.

O   **What is the etiology and correlates of post stroke depression?**

There is evidence to suggest that depression is secondary to the disruption of physiologic pathways for neurotransmitters. Depression has some, but unclear, correlation with the severity of stroke. Some studies suggested that depression is more common in patients with left frontal lobe lesions while others found no correlation.

O   **What is the prognosis of post stroke depression?**

Parikh et al demonstrated poorer recovery in activities of daily living and language in depressed patients. Major depression is usually self-limiting and resolves by 2 years, whereas the prognosis for post-stroke dysthymic depression is frequently unfavorable and often it persists for up to 2 years.

O   **What is the functional recovery outcome for stroke patients?**

One week after stroke onset, 68% to 88% of the patients are dependent in some aspect of self-care and mobility. The percentage decreases to between 40% and 62% by 6 months. At 1 year, only one-third of patients are dependent in self-care and mobility. The rate of recovery of function is fastest in the early weeks to 3 months following the stroke; however, statistically significant recovery continues to occur up to 6 months after stroke onset. Although some patients continue to show improvement up to 1 year following the stroke, this does not reach statistical significance for the group as a whole. Dombovy et al found that 64% of patients maintained their level of function between 1 and 3 years following the stroke. Between 3 and 5 years, many patients experienced increasing disability rather than improvement, perhaps due to comorbidity and increasing age.

O   **What clinical factors influence functional outcome among stroke patients?**

Factors reported to have an adverse effect on functional outcome include coma at onset, severity of the initial impairment, visuoperceptual deficits, poor cognitive function, and incontinence 2 weeks after stroke onset, advanced age, and severe cardiovascular disease. Overall, the level of function on admission to a rehabilitation unit is one of the more reliable predictors of functional status at discharge.

O   **Summarize the mechanisms for stroke recovery:**

Resolution of the ischemic penumbra
Resolution of edema
Resolution of diaschisis
Increased activity through partially spared pathways
Use of ipsilateral pathways
Recruitment of parallel systems and use of distributed networks
Cortical and subcortical reorganization, morphologic plasticity
Pharmacologic/neurotransmitter plasticity
Alternate behavioral strategies
Resolution of the ischemic penumbra

O   **What benefit does carotid endarterectomy offer the at risk stroke patient?**

If they are surgical candidates, patients with asymptomatic carotid artery stenosis of 60% or more should be considered for endarterectomy, as this procedure significantly reduces the risk of stroke over 5 years if the operative morbidity and mortality are less than 3% to 4%.

O   **What is the age association between atrial fibrillation and stroke?**

The prevalence of atrial fibrillation increases with age, and the proportion of strokes attributed to atrial fibrillation also increases with age from 7% for those 50 to 59 years old to 36% for those over 80 years old.

O   **What is the role of anticoagulation therapy in patients with atrial fibrillation at risk for stroke?**

Patients with atrial fibrillation and additional risk factors (valvular heart disease, previous myocardial infarction, enlarged heart chambers, congestive heart failure) should be treated with warfarin anticoagulation regardless of age. Patients over the age of 75 should be monitored closely because of the potential risk of increased intracranial hemorrhage.

O   **What are the risks of seizure complication post stroke?**

The risk of seizures at the onset of stroke is 4% to 5% for patients with infarcts and 15% to 20% for those with intracerebral or subarachnoid hemorrhage.

O   **In Ischemic stroke patients followed over the course of 2-4 years what risks were associated with the occurrence of epilepsy?**

Seizures developed in 6-9% of patients.
Seizures developed in 26% of patients with cortical lesions.
Seizures developed in 2% of patients with subcortical lesions.
Risk factors include the following:
Lobar hemorrhage (acute)
Cortical lesions (chronic)
Persistent paresis (50%)
Other risk factors include the following:
Language function deficit, dysarthria
Visual field defect (20%), hemianopia
Posture and balance deficit
Sensory, cognitive, and perceptual function deficits
Bowel and bladder incontinence
Deconditioning
Congestive heart failure
Hypertension
DM
Dysphasia
Spasticity
Contractures
Heterotopic calcification

○ **What are the recommendations for seizure prophylaxis in stroke?**

In general, anticonvulsants used simply for prophylaxis (i.e., no history of actual seizures) should be discontinued after 3 to 4 weeks after stroke onset.

○ **What neurogenic bladder pattern is most commonly encountered after stroke?**

The neurogenic bladder pattern usually seen in suprapontine stroke is one in which the bladder fills and the detrusor autonomously contracts owing to a loss of central inhibition.

○ **What is the differential diagnosis of hemiparetic shoulder pain?**

Impingement syndrome-Rotator cuff tendonitis
Rotator cuff tear
Bicipital tendonitis
AC joint arthropathy
GHJ arthropathy
SC joint arthropathy
Adhesive capsulitis
CRPS type1/2
Brachial plexopathy
Scapulocostal syndrome

○ **What complications have been reported among stroke patients subsequent to the acute event?**

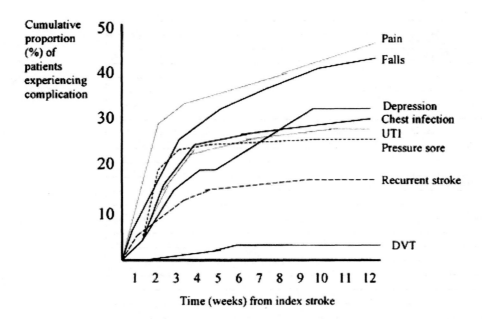

Cumulative proportion (%) of patients experiencing complication

Time (weeks) from index stroke

○ **Is there clinical evidence to support the rehabilitation of language and perceptual deficits?**

Studies generally support the efficacy of therapy for aphasia, although many have been criticized on methodologic grounds. Therapies for neglect and visuoperceptual disorders have shown some promise, particularly instruction in visual scanning techniques.

○ **What are the sexual impairments encountered among stroke patients?**

A significant number of patients with stroke experience sexual dysfunction, including erectile and ejaculatory dysfunction in men; decreased vaginal lubrication and difficulty achieving orgasm in women; as well as decreased sexual satisfaction, decline in libido, and less frequent sexual activity in both. The causes of sexual dysfunction after stroke are multifactorial and include psychological factors, medication, lesion- and disability-related factors, and fear of causing another stroke.

○ **What benefits have been demonstrated for interdisciplinary stroke rehabilitation?**

1. Patients treated on stroke units show more independence in ADLs at discharge and length of hospitalization is shorter, despite similar neurologic deficits between treatment and control groups.
2. Patients from the stroke units have a better functional status than patients from medical wards at 6 weeks and at 1 year as measured by the Barthel index.
3. Patients on stroke units also have decreased mortality as compared to those on the medical wards.
4. A higher percentage of patients are discharged home from stroke units compared to medical wards.

○ **Is fecal incontinence a common problem among stroke patients?**

Fecal incontinence occurs in a substantial proportion of patients after a stroke but clears within 2 weeks in the majority. Continued fecal incontinence signals a poor prognosis. Diarrhea, when it occurs, may be due to medications, initiation of tube feedings, or infection. It can also be due to leakage around a fecal impaction. Treatment should be cause-specific.

○ **Is constipation and fecal impaction more common than incontinence in the stroke patient?**

Constipation and fecal impaction are more common after stroke than incontinence. Immobility and inactivity, inadequate fluid or food intake, depression or anxiety, a neurogenic bowel or the inability to perceive bowel signals, lack of transfer ability, and cognitive deficits may each contribute. Goals of management are to ensure adequate intake of fluid, bulk, and fiber and to help the patient establish a regular toileting schedule. Bowel training is more effective if the schedule is consistent with the patient's previous bowel habits.

○ **What patterns of insomnia may be encountered in the stroke patient?**

Sleep patterns may be altered by the effects of the stroke or by routines of a hospital or nursing facility. Inverted sleep wake rhythms with lethargy during daytime hours and agitation at night, sleep apnea, and reduced sleep efficiency with a suppression of REM sleep and increased non-REM sleep have been reported to result from hemisphere strokes. Depression or anxiety may interfere with sleep. Muscle spasms, pain, inability to move in bed, and urinary frequency or incontinence can interrupt sleep. The unfamiliar environment of a hospital, noise, and awakenings for medications or vital signs also create problems for some patients.

○ **What caution should be exercised in prescribing hypnotic medications to stroke patients?**

If sleep medications are used, side effects such as daytime sedation, paradoxical agitation, confusion, or memory problems need to be carefully monitored. Moreover, there is suggestive evidence that agents such as benzodiazepines may slow sensorimotor recovery, and these agents should be used only if all else fails.

○ **Describe therapeutic strategies for stroke related sensorimotor deficits.**

Sensory deficit:
Teach compensatory strategies. Patient accommodates to diminished sensory input during movement and functional activities.

Range of motion:
Passive and active range of motion. Joint mobilization. Splinting or casting.

Pain:
Positioning (e.g., slings, wheelchair tray, arm supports). Reduction of edema (elevation, pressure gloves or stockings, continuous passive motion, etc.). Modalities (ice, heat, ultrasound, etc.). Proper range of motion (techniques and sequence of exercises to avoid shoulder impingement syndrome).

Force control/Voluntary control:
Facilitory modalities as patient attempts to contract muscles (e.g., quick stretch, vibration, electrical stimulation). Select optimal biomechanical position or position in point of range of motion for patient to initiate movement (e.g., to facilitate hip flexion, have patient assume side lying and place patient's hip in 90 degrees of flexion; also, therapist quick stretches the hip flexors as the patient attempts to contract the muscle). Isometric, eccentric, concentric exercises. Select eccentric exercises prior to concentric exercises. Assistive, active, and resistive exercises. Functional activities (e.g., bridging exercises, sit to stand, dressing, and other daily tasks, etc.). Train the patient in context-specific environments.

Force control/Speed:
Isokinetic exercise training. Functional tasks requiring quick contractions (postural perturbations, kicking a ball, etc.).

Tone/Spasticity:
Stretching, prolonged stretching, passive manipulation by therapists (e.g., slow rhythmic rotation), weight bearing, ice, contraction of muscles antagonistic to spastic muscles, splinting, and casting.

Tone prolonged recruitment and lack of reciprocal inhibition:
Exercise muscle groups antagonistic to muscle that will not turn off with the correct timing. Slow active reciprocal contraction of agonist and antagonist muscles.

○ **Describe therapeutic strategies to enhance synergistic organization in the stroke patient:**

Synergistic Organization: Require increasingly more complex combinations of muscle contractions and sequencing (e.g., ankle dorsiflexion and eversion with hip and knee extended, prehensile patterns of hand with wrist extension, elbow extension, and shoulder flexion). Vary conditions of performance so that patient will be able to adapt to speed and other environmental stresses. Functional use of available controlled movement. Goal is developing a variety of movement patterns and purposeful activities.

○ **Describe therapeutic strategies to enhance mobility in the stroke patient:**

Mobility: Practice moving in bed, rolling, coming to sit, sit to stand, transfers, standing, walking (activities may be done by encouraging as much use of involved extremities as possible, or patient may be taught to compensate with noninvolved extremities).

○ **Describe therapeutic strategies to enhance gait in the stroke patient:**

Gait: Consultation with orthotist to select appropriate orthosis. Select assistive devices. Practice swing, stance, and weight shift components with and without feedback from therapists. Vary conditions of performance (speed, sensory conditions, and different surfaces).

○ **Describe therapeutic strategies to enhance balance in the stroke patient:**

Balance: Weight-shift training with and without feedback. Selecting activities that require automatic weight transfer (e.g., reaching). Practice a variety of activities under different conditions that require sitting, standing, and walking balance (reaching, training, changing directions, carrying objects, going up and down hills, catching, throwing, and reaching in various directions). Patient practices restoring balance as his/her balance is perturbed.

○ **Describe therapeutic strategies to enhance ADLs in the stroke patient:**

Impaired ADL: Practice all basic activities of daily living (patient may be taught compensatory strategies with or without adaptive equipment). Practice all instrumental activities of daily living that the patient needs to be able to do (telephoning, using checkbook, shopping, etc.). Compensatory strategies with or without adaptive equipment. Practice home and community activities (independent walking in the home and community, home management tasks, etc.).

○ **What are examples of eating devices prescribed for stroke patients?**

Built up handles on utensils for weak or incomplete grasp. Rocker knife for one-handed cutting. Nonskid mats to stabilize plate for eating with one hand. Plate guards or scoop dishes for scooping food off the plate when eating one handed. Cups that hold liquid in the upper part and reduce the need to tilt the head when drinking, for patients with a swallowing problem who are at risk of aspiration.

○ **What bathing and grooming devices are prescribed for stroke patients?**

Long handled sponge for limited reach. Washcloth or sponge mitt for patients with a weak grasp. Electric razors with specially adapted heads (e.g., at 90 degrees to the handle). Hand-held shower nozzle. Nonskid mats secured in tub or shower to prevent slipping and falling. A wide selection of grab bars for use in tub or shower that require assessment of the patient's level of need, and the architectural limitations of the bathroom before selecting the design.

○ **What toileting aids are prescribed for the stroke patient?**

Bedside commode, urinal, bedpan. Elevated toilet seat. Toilet seat with rails. Grab bars next to the toilet.

○ **What shower and tub aids are prescribed for the stroke patient?**

Shower and tub seats designed for decreased ability to stand in shower or sit down in or rise from the tub. Shower and tub transfer seats for difficulty with shower and tub transfers and difficulty with standing in shower or sitting in tub. Shower chairs that can be pushed into wheelchair-accessible shower for inability to transfer or stand while showering. Hydraulic and motorized tub lifts if the patient is unable to get into or out of tub; use depends on architecture of bathroom.

○ **What dressing equipment is prescribed for the stroke patient?**

Velcro closures for one-handed dressing. Elasticized shoestrings for one-handed dressing. Long-handled shoe horn when reach *is* limited.

○ **What assistive devices are prescribed for the stroke patient?**

A Cane with a single point of contact that improves stability of gait when leg is weak. The Cane should be fitted to the patient and have a rubber tip to improve traction. A Tripod or quad cane with three or four points of contact provides greater stability but are bulkier and more difficult to handle. A Folding cane chair, allowing the user to walk and then sit and rest. Walkers differ according to structure and purpose but must be lightweight and fold if the patient is to use them outside the home. Adjustable pickup walkers for patients who need support to stand and walk, and are able to lift the walker and maintain balance. Reciprocal walkers are for patients who might lose their balance when lifting a regular walker.

O   **What wheelchair features and modifications are prescribed for the stroke patient?**

Wheelchair and wheelchair cushions Wheelchair. Wheelchair selection is based on body measurements, specific needs (e.g., elevating leg rests), safety, comfort, and maneuverability. A wheelchair for patients with hemiplegia may have a lowered base of support and lowered seat to permit the patient to use the uninvolved foot to propel the wheelchair or a one-armed drive that allows maneuvering with one arm and hand. Wheelchair cushion. This is important for comfort and to prevent skin breakdown; selection is based on the patient's mobility status, body build, nutrition, and skin condition.

O   **What devices are prescribed to facilitate transfers in the stroke patient?**

Plastic or wooden transfer board to assist the patient who is unable to stand to perform bed, chair, shower, tub, or car sliding transfers. Gait/transfer belt for use by caregiver, if indicated. Hydraulic lifts for bed, chair, tub, or car transfers. Hydraulic or electric stair lifts for patients unable to climb stairs. Chairs modified to have higher seats for patients unable to lift out of seat. Electrically or mechanically powered chairs with seats that rise are available but are rarely indicated.

O   **What Leisure and recreation devices are prescribed for the stroke patient?**

Automatic card shufflers, Card holders, Large-faced cards, Books on audio tape, Swimming flotations, Fishing pole harnesses, Gardening tools with built up handles, specially designed golf clubs.

O   **Compare agnosia, aphasia, apraxia and dysarthria:**

Agnosia   An impairment of the ability to perceive and differentiate stimulus patterns although the sensory mechanism is intact; the most fre quently seen types: auditory, visual, and tactile recognition disorders
Aphasia   An acquired impairment of language processes underlying receptive and expressive modalities; caused by damage to areas of the brain that are primarily responsible for the language function
Apraxia of speech An articulation disorder resulting from impairment caused by brain damage to the capacity to program the positioning of speech muscles and the sequencing of muscle movements for the volitional production of phonemes; no significant weakness, slowness, or incoordination of these muscles in reflex and auto nomic acts; prosodic alterations possibly associated with the articulatory problem, perhaps in compensation for it
Dysarthria   A group of speech disorders resulting from disturbances in muscular control: weakness, slowness, incoordination of the speech mechanism caused by damage to the central or peripheral nervous system or both; term encompasses coexisting neurogenic disorders of several or all the basic processes of speech: respiration, phonation, resonance, articulation, and prosody

O   **What are the different types of dysarthrias, agnosias, and aphasias?**

Dysarthria	Flaccid	Lower motor neuron
	Spastic	Upper motor neuron
Ataxic	Cerebellar system	
	Hypokinetic	Extrapyramidal system
	Hyperkinetic	Extrapyramidal system
	Mixed	Upper and lower motor neuron
Agnosia	Visual	Occipital lobe
	Auditory	Temporal lobe
Tactile	Parietal lobe	
Aphasia	Broca's	MCA, frontal lobe
	Wernicke's	MCA, temporal lobe

| Conduction | MCA, arcuate fasciculus |
| Anomic | MCA, angular gyrus |

○ **How are aphasias categorically assessed?**

Fluency, comprehension, repetition, naming, writing, reading

○ **What are the treatment strategies for cognitive and perceptual deficits in stroke patients?**

Treatments for cognitive and perceptual deficits emphasize retraining, substitution of intact abilities, and compensatory approaches. Goals are to remediate the impairment or to reduce the impact of the deficit through repetitive exercises or compensatory treatments that teach patients new methods of response. Evidence of the effectiveness of these techniques is limited to short term effects on outcome measures that share stimulus characteristics with the intervention. Several studies have demonstrated the ability to train patients to improve their visual scanning skills, somatosensory awareness, and visual perception; however, no study has demonstrated that these skills persist or carry over to functional activities. Case studies that have combined skill training with training in a functional activity are inconclusive. Strategies that have been tried for treating neglect include caloric stimulation, eye patching, dynamic stimulation, and optokinetic stimulation; however, there is no evidence of lasting benefits from these.

○ **What are the goals in the treatment of apraxia?**

The goal of treatment for apraxia is to restore the person's ability to perform appropriate habitual or novel movements. Treatments include manually guided movement, graded use of objects and contexts that evoke automatic motor responses, mental imagery, and backward chaining. However, evidence supporting the effectiveness of these treatments is limited.

○ **What are the treatment goals in the rehabilitation of aphasia?**

Goals of treatment for aphasia are to (1) reinstate (remediate) the aphasic patient's ability to speak, comprehend, read, and write; (2) assist the patient in developing strategies that compensate for or circumvent language problems; (3) address associated psychological problems that compromise the quality of life of aphasic patients and their families; and (4) help the family and involved others to communicate with the patient.

○ **What treatment approaches are utilized in aphasia rehabilitation?**

| |
| Traditional stimulus-response modality-specific treatments and drills such as Language Oriented Treatment (LOT), direct stimulus-response treatment, and Melodic Intonation Therapy. |
| Methods that work on deficits that underlie language disorders such as perseveration and difficulties in symbol use, including Treatment of Aphasic Perseveration (TAP). |
| Methods that teach compensatory strategies designed to circumvent language deficits, such as Conversational Coaching and Promoting Aphasic Communicative Effectiveness. |
| Methods that teach alternative and augmentative communication systems to aphasic adults. |
| Developmental methods that represent attempts to apply emerging concepts from cognitive neuropsychology to the remediation of aphasia. |

○ **What treatment methods are utilized for dysarthric patients?**

For dysarthric speakers, indirect treatment methods include sensory stimulation, exercises intended to strengthen speech musculature or modify muscle tone, modifying positioning and posture for speech, and improving respiratory capacity and efficiency. Direct methods include helping dysarthric speakers to produce speech under carefully arranged and controlled conditions. Because speech production typically encompasses respiration, phonation, resonation, articulation, and prosody, each may be the target of direct manipulation and modification.

○ **What treatment strategies are used for apraxic speech?**

Treatment for apraxia of speech focuses on the articulatory aspect of speech production. Emphasis is on relearning articulatory patterns and sequences of gestures, often hierarchically arranged to begin at relatively automatic levels and progress to more purposive communication. Intra- and inter-systemic reorganization of the speech act is a programmatic approach based on learning to intone speech that has been used successfully in apractic speakers.

O   **What are poor prognostic indicators associated with stroke outcome?**

Poor prognostic indicators
Proprioceptive facilitation (tapping) response for more than 9 days
Traction response (shoulder flexors/adductors) in more than 13 days
Prolonged flaccid period
Onset of motion at longer than 2-4 weeks
Severe proximal spasticity
Absence of voluntary hand movement for more than 4-6 weeks

O   **What are salient predictors of outcome in stroke patients engaged in rehabilitation?**

Predictors of outcome
Type, distribution, pattern, and severity of physical impairment
Cognitive, language, and communication ability
Number, types, and severity of comorbid conditions
Level of motivation or determination
Coping ability and coping style
Nature and degree of family and social supports
Type and quality of the specific training and adaptation program provided

O   **What are the clinical findings of Stroke rehabilitation outcome?**

Beginning rehabilitation early correlates with better outcome but may be confounded with case severity. Stroke rehabilitation improves functional ability even in patients who are elderly or medically ill or have severe neurologic/functional deficits. Significant gains achieved are not attributable just to spontaneous recovery. Of patients who survive stroke by more than 30 days, 10% demonstrate complete spontaneous recovery, 10% show no benefit from any treatment, and 80% may benefit.

O   **What impact does stroke rehabilitation have on disposition status?**

Stroke survivors who do not undergo rehabilitation are more likely to be institutionalized. Eighty-five percent of patients went home after 3 months of a stroke rehabilitation program. After 43 days, 80% of patients returned home, 85% were ambulatory, and 50-62% were independent in performance of ADL. Functional state improved in the stroke unit from 6-52 weeks.

SPINAL CORD INJURY

O   **What is the clinical definition for spinal cord injury?**

Spinal cord injury (SCI) is an insult to the spinal cord resulting in a change, either temporary or permanent, in its normal motor, sensory, or autonomic function. The International Standards for Neurological and Functional Classification of Spinal Cord Injury is a widely accepted system describing the level and the extent of injury based on a systematic motor and sensory examination of neurologic function. The following terminology has developed around classification of SCI:
Tetraplegia (replaced the term quadriplegia) - Injury to the spinal cord in the cervical region with associated loss of muscle strength in all 4 extremities
Paraplegia - Injury in the spinal cord in the thoracic, lumbar, or sacral segments, including the cauda equina and conus medullaris

O   **What is the incidence of SCI in the US?**

The incidence of spinal cord injury (SCI) in the United States has been estimated at 30 to 40 cases per million per year.

O   **What is the prevalence of SCI?**

The estimated prevalence is given as between 250,000 and 350,000 Americans, with approximately 10,000 new cases each year.

O   **What are the key demographics for SCI patients?**

According to Model Systems statistics, people with SCI are generally young (between 16 and 30 years of age); with 19 years the most frequent age of injury. Since 2000, the average age at injury is 38.0 years.
Since 2000, 78.2% of spinal cord injuries reported to the national database have occurred among males.

Age (yr.)	Incidence (%)
Birth–10	10
11–20	20
21–30	25
31–40	15
41–50	10
51–60	10
_60	10
Total	100

O   **What are the etiologies of SCI?**

Epidemiology of spinal cord injury. MCA, motor cycle accident; MVA, motor vehicle accident.

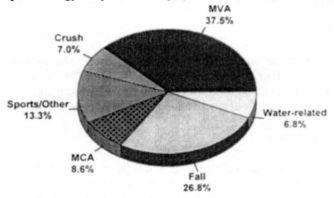

O   **What are additional SCI patient demographics relevant to community reintegration?**

Over one half of the people who experience SCI are single at the time of injury. Individuals with SCI have a reduced likelihood of getting married or remaining married after injury compared with those in the uninjured population. More than 60% of persons are employed at the time of their injury. The employment status appears higher in paraplegic (35%) than in tetraplegic persons (23%) by 10 years after injury. Alcohol or drug abuse, or both, has also been shown to be a contributing factor in approximately 50% of SCIs that result from violence.

O   **What are the demographics with regard to Neurologic level and extent of lesion?**

Since 2000, the most frequent neurologic category at discharge persons reported to the database is incomplete tetraplegia(34.3%), followed by complete paraplegia (25.1%), complete tetraplegia (22.1%), and incomplete paraplegia (17.5%) percent of persons experienced complete neurologic recovery hospital discharge.

Level of Injury	Incidence (%)
Cervical (C1 to C7–T1)	55
Thoracic (T1–T11)	15
Thoracolumbar (T11–T12 to L1–L2)	15
Lumbosacral (L2–S5)	15

O   **What is the mortality associated with SCI?**

Mortality is much higher during the first year than in the succeeding years. This is especially true in patients with severe SCI. According to the SCI Model Systems data, mortality was 3.8% during the first year after injury, 1.6% during the second year, and approximately 1.2% per year over the next 10 years.

○ What prognostic indicators correlate with mortality outcomes?

Prognostic factors related to survival include injury severity (i.e., neurologic level), degree of completeness, ventilatory dependency, and age. Psychological factors such as subjective or overall QOL, decreased activity, dependency, and unemployment have been found to be significant predictors of mortality.

Life expectancy (years) for post-injury by severity of injury and age at injury

Age at Injury	No SCI	For persons who survive the first 24 hours					For persons surviving at least 1 year post-injury				
		Motor Functional at Any Level	Para	Low Tetra (C5-C8)	High Tetra (C1-C4)	Ventilator Dependent at Any Level	Motor Functional at Any Level	Para	Low Tetra (C5-C8)	High Tetra (C1-C4)	Ventilator Dependent at Any Level
20	58.1	53.1	45.7	40.8	36.4	16.6	53.6	46.4	42.0	38.5	23.8
40	39.2	34.6	28.1	23.9	20.5	7.1	35.1	28.7	25.0	22.1	11.4
60	21.9	18.0	13.0	10.2	8.0	1.4	18.4	13.5	10.9	9.0	3.1

○ What are the leading causes of death among SCI patients?

The leading cause of death among persons with SCI initially was related to complications of the urinary tract with eventual renal failure. With diligent management of urinary tract complications, those statistics have improved. Currently, the leading cause of death is pneumonia and other complications related to the respiratory system, including pulmonary emboli in all neurologic levels. The second and third overall leading causes of death are nonischemic heart disease and septicemia, respectively. Among paraplegics, the leading causes of death include septicemia, suicide, heart disease, and cancer.

○ What is the ASIA classification of SCI?

It is a sensorimotor scoring system that establishes the most caudal level of intact spinal cord function according to dermatome and myotome innervation patterns. Motor function is graded in the 0-5 ordinal scale. A muscle must test at ≥ 3 to be scored as intact. Sensation is graded as 0 absent/impaired or 1 intact for either pin prick or light touch.

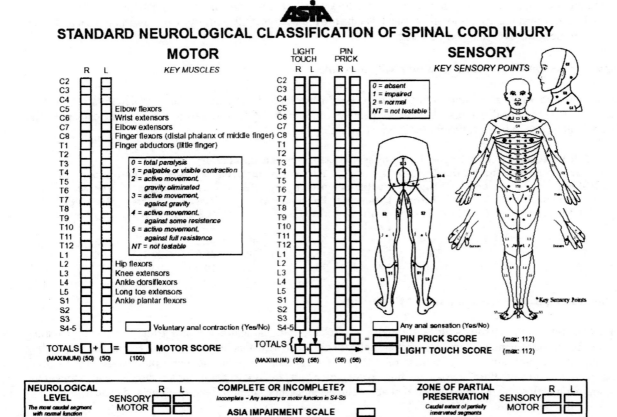

STANDARD NEUROLOGICAL CLASSIFICATION OF SPINAL CORD INJURY

○   **What are the different levels of impairment in the ASIA system?**

ASIA / IMSOP Impairment Scale		Grade D Incomplete	Motor function is preserved below the neurological level, and the majority of key muscles below the neurological level have a muscle grade greater than or equal to 3
Grade A Complete	No motor or sensory function is preserved in the sacral segments S4-S5		
Grade B Incomplete	Sensory but no motor function is preserved below the neurological level and extends through the sacral segments S4-S5	Grade E Normal	Motor and sensory function are normal
Grade C Incomplete	Motor function is preserved below the neurological level, and the majority of key muscles below the neurological level have a muscle grade less than 3		

○   **What is central cord syndrome?**

Central cord syndrome is the most common of the incomplete injury syndromes. It is associated with more significant arm weakness than leg weakness and variable sensory deficits; often, the most affected sensory modalities are pain and temperature because the lateral spinothalamic tract fibers cross just ventral to the central canal. This is sometimes referred to as dissociated sensory loss and is often present in a capelike distribution. Acute traumatic central cord syndrome is typically considered to be caused by a hemorrhage that affects the central part of the spinal cord, destroying the axons of the inner part of the corticospinal tract devoted to the motor control of the hands. The traumatic injury is usually caused by severe neck hyperextension and is characterized by initial quadriplegia replaced over minutes by leg recovery. In addition to the distal more than proximal arm weakness (man-in-a-barrel syndrome), bladder dysfunction, patch sensory loss below the level of the lesion, and considerable recovery occur.

○   **What is the Brown-Séquard syndrome?**

Brown-Séquard syndrome results from an asymmetric cord lesion and is classically thought of as a cord hemisection, although a true hemisection is uncommon with traumatic injuries. The characteristic clinical features include greater ipsilateral motor and proprioceptive loss, with contralateral loss of pain and temperature sensation.

○   **What is the anterior cord syndrome?**

Anterior cord syndrome occurs as a result of interruption of the blood supply to the anterior portion of the spinal cord. It is characterized by motor paralysis with hypoesthesia, hypalgesia, and preservation of posterior column sensory function.

○   **What is the posterior cord syndrome?**

Posterior cord syndrome results in motor paralysis with loss of posterior column sensory function. This very rare syndrome occurs with interruption of the blood supply to the posterior portion of the cord.

○   **How is conus medullaris syndrome differentiated from cauda equina syndrome?**

Clinical Differentiation of Cauda Equina and Conus Medullaris Syndromes

Conus Medullaris (Lower Sacral Cord)	Cauda Equina (Lumbosacral Roots)
Sensory deficit	**Sensory deficit**
Saddle distribution	Saddle distribution
Bilateral, symmetric	Asymmetric
Sensory dissociation present	Sensory dissociation absent
Presents early	Presents relatively later
Pain	**Pain**
Uncommon	Prominent, early
Relatively mild	Severe
Bilateral, symmetric	Asymmetric
Perineum and thighs	Radicular
Motor deficit	**Motor deficit**
Symmetric	Asymmetric
Mild	Moderate to severe
Atrophy absent	Atrophy more prominent
Reflexes	**Reflexes**
Achilles reflex absent	Reflexes variably involved
Patellar reflex normal	
Sphincter dysfunction	**Sphincter dysfunction**
Early, severe	Late, less severe
Absent anal and bulbocavernosus reflex	Reflex abnormalities less common
Sexual dysfunction	**Sexual dysfunction**
Erection and ejaculation impaired	Less common

○   **What are the key muscles for motor level classification in the ASIA scoring system?**

Key Muscles for Motor Level Classification

C5	Elbow flexors
C6	Wrist extensors
C 7	Elbow extensors
C8	Finger flexors (distal phalanx of the middle finger)
T1	Finger abductors (little finger)

T2-LI	No testable myotome and sensory levels are used to determine level
L2	Hip flexors
L3	Knee extensors
L4	Ankle dorsiflexors
L5	Long toe extensors
S1	Ankle plantar flexors

O   What are the key sensory points for sensory level classification in the ASIA scoring system?

Key Sensory Points for Sensory Level
Classification

C2	Occipital protuberance
C3	Supraclavicular fossa
C4	Top of the acromioclavicular joint
C5	Lateral side of the antecubital fossa
C6	Thumb
C7	Middle finger
C8	Little finger
TI	Medial side of the antecubital fossa
T2	Apex of the axilla
T3	Third IS
T4	Fourth IS (nipple line)
T5	Fifth IS (midway between T4 and T6)
T6	Sixth IS (level of xiphisternum)
T7	Seventh IS (midway between T6 and T8)
T8	Eighth IS (midway between T7 and T9)
T9	Ninth IS (midway between T8 and TIO)
T10	Tenth IS (umbilicus)
T11	Eleventh IS (midway between TIO and T12)
T12	Inguinal ligament at midpoint
L1	Half the distance between T12 and L2
L2	Mid-anterior thigh
L3	Medial femoral condyle
L4	Medial malleolus
L5	Dorsum of the foot at the third metatarsophalangeal joint
SI	Lateral heel
S2	Popliteal fossa in the midline
S3	Ischial tuberosity
S4-5	Perianal area (taken as one level)

IS = intercostal space

O   What type of vertebral bony injuries are associated with adult SCI?

Type of Bony Injury	Incidence (%)
Minor fracture (including compression)	10
Fracture dislocation	40
Dislocation only	5
Burst fracture	30
SCIWORA	5
SCIWORET (included cervical spondylosis)	10

SCI-WORA _ spinal cord injury without obvious radiologic abnormality;
SCI-WORET _ spinal cord injury without obvious radiologic evidence of trauma.

O   Compare and contrast adult and pediatric SCI patterns

Spine and Spinal Cord Injuries		
Characteristics	Adult	Pediatric
Mechanism of Injury	Motor vehicle accidents	Pedestrian/falls
Level of Injury		
C1–C3	1–2%	60%

Spine and Spinal Cord Injuries		
Characteristics	Adult	Pediatric
C3–C7	85%	30–40%
Thoracolumbar	10–15%	5%
Type of Injury		
Fracture-dislocation	>70%	25%
Subluxation alone	<20%	>50%
SCIWORA	Rare	Up to 50%
Delayed Neurological	Rare	Up to 50%
Deficits		
SCIWORA, Spinal cord injury without radiological abnormalities.		

O **Summarize the pattern of injuries in traumatic cervical SCI**

HYPERFLEXION INJURY (46-79%)
odontoid fracture
simple wedge fracture (stable)
tear drop fracture
anterior subluxation
bilateral locked facets (unstable)
anterior disc space narrowing
widened interspinous distance
clay shoveler's fracture
HYPEREXTENSION INJURY (20-38%)
anteriorly widened disc space
prevertebral swelling
tear drop fracture
neural arch fracture of C1
subluxation (anterior/posterior)
hangman's fracture
FLEXION-ROTATION INJURY (12%)
unilateral locked facets (stable)
VERTICAL COMPRESSION (12%)
Jefferson fracture
Burst fracture
LATERAL FLEXION/SHEARING (4-6%)
uncinate fracture
isolated pillar fracture
transverse process fracture
lateral vertebral compression
LOCATION (by frequency):
C2, C6 > C5, C7 > C3, C4 > C1

O **What are the two types of SCI pathophysiology?**

Primary and Secondary Mechanisms of Acute Spinal Cord Injury
Primary injury mechanisms
Acute compression
Impact
Missile
Distraction
Laceration
Shear
Secondary injury mechanisms
Systemic effects
Heart rate: brief increase, then prolonged bradycardia
Blood pressure: brief hypertension, then prolonged hypotension
Decreased

Peripheral resistance
Decreased cardiac output
Increased catecholamines, then decreased
Hypoxia
Hyperthermia
Injudicious movement of the unstable spine leading to worsening
compression
Local vascular changes
Loss of autoregulation
Systemic hypotension (neurogenic shock)
Hemorrhage (especially gray matter)
Loss of microcirculation
Reduction in blood flow
Vasospasm
Thrombosis
Electrolyte changes
Increased intracellular calcium
Increased intracellular sodium
Increased sodium permeability
Increased intracellular potassium
Biochemical changes
Neurotransmitter accumulation
Catecholamines (*e.g.*, norepinephrine, dopamine)
Excitotoxic amino acids (*e.g.*, glutamate)
Arachidonic acid release
Free radical production
Eicosanoid production
Prostaglandins
Lipid peroxidation
Endogenous opioids
Cytokines
Edema
Loss of energy metabolism
Decreased adenosine triphosphate production
Apoptosis
Loss of neurotrophic factor support

O   **What neuroprotective effect does Methylprednisolone produce in acute SCI?**

High-dose steroids may improve spinal cord blood flow (SCBF) and microvascular perfusion as well
as clinical neurologic recovery after experimental SCI. They may also provide some cytoprotection through the inhibition of lipid peroxidation, facilitate spinal cord impulse generation, and inhibit prostaglandin-induced vasoconstriction. Because lipid peroxidation begins within the first 5 minutes after an acute SCI, administration of high-dose steroid should occur as close to the time of injury as possible for maximal efficacy. In the clinical situation, high-dose methylprednisolone improves neurologic function if given within 8 hours of an acute SCI however, the improvements noted have been modest with some methodologic problems with the studies.

O   **What is the role of Methylprednisolone in the acute phase of SCI?**

Methylprednisolone has become widely used in the management of acute spinal cord injury and is considered by many to represent a "standard of care." This is largely based on the results of the NASCIS-2 randomized clinical trial and the subsequent NASCIS-3 study. However, these trials have resulted in considerable controversy. Some clinicians have called into question whether the results of NASCIS-2 and NASCIS-3 provide convincing evidence to support the use of methylprednisolone in acute spinal cord injury and have raised concerns regarding potential risks of this intervention.

O   **What is GM-1 ganglioside (Sygen®)?**

GM-1 ganglioside (Sygen®) is a molecule that is abundant in cell membranes, including those of nerve cells, and that has both neuroprotective and neuroregenerative effects in models of central nervous system injury or disease.

O   **What neuroprotective effect does it produce in acute SCI?**

In the Sygen® Multicenter Acute Spinal Cord Injury Study despite a more rapid time course of neurologic recovery in the Sygen® group ($P = 0.01$), the neurologic outcomes at 26 weeks between GM-1 and placebo were similar.

O   **What types of injuries occur with extension trauma?**

Common injuries associated with an extension mechanism include hangman fracture, extension teardrop fracture, fracture of the posterior arch of C1 (posterior neural arch fracture of C1), and posterior atlantoaxial dislocation.

O   **What Common injuries are associated with a flexion mechanism in the cervical spine?**

Simple wedge compression fracture without posterior disruption ; Flexion teardrop fracture ; Anterior subluxation ; Bilateral facet dislocation ; Clay shoveler fracture ; Anterior atlantoaxial dislocation.

O   **What Common injuries are associated with a flexion-rotation mechanism?**

Unilateral facet dislocation and rotary atlantoaxial dislocation.

O   **What are the radiological features of cervical spine instability?**

Vertebral body displacement > 3.5 mm or 50%
Vertebral body compression > 25%
Angulation between vertebra > 11°
Facet joint widening
'Tear drop' fracture
Basal odontoid peg fracture
7 mm lateral displacement of lateral masses of C I on C2
Atlanto-occipital dislocation

O   **What is one example of column theory of spinal instability?**

The thoracolumbar spine can be regarded as three columns: the anterior column consisting of the anterior longitudinal ligament, the anterior annulus fibrosus and the anterior half of the vertebral body; the middle column consisting of the posterior longitudinal ligament, the posterior annulus fibrosus, and the posterior half of the vertebral body; and the posterior column, the facet joints, the supraspinous and interspinous ligaments and the ligamentum flavum. If two of the three columns are disrupted then spinal stability is compromised.

O   **What is the relative instability among cervical spine fractures?**

Trafton has ranked specific cervical injuries based on their degree of mechanical instability. The list below ranks cervical spine injuries in order of instability (most to least unstable):
Rupture of the transverse ligament of the atlas
Fracture of the dens (odontoid fracture)
Burst fracture with posterior ligamentous disruption (flexion teardrop fracture)
Bilateral facet dislocation
Burst fracture without posterior ligamentous disruption
Hyperextension fracture dislocation
Hangman fracture
Extension teardrop (stable in flexion)
Jefferson fracture (burst fracture of the ring of C1)
Unilateral facet dislocation
Anterior subluxation
Simple wedge compression fracture without posterior disruption
Pillar fracture
Fracture of the posterior arch of C1
Spinous process fracture (clay shoveler fracture)

O   **What is the classification of atlas (C1) fractures?**

Four types of atlas fractures (I, II, III, IV) result from impaction of the occipital condyles on the atlas, causing single or multiple fractures around the ring. The first 2 types of atlas fracture are stable and include isolated fractures of the anterior and posterior arch of C1, respectively. The posterior neural arch fracture occurs when the head is hyperextended and the posterior neural arch of C1 is compressed between the occiput and the strong and prominent spinous process of C2, causing the weak posterior arch of C1 to fracture. Anterior arch fractures usually are avulsion fractures from the anterior portion of the ring and have a low morbidity rate and little clinical significance. The third type of atlas fracture is a fracture through the lateral mass of C1. The fourth type of atlas fracture is the burst fracture of the ring of C1 and also is known as a Jefferson fracture.

O   **What is a Jefferson Fracture?**

This fracture is caused by a compressive downward force that is transmitted evenly through the occipital condyles to the superior articular surfaces of the lateral masses of C1. The process displaces the masses laterally and causes fractures of the anterior and posterior arches, along with possible disruption of the transverse ligament. Quadruple fracture of all 4 aspects of the C1 ring occurs.

O   **What are the radiographic findings?**

Radiographically, it is characterized by bilateral lateral displacement of the articular masses of C1. The odontoid view shows unilateral or bilateral displacement of the lateral masses of C1 with respect to the articular pillars of C2; this finding differentiates it from a simple fracture of the posterior neural arch of C1. The lateral projection usually reveals a striking amount of prevertebral soft tissue edema.

O   **How does the radiographic appearance aid in determining injury status?**

When displacement of the lateral masses is more than 6.9 mm, complete disruption of the transverse ligament has occurred, and immediate referral for cervical traction is warranted. If displacement is less than 6.9 mm, the transverse ligament is still competent, and neurologic injury is unlikely.

O   **How are C1 and C2 injuries classified?**

C1 and C2 injuries may present in combination and have been divided into four groups classified according to the presence and type of C1 and odontoid peg fracture.

O   **What are Odontoid peg fractures?**

They are divided into three types:

1.   Type I involves a fracture through the apex of the peg and is a stable injury requiring only a cervical collar to control pain.
2.   Type 2 shows a fracture through the base of the odontoid peg
3.   Type 3 shows a fracture involving the body of the axis and base of the peg.

Types 2 and 3 are unstable injuries which if displaced should initially be reduced with traction. Undisplaced fractures and minimally displaced fractures in those under the age of 40 years can be treated by external immobilization, however, displaced injuries in those over 40 years have a high incidence of non-union and are best treated surgically either by anterior screw fixation or posterior fixation of C1 to C3.

O   **What is a Hangman's fracture?**

The fracture pattern seen in this injury is through both pedicles of C2. The mechanism produced by judicial hanging was one of hyperextension and distraction which inevitably produced cord disruption. The 'modern' traumatic injury results from hyperextension and compression and is uncommonly associated with a neurological lesion although it is an unstable injury. Treatment may be either conservative with reduction of any displacement by traction followed by external immobilization or surgical with posterior fixation of C1 to C3.

O   **What is an extension teardrop fracture?**

A flexion teardrop fracture occurs when flexion of the spine, along with vertical axial compression, causes a fracture of the anteroinferior aspect of the vertebral body. This fragment is displaced anteriorly and resembles a teardrop. For this fragment to be produced, significant posterior ligamentous disruption must occur. Since the fragment displaces anteriorly, a significant degree of anterior ligamentous disruption exists. This injury involves disruption of all 3 columns, making this an extremely unstable fracture that frequently is associated with spinal cord injury. Initial management is application of traction with cervical tongs.

O   **What is a flexion tear drop fracture?**

As with flexion teardrop fracture, extension teardrop fracture also manifests with a displaced anteroinferior bony fragment. This fracture occurs when the anterior longitudinal ligament pulls fragment away from the inferior aspect of the vertebra because of sudden hyperextension. The fragment is a true avulsion, in contrast to the flexion teardrop fracture in which the fragment is produced by compression of the anterior vertebral aspect due to hyperflexion.

O   **What circumstances predispose to a flexion tear drop fracture?**

The fracture is common after diving accidents and tends to occur in lower cervical levels. It also may be associated with the central cord syndrome due to buckling of the ligamenta flava into spinal canal during the hyperextension phase of the injury.

O   **How is it managed?**

This injury is stable in flexion but highly unstable in extension. Initial management is avoidance of iatrogenic extension and cervical traction with tongs.

O   **Describe the distractive flexion injury in the lower cervical spinal column?**

Distractive flexion is the most common injury mechanism producing an unstable injury through failure of the posterior column, and the anterior column with vertebral body displacement in a severe injury. Following reduction the injury should be stabilized by posterior fixation.

O   **What type of injury does compressive extension generate in the lower cervical spine?**

Compressive extension produces an unstable injury due to a bilateral vertebral fracture allowing the vertebral body to displace anteriorly. Both the anterior and posterior columns are disrupted.

O   **What kind of injury does distractive extension generate in the lower cervical spine?**

Distractive extension caused by hyperextension injury may result with failure of the anterior longitudinal ligament. The radiographic clue to this injury is widening of the disc space and a small avulsion fracture from the superior part of the vertebral body. Treatment may be conservative or an anterior vertebral body fusion can be performed.

O   **How are cervical spinal column injuries acutely reduced?**

In cervical spinal column injuries the gold standard technique of initial mobilization is through the placement of Gardner-Wells tongs. The tongs are placed with the pins just above the pinnae of the ears, on an imaginary plane connecting the mastoid processes and the external auditory canals. Once the tongs have been applied under local anesthesia, traction is initiated in a neutral plane. The initial amount of weight to be applied varies considerably with the level of injury and the amount of suspected disruption of the cervical ligaments. If there is significant ligamentous damage, a minimal amount of weight should be used to avoid distraction and potentially significant neurological deterioration. If there is any uncertainty whatsoever, it is best to start with 5 to 6 lb for upper cervical levels and 10 lb for lower levels and then await the initial radiographic evaluation.

O   **What is the primary treatment of choice in nonoperative management of cervical spine instability?**

The halo vest is a primary treatment of choice in nonoperative management of the cervical spine instability. It is a viable treatment alternative for many cases and in some instances it is the only treatment available for the patient, When appropriate identification of fracture classification is made, the surgeon can utilize the halo based upon results of recent research. Except for distractive flexion and compressive flexion type 3 injuries (in which the success rate is 50 per cent), the halo vest im mobilization is successful in over 90 per cent of other fracture types.

O   **What is the most common surgical procedure for spinal column stabilization?**

When halo vest immobilization is not tolerated and if halo-free rehabilitation is desired, posterior surgical stabilization is a safe and effective treatment of cervical instability. Surgical decompression can be performed without significant added risk. From a review of an extremely large series of patients and a review of the literature, it may be argued that a vast majority of destabilizing injuries to the cervical spine respond well to early posterior wiring and fusion. Most frequently it is the primary procedure of choice to achieve surgical stability.

O   **What is the rationale for anterior approach stabilization for spinal column injuries?**

The anterior approach has a primary function in decompressing the cervical spine from bony fragments, disc fragments, osteophytic spurs, or spinal stenosis. In traumatic cases, the patient requires either an initial posterior fusion or a halo vest until the anterior graft incorporates, thus preventing graft dislodgement or late kyphotic deformity. It is the anterior decompression rather than cervical laminectomy that is the procedure of choice to effect relief of compressing elements on the cervical spinal cord and nerve roots.

O   **What is a thoracolumbar (TL) compression fracture?**

The compression fracture results in failure of the anterior and, in severe cases, posterior columns whilst the middle column remains intact. The radiographic feature of this injury is loss of height of the anterior vertebral body in the lateral X-ray. Less than 20%, reduction suggests that the injury will be stable while more than this indicates that the posterior column has been compromised and the injury is therefore unstable.

O   **What are TL burst fractures?**

Burst fractures cause a failure of the anterior and middle columns. The characteristic features are an increase in the inter pedicular distance on the anteroposterior X-ray with retropulsion of fragments of bone into the spinal canal which is best seen by CT scanning.

O   **What are Seatbelt-type injuries?**

This injury includes the classical 'Chance fracture' (Chance 1948) and represents failure the posterior and middle columns generated by flexion and distraction. Radiologically there is an increase in the interspinous distance, fracture of the neural arch or widening of the posterior disc space.

O   **What is the prognosis for ASIA A patients?**

Prediction of functional abilities after SCI generally follows the degree of motor function. In the National SCI Database, the majority (89%) of patients admitted within 24 hours after sustaining complete motor and sensory SCI (ASIA A), remain ASIA A at time of discharge. Approximately 5%, 3%, and 3% of patients will progress to grades B, C, and D, respectively. For patients admitted ASIA grade A greater than 24 hours following injury, 94% remain so at the time of discharge.

O   **What is the prognosis for ASIA B SCI patients?**

Although it is more difficult to predict the long term outcome, the prognosis for incomplete SCI is significantly better than that of complete SCI. In the National SCI Database, approximately 49% of grade B patients remained grade B, 16% progressed to grade C, 28% progressed to grade D, and 5% regressed to grade A.

O   **What is the prognosis for ASIA class C and D SCI patients?**

Prognosis is naturally better for the ASIA grade C and D patients. Of the admission grade C patients in the National Database, 41 % remained grade C, 53% improved to grade D, and 1.3% improved to grade E. In the admission grade D patients, 90% remained grade D and 6.5% improved to grade E. Approximately 64% to 88% of patients with acute SCI and an initial exam grade of ASIA D, and nearly all those initially grade D, have become functional ambulators.

O   **What pattern of neurogenic shock occurs in the acute spinal injury patient?**

When an acute injury occurs in the cervical or high thoracic spinal cord, insufficient sympathetic innervation remains to produce adequate contractions of the heart and constriction of the blood vessels to accommodate changing conditions. Acutely this sympathetic blockage is manifested by hypothermia, hypotension, and bradycardia-the so-called neurogenic shock.

O   **What conservative measures may be utilized to counteract orthostasis?**

As time progresses and when the patient is first allowed to sit, orthostatic hypotension is typically observed. This condition can generally treated by increasing the hydrostatic pressure around the abdominopelvic region and of the legs by applying elastic hose, and around the abdomen with a binder. A Slow, gradual ascent to the sitting position can then in many cases avoid syncopal episodes. This can also be facilitated with a reclining wheelchair and tilt table.

O   **What are the major pulmonary complications that occur during the acute period of SCI?**

Patients are at greatest risk for pneumonia and atelectasis during the first 3 weeks following injury and the risk of these complications is greater in patients with complete injuries. The incidence of atelectasis and pneumonia during the first 30 days is about 50%, and the 4:1 preponderance of left-versus right-sided involvement is hypothesized to be due to preferential direction of the suction catheter toward the right lung.

O   **What therapeutic interventions are recommended for impaired pulmonary function in the acute SCI patient?**

Vigorous pulmonary toilet, including early spine stabilization with facilitation of changes in bed position, deep breathing and incentive spirometry, chest percussion, and manually assisted cough, can decrease the risk of pulmonary complications. Bronchoscopy is frequently used for atelectasis unresponsive to these treatments, but it has not been shown to be superior to chest percussion and bronchodilators. Mechanical exsufflation can produce a peak cough expiratory force that is comparable to a normal cough and greater than a manually assisted cough, and thus is appropriate for management of pulmonary secretions.

O   **What is the incidence of DVT and PE in the acute SCI patient?**

In prospective studies of patients with acute injuries, the incidence of DVT has ranged from 47% to 100%. The risk for DVT is highest in the first 2 weeks following injury, with as many as 62% of patients having positive venographic findings on days 6 to 8 after injury. Retrospective studies found an incidence of PE ranging from 3% to 15%, and the true frequency of PE is undoubtedly higher based on the greater than 50% prevalence of asymptomatic PE in patients with DVT.

O   **What prophylactic treatments are recommended by the 7th ACCP VTE prophylaxis guidelines in acute SCI?**

They recommend that thromboprophylaxis be provided for all patients with acute SCIs. We recommend against the use of LDUH, GCS, or IPC as single prophylaxis modalities. In patients with acute SCI, they recommend prophylaxis with LMWH, to be commenced once primary hemostasis is evident. They suggest the combined use of IPC and either LDUH or LWMH as alternatives to LMWH. They recommend the use of IPC and/or GCS when anticoagulant prophylaxis is contraindicated early after injury. They recommend against the use of an IVCF as primary prophylaxis against PE. During the rehabilitation phase following acute SCI, they recommend the continuation of LMWH prophylaxis or conversion to an oral vitamin K antagonist (VKA) (INR target, 2.5; INR range, 2.0 to 3.0).

O   **What duration of prophylactic treatment is recommended?**

Anticoagulation is continued until discharge from the hospital in ASIA D motor incomplete patients, up to 8 weeks in ASIA C patients, at least 8 weeks in motor complete patients, and 12 weeks for those who are motor complete with additional risk with some physicians choosing to use both pharmacologic and mechanical prophylaxis during the first 2 weeks.

O   **What is the annual incidence of pressure sores in the acute SCI patient population?**

The annual incidence of pressure ulcers in this population is nearly 25%.

O   **What are the major risk factors for pressures in the acute SCI patient population?**

The major risk factors for pressure ulcers in the SCI population include immobility, completeness of SCI, urinary incontinence, older age, cognitive impairment, anemia, and hypoalbuminemia.

O   **What are the most common sites for pressure sore formation?**

According to SCI Model Systems data, the most common sites of ulcer development were the sacrum (37.4%), the heel (15.9%), and the ischium (9.2%). Two years after injury, however, distribution had shifted due to increased time in a sitting position, with 24.3% occurring at the ischium, 20.3% at the sacrum, 12.5% at the trochanter, and 10.9% at the heel.

O   **What pulmonary problems occur in the acute cervical SCI patient?**

Patients with severe high cervical spinal cord injury have impairment of the intercostal muscles and diaphragm, which leads to respiratory compromise. Spinal cord injuries of C1 through C3 are quickly fatal acutely, unless respiratory assistance is provided in the acute setting following the injury. Permanent assisted ventilation or implanted phrenic nerve pacing is required for all C1 and C2, and many C3 patients. A patient with a C4 level may only require nighttime assisted ventilation. Patients with C1-C4 levels usually require tracheostenoses for more comfortable ventilation, and to control tracheobronchial secretions. The tracheostomy can be closed in patients with recovery of paralysis.

O   **Do paraplegics or tetraplegic patients have a higher risk of pressure sores?**

The majority of studies found an increased risk for skin breakdown in paraplegics versus tetraplegics.

O   **Is the cough reflex impaired in the acute SCI patient?**

Whether assisted ventilation is required or not, it is important to remember the pathophysiological changes that cause the impairment of coughing in persons with SCI. The ability to cough is totally impaired in tetraplegics and is partially impaired in paraplegics with thoracic lesions. Because of the paralysis of the abdominal and intercostal muscles, an intrapulmonic pressure that is sufficient to expel secretions cannot be generated. Therefore, substitution for the action of these muscles must be attempted by using a technique called assisted cough.

O   **How is the assisted cough generated?**

External pressure is applied to the abdomen by giving a brief upward thrust with the hands in synchrony with a cough effort by the patient. Functional electrical stimulation (FES) may also be applied to the abdominal muscles to assist in a similar manner. Mechanical insufflator-exsufflator can also help raise secretions in patients whose spasticity is mild.

O   **What is the pneumo belt?**

The pneumo belt can enhance breathing while the patient is seated by inflating during expiration, thereby pushing the abdominal contents toward the thorax and decreasing the residual volume. It deflates during inspiration as the patient's diaphragm descends.

O   **What is the wrap ventilator?**

The wrap ventilator creates a negative pressure external to the chest wall, thereby expanding the chest, and ambient pressure inflates the lung as a result of the negative intrapulmonic pressure.

O   **What is autonomic dysreflexia?**

Autonomic dysreflexia (AD) is a condition marked by paroxysmal hypertension, headache, sweating of the head and torso, piloerection, nasal congestion, and occasionally, reflex bradycardia. Owing to the hypertension, where systolic pressures may quickly reach as high as 300 mmHg, AD should be considered an emergent condition requiring prompt medical attention.

O   **What is the lesion level associated with autonomic dysreflexia?**

In general, AD only affects patients whose lesions are at or above the T6 level, although AD has been observed in patients with lesions below this level.

O   **What is the prevalence estimate for AD?**

The prevalence estimates of AD for the patients at risk vary widely, but in general, about 50% of those at risk will experience at least one episode. AD usually occurs after a patient has recovered from spinal shock. Therefore, it is rare to see it until at least 2 to 6 months after acute injury.

O   **What is the pathophysiology of AD?**

The pathophysiology of AD is related to an alteration in the normal balance of sympathetic and parasympathetic nervous systems caused by the spinal cord lesion. When a patient experiences noxious stimuli from below the level of the lesion, these impulses are transmitted to the sympathetic trunk, causing a reflex sympathetic discharge. Normally, this response is modulated by inhibitory signals from the brain; however, owing to the spinal cord lesion, these signals cannot get through. In addition to the physical blockage of autonomic signals, there are also changes at the neurotransmitter level that worsen symptoms, including an accumulation of substance P and impairment of g-aminobutyric acid (GABA) release. The patient, therefore, experiences the symptoms of sympathetic overload, including headache, piloerection, and hypertension caused by vasoconstriction. The increased blood pressure is detected at baroreceptors. The increased blood pressure is detected at baroreceptors at the carotid sinus and aortic arch, which trigger a parasympathetic response above the level of the lesion. Reflex vasodilation leads to flushing and sweating of the face and trunk and bradycardia.

O   **What symptoms are reported during AD?**

The patient generally gives a history of blurry vision, headaches, Nasal congestion is common. and a sense of anxiety. Feelings of apprehension or anxiety over an impending physical problem commonly are exhibited. No symptoms may be observed, despite elevated blood pressure.

O   **What signs are encountered during AD?**

A sudden significant rise in both systolic and diastolic blood pressures, usually associated with bradycardia, can appear. Normal systolic blood pressure for SCI above T6 is 90-110 mm Hg. Blood pressure 20-40 mm Hg above the reference range for such patients may be a sign of AD. Profuse sweating above the level of lesion, especially in the face, neck, and shoulders, may be noted, but it rarely occurs below the level of the lesion because of sympathetic cholinergic activity. Goose bumps above, or possibly below, the level of the lesion may be observed. Flushing of the skin above the level of the lesion, especially in the face, neck, and shoulders, frequently is noted. Spots may appear in the patient's visual fields.

O   **What complications can occur as a result of AD?**

The elevation of blood pressure may produce significant complications including stroke, seizures, retinal hemorrhages, cardiac dysrhythmias, and rarely even death.

O   **What are the etiologies of AD?**

Bladder distension	Urinary tract infection
Cystoscopy	Urodynamics
Detrusor-sphincter dyssynergia	Epididymitis or scrotal compression

Bowel distension	Bowel impaction
Gallstones	Gastric ulcers or gastritis
Invasive testing	Hemorrhoids
Gastrocolic irritation	Appendicitis or other abdominal pathology trauma
Menstruation	Pregnancy, especially labor and delivery
Vaginitis	Sexual intercourse
Ejaculation	Deep vein thrombosis
Pulmonary emboli	Pressure ulcers
Ingrown toenail	Burns or sunburn
Blisters	Insect bites
Contact with hard or sharp objects	Temperature fluctuations
Constrictive clothing, shoes, or appliances	Heterotopic bone
Fractures or other trauma	Surgical or diagnostic procedures

O   What is the treatment for AD?

The treatment for AD is to remove the noxious stimuli that caused the episode. To avoid further exacerbating the symptoms, local anesthetics should be used during any maneuver that might cause an increase in the stimuli, such as fecal disimpaction or bladder catheterization. If no offending stimuli can be found, and if the patient's blood pressure gets critical, then medication to relieve the hypertension is necessary. Nifedipine and nitroglycerin are common oral agents. If the hypertension is severe and not responsive to oral agents, then intravenous medication may be required.

O   How does muscle tone change after acute SCI?

Spinal shock, usually lasts for a few weeks and is frequently shorter in patients with incomplete injuries, although it can occasionally be as short as 2 days for patients with complete injuries. Velocity dependent hypertonus begins after the return of deep tendon reflexes (DTR)s, and usually it does not become severe until at least 6 to 12 weeks after injury. Noxious stimuli such as urinary tract infections and decubitus ulcers can cause an increase in spasticity, so any rapid increase in spasticity should trigger a search for treatable causes.

O   What are key demographics with regards to hypertonicity in the SCI patient population?

At 1-year follow up, 78% of all patients with SCI and 91% of patients with tetraplegia have findings of increased DTRs, spasticity, or involuntary muscle spasms. By the time of initial discharge from inpatient rehabilitation, 26% of patients are prescribed medications for the treatment of spasticity, and by 1 year after injury, 49% of patients are on anti spasticity medications. During the initial hospitalization, patients with ASIA class B or C are more likely to receive medications for spasticity treatment than are those with ASIA class grade A or D.

O   What are spasms?

The term *spasm* has been defined as involuntary movement of paralyzed muscles without provocative stimuli. Over 95% of patients with chronic SCI report having experienced spasms. The majority of patients who develop spasms note the onset within 2 to 6 months of injury, which is similar to the time of onset for spasticity. Both baclofen and diazepam decrease the frequency and severity of spasms in SCI.

O   What is the rationale for intrathecal baclofen?

This agent, when perfused directly into the intrathecal space, suppresses the unwanted hyperreflexic activity without impairing any residual sensation or voluntary control. Its effects are titratable, reversible, and nondestructive. By adjusting the concentration of the drug in the pump reservoir and the rate of infusion of the solution, control of the spasticity can be set so that the patient can experience just the right amount of spontaneous activity (i.e., enough to keep a salutary effect on muscle bulk but not so much as to interfere with positioning and mobility).

O   **What are salient features of the pump mechanism?**

The pump itself is battery powered, and its motor can be programmed telemetrically to deliver the desired rate, which may be constant or variable, throughout the day. The reservoir contains 18 ml of baclofen, which allows refills to be extended to every 2 to 3 months when the proper concentration and the lowest infusion rate are selected. The battery lasts up to 5 years, provided the pump can be run at a low rate-0.2 ml per day. Tolerance has been noted to occur over the first 2 to 12 months, but after that time, dosage requirements seem to level off and remain constant. These infusion techniques have virtually obliterated the need for both chemically and surgically destructive procedures.

O   **What is the incidence of heterotopic ossification in SCI patients?**

HO has been reported to occur in as few as 16% to as many as 53% of persons with SCI. HO is most frequently detected 1 to 3 months after injury, with most cases being diagnosed at about 2 months after injury.

O   **Where does it occur anatomically?**

The most common location is the hips, followed by the knees, shoulders, and elbows.

O   **What are risk factors for heterotopic ossification in the SCI patient?**

Reported risk factors for HO in patients with SCI include complete neurologic injury, presence of pressure sores, and spasticity.

O   **What gastrointestinal complications occur during the acute phase of SCI?**

During the first 3 weeks of hospitalization, gastrointestinal complications develop in about 6% of patients, with the most common disorders being ileus, peptic ulcer disease, and gastritis. All of these complications are more common in cervical level injuries than in thoracic or lumbar level injuries, and the increased risk of gastrointestinal hemorrhage and gastritis is thought to be due to a loss of sympathetic innervation and an unopposed parasympathetic stimulation of acid secretion.

O   **What other gastrointestinal complications occur during the acute SCI phase?**

Other gastrointestinal complications occurring in the acute period include gastric dilatation, superior mesenteric artery syndrome, and pancreatitis.

O   **What is the superior mesenteric artery syndrome?**

The superior mesenteric artery syndrome, although rare, deserves special consideration because it is preventable. This syndrome results from compression of the third portion of the duodenum by the superior mesenteric artery. It can occur in the patient who has lost the fat layer between the duodenum and the superior mesenteric artery such as after profound weight loss, or in a thin patient who is placed in a body cast in lordosis.

O   **What types of bowel disturbances are encountered in the chronic SCI patient population?**

Investigators evaluating outcomes of bowel management in individuals with chronic SCI, found that 42% of subjects reported constipation, 35% reported gastrointestinal pain, and 27% reported bowel accidents. Constipation was greatest in paraplegics using digital stimulation, with an increased incidence of hemorrhoids seen in those who used suppositories and enemas. Fecal incontinence and diarrhea were diagnosed three times more often in tetraplegics.

O   **What characterizes upper motor neuron pattern of neurogenic bowel?**

The type of neurogenic bowel dysfunction that results from SCI depends on location and completeness of the injury. If the SCI is above the sacral spinal cord segment, an upper motor neuron reflexive bowel pattern develops. Voluntary control with relaxation of the external anal sphincter (EAS) is lost along with the inability to modulate descending inhibitory impulses in the spinal cord. This results in pelvic floor musculature and (EAS) spasticity, which contributes to stool retention. Resting pressure of the (EAS) and internal anal sphincter (IAS) is sustained, which ensures continence most of the time. Reflex coordination of stool propulsion in the colon is preserved because the intrinsic innervation of the colon remains intact.

O   **What characterizes lower motor neuron pattern of neurogenic bowel?**

A complete spinal cord lesion located at or below the sacral segment leads to the development s of a lower motor neuron or areflexic bowel pattern. The sacral defecation center and related nerve supply to the anus and rectum are destroyed. Reflexive peristalsis, which is typically mediated by the spinal cord, is lost. Slow stool propulsion from the c colon into the rectum may lead to impaction. Fecal incontinence is increased due to the laxity of the t anal sphincter as a result of the denervated EAS. Resting anal tone is reduced due to loss of parasympathetic control and reflex innervation of the IAS.

O   **What is the gastrocolic reflex and how does it aid the bowel program?**

Typically, the bowel program is performed shortly after meals to facilitate gastrointestinal motility with the aid of the gastrocolic reflex. This reflex is triggered by eating, especially fatty or protein-rich meals, produces peristalsis in the colon and small intestine. The mechanism is not clearly defined and may include neural or hormonal influences. Studies have been inconsistent in showing a predictable gastrocolic response to meals after SCI.

O   **What are the characteristics of the neurogenic bladder?**

In spinal cord lesions above the sacral cord, a hyperreflexic bladder develops. Sensory nerve input and motor output are preserved; however, function is not under conscious control. A reflexive emptying pattern eventually develops in these patients, and an incontinent state exists. They run the risk for development of detrusor hyperreflexia, which can lead to high bladder pressure and eventual renal damage. In patients with spinal cord lesions at the level of the sacral plexus or below, a lower motor neuron bladder develops with bladder areflexia or a flaccid bladder emptying pattern.

O   **What are the characteristics of bladder function during the acute phase of SCI?**

During the acute phase of SCI, in the presence of spinal shock, flaccid paralysis of the bladder occurs. Urine retention develops, and overflow voiding occurs when the intravesicular pressure is greater than the sphincter. The risk is present for residual atonic bladder if prolonged distention persists. An indwelling Foley catheter is used to provide adequate bladder drainage. During this time the patient is at increased risk for UTI, bacterial colonization, epididymitis, prostatitis, periurethritis, and urethrocutaneous fistula formation if the catheter is used for a prolonged period.

O   **What bladder programs are most frequently used by patients with chronic SCI?**

The majority of patients use the preferred intermittent catheter program or reflex voiding, with the goal of maintaining a balanced bladder, which refers to a low pressure, low postvoiding residual volume, and relative continence. In subsequent years after injury, use of the intermittent catheter program declines in men, with a concomitant increase in the use of external condom catheter drainage. In women, use of intermittent catheterization decreases with the increased use of indwelling urethral catheterization.

O   **How common is bacteruria in patients with chronic SCI?**

Recurrent UTI or bacteriuria is the most frequent secondary medical complication or illness. Inadequate emptying is the major source for the proliferation of bacteria to occur in the bladder. Illness in the form of bacteremia and clinical UTI occurs when bacterial concentration rises to a significant level.

O   **How is bacteruria managed?**

Management may require adequate urinary volume for dilution along with adequate emptying. Appropriate antibiotic treatment for 7-10 days is initiated for symptomatic UTI, that is, urinary incontinence, increased spasticity, fever, general malaise, pain over the bladder, or autonomic dysreflexia. Treatment of asymptomatic bacteriuria remains controversial. Such infections are not treated routinely unless the incidence of bacteriuria is the first occurrence and is accompanied by pyuria, urease-producing organisms are present, or the patient is immunocompromised or has vesicoureteral reflux.

O   **What upper tract renal complications can occur in the chronic SCI patient?**

Upper tract urologic complications can impair long-term health and survival. These complications include hydronephrosis, renal insufficiency and failure, renal calculi, and vesicourethral reflux. Increased frequency of renal calculi, a serious complication, is seen with indwelling catheters. Regular evaluations of the urinary tract (yearly or every few years) are advised to reduce mortality and morbidity and maintain normal renal function.

O   What is central de afferent pain?

The patient with spinal cord injury may experience a form of pain commonly referred to as central deafferentation pain. It is often described as having a burning, stinging, or freezing character, and these sensations are referred to as dysesthesias. Patients with in complete injuries may perceive an augmentation of this altered sensation when the skin of the affected area is touched lightly (allodynia). It is usually diffuse in distribution and often involves the lower extremities, particularly the feet, the rectum, and the genitalia. However, it may also be segmental in distribution, often affecting one or two dermatomes at the transitional zone where sensation changes from normal to abnormal.

O   How prevalent is central deafferent pain?

Estimation of the occurrence of central deafferentation pain varies from 13 to 90% of patients. Its incidence has been reported to be higher among those injured by gunshot wounds and among those with incomplete injuries.

O   What medication interventions may be considered?

See drug table in the section on peripheral neuropathies

O   What imaging studies may prove useful in evaluating reversible causes of deafferent pain?

Magnetic resonance imaging (MRI) or myelography may disclose nerve roots entrapped in scar or glial tissue, particularly in cauda equina injuries. In these cases the pain is often segmental, and freeing up this tissue sometimes improves the situation.

O   How are DREZ lesions useful in treating dysesthetic pain in the SCI patient?

When the pain generator lies within the spinal cord itself and the pain is segmental in distribution, some patients have been helped by use of a surgical procedure known as the dorsal root entry zone (DREZ) lesion. Minute lesions are made by radiofrequency or laser coagulation in the substantia gelatinosa in the dorsal horns of the spinal cord. Although this treatment usually results in a loss of sensation of one or two segments above the original level of injury, it has been found to be quite helpful in relieving the central pain of some patients, particularly lower level paraplegic patients who can adapt to the loss of sensation of one or two dermatomes above their previous sensory level. It is most beneficial in radicular pain patterns; diffuse central deafferentation pain is less likely to respond to DREZ, but may be helped by intrathecal morphine.

O   What regional musculoskeletal pain syndromes are most commonly encountered in SCI patients?

A common site of joint pain in both paraplegics and tetraplegics is the shoulder. While the true incidence of shoulder disorders is unknown, various studies have shown an incidence between 35% and 68% in those with an SCI. These numbers vary, depending on the survey methodology. In general, increasing age and increasing time since injury predispose patients to shoulder problems. Heavy activity such as transfers, outdoor wheelchair ambulation, and moving a wheelchair in and out of a car often exacerbate shoulder symptoms. Both women and men suffer from shoulder problems.

O   What is the pathophysiological basis for shoulder pain in SCI patients?

The pathophysiology of shoulder pain in the SCI patient is likely multifactorial. Some studies implicated high glenohumeral intraarticular pressures during strenuous activities, while others pointed out an imbalance in the shoulder musculature, with relatively weaker shoulder depressors and rotators, leading to a high-riding humerus.

O   What is the differential diagnosis of SCI related shoulder pain?

The differential diagnosis is similar to stroke related shoulder pain, though HO occurs more often in the SCI group. Rotator cuff tendinopathies are most common.

O   **What other upper extremity overuse syndromes are encountered in the SCI patient?**

The wrist is also a common site for overuse syndromes. One study put the incidence of wrist pain in SCI patients at 47%. Very often wrist pain in the SCI patient is due to carpal tunnel syndrome (CTS). Another investigator studied 47 patients with paraplegia and found that while 40% had clinical symptoms of CTS, 64% had electrodiagnostic evidence of it. In addition, ulnar neuropathy at the elbow was a common finding, being diagnosed in 45% of the patients by electromyographic (EMG) criteria. In general, findings were worse over time, and at 30 years after injury, 90% of patients had CTS diagnosed by nerve conduction studies.

O   **How common is syringomyelia in the SCI patient population?**

Prevalence estimates of syringomyelia range from 1% to 5%. It usually occurs within the first few years of an SCI; however, there have been reported cases occurring as early as 2 months and as late as 30 years after injury. Syrinxes may develop at all levels of injury and in those with complete and incomplete lesions. The lesions may remain stable or extend in a rostral or caudal direction in the spinal cord.

O   **What is the diagnostic modality of choice?**

The diagnosis of syringomyelia is best made by MRI . Once the diagnosis is made, the patient should be followed closely for progression of the disorder.

O   **How does syringomyelia present clinically in the SCI patient?**

Patients commonly present with new-onset pain and numbness. Occasionally, weakness can be the presenting complaint; however, this is usually associated with other symptoms including changes in spasticity, hyperhidrosis, Horner syndrome, and orthostatic hypotension. Frequently, symptoms are exacerbated by maneuvers that increase intraabdominal or intrathoracic pressure such as coughing, sneezing, and defecation. The earliest clinical sign of syringomyelia is usually a change in DTRs. In addition, an ascending sensory level and changes in strength may also be noted.

O   **What conservative interventions are recommended?**

Efforts should be made to decrease activities that might worsen the condition (i.e., Valsalva maneuvers). Surgical treatment involves shunting the syrinx to the subarachnoid or intra-abdominal space and is usually reserved for those who have intractable pain and those who have progressive motor loss.

O   **What devices are available to enhance sex function and fertility in male SCI patients?**

Several devices and medical interventions are now available to enhance both sex function and fertility in men with SCI. Erection may be enhanced by the use of vacuum constriction devices, intracorporeal injection of vasoactive agents, or penile prosthesis. Ejaculation may be induced by the use of vibrators or electrical stimulation. Fertility is problematic in the male SCI patient given the compromise of thermal regulation of the gonads. In one study, testicular biopsies revealed abnormalities such as maturation arrest, tubular atrophy, hypospermatogenesis, and interstitial fibrosis in more than 50% of patients. Microsurgical techniques allow retrieval of sperm directly from the vas deferens if other techniques fail. Since electroejaculation is not dependent on reflex activity, it may be used in men with upper motor neuron or lower motor neuron lesions.

O   **What problems are reported by women with SCI?**

Women with SCI may complain of inadequate vaginal lubrication or problems achieving orgasm. Recent data support the hypothesis that women with complete SCI are able to achieve reflex genital vasocongestion but not psychogenic genital vasocongestion.

O   **Do women with SCI lose fertility?**

There are no data to support the loss of fertility in women with SCI, although during the initial few weeks to month's menses may be interrupted temporarily.

○ **What problems are associated with pregnancy in SCI patients?**

Pregnancy may be associated with increased medical problems such as UTIs, pressure sores, and increased spasticity. Although thromboembolic disease is a potential complication given the hypercoagulable state of pregnancy and the immobility of SCI patients, there have been few cases of DVT or PE reported. Pulmonary function in patients with high thoracic or cervical lesions may be impaired with the increased burden of pregnancy or the work of labor, and may cause a need for ventilatory support.

○ **What is the most serious complication associated with pregnancy and delivery in the SCI patient?**

Autonomic hyperreflexia is the most significant potential medical com-plication and may occur during any stage of pregnancy, labor, or delivery, and has even been reported in the early postpartum period.

○ **What is the mode of delivery in SCI patients?**

The mode of delivery is primarily determined by standard obstetric indications. The rate of cesarean delivery is nearly identical to the rate in the general population (23%) and not greatly different from the current rate in the United States (about 25%).

○ **What are the functional expectations for the patient with C3-C4 tetraplegia?**

Power wheelchairs may allow greater independence for the C1-C4 level patients. These chairs operate by chin, mouth, breath, or voice controls. In a similar fashion, environmental control units allow a patient to access a telephone, radio, television, lights, computer, and so forth from one location. These patients are dependent for transfers, feeding, grooming, dressing, bathing, bowel, and bladder routine and therefore require a full-time trained attendant.

○ **What are the functional expectations for the patient with C5 tetraplegia?**

The patient at this level has added antigravity (grade 3/5) strength in the biceps muscle. This allows partial independence in eating skills using splints or other assistive devices such as a mobile arm support. Independence in power wheel chair locomotion is possible. Driving is also possible with specialized equipment and a modified van.

○ **What are the functional expectations for a C6 tetraplegic patient?**

For self-care, dressing requires partial physical assistance. A flexor hinge splint can increase self-care (eating, personal hygiene) and make writing possible. Transfers are now possible. Some patients require a frame over the bed with loops and a sliding board. Some are able to perform transfers with just a sliding board and others may even be able to perform transfers using a "hop-over" technique. With SCI at this level, a manual wheelchair with plastic rims or knobs can be used but a power wheelchair is needed for long distances. Some men are able to perform self catheterization with a splint but are not able to apply a condom catheter. Women are generally not able to perform self-catheterization. The patient with C6 tetraplegia has the highest neurologic level at which driving with hand controls is possible.

○ **What are the functional expectations for a patient with C7/C8/T1 SCI levels?**

Initially, personal hygiene, eating, dressing, writing, transfers, ambulation, and driving are impaired. With extensive treatment, almost all patients in this group become completely independent in all functions but may require assistive devices. Transfers, dressing, and personal hygiene may require partial or standby physical assistance. The patient may be able to live alone. Independent ambulation is with a manual wheelchair. The patient, male or female, with SCI at the C7 level is usually able to perform self catheterization and male patients can apply condom catheters. Clothing may need modification for bladder function.

○ **What are the functional expectations for the SCI patient injury at the T2-T5 level?**

Independent in self care including bladder and bowel function and in wheelchair ambulation can be achieved.

○ **What are the functional expectations for the SCI patient injury at the T6-T12 level?**

Independent bipedal ambulation, if attempted, is usually achieved only for exercise. A walker and a swing to gait pattern is the typical mode of ambulation. Knee-ankle-foot orthoses (KAFOs) are required for bipedal ambulation unless functional electrical stimulation (FES) is used. FES requires appropriate responses to electrical current.

○   **What are the functional expectations for the SCI patient injury at the L1-L3 level?**

Independent bipedal ambulation with KAFOs is possible for short distances. A wheelchair is still needed. An isocentric reciprocating gait orthosis can allow free-standing balance and reduce energy expenditure during gait.

○   **What are the functional expectations for the SCI patient injury at the L1-L3 level?**

Usually ankle foot orthoses are needed plus two canes or crutches. Although prolonged standing may be difficult, a wheelchair is not necessary for short distance ambulation.

TRAUMATIC BRAIN INJURY

○   **Provide a basic working definition of traumatic brain injury?**

Traumatic brain injury (TBI) is one of the leading causes of death and lifelong disability in the United States today. TBI is a nondegenerative, noncongenital insult to the brain from an external mechanical force, possibly leading to permanent or temporary impairments of cognitive, physical, and psychosocial functions with an associated diminished or altered state of consciousness.

○   **What is the incidence of TBI?**

The incidence of mild TBI is about 131 cases per 100,000 people. Incidence of moderate TBI is about 15 cases per 100,000 people. Incidence of severe TBI is about 14 cases per 100,000 people. Inclusion of prehospital deaths increases that figure to 21 cases per 100,000 people.

○   **What is the prevalence of TBI?**

Estimates by the National Institute of Health Consensus Development Panel on Rehabilitation of Persons with TBI showed that 2.5-6.5 million Americans live with TBI-related disabilities. According to statistics from the Centers for Disease Control and Prevention (CDC), out of the estimated 1.5 million yearly survivors of TBI in the United States, approximately 90,000 are left with permanent disabilities. As a result, more than 5 million people are living with TBI-related disabilities. Men are affected 3 times as often as women, with the leading causes of TBI being motor vehicle accidents (MVAs), falls, and violence (CDC, 1999).

○   **What is the gender distribution of TBI?**

Men are approximately twice as likely as women to sustain TBI. This ratio approaches parity as age increases because of the increased likelihood of TBI caused by falls, for which members of both sexes have similar risks in later life. The male-to-female mortality rate for TBI is 3.4:1. However, the cause-specific ratio for firearm-related injuries is 6:1, while that for injuries related to motor vehicle accidents (MVAs) is 2.4:1.

○   **Which age group sustains the highest death rate for TBI?**

Traumatic brain injury (TBI) is one of the leading causes of death and lifelong disability in the United States today. Injury is the leading cause of death among Americans younger than 45 years; TBI is the major cause of death related to injury. The highest mortality rate (32.8 cases per 100,000 people) is found in those aged 15-24 years. The mortality rate in patients who are elderly (65 y or older) is about 31.4 individuals per 100,000 people.

○   **What are the high-risk populations for TBI?**

Some particular segments of the populace are at increased risk of sustaining a TBI, including the following: young people, low-income individuals, unmarried individuals, members of ethnic minority groups, residents of inner cities, men Individuals with previous history of substance abuse individuals with previous TBI.

O   **What association is there between TBI risk and drug use?**

Up to 70% to 75% of individuals who have sustained TBI are under the effects of alcohol or other drugs.

O   **What is the association between previous history of brain injury and subsequent brain injury?**

Investigators have identified increasing risk for subsequent TBI as follows: a threefold increase for another TBI after one brain injury and an eight fold increase in risk for another TBI after more than one brain injury.

O   **Which age group is at greatest risk for TBI?**

The risk of TBI peaks when individuals are aged 15-30 years. The risk is highest for individuals aged 15-24 years. Peak age is similar for males and females. Twenty percent of TBIs occur in the pediatric age group (i.e., birth to 17 y).

Age	Population	% of population	Rate of TBI per 100,000	Number of new injuries in 2000	% of TBI population
0-15	58,629,000	21.2	215	126,000	18.6
15-34	75,736,000	27.5	400	303,000	44.8
34-65	106,173,000	38.6	150	160,000	23.6
65+	34,847,000	12.7	250	88,000	12.9

Estimates of the number of new traumatic brain injuries that will be seen in hospitals in the United States during the year 2000, grouped according to age. This is a conservative estimate, based on TBI surveillance data as recorded by the Centers for Disease Control that requires the injury be of sufficient severity to merit a hospital-based evaluation, and U.S. Census Bureau population estimates for the year 2000.

O   **What is the most common cause of TBI?**

The most common cause of TBI is still the motor vehicle accident, which is also responsible for the highest number of deaths. In the united states motor vehicle accidents account for approximately 50% of all TBIs. Motor vehicle accidents in this case include automobiles, motorcycles, and bicycles. Pedestrians are most likely to sustain TBI and alcohol is a contributing factor in half of all pedestrian versus vehicle collisions.

O   **What preventative measures are taken with regard to motor vehicle safety to reduce the risk of TBI?**

Because of the human and financial cost of TBI, there has been a great deal of emphasis on primary prevention. This may take the form of vehicular equipment such as an airbag, which is estimated to prevent 25% of motor vehicle accident related TBIs. Lap shoulder belts decrease the incidence of fatality and moderate to critical injury from 45% to 50%; with an airbag this is improved to 55% to 60%. Unbelted individuals have more than eight times greater likelihood of TBI with loss of consciousness.

O   **What degree of protection do helmets afford motor cycle drivers?**

The most dramatic impact of equipment related interventions has been with the use of motorcycle helmets: without helmets, riders run a two to three times greater risk of TBI and three to nine times greater risk of fatality. It has been estimated that helmet use would decrease the risk of TBI by 41% and the acute care cost for motorcycle related TBIs by 40%.

O   **What degree of protection do helmets afford bicycle drivers?**

In the case of bicycles, helmets will decrease the incidence of TBI by 74% to 85%.

○   **What is the second leading cause of TBI?**

Falls are the second leading cause of TBI. Falls account for 20-30% of all TBIs. In individuals aged 75 years and older, falls are the most common cause of TBI. The very young also commonly sustain TBI due to falls.

○   **What is the third leading cause of TBI?**

Firearms are the third leading cause of TBI (12% of all TBIs) and are a leading cause of TBI among individuals aged 25-34 years. Gunshot related fatal TBI is higher among men than women and is more prevalent among African Americans than whites.

○   **What are the pathological characteristics of closed primary injury in the brain?**

Closed head injuries do not involve direct penetration of the brain, although some depressed skull fractures may be included within this category. Pathomechanically, there may or may not be an impact injury to the head, but even so, the pathology is largely governed by the velocity, direction, and duration of an acceleration-deceleration inertial load. There is also an effect from the internal anatomy of the skull.

○   **What are the pathological characteristics of penetrating primary injury in the brain?**

Neurologic impairments in penetrating injury are somewhat focal in nature, in that they are confined to the track of the bullet and related to the volume of brain damage as well as the site of injury. Higher velocity missile injuries are associated with greater severity since the percussion force of the bullet produces tissue damage as much as 30 times the diameter of the bullet. Fragments of bone and hair that enter the brain may also be a source of infection. The mortality and severity of disability are closely related to the neurologic status and presence of coma after a missile injury.

○   **What is the basic classification of injury pattern in TBI?**

The pathophysiology of TBI can be separated into primary injury and secondary injury. Primary injury occurs at the time of impact. Secondary injury occurs after the impact secondary to the body's response to primary injury and can be influenced by medical interventions. Primary and secondary injuries can each be subdivided into focal and diffuse types. Focal injuries tend to be caused by contact forces, whereas diffuse injury is more likely to be caused by noncontact, acceleration-deceleration, or rotational forces.

○   **What are the common causes of primary focal TBI?**

Both cortical contusions and intracranial hematomas are common causes of primary focal TBI. Contusions usually occur after direct injuries over bony prominences of the skull, with the most commonly affected areas being the orbitofrontal and anterotemporal regions.

○   **How are intracranial hematomas classified?**

Intracranial hematomas are divided into epidural hematomas, subdural hematomas, and subarachnoid hemorrhages. Epidural hematomas result from rupture of the middle meningeal artery where it crosses the squamous portion of the temporal bone and cause focal injury by increasing pressure over a cortical region of the brain. Subdural hematomas and subarachnoid hemorrhage occur as a result of disruption of the bridging vessels in their respective spaces; both cause focal injury due to increased intracranial pressure (ICP).

○   **What are cerebral contusions?**

Cerebral contusions are hemorrhagic bruises on the surface of the brain over the crest of gyri that typically are distributed to the under surfaces of the frontal and temporal lobes. These most typically occur as the result of acceleration in a sagittal plane, associated with a short pulse duration and directly related to the brain moving en masse over the rough base of the skull. Contusions may be seen as well beneath areas of blunt trauma, particularly in association with depressed skull fractures (which is the only time they are seen in the occipital lobe).

O   **What are Coup contusions?**

Coup contusions are a combination of vascular and tissue damage leads to cerebral contusion. Coup contusions occur at the area of direct impact to the skull and occur because of the creation of negative pressure when the skull, distorted at the site of impact, returns to its normal shape.

O   **What are countrecoup contusions?**

Contrecoup contusions are similar to coup contusions but are located opposite the site of direct impact. Cavitation in the brain, from negative pressure due to translational acceleration impacts from inertial loading, may cause contrecoup contusions as the skull and dura matter start to accelerate before the brain on initial impact.

O   **What factors determine the pattern of the contusion?**

The amount of energy dissipated at the site of direct impact determines whether the ensuing contusion is of the coup or contrecoup type. Most of the energy of impact from a small hard object tends to dissipate at the impact site, leading to a coup contusion. On the contrary, impact from a larger object causes less injury at the impact site since energy is dissipated at the beginning or end of the head motion, leading to a contrecoup contusion.

O   **What are extradural hematomas?**

Extradural hematomas are almost always due to fracture of the skull with laceration of an artery, typically the middle meningeal, in the temporal parietal area. There may be no direct associated damage to the brain, but rather the damage is secondary to the expanding mass from arterial bleeding.

O   **What are subdural hematomas?**

Subdural hematomas are much more common and are caused by bleeding in the subdural space by "bridging veins." These are largely confined to the temporal areas, particularly the temporal tip, and may be associated with intracerebral hematomas. In animal studies, subdural and most intracerebral hematomas are seen with short duration inertial loads and where the angular acceleration is sagittal as opposed to rotatory. This would be exemplified by a fall from a height of less than approximately 15 feet. The degree of permanent neurologic deficits from intracranial hematomas is related to the size and the location of the lesion. Small hemorrhagic areas in key areas such as the brain stem or basal ganglia may lead to severe neurologic deficits. However, even large masses, if they are evacuated rapidly, can leave relatively mild permanent disability.

O   **What is diffuse axonal injury?**

Diffuse axonal injury (DAI) is caused by forces associated with acceleration-deceleration and rotational injuries. This type of injury most commonly occurs during high impact motor vehicle collisions, but these injuries can also be due to contact sports and shaken baby syndrome. DAI is an axonal shearing injury of the axons that is most often observed in the midline structures, including the parasagittal white matter of the cerebral cortex, the corpus callosum, and the pontine mesencephalic junction adjacent to the superior cerebral peduncles.

O   **How is diffuse axonal injury graded?**

Neuropathologic findings in patients with diffuse axonal injury were graded by Gennarelli and colleagues, as follows:
Grade 1 - Axonal injury mainly in parasagittal white matter of the cerebral hemispheres
Grade 2 - As in Grade 1, plus lesions in the corpus callosum
Grade 3 - As in Grade 2, plus a focal lesion in the cerebral peduncle.

O   **What are the causes of secondary brain injury?**

Causes of secondary brain injury include the following: neurochemical and cellular changes, hypotension, hypoxia, increased ICP with decreased cerebral perfusion pressure (CPP) and a risk of herniation, electrolyte imbalances, and ischemia. Recent advances in minimizing secondary injury include minimizing the risk of early hypotension (systolic blood pressure <90 mm Hg) and hypoxia (arterial oxygen <60 mm Hg). In addition, early monitoring for and treatment of elevations in ICP along with the judicious use of pressors has minimized the risk of ischemic injury from low CPP (CPP = mean arterial pressure - ICP).

O   **What molecular events occur in secondary brain injury that contributes to neuro cytotoxicity?**

Initiation of the neuro cytotoxic cascade involves the massive release of excitatory amino acids, particularly glutamate and aspartate. This results in excessive activation of enzyme linked calcium channels and then pathologic influx of calcium into the cell. This influx in turn increases enzymatic activity, which can set off a "self-destruct" program at the nuclear level, produce internal damage to the cell membrane, or significantly disrupt the microtubular system necessary for neuronal viability. There may be associated high levels of reactive oxygen (free radicals) that in turn cause additional damage to the cell membrane.

O   **What role does increased intracranial pressure play as a secondary injury variable?**

Severity of injury tends to increase due to heightened ICP, especially if pressure exceeds 40 mm Hg. Increased pressure also can lead to cerebral hypoxia, cerebral ischemia, cerebral edema, hydrocephalus, and brain herniation.

O   **What role does cerebral edema play as a secondary injury variable?**

Edema may be caused by effects of the above mentioned neurochemical transmitters and by increased ICP. Disruption of the blood brain barrier, with impairment of vasomotor autoregulation leading to dilatation of cerebral blood vessels, also contributes.

O   **What role does hydrocephalus play as a secondary injury variable?**

The communicating type of hydrocephalus is more common in TBI than the noncommunicating type, which frequently is due to the presence of blood products causing obstruction to flow of the cerebral spinal fluid (CSF) in the subarachnoid space and absorption of CSF through the arachnoid villi. The noncommunicating type of hydrocephalus often is caused by blood clot obstruction of blood flow at the interventricular foramen, third ventricle, cerebral aqueduct, or fourth ventricle.

O   **What role does brain injury play as a secondary injury variable?**

Supratentorial herniation is attributable to direct mechanical compression by an accumulating mass or to increased intracranial pressure.

O   **What types of supratentorial herniation are recognized?**

Subfalcine herniation, Central transtentorial herniation, Uncal herniation, Cerebellar herniation.

O   **What is subfalcine herniation?**

The cingulate gyrus of the frontal lobe is pushed beneath the falx cerebri when an expanding mass lesion causes a medial shift of the ipsilateral hemisphere. This is the most common type of herniation.

O   **What is Central transtentorial herniation?**

This type of injury is characterized by displacement of the basal nuclei and cerebral hemispheres downward while the diencephalon and adjacent midbrain are pushed through the tentorial notch.

O   **What is Uncal herniation ?**

This type of injury involves displacement of the medial edge of the uncus and the hippocampal gyrus medially and over the ipsilateral edge of the tentorium cerebelli foramen, causing compression of the midbrain, while the ipsilateral or contralateral third nerve may be stretched or compressed.

O   **What is Cerebellar herniation ?**

This injury is marked by an infratentorial herniation in which the tonsil of the cerebellum is pushed through the foramen magnum and compresses the medulla, leading to bradycardia and respiratory arrest.

O **How does hypoxic-ischemic injury compound the primary injury?**

As a consequence of difficulty in regulating regional blood flow or because of associated shock and hypovolemia or hypoxia, a secondary injury often seen with TBI is hypoxic-ischemic insult. Global hypoxic injury is present in one third of subjects who have had fatal injuries; hypoxia preferentially affects the hippocampus, basal ganglia, and cerebellum. Boundary zone injuries are usually related to perfusion failures and the injury is confined to the overlapping territories of the major cerebral arteries. Hypoxic ischemic encephalopathy accounts for significant disability, particularly in association with other kinds of acquired brain damage.

O **What is the Glasgow coma scale?**

SCORE	
Motor responses	6
Obeys commands	5
Localizing response to pain	4
Generalized withdrawal to pain	3
Flexor posturing to pain	2
Extensor posturing to pain	1
No motor response to pain	
Verbal responses	5
Oriented	4
Confused conversation	3
Inappropriate speech	2
Incomprehensible speech	1
No speech	
Eye opening	4
Spontaneous eye opening	3
Eye opening to speech	2
Eye opening to pain	1
No eye opening	

O **What are the outcomes for severe TBI?**

Severe TBI is associated with a morality rate of more than 50% and those who survive are usually left with significant cognitive impairments and may have residual physical limitations. Only approximately 30% of severe TBI survivors recover to moderate disability or good recovery by 6 months after injury as measured by the Glasgow Outcome Scale (GOS).

O **What are the outcomes for moderate TBI?**

Moderate TBI has a mortality rate of less than 10% and many patients have only mild residual deficits. Approximately 70% of moderate TBI patients attain a GOS rating of moderate disability or good recovery by 6 months.

O **What are the outcomes for mild TBI?**

Mild TBI rarely results in death and the majority of patients return to pre injury levels of functioning. Approximately 95% of mild TBI patients recover to a GOS rating of moderate disability or good recovery by 6 months.

O **What are late complications of TBI?**

Late complications of TBI include chronic subdural fluid collections, abscess, and meningitis from unrecognized dural tears, traumatic fistulas, cavernous sinus thrombosis, and aneurysms.

○ **Describe the prevalence of selected self-reported chronic conditions for TBI versus the US adult general population.**

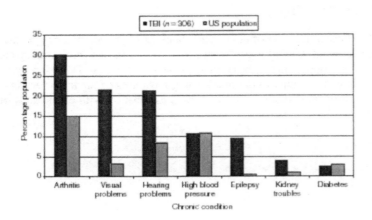

○ **What is the presentation of severe post traumatic amnesia (PTA) and its natural progression?**

The patient in severe PTA is acutely confused, oriented only to personal identity, and shows no ability to acquire new memories. As the patient improves, he or she becomes less distractible and shows evidence of new learning. Orientation to place and at least a superficial understanding of personal circumstances return first while orientation to time is last to recover.

○ **What are the outcome measures most commonly used in TBI rehabilitation?**

The most commonly used measures of global outcome are the GOS, the Disability Rating Scale (DRS), and the Levels of Cognitive Functioning Scale also known as the Rancho Scale. All of these scales have been shown to have adequate reliability and validity. They have been criticized for being insensitive to subtle changes in the patient's functional status and failing to distinguish different areas of patient functioning.

○ **What is the Ranchos Los Amigos Cognitive Scale?**

Ranchos Los Amigos Cognitive Scale
Level I - No response to pain, touch, sound or sight.
Level II - Generalized reflex response to pain.
Level III - Localized response. Blinks to strong light, turns toward/away from sound, and responds to physical discomfort, inconsistent response to commands.
Level IV - Confused/Agitated. Alert, very active, aggressive or bizarre behaviors, performs motor activities but behavior is non-purposeful, extremely short attention span.
Level V - Confused/Non-agitated. Gross attention to environment, highly distractible, requires continual redirection, difficulty learning new tasks, agitated by too much stimulation. May engage in social conversation but with inappropriate verbalizations.
Level VI - Confused/Appropriate. Inconsistent orientation to time and place, retention span/recent memory impaired, begins to recall past, and consistently follows simple directions, goal-directed behavior with assistance.
Level VII - Automatic/Appropriate. Performs daily routine in highly familiar environment in a non-confused but automatic robot-like manner. Skills noticeably deteriorate in unfamiliar environment. Lacks realistic planning for own future.
Level VIII - Purposeful/Appropriate.
Level IX - Purposeful, Appropriate: Stand-By Assistance on Request
Level X - Purposeful, Appropriate: Modified Independent

○ **What pharmacologic agents may enhance neuronal recovery in TBI?**

The drugs that have the strongest evidence for efficacy in improving motor recovery in the experimental animal model, and to some degree in humans, are those that increase norepinephrine. Conversely, those that impede or block norepinephrine, and secondarily dopamine receptors, may retard motor recovery.

O   What post injury factors influence the success of community reintegration?

Post injury factors that are predictive of long term functional outcome include: severity of cognitive deficits, presence of behavioral problems, accuracy of patient self awareness, adequacy of social support, and involvement in litigation. Patients with more severe cognitive deficits have Poorer employment outcome. Patients who exhibit behavioral problems or who are reported by relatives to have a personality change due to TBI also have poorer employment outcome. Impaired self awareness of deficits is a common effect of brain injury. Several studies showed that impaired self awareness contributes to poor long term employment outcome in TBI patients.

O   What are the therapy activities and goals of post acute brain injury?

Therapy activities include training in strategies to compensate for cognitive deficits, counseling regarding emotional response to injury and behavioral functioning, educational services to improve awareness of the effects of TBI, and supervised participation in community based therapy activities designed to transition gains made in the clinic to the patient's real world environments and activities. The goals of therapy are improved community integration as indicated by increased personal independence and participation in productive activities and improved psychosocial and emotional adjustment.

O   What are the characteristics of post traumatic epilepsy?

The incidence of late posttraumatic seizures (LPTS) in individuals with traumatic brain injury (TBI)
ranges anywhere from 5% to 18.9% in civilian populations up to 32% to 50% in military personnel.
The major types of posttraumatic epilepsy include simple partial, generalized, and partial complex seizures; the latter are part of the differential diagnosis for behavioral and cognitive problems after TBI.

O   When should pharmacotherapy be continued for post traumatic epilepsy?

There is no cogent evidence to support the use of prophylactic anticonvulsants beyond the first 2 weeks after injury for patients with a closed head injury. If the patient has late seizures (after the first week), then anticonvulsants should be continued; similarly, clinicians may continue prophylactic anticonvulsants in patients with missile injury or open injury. The preferred medications to manage posttraumatic epilepsy are carbamazepine and valproic acid, largely because of their side effect profile when compared to phenobarbital and phenytoin; however, any of the anticonvulsants can produce significant cognitive impairments.

O   What types of hydrocephalus are encountered in the TBI patient?

Hydrocephalus is characterized as either communicating or noncommunicating on the basis of the location of the causative obstruction. Noncommunicating hydrocephalus occurs secondary to an obstruction within the ventricular system before the exit of cerebrospinal fluid (CSF) from the forth ventricle. Communicating hydrocephalus, which is more common in TBI, occurs when the obstruction is in the subarachnoid space. In TBI, subarachnoid obstruction is commonly caused by inflammation and impaired CSF absorption by arachnoid granulations. The incidence of hydrocephalus is probably no more than 5 percent.

O   What are the symptoms and signs associated with hydrocephalus in TBI?

Clinically, hydrocephalus can occur with nausea, vomiting, headache, papilledema, obtundation, dementia, ataxia, and urinary incontinence.

O   How is hydrocephalus diagnosed?

The diagnosis is made based on clinical suspicion and diagnostic imaging studies, including MRI, CT scanning, and radioisotope cisternography. After a subarachnoid hemorrhage, the development of symptomatic hydrocephalus is predicted by finding cisternal and ventricular blood or hydrocephalus on the initial CT scan.

O   **What is the treatment of hydrocephalus in TBI?**

Acute obstructive hydrocephalus can be a complication of cerebral edema and of blood within the ventricles or the subarachnoid space. A ventricular shunt is indicated.

O   **What are the temporal characteristics of symptomatic nonobstructive or normal pressure hydrocephalus?**

Either condition can develop insidiously over months, even years, after TBI. Ventricular enlargement, however, develops in 30 to 70 percent of patients with severe TBI. Most patients appear to have hydrocephalus ex vacuo, a passive enlargement from the loss of gray and white matter.

O   **What is the definitive treatment for hydrocephalus?**

Ventricular shunting is the definitive treatment; infection, subdural hematoma, and shunt malfunction and obstruction are all potential complications from the procedure.

O   **What forensic evidence is there for endocrine pathology in TBI?**

Autopsy studies in fatal TBI cases demonstrate a fairly high prevalence of hypothalamic and pituitary abnormalities, including anterior lobe necrosis, posterior lobe hemorrhage, and traumatic lesions of the hypothalamic pituitary stalk. Some variability is noted in studies. Anterior pituitary infarction occurred in 9-38% of patients, posterior pituitary hemorrhage occurred in 12-45% of cases, and traumatic lesions of the stalk occurred in 5-30%.

O   **What management approach is appropriate for acute TBI patients with new onset hypertension?**

Hypertension after brain injury occurs as a new condition in 10% to 15% of patients, is related to specific neuroanatomic injury (to baso-orbital frontal area, hypothalamus, or brain stem regulatory structures), and is usually transient. Management is best undertaken with beta-blockers given after the acute phase to avoid detrimental effects on regional cerebral blood flow; calcium channel blockers and other agents may also be effective. Care should be taken in the acute trauma setting as overzealous management of hypertension or tachycardia may have deleterious effects on regional cerebral blood flow.

O   **What is the appropriate diagnostic approach for patients with hyperthermia?**

Hyperthermia, or central fever, is diagnosed after a detailed evaluation for infection. It may be related to anterior hypothalamic injury and is best treated with modalities (cooling blanket, or if severe, iced gastric lavage), nonsteroidal antiinflammatory drugs (NSAIDs) propranolol, or dopamine agonists.

O   **What are diencephalic fits?**

Diencephalic fits are episodes of hypertension, fever, and sweating that may respond to propranolol and dopamine agonists, but often require anticonvulsants.

O   **What is hyperphagia in the context of TBI?**

Hyperphagia is uncommon, and again is often related to hypothalamic or extra hypothalamic dysregulation; management is best undertaken with new classes of selective serotonin reuptake inhibitors (SSRIs) or possibly naltrexone.

O   **What type of pituitary dysfunction is most common in the TBI patient population?**

Pituitary dysfunction is most common in the acute setting and related to disorders of salt metabolism (diabetes insipidus and syndrome of inappropriate secretion of antidiuretic hormone); in both cases the problem is usually transient and a careful evaluation of iatrogenic causes is relevant.

O   **What is cerebral salt wasting (CSW)?**

CSW is caused by impaired renal tubular function, resulting in the inability of the kidneys to conserve salt. The etiology may be attributable to direct neural influence on renal tubular function. Salt wasting with volume depletion is the hallmark of this syndrome. Clinically, patients manifesting CSW are dehydrated, lose weight, have orthostatic hypotension, and demonstrate a negative fluid balance.

O   **What are the comparative features of CSW and SIADH?**

In cases of CSW and SIADH, the laboratory values often are the same for serum/urine osmolalities and electrolytes; however, elevated serum blood urea nitrogen (BUN), serum potassium, and serum protein concentration also are supportive of the diagnosis of CSW. Additionally, serum uric acid is normal in those with CSW and low in those with SIADH.

O   **What are the characteristics of diabetes insipidus in the TBI patient?**

Posttraumatic DI occurs in 2-16% of all cases. The most common etiologies of posttraumatic DI include severe closed head injury, frequently with basilar skull fractures; craniofacial trauma; thoracic injury; post-cardiopulmonary arrest; and intraventricular hemorrhage in neonatal patients. DI frequently is associated with cranial nerve injuries. The usual onset is 5-10 days following trauma.

O   **What is the clinical profile of DI?**

Characteristic features of DI include polyuria, low urine osmolality, high serum osmolality, normal serum glucose, and normal-to-elevated serum sodium. Urine output usually is greater than 90 mL/kg/d, with a specific gravity less than 1.010 and an osmolality of 50-200 mOsm.

O   **What is anterior hypopituitarism (AH)?**

AH is a rare complication following a closed head injury, usually following severe craniocerebral trauma.

O   **What is the etiology of AH in the TBI patient?**

The mechanism of development of AH in patients with severe head injuries is that the major blood supply to the anterior lobe of the pituitary gland is interrupted because of trauma to the unprotected stalk connecting the anterior pituitary to the median eminence of the hypothalamus.

O   **What is the clinical presentation of AH?**

The syndrome of AH may manifest an insidious onset, weeks to months after the original closed head injury. The patient may become progressively lethargic or anorexic and may demonstrate hypothermia, bradycardia, or hypotension with hyponatremia.

O   **What does the diagnostic workup consist of?**

The endocrine workup for AH includes serum hormonal assays (eg, cortisol, testosterone, triiodothyronine (T3), thyroxine (T4), thyroid stimulating hormone [TSH]). Perform a complete blood count (CBC) and serum electrolytes as well.

O   **How does traumatic brain injury affect metabolism in a patient?**

It is apparent that brain injury can stimulate tremendous changes in metabolism, which are inversely related to the Glasgow Coma Scale score, and that these changes may persist throughout the duration of the coma. Autonomic and endocrine alterations, including an increase in catecholamines, steroids, insulin, and glucagon, occur. Increased cardiac Output, hyperventilation, fever, restlessness, posturing, seizures, and secondary infections can cause additional metabolic demands. Several studies have revealed increases of 120 to 200% in resting energy expenditure and twice the normal oxygen consumption in head injured patients. There is also catabolism of endogenous protein, with depletion of lean body mass and excretion of large amounts of nitrogen.

O   **What factors can increase the risk of malnutrition in the head injured patient?**

The likelihood of malnutrition increases when feedings are limited by gastric hypomotility, ileus, diarrhea, emesis, aspiration pneumonia, and a tracheal fistula. The use of corticosteroids and renal and liver failure contribute to this problem. Aphagia accompanies coma and poor attention, jaw and dental injuries, and central and peripheral causes of bulbar dysfunction, such as vocal cord paralysis. Later, during rehabilitation, cognitive and behavioral function and side effects of medications can affect the safety and quantity of oral intake and absorption. Better nutrition may improve functional outcomes. Several studies suggest that early parenteral hyperalimentation is better than nasogastric feeding for supplying needed calories, vitamins, and minerals including zinc in the severely head injured group (GCS score 4-5). Otherwise gastrostomy or jejunostomy enteral nutrition is preferred and successfully implemented in the majority of patients.

How common is dysphagia in TBI patients?

25% of TBI patients overall have dysphagia, with educed cognition a more prominent cause than motor control problems. Eventual progression to safe oral feeding does occur in the vast majority of patients.

What other GI complications occur in the TBI patient population?

Other gastrointestinal complications include gastritis and ulcers (stress related) which may be present in up to 75% of patients. Gastric acid output does increase in the setting of increased intracranial pressure other factors contribute to the risk of mucosal ischemia. Agents often selected for treatment include H2 blockers, proton pump inhibitors and sucralfate. The evidence of efficacy of H2 blockers and sucralfate however, is questionable.

Summarize the traumatic cranial neuropathies

Cranial Nerve	Site of Likely Trauma	Clinical Features	Evaluation	Management	Prognosis
I	Any part of head. More common with occipital than frontal trauma	Decreased or absent sense of smell	Check for possible ethmoid fractures, CSF rhinorrhea, and injury to orbital surface of frontal lobes	Educate patient	Up to 50% of cases, usually during first 3 months but up to 5 years after injury
II	Intracanalicular often associated with a skull base fracture	Decreased or loss of vision. Scotomas, sector, and altitudinal defects can occur	Check visual acuity, fields, and for afferent pupillary defect. CT scan and ultrasound A and B are useful to assess for possible compressive lesions	Controversial for indirect optic neuropathy: include observation, high-dose steroids, and surgery. Surgical decompression often recommended in cases of delayed onset of visual loss	Extremely variable; from 0–100% depending upon the study
III	Where the nerve enters the dura at the posterior end of the cavernous sinus. Uncal herniation much less common	Dilated pupil and turned out eye present in complete palsy. Anisocoria and diplopia in partial lesions	CT and/or MRI scans to look for a compressive lesion	Symptomatic such as eye patch, semitransparent tape to glasses and prisms for diplopia. Muscle shortening procedures may be helpful for permanent diplopia	Recovery begins within 2–3 months when nerve in continuity. Aberrant regeneration often occurs with findings such as lid elevation or pupillary constriction with attempted adduction or depression
IV	Stretching or contusion of the nerve as it exits the dorsal midbrain near the anterior medullary velum	Trauma is the most common cause of trochlear palsies. Bilateral palsies are rather common	Same as above	Same as above	Only 50% recover because of frequent avulsion of the trochlear nerve
V	Trigeminal nerves and branches are commonly injured with facial trauma, especially supraorbital and supratrochlear nerves. The infraorbital nerve is often injured in orbital floor blowout fractures	Injury to the gasserian ganglion and trigeminal trunk is rare after closed head trauma	Imaging studies to exclude underlying fractures	Decompression of the infraorbital nerve in orbital floor fractures. Symptomatic for hyperpathia due to supra- and infraorbital neuropathies with medications such as carbamazepine, tricyclics, and baclofen	Hyperpathia in the distribution of the nerve may be permanent
VI	As the nerve ascends the clivus, in fractures of the	Bilateral palsies are rather common	Same as above	Same as above	Recovery often occurs after 4 months

Cranial Nerve	Site of Likely Trauma	Clinical Features	Evaluation	Management	Prognosis
	petrous bone along with VII and VIII, in the superior orbital fissure along with III and IV, and in its subarachnoid course due to raised intracranial pressure				
VII	Most commonly within the petrous bone but can be injured anywhere along its course	Injured in 50% with a transverse temporal bone fracture. Facial palsy in 25% with a longitudinal fracture, often with a delayed onset	CT scan to evaluate temporal bone trauma. A nerve conduction study 5 or more days after the injury is helpful to assess the degree of nerve injury	Facial nerve decompression is usually indicated for transverse fractures. Artificial tears and eye patch at night to prevent exposure keratitis	Spontaneous recovery usual after longitudinal fractures. When due to transverse fractures, 50% recovery after decompression
VIII	Labyrinthine concussion without a skull fracture is the most common site. Conductive hearing loss follows longitudinal temporal bone fractures in over 50% of cases. Transverse fractures result in vestibular and cochlear nerve laceration in over 80%	Findings associated with a fracture of the petrous portion of the temporal bone include hemotympanum or tympanic membrane perforation with blood in the external canal, hearing loss, vestibular dysfunction, peripheral facial nerve palsy, CSF otorrhea, and ecchymosis of the scalp over the mastoid bone (Battle's sign). Benign positional vertigo occurs in about 25% of patients following head trauma	Examine the external canals and tympanic membranes. An audiogram including pure-tone and speech audiometry, acoustic reflexes, and middle ear function is used to assess hearing loss. An electronystagmogram (ENG) is used to assess vestibular function. CT scan to evaluate temporal bone trauma	A hearing aid may help those with sensorineural hearing loss. Surgical correction is indicated for conductive hearing loss due to ossicular chain disruption. Positioning maneuvers, such as Epley's or Semont's, which move the debris out of the semicircular canal and into the utricle, can be curative for benign positional vertigo	Following temporal bone fractures, patients with low- or high-frequency hearing loss may have some recovery, but those with low- and high-frequency loss usually do not recover. Vertigo due to a labyrinth concussion usually resolves within a year
IX, X, XI, XII	Gunshot or stab wounds occasionally cause injury. A fracture of the occipital condyle, Collet-Sicard syndrome, can injure all four nerves. The peripheral portion of XI can be injured in surgical procedures such as posterior cervical lymph node biopsies. The hypoglossal and recurrent laryngeal nerves can be traumatized in anterior neck operations such as carotid endarterectomy	Lower cranial nerve findings associated with signs of brain stem compression are consistent with an intracranial lesion, whereas the presence of a Horner's syndrome is consistent with an extracranial lesion	A careful clinical examination is mandatory. CT and MRI are both useful, depending upon the case	Treatment of Collet-Sicard syndrome is supportive with elevation of the head for drainage of excess saliva and IV or nasogastric nutrition until normal swallowing returns. Accessory nerve injuries in the neck may require exploration with neurolysis or resection and repair or grafting, depending on the degree of injury	

O   **What concomitant musculoskeletal injuries occur in the TBI patient?**

Occult fractures are a serious problem in TBI, under diagnosed in up to 30%. Appendicular fractures as well as axial fractures occur in the TBI patient population. Pelvic/hip fractures and elbow fractures are associated with a high incidence of heterotopic ossification. The general principles of orthopedic trauma management apply to the TBI patient population. Early reduction and fixation are advocated although the outcome data do not consistently support this practice.

O   **What peripheral nerve injuries are encountered in the TBI patient population?**

An estimated 34% of patients admitted to one rehabilitation unit were diagnosed with previously undetected peripheral nerve injuries. A large majority of the patients were involved in high speed collisions. Ulnar nerve entrapment in the cubital tunnel was found most frequently; brachial plexus injury and common peroneal compression neuropathies were slightly less frequent. Additional nerve injuries include radial, ulnar and median in the forearm, lumbosacral plexus, sciatic, obturator, femoral and pudendal. The diagnosis and management of peripheral nerve injuries is similar to non TBI patients.

O   **What are the distinctive features of heterotopic ossification in the TBI patient population?**

Heterotopic ossification is, perhaps, the most functionally devastating musculoskeletal complication of TBI, occurring in up to 76% of severely injured patients. Unlike spinal cord injury, the most common locations are relatively equally distributed between the hip, shoulder, and elbow. The incidence is higher in association with fractures and spasticity. Treatment can be challenging. While range of motion exercises is the hallmark in spinal cord injury, because of preserved sensation in the affected part, this may prove quite daunting in TBI. Etidronate, NSAIDs, and radiation treatments have been evaluated principally in association with disorders other than TBI. Ultimately, surgical intervention may be necessary, and is timed to coincide with a decrease in serum alkaline phosphatase and "cooling" of the bone scan.

○ **What is the incidence and risk factors for DVT/PE among TBI patients?**

Deep venous thrombosis (DVT) represents a significant source of morbidity and potential mortality for patients with head trauma. Pulmonary embolism from DVT is apparently increasing in importance as a cause of death among inpatients with traumatic brain injury. The National Institutes of Health Consensus Conference estimated the incidence of DVT after severe traumatic brain injury to be approximately 40%. More recent studies have reported a lower incidence of DVT. The incidence of fatal pulmonary embolus is approximately 1 %. The incidence of DVT may be significantly reduced using a specialized approach of prophylactic intervention in conjunction with routine monitoring in high risk patients. High risk factors include (1) advanced age; (2) severe injury; (3) prolonged immobilization; (4) number of transfusions; and (5) elevated thromboplastin time on admission.

○ **What diagnostic and treatment strategies are utilized for DVT/PE among TBI patients?**

The diagnostic modalities include D-Dimer, Doppler-ultrasound, IPG and venography for DVT; D-Dimer, V/Q scans and pulmonary arteriography for PE. The emphasis in prevention is on mechanical and pharmacological prophylaxis.

○ **What is the most common medical complication after TBI?**

Hypoxemia and respiratory failure.

○ **Is the TBI patient at an increased risk for pneumonia?**

Approximately 34% of traumatic brain injury survivors develop respiratory complications that predispose to pulmonary infections. Poor ventilation with secondary atelectasis is thought to be the most common pulmonary complication of trauma and a potential forerunner of pneumonia. Tissue necrosis secondary to lung trauma with subsequent formation of a pulmonary cavity also may predispose the patient to secondary lung infections. Endotracheal or tracheostomy tubes predispose patients to bacterial colonization and a greater risk of secondary lung infection. Finally, tubes used for enteral feeding increase the probability of aspiration pneumonia by as much as 25%.

○ **What are risk factors for pneumonia?**

In addition to the usual risk factors for pneumonia in ICU patients, such as impaired airway reflexes, aspiration, and more than 24 hours of ventilatory support, head injured patients having alcohol toxicity, ICP monitoring or receiving barbiturates or steroid therapy for intracranial hypertension are also at risk.

○ **What cardiac abnormalities can occur in association with TBI?**

Myocardial injury may occur in up to 50% of head injured patients, even in the absence of coronary artery disease. Although well described in adults, myocardial dysfunction can occur in children as well. The lesions produced are similar to those seen after acute myocardial infarction, pheochromocytoma, or catecholamine infusions. The myocardial injury may be induced by blunt trauma and ECG changes may be secondary to central vasomotor abnormalities.

○ **What is the incidence of UTI's in the TBI patient population?**

Urinary tract infections affect approximately 40% of traumatic brain injury survivors during the rehabilitation phase of recovery.

○ **What are the major motor deficits encountered in the TBI patient population?**

The major deficits encountered with TBI pertain to hyperactive deep tendon reflexes, increased tone, motor weakness, and decreased control and primitive patterns of movement dominating and impeding skilled functions.

○   **What are the consequences for spasticity and upper motor neuron (UMN) syndrome for the TBI patient?**

The consequences of spasticity and UMN syndrome to TBI is that in the acute setting, it may increase metabolic demand and potentially impact on intracranial pressure. It is also a significant etiology for early and severe contracture formation.

○   **What interventions are used to manage spasticity in the TBI patient?**

Range of motion and stretching exercises and modalities play a role, but the principal medical rehabilitative interventions are the use of casting, tone inhibiting orthotics, specific physical and occupational therapeutic techniques both to inhibit abnormal tone and movements and to facilitate normal skilled movement, and medications. Caution must be exercised with the medications since TBI patients may be more susceptible to cognitive ide effects; hence, dantrolene is the preferred systemic medication.

○   **What other selective motor control treatments are available?**

Increasingly, specific muscles and patterns are targeted, using clinical evaluation and motion analysis for treatment with either phenol neurolysis/motor point blocks or botulinum toxin injection. These injections are temporary and may be employed in the rehabilitation setting to specifically assist in the prevention of spastic contractures (e.g., heel cord). Another useful strategy in the acute setting is the use of intravenous dantrolene, which is subsequently given in enteral form; this can significantly reduce tone and posturing and the consequent risk for contracture formation.

○   **What options are available during the chronic phases of recovery?**

In the more chronic phase of recovery, consideration may be given to surgical intervention to control spasticity, such as placement of a baclofen pump, neurosurgical ablative interventions, or orthopedic tendon lengthening procedures.

○   **What other movement disorders are encountered in the TBI patient population?**

Other movement disorders after TBI include rigidity including a parkinsonian-like disorder, tremors, akathisia, ataxia, myoclonus (particularly palatal myoclonus), and dystonias including athetosis, ballism, and chorea. The relative incidence of these disorders after TBI is unknown; Pharmacologic intervention is with dopamine agonists and potentially anticholinergic agents, although the latter may impact on already dysfunctional memory. Essential tremors often respond to propranolol; clonazepam may also help but is variably tolerated, again because of sedation and cognitive side effects. Botulinum toxin has also been used with some success.

○   **What treatment options are available for the patient with ataxia, ballism and chorea and focal dystonias?**

Ataxia is an extremely difficult problem to treat with either therapies or medication; medications that have been tried include beta blockers, baclofen, clonazepam, and acetazolamine, thyrotropin releasing hormone, and serotonin agonists. Athetosis, ballism, and chorea are also difficult to treat; the armamentarium includes anticonvulsants as well as potential surgical intervention. Botulinum toxin is commonly utilized for other dystonias including torticollis.

○   **What factors determine the pattern of cognitive and behavioral impairments in brain injury?**

The residual pattern of cognitive and behavioral impairments after TBI depends on the initial severity of injury, the combination of diffuse and focal brain lesions, the occurrence of medical complications affecting brain function, the patient's pre injury level of functioning, and numerous other factors.

○   **What pattern is encountered in patients with diffuse brain injury?**

Patients who have suffered blunt head trauma and have diffuse injuries with no large focal lesions show a typical pattern of cognitive deficits in the areas of arousal, attention, resistance to distraction, speed of cognitive processing, memory, abstract reasoning, cognitive flexibility, initiation, and self awareness. Severe aphasia or visual/perceptual disorders are uncommon in such patients. Patients who have had penetrating head wounds may show aphasia, neglect, or other signs of focal brain lesions.

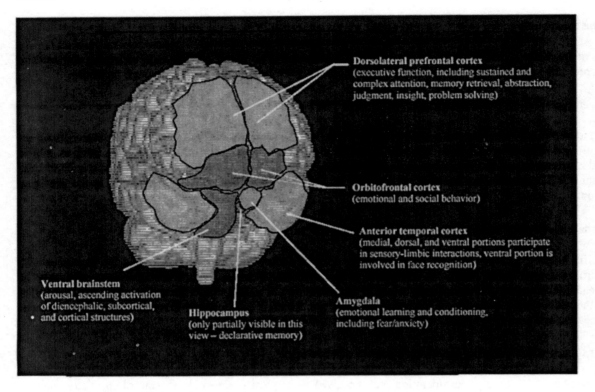

○   **Over what period of time does cognitive recovery occur in brain injury?**

Cognitive recovery continues for 6 to 18 months after moderate and severe TBI.

○   **What kind of behavioral and psychosocial adjustment issues occur subsequent to TBI?**

Behavioral deficits and psychosocial adjustment issues after TBI include depression, poor social awareness, impaired self awareness, and disorders of initiation, agitation, and aggressive behavior. These difficulties appear to be more severe in patients who have more damage to the frontal lobes, though similar problems are seen in patients with no evidence of focal frontal lesions. In contrast to the generally improving course for cognitive deficits during the period from 6 to 12 months after injury, behavioral and personality functioning, as judged by family member ratings, may decline over this period. These findings have led some clinicians to argue that the psychosocial consequences of TBI are more handicapping than the residual cognitive and physical deficits.

○   **How does coma compare with persistent vegetative state?**

True coma is a transient phenomenon, evolving into death or one of the following categories. The vegetative state is distinguished from coma by the presence of eye opening, intact basic autonomic functions, sleep-wake cycles, and possible responsiveness to optikokinetic stimulation. The additional adjective persistent has been the subject of considerable controversy. For nontraumatic brain injury, 3 months is the interval after which significant improvement is not expected; for trauma the interval is currently considered to be 12 months.

○   **What is the underlying pathology behind PVS?**

It is currently believed that the pathology responsible for PVS, severe bilateral hemispheric damage with relative preservation of the brain stem, occurs in the injury period. Whereas some individuals who present behaviorally as vegetative do have some reversible neuronal dysfunction, those destined to be in a PVS are not likely to respond to medical or therapeutic intervention to reverse or correct the process; it is, however, impossible to identify these individuals immediately at the time of injury.

O   **What is locked in syndrome?**

Locked-in syndrome is a specific condition secondary to injury in the pons or lower mesencephalon whereby eye opening is present, vertical eye movement is present volitionally, and there is severe quadriplegia, acutely involving bulbar musculature as well as the body (corporeal sensation may be preserved). Cognitive function may be intact.

O   **What is akinetic mutism?**

Akinetic mutism is a disorder classically related to a bilateral midline lesion in the area of the third ventricle (mesencephalon, cingulate gyrus, basal or mesial frontal lobe). Eye opening is present with spontaneous environmental tracking; patients follow commands inconsistently, initiation is profoundly impaired, and speech and movement are severely deficient.

O   **What is the minimally responsive patient?**

Finally, the minimally responsive patient resembles the patient with akinetic mutism but may have a slightly greater ability to follow commands, or their limitations can be explained by concomitant associated neurologic impairments (double hemiplegia). Latencies of response are often markedly prolonged, but a meaningful response is elicitable. These patients may respond to dopamine agonists.

O   **What are reversible causes of impaired arousal in the minimally responsive patient?**

Specific problem areas include the presence of hydrocephalus or other intracranial space occupying lesion, undiagnosed seizures, iatrogenic problems typically from medications, disorders related to other organ systems (hypoxemia), metabolic disorders (sodium balance), and fever.

O   **What rehabilitation strategies are utilized with the minimally responsive patient?**

Rehabilitation strategies include efforts to minimize complications from bed rest and are largely passive, but valuable. These include appropriate attention to skin care, bowel and bladder dysfunction, nutrition and the securing of an appropriate route for chronic enteral feeding, pulmonary care, eye care, and management of neuroendocrine and autonomic dysfunction. The patients should be taken out of bed and placed in an appropriate wheelchair, which in part can be used as a "truncal orthosis" and can facilitate some prophylaxis from the effects of chronic bed rest. Spasticity should be managed aggressively and provision of appropriate orthotics and appliances to prevent or reverse contractures is fundamental to the care of the minimally responsive patient. Heterotopic ossification should also be addressed as appropriate.

O   **What approaches are used to ameliorate the level of arousal in the minimally responsive state?**

One approach is pharmacologic, principally using dopamine agonists, including L-dopa, amantadine, or bromocriptine, or psychostimulants such as methylphenidate or modafinil. The psychostimulants may be particularly effective for patients who are not "minimally responsive" but who are at the higher end of the attention arousal spectrum. Antidepressants have also been used to facilitate improved arousal and initiation after TBI. Animal studies indicate that pharmacologic intervention can facilitate recovery after experimental brain injury and such intervention is rational, supporting the human data.

O   **What is the role of sensory stimulation?**

A second approach involves structured sensory stimulation. There are animal data to suggest that enriched therapeutic environments, when contrasted to impoverished environments, facilitate neurologic recovery after experimental brain injury. However, the few reports on the use of therapeutic sensory stimulation do not corroborate its effectiveness in humans who are minimally responsive, although the data are complicated by small sample size, poor outcome measures, and inconsistencies in technique and causes of cerebral injury. This is not tantamount to discrediting the use of structured sensory stimulation or assessment as a "diagnostic" modality to assess the effectiveness of pharmacologic and other interventions. Indeed, given the severity of neurologic impairments, latencies of responses, and the like, this kind of structured interdisciplinary assessment is likely to be more sensitive to subtle changes in the minimally responsive patient than is a quick bedside check.

O   **What family counseling should be considered for the minimally responsive patient?**

Family counseling regarding the prognosis for the minimally responsive or vegetative patient is important to the family's adjustment and eventual ability to care for the patient. It is usually beneficial for the family to play a role in providing the patient's care as early as possible. This involvement gives family members the sense that they can make some contribution to the patient's comfort and provides an opportunity for rehabilitation staff to train family members in skills that they will need to care for the patient after discharge.

O   **What medical complications may serve as the etiology for agitation?**

Possible medical complications such as electrolyte imbalance, seizure activity, sleep disturbance, discomfort due to musculoskeletal injury, or post traumatic hydrocephalus that may be exacerbating the patient's confusion should be searched for and treated.

O   **What is agitated behavior in the TBI patient?**

As TBI patients progress from the non responsive state to resolution of PTA, many exhibit agitated and restless behavior. This agitation is characterized by confusion, emotional lability, excessive motor activity, and in some cases, aggression. The period of agitation is generally relatively brief, with resolution coming as the patient becomes better oriented and regains some ability to retain new memories. Nonetheless, agitation is a concern as it may be a manifestation of an underlying medical problem and agitated patients are often noncompliant with therapy.

O   **What initial management is appropriate for agitation in the TBI patient?**

The initial management of agitation involves ensuring that the patient does not injure himself or herself or others. Such patients may pull out tubes; strike out at staff during dressing, bathing, or therapy activities; or attempt to elope. If possible, physical restraints should be avoided as these frustrate the patient and result in increased agitation. Preferred management techniques include reducing stimulation and increasing the structure and familiarity of the patient's environment. Agitation will generally decrease if the patient is in a quiet room and primarily interacts with staff with whom he or she is familiar. Only one person should address the patient at a time and the tone of voice should be calm. Some patients respond to familiar music or pictures of family members. Craig beds or net beds that allow the patient to move but guard against self injury may be helpful.

O   **What counseling should be given to families of head injured patients?**

Family members should be instructed regarding appropriate agitation management so that they do not inadvertently overstimulate the patient. Counseling regarding the recovering course of agitation is reassuring to family members, as the patient's physical and verbal outbursts can be quite upsetting. Sedating medicines such as neuroleptics and benzodiazepines may be necessary for the few patients who would otherwise injure themselves or others, but these should be avoided if at all possible as they will increase confusion and may have other adverse effects.

O   **What are the most common correctible medical etiologies of agitation in the TBI patient?**

While epilepsy or space occupying lesions are possible problems, particular attention should be paid to hypoxemia, fever, and iatrogenic causes from medication. The environment of most hospitals, especially the intensive care unit, is not typically conducive to orientation of confused and fearful individuals. Sleep disturbances should also be addressed; trazodone may be an effective agent for inducing sleep and nortriptyline for sustaining sleep. Ambien® (zolpidem tartrate) or Sonata®/Zaleplon may also be effective without the "hangover" associated with some benzodiazepine derivatives, although rebound insomnia is still possible. Sources of pain should be evaluated and treated while guarding against impediments to cognition.

O   **Summarize pharmacotherapy for mood, cognitive and behavioral disorders in TBI**

Drug	Depression	Affective Lability and/or Irritability	Mania	Psychosis	Agitation or Aggression	Anxiety	Apathy	Cognition	Risk of Adverse Events
Nortriptyline	++	+	-					-	+
Desipramine	++	+	-					-	+
Amitriptyline	+		-		+++				+++

Protriptyline	+	+	-				++	-	+
Fluoxetine	+++	+++	-		++				++
Sertraline	+++	+++	-		++				+
Paroxetine	++	+++	-		++				+
Lithium		+	+		++			-	+++
Carbamazepine		+	++		+++			--	++
Valproate		++	+++		+++				+
Benzodiazepines						+			+++
Buspirone	+	++			+	+			+
Typical Antipsychotics				++	+			--	+++
Atypical Antipsychotics				+++	+			-	+
Methylphenidate	++	++			++		++	++	
Dextroamphetamine	++						++	++	
Amantadine	+	++			++		+	+	
Bromocriptine			-	-			++	+	+
L-dopa/carbidopa			-	-			+	+	+
Beta-blockers	--				+++		-	-	-
Donepezil								+	+

O **Summarize the dosing of these drugs in the TBI patient**

Medication	Adult Dose Range (mg/day)	*Typical Dosing Schedule*
Nortriptyline	25 – 150	Q hs
Desipramine	25 – 300	Q hs
Amitriptyline	25 – 150	Q hs
Protriptyline	15 – 60	Q AM
Fluoxetine	10 – 40	Q AM or Q hs depending on medication-related activation or sedation
Sertraline	25 – 200	Q AM or Q hs depending on medication-related activation or sedation
Paroxetine	5 – 50	Q AM or Q hs depending on medication-related activation or sedation
Lithium	150 – 1500	QD to TID
Carbamazepine	200 – 1000	QD to TID
Valproate	125 – 1500	QD to TID
Buspirone	15 – 90	TID to QID
Haloperidol	0.5 – 5	QD
Risperidone	0.5 – 4	QD
Olanzapine	2.5 – 10	QD
Methylphenidate	5 – 60	BID to TID
Dextroamphetamine	5 – 60	BID to TID
Amantadine	50 – 400	QD to BID
Bromocriptine	2.5 – 20	TID

L-dopa/carbidopa	10/100 – 25/250	BID to QID
Propranolol	80 – 400	BID to QID
Donepezil	5 – 10	QD

○ **What medications may be helpful for hyperphagia?**

Aggressive hyperphagia may be managed with SSRIs or naltrexone.

○ **What medication may be warranted for aggressive sexual behavior?**

Rarely, aggression with a sexual resonance may require medroxyprogesterone acetate (Depo-Provera) or the equivalent of chemical castration.

○ **What are some of the common areas of cognitive impairment after TBI?**

COMMON AREAS OF COGNITIVE IMPAIRMENT AFTER TRAUMATIC BRAIN INJURY

Attention
  Alertness Mental processing (slow)
  Selective attention during distraction
  Divided attention
  Sustained attention
  Awareness of disability and impairment
Perception
  Visual
  Auditory
  Visuospatial
Memory
  Retrograde, anterograde Immediate, delayed, cued, and recognition recall
  Visual and verbal learning
Executive Functions
  Planning, Initiation
  Maintaining goal or intention
  Conceptual reasoning
  Hypothesis testing and shifting response
  Self-appraisal
  Self-regulation
Intelligence
  Verbal expression
  Performance
  Problem solving
  Abstract reasoning
Language
  Speech (aphasia; vague, tangential,
  confabulatory speech; verbose or
  impoverished speech)
  Affective expression

○ **What are the practical cognitive assessment instruments that are often selected in the TBI patient population?**

Efforts have been made to identify the least number of tests done in the acute period that can provide the greatest amount of relevant, prognostic information for 3 and 6 month outcomes. Four tests have been identified: Controlled Oral Word Association, Grooved Pegboard, Trail making Part B, and the Rey-Osterrieth Complex Figure Delayed Recall.

○ **What have serial neuropsychological tests revealed about cognitive recovery?**

Serial neuropsychological test data have found that information processing speed, memory skills, and simultaneous processing abilities are related to the level of functional outcome. Investigators report that impairment in memory and slowness of information processing are common 1 year after severe TBI, but language and visuospatial ability often recover to a normal range. Five years after injury 50% of severe, 14.3% of moderate, and 3.1% of mild injuries still demonstrate cognitive impairments (slow speech or reaction time) and attention and comprehension problems.

O   **What have cognitive screening studies revealed about cognition in the TBI patient population?**

Cognitive screening finds that memory, followed by attention and reasoning abilities are the areas most frequently affected in the mild TBI patient. Patients with a GCS score of 13 or 14 had more problems identified on the screening tests when compared to the patients with a GCS score of 15. Cognitive screening provides data that can assist in the early planning of appropriate rehabilitation programs, and subsequent follow up studies can contribute further information to help with predicting functional recovery and long term prognosis.

O   **What are the results of community reintegration programs in the TBI patient population?**

A greater emphasis is being placed on community re-entry and vocational rehabilitation after TBI, with specialized postacute rehabilitation programs being developed to help patients achieve their maximum potential. These programs have reported that 56% of the patients gain independence in work, school, or homemaking compared to 43% of the patients that were not participating in a specialized re-entry program. Formalized case management systems have been suggested as a way to facilitate the start of vocational and rehabilitation services after a brain injury. Factors that can help predict a return to work or school include the patient's age, verbal intellectual power, information processing speed, performance IQ, emotional disturbances, and the presence of vocational services.

O   **What is the rationale behind cognitive remediation?**

Cognitive remediation has many nuances but it usually includes a cognitive process specific approach that articulates subroutines of a mental process. Therapists aim to ameliorate impairments in problem solving, they often use feedback, and they consider that the therapeutic methods used may reorganize the function of the patient's cognitive neural networks. The approach targets distinct, if theoretic, components of separable cognitive processes. Repetition of a task at one level of difficulty or related to one sub component of the cognitive process continues until the goal is reached. Then the task is enlarged within its presumed hierarchic organization. For example, once two dimensional constructions are copied, three dimensional drawings may be undertaken. Once auditory attention is learned, auditory encoding is practiced. Gains are expected to generalize to related tasks and to transfer into real world functioning.

O   **Compare retrograde vs. anterograde amnesia:**

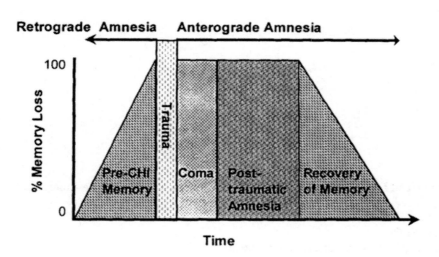

O   **Describe aids and strategies to compensate for memory impairment?**

AIDS AND STRATEGIES FOR COPING WITH MEMORY IMPAIRMENT

External
Reminders by others
Tape recorder
Notes written on hand
Time reminders
Alarm clock/phone call
Personal organizer/ diary; calendar/wall planner
Orientation board
Place reminders
Labels; codes: colors, symbols Person reminders
Name tags
Clothes that offer a cue Organizers
Lists; items grouped for use
Electronic or written calendar organizer
Posted numbered series of reminders Radio pagers

Internal
Mental retracing of events; rehearsal
Visual imagery
Alphabet searching; first-letter mnemonics
Associations with items already recalled
Chunking or grouping of items

O **What are common changes in behavior and personality after TBI?**

COMMON CHANGES IN BEHAVIOR AND PERSONALITY AFTER TRAUMATIC BRAIN INJURY

Disinhibition
Impulsiveness
Aggressiveness
Irritability
Lability
Euphoria
Paranoia
Lack of self-criticism and insight
Irresponsibility, childishness
Egocentricity, selfishness
Sexual deviation, inappropriateness
Substance abuse
Self abuse
Poor personal habits
Indecision
Lack of initiation
Blunted emotional responses
Poor self worth
Apathy, inertia
Indifference
Passive dependency

O **How is mild TBI defined by the Head Injury Interdisciplinary Special Interest Group of the American Congress of Rehabilitation Medicine?**

1. Any period of loss of consciousness (LOC),
2. Any loss of memory for events immediately before or after the accident,
3. Any alteration in mental state at the time of the accident,
4. Focal neurologic deficits, which may or may not be transient."

○ **What other criteria for defining mild TBI are considered?**

1. GCS score greater than 12
2. No abnormalities on CT scan
3. No operative lesions
4. Length of hospital stay less than 48 hours

○ **What are the DSM-IV criteria for mild TBI?**

1. a period of unconsciousness lasting more than 5 minutes, and
2. a period of post traumatic amnesia lasting more than 12 hours subsequent to the closed head injury, and
3. a new onset of seizures or marked worsening of pre-existing seizure disorder that occurs within the first six months.

○ **What additional criteria are considered in the DSM IV criteria?**

In addition a further criterion is that, on neuropsychological testing, difficulties in attention and memory must be demonstrated. The definition also includes that three or more symptoms persist for at least three months, and that these include:

1. becoming easily fatigued,
2. disordered sleep,
3. headache,
4. vertigo or dizziness,
5. irritability or aggression on little or no provocation,
6. anxiety,
7. depression or affective lability,
8. changes in personality (e.g., social or sexual inappropriateness),
9. apathy or lack of spontaneity.

○ **What proportion of TBI patients present with mild neurological injury?**

Approximately 80% of patients who sustain TBIs have had mild TBI as judged by GCS criteria, and of TBI patients who survive, 86% had mild injuries. The majority of these patients make excellent neurobehavioral recovery, but some have persistent and disabling symptoms.

○ **What is the pathogenesis of mild TBI?**

Pathologically, the lesion in mild TBI patients may show little to no structural discontinuity; although in animal studies axonal disruption may be evident, especially in the hippocampus. The injury is likely to be largely due to the pathologic neurochemical cascade, but is insufficient to produce widespread neuronal dysfunction or the axonal disruption that characterizes more severe cerebral pathology.

○ **How does the site of neuropathology correlate with the clinical syndrome in mild TBI?**

The pathology is centripetally distributed however, and may explain some of the characteristic post concussive symptomatology: Surface lesions result in amnesia, impairments to short term memory or attention, or other transient focal neurologic dysfunction; medullary injuries can result in nausea, vomiting, or respiratory or cardiac irregularities (all transient in the immediate post injury period); pontine and mesencephalic involvement may produce the classic concussion with associated brief loss of consciousness.

○ **What are the most common cognitive complaints subsequent to mild TBI?**

The most common cognitive complaints after mild TBI are impaired memory, increased distractibility, and slowed speed of cognitive processing. These areas of cognitive function can be assessed quickly with a battery of tests. These tests are outlined in the section on behavioral medicine section. In patients in whom malingering is a suspected, additional test that has been shown to be sensitive to malingering and should be added to the battery. Examples of such tests include the

Seashore rhythm test, the recognition memory test, the digit span test, the Knox cube test, Portland digit recognition test, the test of memory malingering , the Rey 15 item visual memory test.

○   **What other neurobehavioral symptoms are reported?**

Emotional and behavioral symptoms reported after mild TBI include depression, anxiety, and irritability. Personality inventories such as the Minnesota Multiphasic Personality Inventory-2 and behavioral rating scales such as the Neurobehavioral Rating Scale and the Portland Adaptability Index are useful in evaluating these complaints.

○   **To what degree does litigation influence outcome in brain injury?**

Studies are divided in their findings with regard to whether concurrent litigation influences prognosis and treatment response.

○   **What medical forensic evidence is used to help establish organicity of the mild TBI?**

Careful review of patient information including initial medical records (GCS, CT or MRI findings, length of PTA, etc.), premorbid medical history (previous head injury or other neurologic illness or injury, alcohol and substance abuse, etc.), premorbid functioning (educational level, history of developmental or learning disability, employment history, psychiatric history, etc.), post morbid medical status (medications, possible seizures or other complications, etc.), and post morbid functional status (course of cognitive recovery, neuropsychological test findings, emotional and behavioral problems, interview with significant other, etc.) will generally reveal whether the patient's symptoms are consistent with the expected course of recovery.

○   **What are the sequelae of post concussive disorder?**

Cranial nerve symptoms and signs

Dizziness
   Vertigo
   Tinnitus
   Hearing loss
   Blurred vision
   Diplopia
   Convergence insufficiency
   Light and noise sensitivity
   Diminished taste and smell

Cognitive impairment

Memory dysfunction
   Impaired concentration and attention
   Slowing of reaction time
   Slowing of information processing speed

Rare sequelae

Subdural and epidural hematomas
Cerebral venous thrombosis
Second impact syndrome
Seizures
Nonepileptic post-traumatic seizures
Transient global amnesia
Tremor
Dystonia

Psychological and somatic complaints

Irritability
   Anxiety
   Depression
   Personality change
   Post-traumatic stress disorder
   Fatigue
   Sleep disturbance
   Decreased libido
   Decreased appetite
   Initial nausea/vomiting

○   **What is the differential for post traumatic headache?**

Muscle contraction or tension type
Cranial myofascial injury
Secondary to neck injury (cervicogenic)
Myofascial injury
Intervertebral discs
Cervical spondylosis
C2-3 facet joint (third occipital headache)

Secondary to temporomandibular joint injury
Greater and lesser occipital neuralgia
Migraine with and without aura
Footballer's migraine
Medication rebound
Cluster
Supraorbital and infraorbital neuralgia
Due to scalp lacerations or local trauma
Dysautonomic cephalgia
Orgasmic cephalgia
Carotid or vertebral artery dissection
Subdural or epidural hematomas
Hemorrhagic cortical contusions
Mixed

O **What neurodiagnostic testing may be utilized in post concussive disorders?**

Neurodiagnostic Testing for Specific Post-concussive Sequelae

Posttraumatic Sequelae	Neurodiagnostic Procedure
Attentional deficits	Cognitive evoked potentials
Balance dysfunction	Posturographic assessment
Cerebral perfusion changes	Single-photon emission computerized tomography (SPECT)*
Cerebral metabolic changes	Positron emission tomography (PET)*
Electroencephalographic abnormalities	Sleep-deprived electroencephalography (EEG), 24-hour Holter EEG, video EEG, brain electrical activity mapping
(BEAM/QuantEEG)	magnetoencephalography (MEG)*
Erectile dysfunction	Nocturnal penile tumescence monitoring
Eye movement disorders	Electrooculography, rotary chair
Focal and/or diffuse brain dysfunction	Magnetic source imaging (MSI)
Neuralgic scalp pain, including cervical roots	Diagnostic/therapeutic local anesthetic block
Olfactory and gustatory dysfunction	Chemosensory evaluation for smell and taste
Perilymphatic fistula	Platform fistula test* on posturography, surgical exploration
Regional blood flow alterations	Transcranial color duplex/Doppler JCD)
Sensorineural and conductive hearing loss	Audiologic evaluation, brainstem auditory evoked responses (BAERs), electrocochleography
Sleep disturbance	Polysomnography with median sleep latency test
Structural parenchymal changes	Magnetic resonance imaging
Vascular injury	Magnetic resonance angiography (MRA), angiography
Vestibular dysfunction	Electronystagmography with calorics, BAERs

O **What pharmacological interventions are appropriate for common post traumatic sequelae?**

Common Posttraumatic Sequelae	Pharmacologic Intervention
Anxiety	Serotonergic agonists: buspirone, sertraline, paroxetine, trazodone
Basilar artery migraine (BAM)	Antimigraine regimens psychotropic anticonvulsants catecholaminergic
Cognitive dysfunction	agonists, cholinergic agonists and/or precursors, neuropeptides,* vasoactive agents*
Depression	Tricyclic antidepressants (TCA's), selective serotonin reuptake inhibitors (SSRIs), venlafaxine, monoamine oxidase inhibitors (MAOIs), lithium carbonate, carbamazepine
Emotional lability and/or	
Irritability trazodone	SSRIs, psychotropic anticonvulsants, TCA's, lithium carbonate,
Fatigue	Catecholaminergic agonists: Methylphenidate

	Amantadine
	Dextroamphetamine
	Caffeine
Libidinal alteration:	
Decreased	Noradrenergic agonists, hormone replacement if low to borderline low
Increased	SSRIs, trazodone, hormones-cyproterone or medroxyprogesterone acetate
Myofascial pain/dysfunction	NSAIDs, TCA's, SSRIs, mild muscle relaxants, capsaicin
Neuralgic and neuritic pain	Capsaicin, TCA's, SSRIs (?), carbamazepine and other antiepileptic drugs, NSAIDs, local anesthetic blockade
Posttraumatic stress disorder	Antidepressant medications, psychotropic anticonvulsants, propranolol, clonidine, MAOls, lithium, benzodiazepines
Sleep initiation problems	Serotonergic agonists-trazodone, doxepin, and amitriptyline
Sleep maintenance problems	Catecholaminergic agonists-nortriptyline
Tinnitus	Gingko biloba * tocainide,* anti-migraine medications*
Vascular headache	Antimigraine regimens:
	Symptomatic
	Abortive
	Prophylactic
	Atypical agents: valproic acid

MULTIPLE SCLEROSIS (MS)

O   **What is the incidence of multiple sclerosis?**

MS appears between the ages of 10 and 50, the average age being about 30 at the time of diagnosis. Symptoms usually begin during young adulthood, with the peak onset at age 24. The risk of MS after the age of 60 is minimal. The incidence of MS is higher for women than for men. A longitudinal and comprehensive review of cases from Olmsted County in Rochester, Minnesota, found that over an 80 year period, the age adjusted incidence rates were 3.0 and 7.0 per 100,000 population for males and females, respectively. It affects millions worldwide and approximately 250,000 to 350,000 in the United States alone

O   **What is the geographic predilection of MS?**

MS is rare in tropical areas, and the prevalence increases proportional to the distance from the equator, excluding polar regions. The prevalence is less than 5 cases per 100,000 in tropical areas; in high prevalence areas it can be higher than 30 per 100,000, reaching up to 100/100,000 in selected areas.

O   **What evidence is there for environmental factors in MS?**

Perhaps the most incriminating evidence for the role of environmental factors in the development of MS is the changing risk with migration and the occurrence of MS clusters and epidemics. Immigrant populations tend to acquire the MS risk inherent to their new place of residence.

O   **Is there a genetic risk factor for MS?**

The only definitive genetic association in MS is with the serologically defined human leukocyte antigen (HLA) DR15, DQ6. This is one of the DR2 haplotypes. This gene is found in many Northern Europeans and is also found in many people with MS. The presence of this gene does not guarantee the development of MS.

○ **Is there a viral etiology for MS?**

It is possible that MS is triggered by a viral infection that initiates an immune response. T lymphocyte clones from MS patients that are specific for a myelin basic protein (MBP) peptide also recognize several common viruses. Viruses may cause demyelination directly, such as in postinfectious encephalomyelitis. However, specific viruses have not been consistently found in people with MS.

○ **How may the diagnosis of multiple sclerosis be described?**

MS for diagnostic purposes may be defined as involving objective neurologic deficits in two or more areas, primarily reflecting white matter involvement. These deficits should occur at two or more points in time lasting longer than 24 hours and separated by more than 1 month, or in a slow progression of more than 6 months' duration. MS occurs between the ages of 10 and 50 years with a pattern of signs and symptoms that should not be better attributable to an alternative diagnosis.

○ **What are the clinical features more suggestive of multiple sclerosis?**

Clinical Features Suggestive of MS	Clinical Features Not Suggestive of MS *
Onset between ages 15 and 50	Onset before age 10 or after 55
Relapsing-remitting course	Continued progression from onset without relapses
Optic neuritis	
Lhermitte's sign	Early dementia
Partial transverse myelitis	Seizures
Internuclear ophthalmoplegia	Aphasia
Sensory useless hand	Agnosia
Acute urinary retention (especially in young men)	Apraxia
	Homonymous or bitemporal hemianopia
Paroxysmal symptoms	
Diurnal fatigue pattern	Encephalopathy
Worsening symptoms with heat or exercise	Extrapyramidal symptoms
	Uveitis
	Peripheral neuropathy

*Whereas features listed in the right column may be seen in MS, they are atypical and should prompt consideration of alternate explanations.

○ **What is the differential diagnosis of MS?**

Differential Diagnosis of Multiple Sclerosis	
Other inflammatory demyelinating CNS conditions	Lymphoma
Acute disseminated encephalomyelitis	Paraneoplastic syndromes
Neuromyelitis optica	Metabolic disorders
Systemic or organ-specific inflammatory diseases	Vitamin B_{12} deficiency
Systemic lupus erythematosus	Vitamin E deficiency
Sjögren's syndrome	Central (or extra) pontine myelinolysis
Behçet's disease	Leukodystrophies (especially adrenomyeloneuropathy)

Inflammatory bowel disease	Leber's hereditary optic neuropathy
Vasculitis	Structural lesions
Periarteritis nodosa	Spinal cord compression
Primary CNS angiitis	Chiari malformation
Granulomatous diseases	Syringomyelia/syringobulbia
Sarcoidosis	Foramen magnum lesions
Wegener's granulomatosis	Spinal arteriovenous malformation/dural fistula
Infectious disorders	Degenerative diseases
Lyme neuroborreliosis	Lymphoma
Syphilis	Hereditary spastic paraparesis
HTLV-1 associated myelopathy	Spinocerebellar degeneration
Viral myelitis (HSV, VZV)	Olivopontocerebellar atrophy
Progressive multifocal leukoencephalitis	Psychiatric disorders
Subacute sclerosing panencephalitis	Conversion reactions
Cerebrovascular disorders	Malingering
Multiple emboli	Hereditary spastic paraparesis
Hypercoagulable states	Spinocerebellar degeneration
Neoplasms	Metastasis

HTLV-1, Human T-cell lymphotropic virus type 1; HSV, herpes simplex virus; VZV, varicella-zoster virus; CNS, central nervous system.

○ **What problems do MS patients typically report?**

Frequent problems included fatigue, difficulty with balance, weakness, paresthesias, bladder dysfunction, and spasticity, in decreasing order of frequency, although paresthesias were listed less frequently as a problem in terms of impact on ADLs.

○ **What findings are common after the diagnosis of MS is made later in the course of the disease?**

Predominant findings were abnormal sensation and spastic paresis, with the percentage of patients having these findings roughly doubling over the 5 years, but more dramatic progression was seen for brain stem and cerebellar findings with ataxia, with the percentage of patients having these increasing approximately threefold and fourfold. Once thought uncommon, cognitive disorders are now known to be present in 40 to 70 percent of MS patients.

○ **What are the new multiple sclerosis diagnostic criteria?**

New multiple sclerosis diagnostic criteria		
Clinical (attacks)	**Objective Lesions**	**Additional Data Needed for MS Diagnosis**
Two or more attacks	Two or more	None
Two or more attacks	One	Dissemination in space, by MR imaging or positive CSF, and two or more MR imaging lesions consistent with MS or further clinical attacks implicating different sites
One attack	Two or more	Dissemination in time, by MR imaging or second clinical attack
One attack (monosymptomatic presentation)	One	Dissemination in space, by MR imaging or positive CSF, and two or more MR imaging lesions consistent with MS and dissemination in time, by MR imaging or second clinical attack
Neurologic progression from onset,	One	Positive CSF and dissemination in space, by

New multiple sclerosis diagnostic criteria		
Clinical (attacks)	**Objective Lesions**	**Additional Data Needed for MS Diagnosis**
suggestive of MS		
		1) Nine or more T2 brain lesions or
		2) Two or more cord lesions or
		3) Four to eight brain lesions plus one cord lesion or
		4) Abnormal VEP with four to eight brain lesions, or
		5) Abnormal VEP with less than four brain lesions and one spinal cord lesion
		And dissemination in time, by MR imaging or continued progression for one year

CSF = cerebrospinal fluid; MS = multiple sclerosis; VEP = visual evoked potential.
Adapted from McDonald, et al: Recommended diagnostic criteria for multiple sclerosis: Guidelines from the International Panel on the Diagnosis of Multiple Sclerosis.

○ **What are the four categories of MS?**

The temporal course of MS can be described by one of four categories: relapsing-remitting (RR), secondary progressive (SP), primary progressive (PP), and progressive relapsing (PR).

○ **What is relapsing remitting MS (RRMS) ?**

Patients who improve after acute attacks have relapsing remitting MS (RRMS). However, during the natural course of RRMS, approximately 75-85% of patients enter a stage referred to as secondary progressive MS (SPMS). Patients who have RRMS but accumulate disability between and during attacks can be defined as having relapsing progressive disease (RPMS), a term not widely used by neurologists.

○ **What is primary progressive MS (PPMS) ?**

Patients with primary progressive MS (PPMS) tend to accumulate disability without interruption (i.e., without remissions). Some of these patients first present with weakness of only one limb, which gradually progresses to involve other limbs and culminates in total paralysis. Patients with PPMS typically respond poorly to the current therapeutic options for MS, accumulate disability faster than other patients, and tend to have more weakness of the legs as well as incontinence (a reflection of greater spinal cord involvement). Patients with PPMS tend to have more involvement of the spinal cord by demyelinating plaques. These cases must be differentiated from SPMS.

○ **What is Progressive-relapsing (PR) MS?**

It is a continuous progressive form of MS from onset, in which there are clearly defined subsequent superimposed relapses with or without some recovery between the relapses.

○ **What is the prognosis of MS?**

Prognostic factors in MS	
Favorable Prognostic Factors	**Unfavorable Prognostic Factors**
Female gender	Male gender
Young age at onset	Old age at onset
Few symptoms at onset	Multiple symptoms at onset
Optic neuritis or sensory deficits at onset	Motor or cerebellar/brain stem symptoms at onset

Prognostic factors in MS	
Favorable Prognostic Factors	**Unfavorable Prognostic Factors**
Long intervals between the initial attacks	Short interval between the initial and the second attack
Low relapse rate **in** early years	High relapse rate **in** early years
Complete recovery after the initial attacks	Incomplete remission after the first relapses
No disability **in** early years	Early disability, clinical progressive course
Few lesions on MR imaging of the brain	High lesion load detected by early MR imaging of the brain

O   **What functional instruments are used in MS?**

The most widely accepted clinical rating scale is the 10 point Kurtzke Expanded Disability Status Scale (EDSS), developed originally in 1955 as the Disability Status Scale (DSS). These criteria have been revised over the years and remain the standard scale by which patients may be compared. The scale ranges from 0-10 in 0.5 increments. The scores from grades 0-4 are derived from Functional System (FS) scales that evaluate dysfunction in 8 neurologic systems, including pyramidal, cerebellar, brainstem, sensory, bladder and bowel, vision, cerebral, and "other."

O   **What are the advantages of the Expanded Disability Status Scale (EDSS)?**

Advantages of this scale are that it is widely used clinically, is easy to administer, and requires no special equipment.

O   **What are limitations of the EDSS?**

Limitations of the EDSS are that it (1) is heavily dependent on mobility; (2) is somewhat subjective in certain areas (eg, bowel and bladder function); (3) is insensitive to small changes; and (4) does not present an accurate picture of the patient's cognitive abilities and functional abilities in performing activities of daily living (ADL).

O   **What is the basic pathology in MS?**

Multiple sclerosis (MS) is an inflammatory, demyelinating disease of the central nervous system (CNS). MS lesions, characterized by perivascular infiltration of monocytes and lymphocytes, appear as indurated areas in pathologic specimens; hence, the term "sclerosis in plaques."

O   **What is the role of immune cells in the pathogenesis of MS?**

Lymphocytes, macrophages, and plasma cells access the CNS, and proinflammatory cytokines are released. In MS, activated T cells may adhere to the endothelial wall of the BBB, cross the BBB, and invade the CNS. T cells are activated by cytokines secreted by macrophages and other cells. Proinflammatory cytokines may further contribute to a leaky BBB. Lymphocytes and macrophages are recruited, and myelin break down ensues. This T cell–mediated immune response destroys the oligodendrocytes. Additionally, plasma cells (B cells) are activated to produce antibodies against oligodendrocytes and myelin.

O   **What is the distinction of acute versus chronic plaques?**

A plaque is formed as myelin is destroyed. Active plaques are edematous, with leakage of plasma proteins from the capillary beds around the plaques. These lesions are infiltrated by inflammatory cells such as lymphocytes and macrophages. An old plaque is formed as oligodendrocytes become damaged and lost, and astrocytes proliferate. Loss of oligodendrocytes decreases the chance of re myelination. Multiple areas of gliosis form, which explains how MS was named.

O   **Where are plaques commonly seen in the CNS of MS patients?**

The plaques of MS are often seen around the ventricles, optic tracts, and cerebellum. Other areas may include the basal ganglia, the gray matter, and the white matter of any lobe of the brain. The cervical region of the spinal cord is more affected than the thoracic area. The plaques and demyelination can cause disruption of nerve conduction.

○ **What is the role of myelin and what are the consequences of injury to it in MS?**

Myelin, composed of MBP and lipids, facilitates signal transmission in the axons by increasing the speed of conduction and allowing for saltatory conduction. Compromise of myelin causes decreased conduction velocity, conduction block, and the symptoms of MS. Sodium and potassium channels are important to the pathophysiology of demyelinated axons: "Unmasked" potassium channels interfere with conduction in demyelinated axons. This is the basis of clinical trials using potassium channel blockers such as 4-aminopyridine and 3, 4 diaminopyridine. Factors that further decrease conduction velocity, such as elevated temperature, may make symptoms worse.

○ **What role do VEPs play in the diagnosis of MS?**

Visual evoked potentials (VEPs), obtained by stimulation with a checkerboard pattern or strobe, may be abnormal in 75% of patients with definite MS. VEPs can help establish abnormalities in the optic nerve and tract, and therefore are helpful diagnostically. While such abnormalities are common in MS, they also occur in other diseases such as compressive lesions of the visual pathways and spinocerebellar degeneration.

○ **What are the most common presenting signs and symptoms in MS?**

Disturbances of gait and vision and sensory symptoms are the most common symptoms at the time of initial presentation. The most common presenting signs in MS include abnormal reflexes, Babinski sign, ataxia, and decreased vibration sense.

○ **What other evoked potential studies may be used in elucidating the diagnosis of MS?**

Brain stem auditory evoked potentials (BAEPs) assess the pons and midbrain using auditory stimulation, and may be very effective in identifying subclinical lesions.

○ **What is the preferred imaging technique to support a diagnosis of MS?**

MRI is currently the preferred imaging technique to support the diagnosis of MS, and the findings are positive in 70% to 95% of patients with MS. MRI is more sensitive than CT in the diagnosis of MS, and it may visualize subclinical lesions.

○ **Where are plaques commonly imaged in MRI?**

Plaques are found characteristically in the periventricular location, but may also be commonly found in other areas of the white matter. Gadolinium enhanced MRI may identify active disease and may distinguish new versus old lesions by identifying areas of BBB breakdown.

○ **What effect does corticosteroid therapy have on MS?**

The recovery from acute exacerbations of MS is hastened, but there does not appear to be any prevention of further attacks or progression of disease. Steroids also may be used to treat optic neuritis. Intravenous steroids such as methylprednisolone may decrease the rate of development of subsequently diagnosed MS in patients with optic neuritis.

○ **What is glatiramer acetate?**

This chain of four amino acids is immunologically cross reactive with MBP. It appears to inhibit T-cell responses to MBP. There are several theories on how glatiramer acetate may work, such as desensitization, suppressor T-cell production, and competition for MHC class II binding sites for MBP. Glatiramer acetate has been approved by the Food and Drug Administration (FDA) for use in treating R-R MS. It is given by subcutaneous injection each day. It could decrease the relapse rate of R-R MS by 32% after 2 years. Side effects include injection site reactions and postinjection reactions of flushing and chest tightness. The latter is self limited and transient, with no long term consequences reported.

○ **What is Betaseron?**

Interferon beta-1b (Betaseron), the first drug to be approved by the FDA, altered the course of the disease in a controlled clinical trial. Betaseron is made using recombinant technology in *Escherichia coli* bacteria and has an amino acid sequence that differs from the natural interferon by only one amino acid. It is typically given subcutaneously every other day. The precise mechanism of action is unclear. It may decrease T-cell production; block interferon-g secretion; block the action of interferon-g decrease tumor necrosis factor, which has been shown to injure oligodendrocytes; and restore suppressor T-cell function.

○   **What clinical efficacy has Betaseron shown in MS?**

Interferon beta-1b reduced the exacerbation rate in MS patients by 35% compared with placebo. MRI showed a significant reduction in disease activity in treated patients. The most common adverse effects include flu-like symptoms and injection reactions. Antibodies may develop with continued use. In the one third of patients estimated to develop antibodies after 1 year of treatment, the benefits of interferon beta may be lost.

○   **What is Avonex?**

Interferon beta-1a (Avonex) is also made by recombinant technology, is produced in mammalian cells, and has the same amino acid sequence and glycosylation that is found in naturally occurring interferon-b. It is administered intramuscularly once weekly, and has been approved by the FDA for relapsing forms of MS.

○   **What efficacy has Avonex demonstrated in MS?**

Clinical trials demonstrated a 32% reduction in exacerbations, a decrease in the number and volume of MRI lesions, and an increase in time to sustained worsening of disability in that taking interferon beta-1a. The risk of progression of disability was reduced by 37% over 2 years. Side effects include flu-like symptoms such as fever, chills, muscle aches, and fatigue. Antibodies to interferon beta-1a may develop.

○   **What is the efficacy of rehabilitation for patients with MS related disability?**

Studies of patients with progressive MS, nonambulatory (higher EDSS) and ambulatory patients (EDSS 3.0-6.5), showed a positive effect of a rehabilitation program on disability and negligible effect on impairment. Ambulatory patients with MS benefited from aerobic exercises. They had decreased fatigue and increased quality of life. The rehabilitation interdisciplinary assessment, which identifies areas of potential functional improvement, is important in setting short term and long term goals and measurement of outcomes.

○   **What acute and chronic neuropathic pain disorders occur in patients with MS?**

The acute pain disorders typically involve paroxysmal symptoms, with half of patients diagnosed as trigeminal neuralgia. These symptoms respond best to treatment with anticonvulsant medications. Baclofen may also be useful as an alternative. Chronic symptoms are most often dysesthesias involving the extremities or back. Dysesthesias respond to treatment with tricyclic medications, with improvement noted by more than 50% of patients.

○   **What pattern of dysfunction is most responsible for MS disability?**

Motor dysfunction, including weakness and ataxia, is the major cause of disability in MS.

○   **What motor dysfunction characterizes MS patients?**

Movement disorders such as Parkinsonism, dystonia, and myoclonus are relatively infrequent compared to ataxia and tremor.

○   **When is treatment of spasticity in MS indicated?**

Treatment of spasticity in MS is indicated when its disadvantages outweigh any potential advantages.

○   **What rehabilitation strategies may be utilized in MS patients with motor dysfunction?**

Two studies noted responses to treatment using rehabilitation therapies and medications. Motor training with biofeedback and Frenkel exercises can be incorporated with weights to dampen the oscillation of ataxia. Orthotic intervention and bracing to improve motor control and stability may be helpful; for example, a soft cervical collar may increase head control. Training may be limited by an increased difficulty

O   **What general measures should be considered in the patient with MS?**

Good general care is the cornerstone of prevention and initial treatment: Proper skin care, pressure relief, early treatment of symptomatic bladder infections, good bowel programs, prevention of deep venous thrombosis, and avoidance of any noxious stimuli all help minimizes spasticity.

O   **What other interventions may be considered to manage spasticity in MS?**

Proper posture and positioning, effective seating, and orthotics or splinting is also important. Active and passive range of motion exercises should be part of an active rehabilitation program, and may lead to relief of spasticity. Topical cold therapy may also be effective, and may have the added benefit of dissipating heat in MS patients who are heat intolerant.

O   **What medication is considered first choice in the management of MS related spasticity?**

Baclofen is usually the first drug of choice for patients with MS. It is most useful in treating spasticity from spinal lesions such as those seen in spinal cord–injured patients and MS patients. It acts, in part, by interfering with the release of excitatory transmitters. While some patients with MS report weakness as a side effect, the weakness may simply be the perception of less resistance to muscle contraction in patients with MS. Baclofen should be titrated with careful attention to efficacy, side effects, and function. It should not be discontinued abruptly.

O   **What other drugs can be used to manage spasticity in MS patients?**

Benzodiazepines, dantrolene.

O   **What is tizanidine role in managing spasticity in MS patients?**

Tizanidine, an imidazoline derivative, also has alpha-adrenergic agonist activity. It has been approved by the FDA for the treatment of spasticity. Tizanidine shows promise in providing comparable or superior results to baclofen, and may be better tolerated in some patients. Its side effects include hypotension, sleepiness, dry mouth, and weakness. Tizanidine can reduce spasms and clonus in MS.

O   **What is the role of intrathecal baclofen?**

For patients with MS whose spasticity is poorly controlled with conservative treatment and oral medications, intrathecal baclofen should be considered before ablative surgical options. Intrathecal baclofen can control severe spinal spasticity and improve function. Computerized telemetry allows precise titration and treatment, since the pump can deliver different doses at various times of the day.

O   **What are the advantages of intrathecal baclofen in the management of MS related spasticity?**

Although intrathecal baclofen is not as effective for spasticity in the upper extremities as for the lower extremities, the low frequency of cognitive dysfunction associated with its use makes it a valuable option for the appropriate individual with MS. Additionally, it often allows a patient to take significantly less anti spasticity medication, and in some cases may eliminate the need for oral agents. This reduced need is of particular benefit to MS patients who may enjoy improved function and QOL by avoiding the medications that can sedate and add cognitive dysfunction.

O   **How common is fatigue in MS?**

Fatigue is the most common symptom **in** MS and usually affects the quality of life. Overall, 75% to 90% of patients with MS report having fatigue, and 50% to 60% report it as the worst symptom of the disease.

O   **What medications may be considered in patients with MS related fatigue?**

Management strategies include education, pharmacologic agents, and energy conservation techniques. The pharmacologic agents, amantadine, pemoline, modafinil, and selective serotonin reuptake inhibitors (SSRIs), are used to treat MS related fatigue with modest success.

○ **What is the extent of cognitive dysfunction in patients with multiple sclerosis?**

The problems are often subtle and may not be detected on standard mental status evaluation. The pattern of cognitive decline is typified by decrease of episodic memory, processing speed, verbal fluency, and difficulty with abstract concepts and complex reasoning. To a lesser extent, executive functioning and visual perception, semantic memory, and attention span may also be also decreased. General intelligence is not typically affected.

○ **Is there any correlation between cognitive impairment and other MS disease parameters?**

Age, duration of MS, and physical disability do not predict the presence of cognitive dysfunction, but the total lesion load seen on MRI does seem to correlate with the degree of cognitive decline. Brain atrophy, enlarged ventricles, and thinning of the corpus callosum also portend symptoms of cognitive dysfunction.

○ **What are some of the patterns of cognitive impairment associated with MS?**

Retrieval of information is often delayed in patients with MS, and information processing is slowed. Conceptual reasoning may be impaired, and perseveration is not unusual. Recent memory and abstract reasoning are less affected than verbal intelligence, language, and memory sparing. The dementia seen in MS is often, but not always, "subcortical" in nature, with decreased insight, cognitive slowing, impaired memory, and dysarthria as the primary findings.

○ **What is the impact of cognitive impairment in MS on QOL?**

The impact of cognitive dysfunction on psychosocial functioning is pervasive: Cognitively impaired patients with MS are less likely to be working, engage in fewer social and avocational activities, report more sexual dysfunction, and have greater difficulty with household tasks.

○ **What are the benefits of neuropsychological testing in patients with MS?**

Information from neuropsychological testing is helpful for clinical monitoring and has direct clinical value for rehabilitation. Specific findings may be utilized for patient and family counseling, vocational and avocational intervention, and rehabilitation designed to improve function, independence, and QOL. Detailed information on cognitive processes is invaluable to the treating rehabilitation team members, who can individualize treatment based on patient needs.

○ **How can neuropsychological assessment aid clinicians in rehabilitation of patients with MS?**

Therapists may modify their remediation, compensation training, and adaptation techniques based on a patient's skills and deficits. Psychologists and social workers find neuropsychological testing helpful in their treatment and support of the individual. For example, socialization, relations, depression and other affective disorders, defenses, and coping strategies are all impacted greatly by cognitive deficits.

○ **How may vision problems in MS be characterized?**

Vision problems can be characterized into four areas: loss of acuity, field deficits, loss of color or contrast sensitivity, and oculomotor dysfunction such as diplopia and nystagmus.

○ **What treatment options exist for the patient with diplopia and nystagmus?**

Treatment for diplopia and nystagmus includes the use of alternating eye patches or a trial with medication such as clonazepam or baclofen. Loss of acuity and reduced sensitivity for color and contrast are most frequently seen with optic neuritis.

O   **What are the most common bladder symptoms in MS?**

The most common bladder symptoms are frequency and urgency (80%–90%), followed by hesitancy or actual incontinence (50%–70%).

O   **What are the associated bladder disorders encountered among MS patients?**

The associated bladder disorders can be categorized into three types based on function and neurogenic status: disorders of storage, of emptying, and a combination, correspond respectively to hyperreflexic, hyporeflexic, and dyssynergic conditions.

O   **What is the distribution of the above bladder function disorders?**

Over 50% of patients are hyperreflexic and as many as half of them have detrusor–external sphincter dyssynergia (DSD).

O   **What is the major risk of urinary tract disease in these patients?**

The risk in these patients is from vesicoureteral reflux due to raised intravesicular pressures above 40 cm H_2O. The high bladder pressure and reflux can cause upper tract problems over time, including hydronephrosis and renal failure.

O   **What therapy options are available for problems of storing urine?**

If the patient is unable to store urine adequately, has low PVR volume, and has frequency due to hyperreflexia, the anticholinergics such as oxybutynin or propantheline can be useful to reduce bladder tone.

O   **What options are available for patients that have difficulty with voiding?**

If there is difficulty voiding and elevated PVR volumes, then the risk of infection increases as a result of difficulty clearing the urine. Difficulty clearing the urine can be due to ineffective bladder emptying with hyporeflexia or due to obstruction with external sphincter spasticity resulting in dyssynergia with a hyperreflexic bladder. In both cases assisted drainage using a catheter is necessary. Intermittent catheterization remains the best form of management along with regulation of fluid intake. An indwelling catheter may be necessary for some individuals who have difficulties with intermittent catheterization. Surgical treatment can include a suprapubic cystostomy, sphincteroplasty, and bladder augmentation. Sphincter problems can be managed with medications. Adrenergic agents or alpha-blockers can be utilized to reduce spasticity. Alpha agonists can be used for sphincter insufficiency such as with stress incontinence if there is no hyperreflexia.

O   **What patterns of bowel dysfunction occur in patients with MS?**

Bowel dysfunction occurs in two thirds of patients with MS. Bowel function is compromised by lesions affecting motor and autonomic pathways. The gastrocolic reflex may be compromised. Colonic transit time is decreased, and sensation may be decreased. Symptoms of bowel dysfunction includes constipation, incontinence of bowel, and fecal urgency.

O   **What conservative measures can maintain colonic motility and a bowel program in MS patients?**

Timing the bowel program after a meal utilizes the gastrocolic reflex as much as possible. The consistency of the stool can be managed with stool softeners, if necessary. Oral laxatives, such as senna (Senokot®), may be taken at the appropriate time before the scheduled bowel program (i.e., at noon for an evening program). Fiber and exercise can also increase colonic motility.

O   **How may sexual dysfunction be addressed in the MS patient?**

Sexual dysfunction may be tactfully addressed using the acronym PLISSIT model. *P* stands for permission to discuss the issues as a first step so patients are as comfortable as possible. Permission establishes that it is appropriate to discuss sexual dysfunction as much as one is comfortable doing so. *LI* stands for limited information that can be given regarding possible interventions. *SS* stands for specific suggestions, referring to individually based interventions such as devices. *IT*, or intensive therapy, is necessary when there are complex issues requiring a trained therapist.

O **What affect does MS have on libido?**

A decreased libido has been described in patients with MS. Both libido and sexual dysfunction may fluctuate with disease activity.

O **How common is sexual dysfunction among patients with MS?**

Erectile dysfunction is a common complaint in up to 80% of men, and 10% have ejaculatory problems. Decreased penile sensation, inability to reach orgasm, premature ejaculation, inability to ejaculate, and trouble with achieving and maintaining erections have been reported. Neurophysiological testing indicates the presence of supra sacral spinal cord lesions in most men with sexual dysfunction.

O **What is the treatment for erectile dysfunction in MS patients?**

Treatment may include intracavernous injections of vasoactive agents, vacuum devices, penile prosthesis, and sexual counseling.

O **What are the characteristics of sexual dysfunction in female MS patients?**

Sexual dysfunction is reported in up to 75% of women. It may also be a presenting symptom. In some individuals, the most common problem related to sexual function is fatigue. Decreased vaginal lubrication and decreased maintenance of lubrication, decreased vaginal sensation, and lack of orgasms are most commonly reported. Other findings include decreased libido, severe external dysesthesia, and vaginal dyspareunia. Changes in sexual function in women are related to weakness of the pelvic floor as well as bowel and bladder dysfunction. Pudendal evoked potentials may be abnormal, as well as urodynamic studies, anal reflexes, and sensation.

O **What treatment strategies may be employed in these patients?**

Treatment principles include correcting as many of the contributing factors as possible (i.e., spasticity, fatigue, etc.). Sensory dysesthesia may be amenable to pharmacological intervention with low dose tricyclic antidepressants. Water soluble vaginal lubricants may be helpful. Estrogen supplements may also help in post menopausal women.

O **How common are affective disorders among patients with MS?**

Affective and psychiatric disorders are common in MS. Up to 30–40% of patients in the early stages of MS may have depression. As many as 75% of patients may experience depression at some time during their illness. Unfortunately, the suicide rate is 7.5 times higher in patients with MS than in the general population. Affective disorders may be related to lesions in the temporal lobes in patients with MS. Bipolar disease is estimated to be 13 times higher in MS.

O **What makes the diagnosis of depression difficult in the MS patient?**

The symptoms of depression, such as fatigue, sleep disturbance, lethargy, and cognitive deficits, may be similar to those seen frequently in MS. Fatigue can independently contribute to depression. These factors may lead to under diagnosis of depression. Patients with cerebral involvement of disease are more likely to be depressed than those with cord involvement. Depression correlates with the degree of neurologic impairment.

O **What other affective manifestations occur in MS patients?**

Emotional lability and euphoria may be observed in patients with MS. Pathological crying and laughing may be treated with amitriptyline. Euphoria may increase as the patient's condition worsens.

O **What are the characteristics of dysphagia in MS patients?**

Swallowing difficulty (dysphagia) may occur in patients with MS. Approximately 33% of patients with MS have impaired chewing or swallowing. Swallowing impairment may be the consequence of plaques involving the corticobulbar fibers in multiple areas of the brain or from demyelination in the brain stem. The swallowing process involves an oral phase, a pharyngeal phase, and an esophageal phase. Reduced pharyngeal peristalsis and delayed swallowing reflex are the most common features in MS.

O   **What are the characteristics of speech disorders are encountered in MS patients?**

Speech is a motor activity, innervated and controlled by the speech and articulatory centers located mostly in the left hemisphere, brain stem, and lower cranial nerves. About 44% of patients with MS have impaired speech. Sixteen percent reported that speech was one of their greatest problems. Dysarthria, dysphonia, and aphasia are impairments that may be seen in patients with MS. Dysarthria is more common in patients with MS, and aphasia is a rare occurrence. The most common type of dysarthria in patients with MS is ataxic dysarthria.

O   **What techniques may be used to treat dysarthria, dysphonia and dysphagia?**

Brain stem findings as a whole are the third most common functional system to be affected as noted by Kurtzke scale reports. Treatment commonly centers on training exercises to improve breath control, pacing, and bolus control. The use of compensatory techniques such as head tilt and a modified diet can be incorporated with dietary counseling. Further adaptive techniques may include the use of a palatal lift, Teflon injections to stiffen the vocal cord, and the use of tubes for feeding.

O   **What techniques may be used to treat speech/language disorders?**

Patients with speech abnormalities secondary to MS are encouraged to maximize their functional communication by paying attention to the clarity and precision of their speech. At times, patients with MS need to modify their speaking patterns by controlling rate, consonant emphasis, and number of words per breath.

PARKINSON'S DISEASE

O   **What is the classification of Parkinson's disease?**

Idiopathic Parkinson's disease is the most common variant of Parkinsonism, accounting for over 80% of all Parkinson syndromes seen in the general population. Neuroleptic induced Parkinsonism, also known as drug induced Parkinsonism, is now the second most common variant in the general population, and accounts for 7-9% of parkinsonian patients. Multiple system atrophy, which includes Shy-Drager syndrome, striatonigral degeneration, and olivopontocerebellar degeneration, accounts for approximately 2.5%, while progressive supranuclear palsy and vascular Parkinson syndrome are seen at approximately 1.5% and 3% of all Parkinson patients. Rare causes of Parkinson syndrome are MPTP-induced Parkinsonism, carbon monoxide poisoning, manganese poisoning, recurrent head trauma, etc. It is of note that no new cases of postencephalitic Parkinsonism have been reported since the 1960s.

O   **What is the incidence of Parkinson's disorder?**

The incidence of Parkinson syndrome and Parkinson's disease rises with age, and has been reported at between five and twenty four cases per hundred thousand. The best available incidence studies- those from the Rochester, Minnesota, database suggest the incidence of Parkinson syndrome in the U.S.A. is 20.5 per 100,000 population. Because the population is slowly aging, and the recognition of Parkinson's is improving, it is expected that the incidence will slowly rise.

O   **What is the prevalence of Parkinson's disease?**

Estimates of PD prevalence range from 18-328 per 100,000 population, with most studies yielding a prevalence of approximately 120 per 100,000.

O   **What are the chronological characteristics of Parkinson's disease?**

A review of 934 patients found the onset of Parkinson syndrome was at age 61.6, while the onset of Parkinson's disease was at age 62.4 years. Parkinsonism is very rare before age 30 and only 4-10% of the cases have onset before the age of 40 years.

O   What is the natural history of Parkinson's disease?

As a rule, Parkinson syndromes are progressively disabling, except for drug induced parkinsonism or parkinsonism due to a single event such as a stroke, and there are wide variations in the course of progression. The rate of disability is more rapid where the pathology is widespread, such as in multiple system atrophy or progressive supranuclear palsy. In general, the prognosis for life expectancy is better in the non-demented, tremor dominant Parkinson's disease cases than in the other variants of Parkinson syndrome.

O   What is the mean life expectancy after the onset of parkinsonism?

It is estimated that mean survival after onset of parkinsonism today is approximately 15 years. Survival is longer in those patients who at the first clinical assessment were non-demented. Survival has significantly improved since the widespread use of levodopa, provided the drug is started before the patient reaches Unified Parkinson's disease scale 9 (UPDRS- see below) stage 2.5. The survival in Parkinson's disease is longer than it is in multiple system atrophy or progressive supranuclear palsy. The most common causes of death are pulmonary infection/aspiration, pulmonary embolism, urinary tract infection, and complications of falls and fractures.

O   What do the following pathology specimens represent?

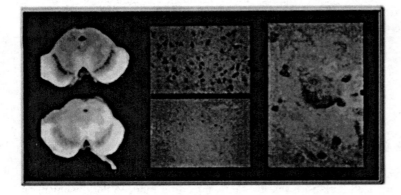

Changes in the substantia nigra in Parkinson's disease and Lewy bodies

O   What is the apoptosis theory of Parkinson's disease?

The current evidence indicates that the pathogenetic process of PD is probably apoptosis. It is hypothesized that there is excessive oxidative stress in the substantia nigra, and there is reduced antioxidant capacity in Parkinson's disease. There is evidence that free radical formation is increased and Complex I levels are reduced in the substantia nigra compacta, though they are not specific for Parkinson's disease. There is also evidence of reduced glutathione in the substantial nigra compacta which normally neutralizes hydrogen peroxide.

O   What alternative theories of pathogenesis have been postulated?

The other theory is that there is slow or weak excitotoxic activity occurring over a long period of time. ATP is required to maintain normal membrane potential. A decline in membrane potential from -90 to -60 or greater produces persistent activation of NMDA receptors. That leads to influx of calcium and formation of nitric oxide, superoxide, and peroxynitrite which lead to neuronal death. The other possibility is that there is inadequate neurotrophic factor or factors that are necessary to maintain normal physiological and anatomical integrity of the substantia nigra neurons.

O   What is the Hoehn & Yahr staging system for Parkinson's Disease?

Stage One

1.   Signs and symptoms on one side only

2.   Symptoms mild
3.   Symptoms inconvenient but not disabling
4.   Usually presents with tremor of one limb
5.   Friends have noticed changes in posture, locomotion and facial expression

Stage Two

1.   Symptoms are bilateral
2.   Minimal disability
3.   Posture and gait affected

Stage Three

1.   Significant slowing of body movements
2.   Early impairment of equilibrium on walking or standing
3.   Generalized dysfunction that is moderately severe

Stage Four

1.   Severe symptoms
2.   Can still walk to a limited extent
3.   Rigidity and bradykinesia
4.   No longer able to live alone
5.   Tremor may be less than earlier stages

Stage Five

1.   Cachectic stage
2.   Invalidism complete
3.   Cannot stand or walk
4.   Requires constant nursing care

O   **Describe the Unified Parkinson's disease scale**

The UPDRS is a rating tool to follow the longitudinal course of Parkinson's Disease. It is made up of the 1) Mentation, Behavior, and Mood, 2) ADL and 3) Motor sections. These are evaluated by interview. Some sections require multiple grades assigned to each extremity. A total of 199 points are possible. 199 represents the worst (total) disability), 0--no disability.

O   **What are the four cardinal features of Parkinson's disease?**

The four cardinal features or characteristics of Parkinson's disease include resting tremor, bradykinesia, rigidity, and postural instability. Resting tremor occurs with the hands at rest in the lap and classically is described as a tremor of the hand and fingers in a "pill rolling" type movement. The tremor may also affect the face, lips, tongue, neck, and lower extremities. Resting tremor should be distinguished from the postural, action tremor of essential tremor.

O   **What is bradykinesia?**

Bradykinesia, or slowness of movement, is often the most disabling of the cardinal signs of Parkinson's disease. The slowness of movement can result in a reduction in the patient's ability to perform activities of daily living, and impair a patient's ability to regain balance or catch himself to prevent injury from a fall.

O   **What is rigidity?**

In contrast to tremor and bradykinesia, rigidity is rarely a patient reported symptom. Assessment of rigidity involves passive movement of the neck, upper limbs, and lower limbs, to assess for an increase in tone throughout the range of motion. In mild cases, rigidity may be increased by "activation" of the contralateral limb by opening and closing the hand, or other repetitive tasks. Rigidity should be distinguished from spasticity because this increase in tone is more prominent with initiation of movement and is greater in one direction than the other; it is also not velocity dependent.

O   **What is postural instability?**

Although usually not an early sign or symptom of idiopathic Parkinson's disease, postural instability emerges with disease progression. On examination, the examiner should stand behind the patient and ask the patient to maintain their balance when pulled backwards. The examiner should pull back briskly to assess the patient's ability to recover, being careful to prevent the patient from falling.

O   **What are other symptoms and signs associated with Parkinson's disease?**

There are numerous other signs and symptoms of Parkinson's Disease that are often brought to the physician's attention by the patient or family members. Micrographia is a common early sign, characterized by a slowness or smallness to the handwriting. Mask facies is another bradykinetic symptom characteristic of Parkinson's disease. Slowing of activities of daily living occurs, including such activities as dressing, bathing, turning in bed, getting in and out of a chair, or in and out of a car. Bulbar symptoms include bradykinetic or hypophonic speech, which may require the patient to repeat himself frequently. Drooling is common. Choking may occur. Although nonspecific, the loss of the sense of smell, or anosmia, has been well documented in Parkinson's disease.

O   **What are the characteristics of gait in PD?**

Gait is often characterized by some shuffling or dragging of a leg, and the posture may be stooped with flexion of the knees, hips, trunk, and neck. Some patients will present with a foot dystonia in which the foot will turn in and there will be involuntary curling of the toes, especially in the morning.

O   **Are there variants of Parkinson's disease to be aware of?**

Besides PD, there are many other causes of parkinsonism. The second most common group is the parkinsonism-plus syndromes (12 percent), a conglomerate term for a large number of degenerative disorders in which parkinsonism is one of several neurological features. Drug-induced parkinsonism (8 percent) and heredodegenerative conditions, such as juvenile Huntington's disease, are less frequent.

O   **What is progressive supranuclear palsy (PSP)?**

The hallmark signs of supranuclear downgaze palsy and square wave jerks are often late stage symptoms, but should always be looked for in patients with parkinsonism. Unlike the stooped posture of a Parkinson's disease patient, PSP patients are often quite upright. Furthermore, when these patients sit in a chair, rather than carefully sitting to protect themselves like PD patients, PSP patients will almost fall into the seat, sometimes striking their heads on the wall with their feet leaving the ground. PSP patients also exhibit pseudobulbar emotionality, or laughing or crying somewhat inappropriately and often uncontrollably. Finally, the classic PSP type facial expression is one of a furrowed brow and a significant stare with a lack of eye blinks and a lack of the ability to move the eyes. Early in the course of PSP, patients may respond fairly well to dopaminergic medications, but the response usually wanes.

O   **What is Corticobasal degeneration?**

Corticobasal degeneration, also known as corticobasal ganglionic degeneration, is a neurodegenerative parkinsonian disorder often associated with a very coarse unilateral tremor. The pathognomonic clinical sign of corticobasal degeneration is a limb apraxia, usually of one upper limb. The arm is often held in a dystonic posture, and the arm may move seemingly on its own and under poor control by the patient, the "alien limb" sign. This condition does not respond to anti-PD medications, but the dystonic posture may benefit from botulinum toxin injections.

O   **What other syndromes should be differentiated in Parkinson's disease?**

Other neurodegenerative disorders that present with parkinsonism are the various types of multiple system atrophy. As the name implies, these are disorders in which multiple neuronal systems have degenerated.

In patients with Shy Drager syndrome, the main characteristic differentiating it from Parkinson's disease is an autonomic disturbance, such as orthostatic hypotension, impotence, and bowel and bladder incontinence. Although the parkinsonian features respond poorly to anti-PD medications, low blood pressure symptoms respond to midodrine and fludrocortisone. Striatonigral degeneration is clinically similar to idiopathic PD, but tremor is not a prominent feature, and has a limited response to anti dopaminergic medications.

Patients with olivopontocerebellar atrophy, or OPCA, have cerebellar signs that differentiate it from idiopathic Parkinson's disease. There are currently no treatment options for these patients, although one recent study reports some benefit from amantadine.

O   **What is normal pressure hydrocephalus?**

Patients with normal pressure, communicating, or obstructive hydrocephalus can have parkinsonian symptoms. The clinical triad that patients develop is a parkinsonian gait disorder, incontinence, and dementia. The diagnosis is usually made by CT or MRI scan showing the hydrocephalus. In some instances, nuclear medicine cisternography, looking for abnormalities in CSF flow, is helpful. Hydrocephalus induced parkinsonism may improve if the underlying cause of hydrocephalus is determined and treated. Additionally, patients with normal pressure hydrocephalus may benefit from ventriculoperitoneal (V-P) shunting. Often, lumbar puncture with removal of 15-25 cc of CSF on three consecutive days may produce a self limiting improvement in gait, and is a useful "diagnostic" test prior to V-P shunting. However, some cases in which no improvement is seen after serial lumbar puncture may improve after ventriculoperitoneal shunting.

O   **How is Parkinson's disease differentiated from essential tremor (ET)?**

Patients with essential tremor should have tremor alone with no signs of parkinsonism, or any of the other neurologic signs mentioned above, such as hyperreflexia, weakness, and sensory loss. Both disorders may have both a kinetic and rest component, although traditionally patients with essential tremor have more of a postural and kinetic tremor with dampening upon rest, whereas Parkinson's disease patients more often have a rest tremor that dampens with action. In addition, ET patients may exhibit mild signs of bradykinesia and cog wheeling when examined for rigidity. In the early tremor patient, the historical findings of family history suggesting an autosomal dominant inheritance, a long history of tremor without progression of motor difficulties, and tremor response to alcohol, are helpful in the diagnosis of essential tremor. Lastly, ET does not respond to anti-PD drugs, but may improve with proprandol, primidone, benzodiazepines, and other agents.

O   **What differentiates parkinsonian gait?**

In the normal walking cycle, the pelvis and thorax rotate in opposite directions in the horizontal plane. In the parkinsonian patient, the trunk and pelvis tend to rotate together (en bloc) as a single unit rather than in the thoracopelvic reciprocal pattern. However, the pattern tends to be normal in some, presumably less severely affected patients. Parkinson patients have decreased hip flexion and excursion, which worsens as the disease progresses.

O   **What is the corner stone of symptomatic management in Parkinson's disease?**

Dopaminergic therapy with levodopa or dopamine agonists is the cornerstone of symptomatic management of Parkinson's disease. Levodopa replaces dopamine presynaptically, while dopamine agonists act directly on receptors postsynaptically. Levodopa is administered with a peripheral decarboxylase inhibitor, either benserazide or carbidopa. The newest class of drugs, the COMT inhibitors, also increases the bioavailability of levodopa, by inhibiting peripheral or central catechol O-methyl transferase. Other agents are anticholinergics, the MAO-B inhibitor selegiline, and the antiviral amantadine.

O   **Diagram the sites of drug specificity in Parkinson's disease**

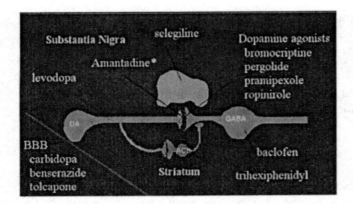

○   **What is the role of anticholinergic medications in Parkinson's disease?**

Although the exact mechanism of action is unknown, it is believed that dopamine depletion leads to an overactivity of acetylcholine in the striatum, and that reduction of this relative overactivity is responsible for improvement in parkinsonian symptoms. Anticholinergics may also inhibit dopamine reuptake in the striatum. Clinical studies have shown that cholinergics are mainly effective for tremor and rigidity and do not help with other parkinsonian symptoms. The commonly used anticholinergics include trihexyphenidyl, benztropine, and ethopropazine. The anticholinergics should be started at very low doses, and then gradually increased. Anticholinergics are usually not recommended in older patients because of higher propensity to cause adverse effects. Common side effects of anticholinergics include dry mouth, sedation, delirium, confusion, hallucinations, constipation, and urinary retention.

○   **What is amantadine?**

Amantadine was initially introduced as an antiviral agent, and was first reported to be useful in the treatment of parkinsonian symptoms in 1969. It has weak antiparkinsonian benefits for the cardinal manifestations of tremor, bradykinesia, and rigidity. Recently, amantadine has been shown to be effective for levodopa induced dyskinesias. The exact mechanism of action of amantadine is unknown, but there are several possibilities.

○   **What are the pharmacodynamics of amantadine?**

Presynaptically, it functions by enhancing the release of stored catecholamines from intact dopaminergic terminals and by inhibiting catecholamine reuptake processes in the presynaptic terminals. Postsynaptically, it acts by directly activating the dopamine receptor, and inducing changes in the dopamine receptor conformation that fix the receptor in a high affinity configuration. Recently, it has also been proposed that amantadine may be mediated in part by NMDA receptor blockade, which may explain its antidyskinetic properties.

○   **How is amantadine dosed?**

The usual recommended dose of amantadine is 100 milligrams twice a day, although, in some patients, up to 300 milligrams a day may be used.

○   **What are the side effects of amantadine?**

The side effects are similar to anticholinergics such as dry mouth, difficulty concentrating, confusion, insomnia, nightmare, agitation, and hallucinations. Symptoms of orthostatic hypotension such as lightheadedness might also be seen. Peripheral edema and livedo reticularis (mottled skin) are common undesirable side effects at therapeutic doses. Patients with renal insufficiency will require the dose to be reduced significantly.

○   **What is Selegiline?**

Selegiline is the prototype MAO-B inhibitor for the treatment of Parkinson's disease. The question of selegiline putative neuro protection has been controversial since its development. Selegiline is dosed at 5 mg twice daily, at breakfast and lunch. Selegiline side effects include hallucinations, orthostatic hypertension, insomnia and, on occasion, nausea. There is also potential for a serious reaction with certain antidepressants, known as the serotonin syndrome, in which patients may develop extremely high blood pressure and other associated symptoms.

○   **What are the formulations of levodopa?**

Levodopa is available in three different formulations. The controlled release preparation has a longer latency to onset than the immediate release preparation, and evens out plasma concentrations somewhat. The primary advantage of this drug is that, for those with early disease, it can be given twice daily as opposed to the TID dosing recommended in the immediate release form of levodopa. The use of controlled release formulations may lengthen the "on" state in patients who have motor fluctuations. But on the down side, this particular type of levodopa might be less effective in patients with particularly advanced disease. These patients often complain that the controlled release formulation is not as reliable or as effective as the immediate release form of levodopa. The liquid preparation is available for patients requiring more rapid onset of effect.

○   **What is the role of levodopa in PD?**

Levodopa was first introduced as a therapeutic agent for Parkinson's disease in the late 1960s, and rapidly became the drug of choice for treatment. Despite the development of many more treatment options, it remains the mainstay of therapy for most patients. It is by far the most clinically effective drug for the symptoms of Parkinson's disease, being capable of alleviating virtually all of the cardinal symptoms including bradykinesia. Since bradykinesia is among the most disabling features of this disorder, the effectiveness of levodopa for this problem cannot be over emphasized. When this drug is started early in the course of Parkinson's disease it can produce a smooth and dramatic clinical response leading to virtually normalization of symptoms. This smooth response typically lasts for several years before problems with therapy develop.

○   **What are the side effects?**

Nausea and vomiting are probably the most common side effects, with occurrence of nausea in as many as 20% of patients when first started on levodopa. In most cases, this nausea is due to insufficient blockade of peripheral decarboxylase, and therefore the administration of supplemental carbidopa can be very effective at controlling this kind of nausea. Carbidopa is now available for prescription in the United States under the trade name Lodosyn®.

○   **What problems can arise with levodopa?**

Other patients may develop postural hypotension when levodopa is added and this may reflect the mild autonomic insufficiency, which patients with Parkinson's disease develop. Dyskinesias and motor fluctuations are late effects seen with increased loss of dopaminergic neurons.

○   **How is levodopa absorbed?**

Levodopa is actively transported across the gut barrier and the blood-brain barrier via the large neutral amino acid carrier. It is believed to be subsequently taken up by the presynaptic nigral neuron, where it is converted into dopamine and can then be released in a physiologic fashion into the synaptic cleft.
When levodopa is administered along with other dietary amino acids, competition will exist for transport across both the gut and the blood-brain barriers. This is the primary reason why administration with food is generally not advised, since levodopa will not be fully absorbed when administered in this fashion.

○   **How is it metabolized in the circulation?**

In the peripheral circulation, levodopa is rapidly decarboxylated into dopamine, where it is then quickly degraded. Dopamine itself does not cross the blood brain barrier, and can stimulate the area postrema, causing significant nausea and vomiting.

○   **Why are decarboxylase inhibitors needed?**

A few years after levodopa was brought into clinical practice, a decarboxylase inhibitor was developed which prevents peripheral degradation of dopamine, thereby enabling a much larger percentage of levodopa to actually cross the blood brain barrier into the central compartment. There are a number of decarboxylase inhibitors available around the world, the two most common being carbidopa in the United States and benserazide in Europe and elsewhere. With a decarboxylase inhibitor, the drug is rapidly absorbed into the brain, usually 30 to 45 minutes after oral ingestion, and once in the central nervous system the drug has a half life of about 60 to 90 minutes.

○ **What are the COMT inhibitors?**

The COMT inhibitors are the newest class of antiparkinsonian drugs. COMT stands for catechol O-methyltransferase, which is the second major enzyme involved in the peripheral degradation of levodopa. COMT acts on levodopa to create an inactive metabolite, CO methyldopa. This particular metabolite competes with levodopa itself for active transport across the blood brain barrier and therefore reduces levodopa absorption. Drugs that block formation of this metabolite therefore potentiate the effect of levodopa and lengthen its half life. The COMT inhibitors have been positioned as particularly useful for patients with brittle Parkinson's disease who experience rapid and frequent motor fluctuations. The current examples of COMT inhibitors available world wide include tolcapone and entacapone.

○ **What is tolcapone?**

Tolcapone was the first inhibitor to be licensed in the United States. It is available in 100 and 200 milligram tablets intended for 3 time's daily administration. Tolcapone has a relatively long half life compared to entacapone and can thus be given three times daily. Patients starting out on COMT inhibitors generally require a mild levodopa dose reduction to avoid accentuation of levodopa induced side effects such as dyskinesias or nausea.

○ **What is the mechanism of action of dopamine agonists?**

Dopamine agonists act on postsynaptic dopamine receptors, obviating the need for conversion to dopamine by nigrostriatal neurons. They also do not compete with dietary amino acids for uptake from the gastrointestinal tract or for transport across the blood-brain barrier. Dopamine agonists have longer half lives than levodopa–four to eight hours or more, compared to approximately one hour for levodopa.

○ **How are they used clinically?**

Dopamine agonists may be used as monotherapy in Parkinson's patients with functional disabilities who are not presently on levodopa. They are also used as adjunctive therapy for stable Parkinson's disease patients who are on levodopa or other medications to enhance the antiparkinsonian benefits.

○ **What are the dopamine agonists?**

Dopamine agonists differ significantly in their serum half lives, with resulting differences in dosing schedules. All dopamine agonist should be started at very low doses and gradually increased until a therapeutic response is obtained or the patient has an adverse effect related to the medications. Starting dopamine agonists at very low doses prevents adverse effects like nausea, vomiting, lightheadedness, and dizziness. The information provided here refers to monotherapy with dopamine agonists.

○ **What is the dosing of bromocriptine?**

Bromocriptine should be started at 1.25 milligrams per day and every 3rd to 7th day 1.25 milligrams should be added until there is a therapeutic response. The usual recommended dose for bromocriptine is 10-16 milligrams per day in equally divided doses.

○ **What is the dosing of pergolide?**

Pergolide should be initiated at 0.05 milligrams once a day and gradually increase every three to four days by 0.1 to 0.15 milligrams until the patient is on 0.25 milligrams 3 times a day. Further increases should be made depending on the response.

○ **What is the dosing of Pramipexole?**

Pramipexole is usually started at 0.125 milligrams 3 times a day, and increased to 0.25 milligrams 3 times a day in the second week, and 0.5 milligrams 3 times a day by week three.

○   **What is the dosing for Ropinirole?**

Ropinirole is initiated at 0.25 milligrams 3 times a day and increased by 0.25 milligrams every week until the patient is on 1 milligram 3 times a day, and further increases are made depending on the efficacy.

○   **What are the side effects of the dopamine agonists?**

Common adverse effects of dopamine agonists include nausea, vomiting, orthostatic hypotension, headaches, dizziness, drowsiness, dyskinesias, confusion, hallucinations and paranoia. More rare adverse effects include diplopia, abnormal vision, rash, weight gain or loss, erythema, dry mouth, constipation, and diarrhea. Erythromelalgia, pulmonary and retroperitoneal fibrosis, plural effusion and plural thickening, and Raynaud's phenomenon are rare adverse effects, which are believed to be more common with ergotamine dopamine agonists. However, some of these same adverse effects have also been reported in a patient using the non ergot dopamine agonist ropinirole.

○   **What are the physical rehabilitation goals for the patient with Parkinson's disease?**

1.   To maintain or increase active and passive range of motion, especially extension, and to prevent contractures by stretching tight muscles
2.   To improve speed, flexibility, dexterity, and coordination of motor movements and repetitive tasks
3.   To enhance awareness of posture and balance losses and correct where possible
4.   To restore chest expansion/contraction not only as an end in itself, but to encourage relaxation and increase voice volume
5.   To review gait with particular emphasis on increasing step length, widening the base of support, increasing the range of hip flexion, enhancing reciprocal arm movements, and improving stops, starts, and turns
6.   To upgrade activities of daily living, teach simplification of tasks and conservation of energy techniques for the patient and caregiver

○   **What happens to speech production in Parkinson's disease?**

In Parkinson disease, there is a breakdown of prosody and its component features. Vocal tone can be "breathy," harsh, and low pitched. There can also be incomplete glottal closure and faulty abduction and adduction of the vocal cords. In the early stages of the disease, with mild impairment, there is prompt abduction for inspiration and slow adduction for phonation. In the later severe stages, there is overall decreased vocal cord motion and associated tremor.

○   **What other communication problems occur in Parkinson's patients?**

Another significant problem in Parkinson patients is dysprosody. It has been reported that parkinsonian patients are unable to appreciate the prosodic features of speech in themselves or in others. This especially involves intonation and its affective import. They seem to have the greatest difficulty in recognizing and producing interrogative or angry statements. They also have difficulty recognizing and interpreting facial expression, which is believed to be an adjunctive component of their overall communication difficulty.

○   **Can speech therapy be effective in patients with Parkinson's disease?**

Studies have shown that intensive 2 week speech therapy programs could produce sustained improvements in speech, especially prosody and its component parts (variation of intonation, pitch, volume, rate, and rhythm) for up to 3 months and sometimes up to 6 months.

○   **What oropharyngeal disorders occur among Parkinson's disease (PD) patients?**

Dysphagia and sialorrhea together make oropharyngeal problems the most common gastrointestinal difficulties in Parkinson disease. Although the term sialorrhea implies excessive secretion of saliva, this is not the case. Impaired swallowing underlies the excessive oral pooling of saliva. The earliest signs of sialorrhea are drooling at night, then daytime drooling. Anticholinergic medications work well on this symptom, but dry mouth can result, making swallowing more difficult. Sialorrhea has been reported in at least 70% of patients.

○   **How common is dysphagia among PD patients?**

Dysphagia occurs in at least 50% of patients versus 6% of age matched controls. The numbers vary among studies. In Parkinson disease, it also seems to affect solids more than liquids.

O   **What are the characteristics of dysphagia in PD patients?**

In Parkinsonian patients, these tongue segments do not elevate sufficiently to move the bolus effectively to the back of the throat. Instead, there is a "rocking-like motion". It usually takes two to five such motions to finally propel the food into the pharynx. When rocking propels small parts of the single bolus posteriorly, it produces a relatively inefficient "piece meal" deglutition. Repetitive tongue pumping describes abnormal tongue motion in progressing the bolus. The patient requires several lingual pumps to push portions of the food posteriorly, rather than one single efficient action transferring the entire bolus posteriorly.

O   **What techniques have been recommended to PD patients with dysphagia?**

The supraglottic swallow and thermal stimulation

O   **What medication has proven helpful in PD patients with chronic constipation?**

Apomorphine

O   **What are the most common urological problems in PD patients?**

The major urologic abnormality in Parkinson disease is detrusor hyperreflexia. The usual symptoms are urgency incontinence, followed by hesitancy with a poor stream.

O   **What is the proposed etiology of sexual dysfunction in PD patients?**

Autonomic dysfunction

O   **What is the incidence of dementia in PD patients?**

Overt dementia may occur in 30% to 40% of Parkinson's disease (PD) patients, and more subtle intellectual impairment is seen in the majority of patients. The incidence rises such that by the age of 85 years, the incidence of dementia in Parkinson disease is 65%. The dementia in PD might be explained by the co-occurrence of AD in some cases. However, in many cases the cholinergic system is prominently affected in the absence of cortical Alzheimer's pathology. Several trends have been noted comparing demented versus non-demented parkinsonian patients. The demented group generally had later onset of symptoms, increased incidence of dystonic dyskinesia, and a worsened response to levodopa.

O   **What are therapeutic options for patients with dementia associated with PD?**

There have been a few small studies examining the effects of Acetylcholinesterase inhibitors (AChEIs) on the treatment of dementia associated with PD. Donepezil was significantly better than placebo in improving cognitive performance, with no increase in Parkinsonian symptoms during treatment. The role of other AChEIs remains to be established.

O   **Is depression a common problem among PD patients?**

Depression has been estimated to occur in 47% of the Parkinson population. While some authors felt that it may contribute to cognitive dysfunction, most other studies of parkinsonian dementia stated that depression appears to be an independent variable. The male-female ratio is 7: 2. Limited studies suggest that tricyclic and selective serotonin reuptake inhibitor (SSRI) antidepressants have efficacy in depression in this setting. SSRIs occasionally can exacerbate motor symptoms of PD.

O   **What problems can the patient with Parkinson's disease experience with regard to psychosis?**

Psychotic symptoms are common in patients suffering from Parkinson's disease (PD). Visual hallucinations are the most common manifestation, occurring in approximately 30% of patients with PD. Multiple risk factors for PD related hallucinations have been identified. Psychotic symptoms usually occur in cases of advanced, chronically treated PD. Chronic exposure to multiple anti-PD medications appears to be a particularly potent risk factor for their occurrence Additionally, the use of all anti-PD medications, without exception, has been implicated in the development of hallucinations.

○   **What are the therapeutic agents appropriate for psychosis associated with PD?**

Clozapine is the only antipsychotic agent for which there are randomized, controlled trials with positive data specifically in PD, thus actually being the first line choice for the treatment of drug induced psychosis in PD, albeit at very low doses (12.5–25 mg/day). Quetiapine also may be a reasonable alternative. Risperidone and olanzapine may worsen motor symptoms of PD and are thus not drugs of first choice. Atypical antipsychotic agents such as clozapine, quetiapine and olanzapine should therefore be started at very low doses that are increased gradually. Cholinomimetic therapy may prove to be helpful in the prevention and treatment of psychotic manifestations in Parkinson's disease patients, given the effects observed in patients suffering from dementia with Lewy bodies.

○   **What is the role of exercise therapy in PD patients?**

Regular physical exercise can influence the survival rate in Parkinson's disease by preventing decline from disuse. Individuals with mild to moderate Parkinson's disease can maintain normal exercise capacity with regular aerobic exercise such as walking or cycling. Support to maintain an active lifestyle, incorporating physical activity, is important in relation to the tendency to reduce physical activity, specific difficulties encountered with several common activities, and maintaining optimal drug effect while exercising.

○   **What are the benefits of specific exercise programs in PD patients?**

An individualized home exercise program focusing on trunk and lower limb function can improve functional activities. Strengthening exercises specific to the trunk and incorporated into a course of aerobic exercise classes can improve trunk muscle performance. A 10 week individualized exercise program designed to promote spinal flexibility demonstrated improvements in axial mobility and functional performance. A 10 week balance and lower limb strength training program demonstrated improvements in equilibrium and reduction in falls.

○   **What are the Typical components of a general therapeutic exercise program, whether delivered individually or in a group format ?**

1)exercises for the trunk, upper and lower limbs and face in lying, sitting and standing
2)speech and breathing exercises
3)gait training
4)balance training
5)transfer training
6)relaxation

○   **What are the requirements for locomotion and motor deficits in Parkinson's Disease?**

Requirements for Locomotion and Motor Deficits in Parkinson's Disease	
Task	**Impairments**
Initiation and termination of locomotion	Freezing before walking or after turn of direction Reduced muscle-force production Loss of heel strike, which impairs braking Impairment of ballistic movements
Generation and maintenance of continuous movement toward destination	Reduced speed forward caused by diminished stride length and increased double-limb support phase Instability of upper trunk caused by lack of transverse pelvis rotation Fixed shoulder-elbow position
Adaptation to a changing environment or to concurrent tasks	Difficulties in performing two tasks at the same time Insufficient function of sensory-motor association cortex, less focused cortical activity

○   **What strategies may be employed to improve specific deficits in Parkinson's Disease?**

Strategies to Improve Specific Deficits in Parkinson's Disease

Deficit	Corrective Exercise
Initiation of movements	Polysensory cueing
Hastening	Selection of cueing frequencies Gait preparation exercise with different gait types (forward, backward, sideways) Position change (lying to sitting or sitting to standing)
Braking	Alternate gait types (forward, backward, walking on toes and heels)
Muscle rigidity	Stretching exercises to aid flexibility Exercises in warm water to aid relaxation
Trunk stiffness	Rotational and straightening-up exercises
Complex and compound movements, dual and/or sequential tasks	Training with simple motor sequences
Simultaneous movements and coordination	Forming complex and simultaneous movements from simple motor sequences
Miscalling of movements	Training of large-amplitude movements
Balance	Roll exercises, reach exercises Pezzi ball (also called gymnastic ball or physiotherapy ball) exercises Pool exercises with paddles and swim noodles
Strength	Isometric exercises in supine, prone, and quadruped positions Rollover exercises Training against water resistance

CEREBRAL PALSY

○   **What is cerebral palsy (CP)?**

Cerebral palsy (CP) is a diagnostic term used to describe a group of motor syndromes resulting from disorders of early brain development. CP is caused by a broad group of developmental, genetic, metabolic, ischemic, infectious, and other acquired etiologies that produce a common group of neurologic phenotypes. Although it has historically been considered a *static encephalopathy*, this term is now inaccurate because of the recognition that the neurologic features of CP often change or progress over time. In addition, although CP is often associated with epilepsy and abnormalities of speech, vision, and intellect, it is the selective vulnerability of the brain's motor systems that defines the disorder. Many children and adults with CP function at a high educational and vocational level, without any sign of the type of cognitive dysfunction that is generally implied by the term *encephalopathy*.

○   **How is CP classified?**

The subtypes of cerebral palsy are defined according to the predominant muscle tone abnormality, its distribution and severity. There is widespread agreement that CP subtypes should be divided into the following groups. Spastic subtypes (hemiplegia: unilateral asymmetric spasticity; diplegia: bilateral symmetric spasticity, lower limbs more affected than upper limbs; quadriplegia: bilateral symmetric spasticity, upper and lower limbs affected equally), dystonic or athetotic type; and other miscellaneous types: hypotonic, mixed types, etc. The relative distributions are as follows:
1.   Quadriplegia (10-15%): All 4 extremities are affected equally along with the trunk.
2.   Diplegia (30-40%): Lower extremities are affected to a greater degree than the upper extremities.
3.   Hemiplegia (20-30%): Involvement is observed on 1 side of the body, including an arm and a leg.
4.   Monoplegia (rare): Involvement is noted in 1 limb, either an arm or a leg.
5.   Dyskinetic, 10-15% of cases
6.   Ataxic, <5% of cases

○   **Summarize in table format**

Classification of Cerebral Palsy and Major Causes

Motor Syndrome	Neuropathology	Major Causes
Spastic Diplegia	Periventricular Leukomalacia (periventricular leukomalacia [PVL])	Prematurity Ischemia Infection Endocrine/metabolic (e.g., thyroid)
Spastic quadriplegia	PVL Multicystic encephalomalacia Malformations	Ischemia Infection Endocrine/metabolic Genetic/developmental
Hemiplegia	Stoke: in utero or neonatal	Thrombophilic disorders Infection Genetic/developmental Periventricular hemorrhagic infarction
Extrapyramidal (athetoid, dyskinetic)	Basal ganglia Pathology: putamen, globus pallidus, thalamus	Asphyxia Kernicterus Mitochondrial Genetic/metabolic

O   **What is the pathophysiology of CP?**

CP is caused by an insult to the immature brain at any time prior to birth up to 2 years of age. Cerebral insult produces alterations in muscle tone, muscle stretch reflexes, primitive reflexes, and postural reactions. Other associated symptoms may be involved secondary to the neurological insult (eg, mental retardation, vision and hearing problems, seizures). The etiology of such cerebral insults includes vascular, hypoxic-ischemic, metabolic, infectious, toxic, teratogenic, traumatic, and genetic causes. The pathogenesis of CP involves multifactorial causes, but much is still unknown. Different mechanisms of CP pathogenesis have been associated with preterm and term births.

O   **What is the incidence of CP?**

The incidence of CP in Europe, North America and Australasia is estimated to be 2.5 per thousand live births.

O   **What age range is affected?**

Initial insult occurs between birth and age 2 years, but children usually are not diagnosed until after 1 year of age, as they fail to meet developmental milestones.

O   **What history does the CP patient typically present with?**

The child with CP can present after failing to meet expected developmental milestones or failing to suppress obligatory primitive reflexes. Abnormal muscle tone is the most frequently observed symptom. The child may present as either hypotonic or hypertonic with either decreased or increased resistance to passive movements, respectively. Children with CP may have an early period of hypotonia followed by hypertonia. Definite hand preference before the age of 1 year is common (especially in hemiplegic patients). Asymmetric crawl or failure to crawl also may suggest CP. Growth disturbance also is noted in children with CP.

O   **What physical findings are encountered in the patient with CP?**

Joint contractures secondary to spastic muscles, hypotonic-to-spastic tone, and growth delay; persistent primitive reflexes (eg, Moro reflex, asymmetric tonic neck, symmetric tonic neck, palmar grasp, tonic labyrinthine, foot placement) are noted. Moro reflex & tonic labyrinthine should extinguish by the time the infant is aged 4-6 months, palmar grasp by 5-6 months, asymmetric & symmetric tonic neck by 6-7 months, and foot placement before 12 months.

O   **What observations are made with regard to gait?**

Hip - Assess for excessive flexion, adduction, and femoral anteversion.
Knee - Flexion and extension with valgus or varus stress.
Foot - Equinus or toe walking and varus or valgus of the hindfoot.
Gait abnormalities may include crouch position with tight hip flexors and hamstrings, weak quadriceps, and/or excessive dorsiflexion.

O   **What are the physical attributes of Spastic quadriplegia?**

It is the most severe form of CP because of marked motor impairment of all extremities and the high association with mental retardation and seizures. Swallowing difficulties are common as a result of supranuclear bulbar palsies, often leading to aspiration pneumonia. The most common lesions seen on pathologic examination or on MRI scanning are severe PVL and multicystic cortical encephalomalacia. Neurologic examination shows increased tone and spasticity in all extremities, decreased spontaneous movements, brisk reflexes, and plantar extensor responses. Flexion contractures of the knees and elbows are often present by late childhood. Associated developmental disabilities, including speech and visual abnormalities, are particularly prevalent in this group of children. Children with spastic quadriparesis often have evidence of athetosis and may be classified as having mixed CP.

O   **What are the physical attributes of dyskinetic CP?**

Athetoid CP, also called *choreoathetoid* or *extrapyramidal* CP, is less common than spastic cerebral palsy. Affected infants are characteristically hypotonic with poor head control and marked head lag and develop increased variable tone with rigidity and dystonia over several years. Feeding may be difficult, and tongue thrust and drooling may be prominent. Speech is typically affected because the oropharyngeal muscles are involved. Speech may be absent or sentences are slurred, and voice modulation is impaired. Generally, upper motor neuron signs are not present, seizures are uncommon, and intellect is preserved in many patients. This form of CP is also referred to as dyskinetic CP in Europe and is the type most likely to be associated with birth asphyxia. Extrapyramidal CP secondary to acute intrapartum near total asphyxia is associated with bilaterally symmetric lesions in the posterior putamen and ventrolateral thalamus. Athetoid CP can also be caused by kernicterus secondary to high levels of bilirubin, and in this case the MRI scan shows lesions in the globus pallidus bilaterally.

O   **What clinical features are encountered in the patient with spastic diplegia?**

Spastic diplegia is bilateral spasticity of the legs greater than in the arms. The first indication of spastic diplegia is often noted when an affected infant begins to crawl. The child uses the arms in a normal reciprocal fashion but tends to drag the legs behind more as a rudder (commando crawl) rather than using the normal four limbed crawling movement. If the spasticity is severe, application of a diaper is difficult because of the excessive adduction of the hips. Examination of the child reveals spasticity in the legs with brisk reflexes, ankle clonus, and a bilateral Babinski sign. When the child is suspended by the axillae, a scissoring posture of the lower extremities is maintained. Walking is significantly delayed, the feet are held in a position of equinovarus, and the child walks on tiptoes. The prognosis for normal intellectual development is excellent for these patients, and the likelihood of seizures is minimal.

O   **What clinical features are encountered in the patient with spastic hemiplegia?**

Infants with *spastic hemiplegia* have decreased spontaneous movements on the affected side and show hand preference at a very early age. The arm is often more involved than the leg and difficulty in hand manipulation is obvious by 1 yr. of age. Walking is usually delayed until 18–24 mo, and a circumductive gait is apparent. Examination of the extremities may show growth arrest, particularly in the hand and thumbnail, especially if the contralateral parietal lobe is abnormal, because extremity growth is influenced by this area of the brain. Spasticity is apparent in the affected extremities, particularly the ankle, causing an equinovarus deformity of the foot. An affected child often walks on tiptoes because of the increased tone, and the affected upper extremity assumes a dystonic posture when the child runs. Ankle clonus and a Babinski sign may be present, the deep tendon reflexes are increased, and weakness of the hand and foot dorsiflexors is evident. About one third of patients with spastic hemiplegia have a seizure disorder that usually develops during the first year or two, and approximately 25% have cognitive abnormalities including mental retardation.

O   **What does brain imaging reveal in these patients?**

A CT scan or MRI study may show an atrophic cerebral hemisphere with a dilated lateral ventricle contralateral to the side of the affected extremities. An MRI is far more sensitive than CT for most lesions seen with CP, although a CT scan may be useful for detecting calcifications associated with congenital infections.

O   **What are risk factors selective to spastic hemiplegia?**

Focal cerebral infarction secondary to intrauterine or perinatal thromboembolism related to thrombophilic disorders, especially anticardiolipin antibodies, is an important cause of hemiplegic CP. Family histories suggestive of thrombosis and inherited clotting disorders may be present and evaluation of the mother may provide information valuable for future pregnancies and other family members.

O   **What are the prenatal causes of CP?**

Intrauterine infections, Congenital malformations, Toxic or teratogenic agents, Multiple births, Abdominal trauma, Maternal illness.

O   **What are the causes of neonatal CP?**

Prematurity (less than 32 weeks gestation), Birth weight less than 2500 g, Growth retardation, Intracranial hemorrhage, Trauma, Infection, Bradycardia and hypoxia, Seizures , Hyperbilirubinemia , Abnormal birthing presentations.

O   **What are postnatal causes of CP?**

Trauma, Infection, Intracranial hemorrhage, Coagulopathies.

O   **What laboratory tests are indicated for the patient with suspected CP?**

Thyroid studies, Lactate level, Pyruvate level, Organic and amino acids, Chromosomes, Cerebrospinal protein levels may assist in determining asphyxia in the neonatal period. Protein levels can be elevated along with an elevated lactate to pyruvate ratio.

O   **What Imaging Studies are indicated for the patient with suspected CP?**

Neuroimaging studies can help to evaluate brain damage and to determine those at risk of developing CP.. Ultrasound in the neonate provides information about the ventricular system, basal ganglia, and corpus callosum, as well as diagnostic information on intraventricular hemorrhage and hypoxic-ischemic injury to the periventricular white matter. Periventricular leukomalacia initially is an echodense area that converts to an echolucent area when the patient reaches the approximate age of 2 weeks. Computed tomography (CT) scan provides information to help diagnose congenital malformations, intracranial hemorrhages, and periventricular leukomalacia, especially in the infant. Magnetic resonance imaging (MRI) is most useful after 2-3 weeks of life. MRI is the best study for assessing white matter disease in an older child.

O   **What is the role for electrodiagnostic testing in CP?**

Evoked potentials are used to evaluate the anatomic pathways of the auditory and visual systems. Electroencephalogram (EEG) is useful in evaluating severe hypoxic-ischemic injury. Initially, evidence of marked suppression of amplitude and slowing is followed by a discontinuous pattern of voltage suppression with bursts of high-voltage sharp and slow waves at 24-48 hours.

O   **What other tests are indicated?**

Hearing and vision screens.

O   **What therapeutic exercises are appropriate for the patient with CP?**

Daily ranges of motion (ROM) exercises are important to prevent or delay contractures secondary to spasticity and to maintain mobility of joints and soft tissues. Stretching exercises are performed to increase motion. Teach progressive resistance exercises to increase strength. Age appropriate play and adaptive toys and games using the desired exercises are important to elicit the child's full cooperation. Strengthening knee extensor muscles helps to improve crouching and stride length. Postural and motor control training is important following the normal developmental sequence of children (i.e., achieve head and neck control if possible before advancing to trunk control).

O   **What are the rehabilitation goals in CP?**

Treatment is aimed at improving infant-caregiver interaction, giving family support, supplying resources, and parental education, as well as at promoting motor and developmental skills. Teach the parent or caregiver the exercises or activities necessary to help the child reach his or her full potential.

O   **What rehabilitation strategies are taken into consideration when devising a treatment plan?**

Always keep the child's developmental age in mind and use adaptive equipment as needed to help attain these milestones. For example, if a child is developmentally ready to stand and explore the environment but is limited by lack of motor control, encourage use of a stander to enable them to facilitate achievement of milestones. Encourage performance at a level of success to maintain the child's interest and cooperation. Order assistive devices and durable medical equipment to attain function that may not be possible otherwise. Orthoses frequently are required to maintain functional joint position especially in the non-ambulatory or hemiplegic patients. Frequent reevaluation of orthotic devices is important as children quickly outgrow them and can undergo skin breakdown from improper use of orthotic devices.

O   **What is Hippo therapy?**

Hippo therapy (horseback riding therapy) is frequently a well-liked therapy of parents and patients alike to help work on tone, ROM, strength, coordination, and balance. Hippo therapy offers many potential cognitive, physical, and emotional benefits.

O   **What is the role for speech therapy in regard to the CP patient?**

Many children with dyskinetic CP have involvement of the face and oropharynx causing dysphagia, drooling, and dysarthria. Speech therapy can be implemented to help improve swallowing and communication. Some children benefit from augmentative communication devices if they have some motor control and adequate cognitive skills. Those patients with athetoid CP may benefit the most from speech therapy as most have normal intelligence and communication is an obstacle secondary to the athetosis affecting their speech. Adequate communication is probably the most important goal for enhancing function in the athetoid CP patient.

O   **What pulmonary complications may arise in the CP patient?**

Pulmonary complications eg, aspiration, oro motor dysfunction may be encountered. Bronchopulmonary dysplasia may be seen in premature infants.

O   **What dental problems may arise in the CP patient?**

O   Dental problems (eg, enamel dysgenesis, malocclusion, caries, and gingival hyperplasia).

O   **What gastrointestinal problems may arise in the CP patient?**

Gastrointestinal symptoms (eg, reflux, constipation) and/or dysphagia may cause failure to thrive, resulting in growth failure. Patients may require a gastrostomy tube (G-tube) or a jejunostomy tube (J-tube) to augment nutrition.

O   **What nutritional problems may arise in the CP patient?**

Nutrition consultation should be done early and periodically to ensure proper growth. Parents and the medical professionals must keep on top of the potential nutritional difficulties in these children.

O   **What other CNS problems are encountered in the CP patient?**

Mental retardation is seen in 30-50% of children with CP, most commonly associated with spastic quadriplegia. Hearing loss is encountered in children with hyperbilirubinemia.

O   **What orthopedic surgical procedures may be indicated in the patient with CP?**

Scoliosis repair, Hip relocation surgery for dislocations, Tendon lengthening or transfer to decrease spastic muscle imbalance and deforming forces, Osteotomy to realign limb (eg, femoral neck, tibia, calcaneus).

O   **What is the role for Intrathecal baclofen pump therapy?**

Appropriate candidates for intrathecal infusion should have an Ashworth score of 3 or higher in the lower extremity and must have enough body mass at a minimum age to support the pump. Although these are estimated at 40 pounds and 4 years, younger age groups and patients with less weight have been successfully implanted. The development of subfascial placements has contributed to this wider indication. Patients who benefit from ITB include those who have poor underlying strength whose extremity movements are impeded by spasticity, nonambulatory spastic quadriparetics whose spasticity interferes with daily living skills, nonfunctional patients for whom the goal is to enhance quality of caregiving, and patients who have dystonia or other movement disorders.

O   **When is Selective posterior rhizotomy utilized?**

The best candidates are children 3 to 7 years old who have spastic diplegia, good trunk control, and isolated leg movements. These individuals typically have significant weakness after the procedure and require extensive therapy. If they have significant underlying weakness beforehand and the spasticity is removed, they do not have functional improvement.

O   **What is the role for chemo denervation inpatients with CP?**

Phenol intramuscular neurolysis and botulinum toxin intramuscular blocks reduce spasticity for 3-6 months. The botulinum toxin is dose-limiting to 12 mg/kg per visit. The larger muscles may not respond to this limiting dose, or quite often, patients need several muscles done at each visit. Phenol can be used for some of the larger muscles or when doing several muscles, but is more difficult to perform, and in certain nerves, phenol can cause unpleasant sensory dysesthesias.

O   **What seating/locomotion considerations are necessary in the patient with CP?**

A manual wheelchair may be needed with seating adaptations to keep the back straight and the hips from excessive adduction or abduction. The early introduction of independent mobility is important, as the ability to explore one's environment has been demonstrated to improve self-esteem. A power wheelchair may be needed for children with severe spasticity or athetosis. A power wheelchair can be introduced to children aged 3 years with normal intelligence. Walkers also may be prescribed to enhance mobility. Any child with the ability and/or desire to ambulate should be given every chance. A posterior walker promotes a more upright posture than the traditional walkers.

O   **What are the benefits of serial casting in patients with CP?**

Casting and splinting for 2-3 months can improve ROM of a joint and decrease tone for 3-4 months. This is particularly completed at the ankles to help with plantar flexion contractures, but it also can be done on any contracted joint to provide a slow progressive stretch.

O   **What is the prognosis for Spastic quadriplegic patients?**

Twenty five percent of patients have minimal or no functional limitation in ambulation and self care. Fifty percent of patients have moderate impairment and are not independent but are able to function. Twenty five percent of patients are impaired severely, require complete care, and are not ambulatory.

O   **What is the prognosis for Dyskinetic patients?**

Fifty percent of patients are ambulatory.

O   **What is the prognosis for Hemiplegic patients?**

Most patients with CP become independent in activities of daily living (ADL) but may need assistive devices; most become ambulatory.

O   **What is the prognosis for Spastic diplegic and quadriplegic patients?**

Molnar's study (1976) reports that patients with CP who sat by the age of 2 years eventually walked. Suppression of obligatory primitive reflex activity by 18-24 months provides a sensitive indicator to distinguish children who ultimately walked from those who would not be expected to walk.

O   **What clinical problems occur among CP patients during adulthood?**

The general health of persons aging with CP is reported to be fairly good. However, an increased incidence of bowel and bladder dysfunction with urinary tract infections (UTIs),oral motor and dental disorders, fractures fatigue, gastroesophageal reflux, problematic spasticity, pain, progressive musculoskeletal deformity and dysfunction deterioration of functional ambulation, and progressive cervical spine degeneration complicated by radiculopathy or myelopathy have been noted as people age.

MYELOMENINGOCELE

O   **What is myelomeningocele?**

Myelomeningocele is a complex malformation of the spinal cord, nerve roots, meninges, vertebral bodies, and skin. This neural tube defect is a common congenital anomaly and typically is referred to as spina bifida. This condition results from failure of the neural tube to close in the developing fetus. Medical, surgical, and rehabilitation issues arise in the patient with myelomeningocele from birth through adulthood.

O   **What is the pathophysiology of myelomeningocele?**

Myelomeningocele is the result of a teratogenic process causing failed closure and abnormal differentiation of the embryonic neural tube during the first 4 weeks of gestation. Abnormal development of the posterior caudal neural tube produces spinal cord damage, or myelodysplasia. The anatomic level of the spinal cord lesion roughly correlates with the patient's neurologic, motor, and sensory deficits. Abnormal development of the cephalic anterior tube gives rise to central nervous system (CNS) anomalies.

O   **What is the Arnold Chiari Type II malformation ?**

The Arnold Chiari Type II malformation is characterized by cerebellar hypoplasia and varying degrees of caudal displacement of the hindbrain into the upper cervical canal through the foramen magnum. This deformity impedes the flow and absorption of cerebrospinal fluid (CSF) and causes hydrocephalus, which occurs in more than 90% of infants with myelomeningocele.

O   **What other neuropathological findings can occur?**

Cerebral cortex dysplasia, including heterotopias, polymicrogyria, abnormal lamination, fused thalami, and corpus callosum abnormalities, also occurs frequently.

O   **What other anomalies occur with myelomeningocele?**

Myelomeningocele often occurs with multiple system congenital anomalies. Commonly associated anomalies are facial clefts, heart malformations, and genitourinary tract anomalies. Urinary tract anomalies, such as solitary kidney or malformed ureters, may contribute to increased morbidity in the presence of neurogenic bladder dysfunction. Mesodermal structures surrounding the neural tube, such as the vertebra and ribs, also may be malformed. Mesodermal structure anomalies may lead to congenital or early onset kyphotic and scoliotic deformities.

O   **What is the incidence of myelomeningocele?**

Myelomeningocele is the most common major birth defect. Birth prevalence of the disease was reported to be 4.4-4.6 cases per 10,000 live births from 1983-1990. The highest estimated rates of myelomeningocele in the US are found in Appalachia.

O   **What morbidity and mortality occur with myelomeningocele?**

In the US, the leading identified cause of infant death is birth defects, and myelomeningocele is one of the most common birth defects. Mortality rates reported for infants who are untreated for myelomeningocele range from 90-100% based on several series of studies dating from the turn of the century through recent years. Most untreated infants die within the first year of life. Death in the first 2 years of life for those untreated usually results from hydrocephalus or intracranial infection. The likelihood that a 2-month-old infant untreated for myelomeningocele lives to be 7 years is only 28%.

O   **How have survival rates improved?**

Survival rates for infants born with myelomeningocele have improved dramatically with the introduction of antibiotics and developments in the neurosurgical treatment of hydrocephalus. Early death in both treated and untreated patients is associated with advanced hydrocephalus and multiple system congenital anomalies. In the US, antibiotics, sac closure, and ventriculoperitoneal shunt placement are the standard of care and are implemented in the perinatal period in 93-95% of patients. Supportive care only may be recommended in cases where there is an irreparable sac; active gross CNS infection or bleeding; and/or other gross congenital organ anomalies causing life-threatening problems.

O   **What neurological morbidity is encountered in patients with myelomeningocele?**

Paraplegia from the myelodysplasia typically causes some impairment of mobility along with neurogenic bowel and bladder. Other neurologic deficits may present acutely or chronically at birth or later. These deficits can be related to hydrocephalus, Arnold Chiari II malformation, or a variety of intraspinal pathologies. Seizures occur in 10-30% of affected children and adolescents. These seizures can be related to brain malformation, or they may be a sign of shunt malfunction or infection.

O   **What additional systemic morbidity occurs in patients with myelomeningocele ?**

Musculoskeletal deterioration may be caused by progressive bony and joint deformities, pathologic fractures, and muscle deterioration. Renal compromise occurs because of problems related to neurogenic bladder. Despite advances in the management of neurogenic bladder, renal failure is still the leading cause of death in patients with myelomeningocele after the first year of life.

O   **What physical findings are evident at birth?**

At birth, a midline defect in the posterior elements of the vertebrae is noted with protrusion of the meninges and neural elements through an external dural sac. The obvious physical manifestation of myelomeningocele is paraplegia caused from spinal cord malformation. Myelomeningocele patients frequently are described as belonging to certain groups, based on the motor or neurosegmental lesion level. This approach is useful for general functional prognosis and anticipation of specific musculoskeletal complications.

O   **What are the findings in the thoracic group of myelomeningocele?**

In the thoracic group, innervation of the upper limb and neck musculature and variable function of trunk musculature are present with no volitional lower limb movements. Patients with thoracic malformations tend to have more involvement of the CNS and associated cognitive deficits.

O   **What are the findings in the high lumbar group of myelomeningocele?**

In the high-lumbar group, variable hip flexor and hip adductor strength is characteristic, and absence of hip extensors, hip abductors, and all knee and ankle movements are noted.

○ **What are the findings in the low lumbar group of myelomeningocele?**

In the low-lumbar group, hip flexor, adductor, medial hamstring, and quadriceps strength is present; strength of the lateral hamstrings, hip abductors, and ankle dorsiflexors is variable; and strength of the ankle plantar flexors is absent. In the sacral level group, strength of all hip and knee groups is present, and ankle plantar flexor strength is variable.

○ **What characterizes the muscle tone in myelomeningocele?**

Muscle tone in any of these groups of patients with myelomeningocele usually is flaccid; however, up to two thirds exhibit some upper motoneuron signs, with only 9% demonstrating a true spastic paraparesis.

○ **What is responsible for the presence of impaired upper extremity coordination?**

Lack of upper limb coordination is common, especially in patients with hydrocephalus. This lack of coordination also may be related to Arnold Chiari II malformation, motor-learning deficits, and/or delayed development of hand dominance. Affected children have problems with fine motor tasks, particularly when timed. New onset weakness in the upper extremities may be a hallmark of progressive neurologic dysfunction.

○ **Are spinal and lower extremity deformities occur in myelomeningocele?**

Spinal and lower extremity deformities and joint contractures are prevalent in children with myelomeningocele. Multiple factors may be involved, including intrauterine positioning, other congenital malformations, muscle imbalances, progressive neurologic dysfunction, poor postural habits, and reduced or absent joint motion.

○ **What musculoskeletal deformities occur in the patient with myelomeningocele?**

The musculoskeletal deformities that occur are related to the functional level of the lesion. Thoracic and high-lumbar groups tend to have increased incidence of lumbar lordosis, hip abduction and external rotation contractures, knee flexion, and equinus contractures of the ankles. Unopposed hip flexion and adduction contractures in the high-lumbar group frequently result in dislocated hips. The mid and low lumbar groups often have hip and knee flexion contractures, increased lumbar lordosis, genu and calcaneal valgus malalignment, and over pronated feet. Patients in the sacral group often exhibit mild hip and knee flexion contractures and increased lumbar lordosis with various ankle and foot positions.

○ **Does scoliosis occur in patients with myelomeningocele?**

Scoliosis can be congenital or acquired. The congenital form is associated with underlying vertebral anomalies. The acquired form develops in 40-60% of children with myelomeningocele and is related to muscle imbalances. Increased lumbar lordosis and kyphosis of the entire spine or localized to the lumbar region also are observed. All the spinal deformities occur more frequently in groups with higher spinal lesions.

○ **Are cranial nerve palsies encountered in patients with myelomeningocele?**

Ocular muscle palsies, swallowing and eating problems, and abnormal phonation are signs of cranial nerve dysfunction. These symptoms may be related to Arnold Chiari II malformation, hydrocephalus, and/or brainstem dysplasia. Thus the cranial nerve palsies include IV, IX, X.

○ **What is the pathogenesis of myelomeningocele?**

The etiology in most cases of myelomeningocele is multifactorial, involving genetic, racial, and environmental factors. Other offspring in a family with one affected child are at increased risk of neural tube defect than children without affected siblings. The risk is 1 in 20-30 for subsequent pregnancies, and if 2 children are affected, the risk becomes 1 in 2. Most infants born with myelomeningocele are born to mothers with no previously affected children. A small number of cases are linked to specific etiologic factors. Up to 10% of fetuses with a neural tube defect detected in early gestation have an associated chromosome abnormality. Associated chromosome abnormalities include trisomies 13 and 18, triploidy, and single gene mutations. Maternal risk factors include insulin-dependent diabetes mellitus (IDDM) and hypothermia. Intrauterine drug exposures to valproate, carbamazepine, and drugs to induce ovulation are identified risk factors.

○ What is the association between folic acid and neural tube defects?

Prior to 1991, most neural tube defects occurred without identification of a specific cause. Research in the 1980s showed correction of folic acid deficiency as an effective means of primary and recurrent prevention. After 1991, 50% of cases of neural tube defects are related to a nutritional deficiency of folic acid and, thus, are preventable .In September 1992, the US Public Health Service (USPHS) recommended intake of folic acid at a dosage of 0.4 mg/d for all women anticipating pregnancy .In February 1996, the USPHS announced mandatory folic acid fortification of enriched cereal grain, a measure expected to increase the daily intake of folic acid in women of reproductive age by approximately 100 mcg/d. The ACOG recommends 0.4 mg folate daily, beginning at least 1 month prior to conception. In women who have had a child with a prior NTD, 4 mg daily is recommended.

○ What laboratory studies are indicated in patients with myelomeningocele?

Laboratory screening tests for neural tube defects can be performed through 2 methods, blood tests and amniocentesis, typically used in combination. Myelomeningocele can be detected in 99% of affected fetuses through combined use of these tests. Perform urinalysis, urine culture, and serum urea nitrogen creatinine test at birth to evaluate renal function. Recommend regular bacterial urinary cultures for children who have vesicoureteral reflux or signs and symptoms of urinary tract infection.

○ What role does ultrasound play in the assessment of myelomeningocele?

Some centers use fetal ultrasound as the primary screening tool for neural tube defects, usually at approximately 18 weeks gestational age. This trend reflects the increasing sophistication of fetal ultrasonographic technology. The procedure avoids the roughly 1% risk of abortion following amniocentesis, but accurate diagnosis depends on the skill and experience of the operator and the quality of the equipment. With ultrasonography, myelomeningocele may be detected during scanning of the fetal head for subtle changes in the cranial and cerebellar configurations.

○ What are the limitations of ultrasound in the diagnosis of myelomeningocele?

Currently, ultrasonography is not sensitive enough to provide reliable and accurate detection of the level of the defect. After confirmation of fetal myelomeningocele; clinicians at most tertiary care centers perform weekly ultrasonographic examinations to observe the growth and development of the fetus. More recent studies suggest that most cases are diagnosed either after the 24th week of gestation or they remain undiagnosed until after birth.

○ What value is there in performing a caesarian section?

A caesarean section before rupture of the amniotic membranes and onset of labor has been shown to reduce the degree of paralysis in fetuses with myelomeningocele. Improving ultrasound accuracy for detection of the defect level may help identify mothers and infants most likely to benefit from an elective caesarean section.

○ What strategies are considered in the physical rehabilitation of the patient with myelomeningocele in the first year?

General functional expectations have been developed for patients in each lesion-level group to help direct physical therapy goals within an appropriate developmental context from infancy through adulthood. In managing the cases of newborns with myelomeningocele, the physical therapist establishes a baseline of muscle function. As the child develops, the physical therapist monitors joint alignment, muscle imbalances, contractures, posture, and signs of progressive neurologic dysfunction. The physical therapist also provides caregivers with instruction in handling and positioning techniques and recommends orthotic positioning devices to prevent soft tissue contractures. The therapy programs should be designed to parallel the normal achievement of gross motor milestones. Provide the infant with sitting opportunities to facilitate the development of head and trunk control.

O   What strategies are considered in the physical rehabilitation of the patient with myelomeningocele after the first year?

Near the end of the first year of life, provide the child with an effective means of independent mobility in conjunction with therapeutic exercises that promote trunk control and balance. For patients who are not likely to become ambulatory, place emphasis on developing proficiency in wheelchair skills. For patients who are predicted to ambulate, pre gait training should begin with use of a parapodium or swivel walker. Exercise or household distance ambulation may be pursued with use of traditional long leg braces (eg, hip-knee-ankle-foot orthosis, knee-ankle-foot orthosis) or the reciprocating gait orthosis [RGO]). Teach the school-aged child community-level wheelchair mobility skills, emphasizing efficiency and safety. The physical therapist assists with assessment of the community, home, and school environments to determine whether architectural barriers exist that may interfere with the child's daily activities.

O   What treatment strategies are used in patients with urinary tract pathology?

Treatment strategies are designed both to prevent deterioration of renal function and to establish infection free social continence. These goals can be accomplished by several different methods of bladder drainage, including vesicostomy, intermittent catheterization, and placement of indwelling catheters. Long term maintenance of low bladder pressures may require the adjunctive use of medications to reduce bladder pressures and/or decrease spastic or hypotonic sphincter function. The success rate of intermittent catheterization and/or anticholinergic medications in achieving continence is estimated to reach 70-80%.

O   Is there a role for intrauterine repair of a myelomeningocele?

Studies of intrauterine repair of the myelomeningocele suggest that this procedure may decrease development of hindbrain herniation and significant hydrocephalus without changing the motor outcome, despite decreased exposure injury to the dysplastic cord.

O   What strategies are considered in the occupational therapy of the patient with myelomeningocele after the first year?

Fine motor skills and independence with activities of daily living (ADL) often are impaired. Initiate training early to compensate for these deficits and progress along the developmental sequence as closely as possible. Upper extremity stabilization and dexterous hand use require adequate postural control of the head and trunk. In the first year of life, encourage development of these postural mechanisms or substitute passive support, if necessary, to promote eye-hand coordination and manipulatory skills. When adequate fine motor skills have been achieved, the occupational therapist provides instructions for use of adaptive equipment and alternative methods for self-care and other ADL for preschool and school-aged children.

O   What impact does myelomeningocele have on genitourinary function?

Disruption of the neural axis between the pons and the sacral spinal cord by the myelomeningocele may cause uninhibited detrusor contractions or dyssynergia, a lack of coordination of the external bladder sphincter that causes involuntary sphincter activity during detrusor contraction. Myelomeningocele in the sacral area can produce a lower motor neuron lesion, resulting in detrusor areflexia. These abnormalities may occur singly or in combination and typically result in incontinence and impaired bladder emptying that can lead to vesicoureteral reflux and high-voiding pressures. If untreated, this condition can lead to potentially more serious complications, including frequent infections, upper urinary tract deterioration, and, ultimately, renal failure.

O   What is the most common urinary tract problem in patients with myelomeningocele?

A high incidence of vesicoureteral reflux and ureteral dilation is found in patients with myelomeningocele whose leak-point pressures were greater than 40 cm H_2O. High pressures may result from increased outlet resistance or decreased bladder wall compliance. Increased outlet resistance may be caused by sphincter dyssynergia or fibrosis of a denervated sphincter. Decreased bladder wall compliance is associated with areflexia of the detrusor. Any of these urologic dysfunctions can occur in myelomeningocele, but manifestations may vary over time because of the changing neurologic status in some of these patients.

O   **What bowel problems occur in patients with myelomeningocele?**

Abnormal anal sphincter function and anorectal sensation are associated with myelomeningocele involving spinal segments S2-S4. Many individuals with myelomeningocele, therefore, do not have the sensation and control needed to defecate volitionally. The result is bowel incontinence, often with related problems of constipation and impaction. Fecal incontinence can become a serious barrier in attending school, obtaining employment, or sustaining an intimate relationship.

O   **What do assisted bowel programs achieve in patients with myelomeningocele?**

Assisted bowel programs designed to empty the bowels regularly can establish social continence and prevent constipation. Develop a regimen for bowel movements, usually on a daily or every other day basis. These programs typically attempt to take advantage of the gastrocolic reflex by timing the bowel movement after a meal, typically breakfast or dinner. Some patients are able to use the Valsalva maneuver to defecate, but some may need the assistance of digital stimulation, a stimulant suppository, and/or an expansion enema. Use of these techniques can help to achieve proper timing of the bowel movement and complete evacuation. A high-fiber diet, sometimes in combination with use of stool softeners, may help to optimize stool size and consistency.

O   **When is surgical closure of the myelomeningocele performed?**

Closure of the myelomeningocele is performed immediately after birth if external CSF leakage is present and typically within the first 24 - 48 hours in the absence of CSF leakage. The surgery can be delayed for several days without additional morbidity or mortality. A delay gives families more time to deal with the shock and learn about the condition to enable them to participate to a greater degree in the decision-making process.

O   **What does the surgery accomplish?**

Steps in the closure procedure include extensive undermining of the skin, dissection of the neural plaque that is replaced into the spinal canal, and meticulous watertight closure of the dura, fascia, subcutaneous tissues, and skin.

O   **What are the surgical complications?**

Perioperative complications include wound infection, CNS infection, delayed wound healing, CSF leakage, additional neurologic damage to the cauda equina, and acute hydrocephalus. Long term complications include cord tethering and progressive hydrocephalus.

O   **Do patients with myelomeningocele develop hydrocephalus?**

Approximately 25-35% or more of children with myelomeningocele are born with hydrocephalus, and an additional 60-70% of patients with myelomeningocele develop hydrocephalus after closure of the back lesion. Hydrocephalus can cause expansion of the ventricles and loss of cerebral cortex and is associated with a considerable decline in intellectual function.

O   **Is shunting required?**

In a few cases, the hydrocephalus arrests spontaneously, but, in most cases, shunting is required. Ventriculoperitoneal shunting is the preferred modality. Alternatives include ventriculoatrial and ventriculopleural shunting.

O   **What are the perioperative complications?**

Perioperative complications include intracerebral and/or intraventricular hemorrhage, bowel perforation, and infection. Long-term complications include infection, overdrainage or under drainage, and obstruction of the shunt system.

O   **What concerns are there for patients with the Patients with the Arnold Chiari Type II malformation?**

Arnold Chiari Type II may present with signs and symptoms of acute or subacute brainstem and/or upper cervical cord compression. Surgical intervention for Arnold Chiari Type II malformation necessitates an occipital craniotomy and cervical laminectomy.

O   **What hip pathology can occur in myelomeningocele patients?**

Paralytic muscle imbalance around the hip joints may lead to progressive hip dislocation, which typically occurs in early childhood in patients with high- and mid-lumbar lesions and in late childhood or adolescence in children with low-lumbar lesions. The literature evaluating the benefits of surgical relocation of hips reflects ongoing controversy surrounding the topic. For bilaterally dislocated hips, questionable functional benefit of surgery exists for patients with L3 and L4 lesions. Surgery for unilateral dislocation of the hip may not be indicated for patients who are nonambulatory or have high-level lesions.

O   **What spinal malformations occur in myelomeningocele?**

Spinal deformities are common, and progressive kyphosis or scoliosis may lead to decline in functional status, as well as increased risk for development of decubiti and potential cardiopulmonary compromise. Spinal stabilization is necessary to correct kyphosis, which may be related to congenital vertebral malformation or may be a result of the collapsing spine in high-thoracic paraplegia. Paralytic scoliosis develops in 40-60% of children with spinal deformities caused by myelomeningocele and may be the result of asymmetric muscle forces, unilateral hip dislocation and pelvic obliquity, or an underlying progressive neurologic process such as syringohydromyelia. Intervention to introduce use of orthotic devices may serve as a temporizing measure, but growing children with spinal curves greater than 30-35° require surgical fusion.

O   **What knee problems occur in myelomeningocele patients?**

Common knee deformities include flexion and extension contractures, usually related to a capsular contracture. Surgery is indicated when the contracture causes a functional problem. Types of surgery include a simple tenotomy of the knee flexor tendons in the child with a high-level lesion or lengthening of the tendons in the child with a low-lumbar or sacral level lesion, for which preservation of hamstring function is important. Extension contractures are less common, but they interfere with sitting and are associated with hip dislocation and clubfoot. If the contracture is not amenable to conservative measures (eg, serial casting), an extensor tendon release is performed.

O   **What is tibial torsion and how is it managed?**

The most common rotational deformities seen in myelomeningocele are internal and external tibial torsion. Some malformations improve with growth and/or use of bracing. If improvement is not noted by the age of 6 years, recommend derotation osteotomy with plate fixation, but complications (eg, nonunion, delayed union, infection) are common. Postoperative care requires immobilization for 6-8 weeks.

O   **What foot and ankle deformities occur in myelomeningocele patients and how are they managed?**

In the case of clubfoot, most patients need surgical correction in the first year of life, usually involving multiple soft tissue release procedures with tendon excisions. In older children, other types of deformities (eg, adduction, calcaneovarus, and calcaneovalgus) may require muscle tendon transfer, tenotomy, and/or osteotomy to decrease the paralytic muscle imbalances and achieve a supple plantigrade foot that can tolerate a brace. Triple arthrodesis rarely is indicated but may be necessary in cases of ankle instability.

O   **What is the tethered cord syndrome?**

Tethered cord syndrome is related to the tendency for the spinal cord to adhere to the meningocele repair and prevent the normal cephalad migration of the cord during growth.

O   **What are the clinical symptoms of tethered cord syndrome?**

Magnetic resonance imaging (MRI) shows signs of tethering of the spinal cord in most children with myelomeningocele, but only approximately 30% have clinical manifestations. Symptoms can include pain, sensory changes, spasticity, and progressive scoliosis.

O   **What are the clinical signs associated with tethered cord syndrome?**

Clinical signs are variable, but the most consistent are (1) loss of motor function, (2) development of spasticity in the lower extremities, primarily the medial hamstrings and ankle dorsiflexors and evertors, (3) development of scoliosis before the age of 6 years in the absence of congenital anomalies of the vertebral bodies, (4) back pain and increased lumbar lordosis in an older child, and (5) changes in urological function. MRI and, if necessary, computed tomography (CT), as well as myelographic evaluation, should be performed in any child suspected of having a tethered cord syndrome.

○ **What is the role of surgery in tethered cord syndrome?**

Surgical release is performed to attempt to return to previous level of function and prevent further loss. If clinical signs are documented, surgical treatment is indicated to prevent further deterioration of the motor function and to diminish the progress of spasticity and scoliosis. It is important to make an early diagnosis and start treatment because surgical release of the tethered cord rarely provides complete return of lost function.

○ **What integumentary problems occur in patients with myelomeningocele?**

Skin breakdown occurs in 85-95% of children with myelomeningocele before young adulthood. Recurrent decubiti can lead to prolonged morbidity and functional disability. Healing can occur if the precipitating mechanical factors are eliminated. Plastic surgical correction may be necessary in severe cases and may involve orthopedic correction of underlying postural abnormalities.

○ **What skin sites are vulnerable to breakdown?**

The sites and causes of skin breakdown vary by age and lesion level. Skin breakdown on the lower limb occurs in 30-50% of cases in all lesion level groups. The most common areas of breakdown in the thoracic level group are the perineum and above the apex of the kyphotic curve. Overall, tissue ischemia from pressure necrosis is the most common etiology. Other frequent causes more prevalent in the younger child include casts or orthotic devices, skin maceration from urine and stool soiling, friction, shear, and burns.

○ **What skin sites are vulnerable to breakdown in older children?**

Older children may have higher risk of skin breakdown because of increased pressure of a larger body habitus, asymmetric weight bearing from acquired musculoskeletal deformities, and lower limb vascular insufficiency or venous stasis.

○ **Are these patients at risk for osteoporosis?**

Bone mineral density is decreased in patients with myelomeningocele. Markers of bone reabsorption were found more frequently in both limited ambulators and nonambulators than in children who ambulated regularly. Children with myelomeningocele are at higher risk of lower extremity fractures. Reduced muscle activity in the paralyzed limb and decreased weight-bearing forces result in decreased bone mass. In addition, many fractures occur after orthopedic interventions, especially after procedures associated with cast immobilization.

○ **What are the characteristics of fracture healing in myelomeningocele patients?**

Fractures in myelomeningocele tend to heal quickly, and excessive callus formation often is seen. Relative immobilization (i.e., short casting times and early weight bearing) is the standard recommendation for healing after fractures. The goal is maintaining functional alignment and rotation without compromising the patient's ability to stand and ambulate.

○ **Is obesity an acquired morbidity in myelomeningocele patients?**

Obesity is prevalent in children with myelomeningocele, especially those with high-lumbar and thoracic-level lesions because of reduced capacity for caloric expenditure. The decreased muscle mass of the lower body musculature results in a lower basal metabolic rate. In addition, activity levels generally are lower than in unaffected children, both as a direct result of lesion-related mobility deficits and as an indirect result of decreased opportunities for disabled children to participate in physical play. Obesity can exert negative impact on self-image and further perpetuate a cycle of inactivity and overeating. Because of their decreased linear limb growth and spine growth, patients with myelomeningocele should be monitored for weight using arm span measurements, as opposed to ratios of height versus weight.

○   **What are the prognostic indicators for the prediction of ambulatory ability?**

Recent studies of children with prenatally diagnosed myelomeningocele suggest that less severe ventriculomegaly and a lower anatomic level of lesion on prenatal ultrasound predict better developmental outcomes in childhood. The level of the lesion and associated strength of the lower extremity muscles are the most important factors influencing the achievement of ambulation in children with myelomeningocele.

○   **What are the neuromuscular findings to predict a favorable ambulatory prognosis?**

Several studies have shown that ambulation in patients with myelomeningocele is related to the strength of certain key muscles, including the iliopsoas, gluteus medius, hamstrings, and/or quadriceps. Specifically, a motor neurologic level of L5 or quadriceps strength graded as good in the first 3 years of life is predictive of a good prognosis for community ambulation. Gluteus medius strength was the best predictor of a need for gait aids and orthoses.

○   **What are the ambulatory characteristics for patients with myelomeningocele?**

Approximately 50% of patients ambulate household or community distances, with about 20% of these patients using some orthotic or assistive device. The other 50% of patients use wheelchairs as their primary form of mobility. Approximately 20% of these individuals ambulate with orthotics and assistive devices as a form of therapeutic exercise.

○   **What is the prognosis for renal function in myelomeningocele patients?**

With proper urologic management, more than 95% of children with myelomeningocele continue to have normal renal function. The psychosocial consequence of bowel and bladder incontinence can have a dramatic impact on children with myelomeningocele, especially in adolescence. The extent of achievement of acceptable social continence varies, with studies reporting 40-80% achievement of bladder continence and 30-40% achievement of bowel continence. Approximately 25% of patients are continent of both bowel and bladder. The likelihood of social continence improves when training is instituted before the age of 7 years.

○   **What are the prospects for the adult patient with myelomeningocele in the community?**

Studies of adults with myelomeningocele have shown that about 20% secure gainful employment, but most patients continue to live with their parents, many in total social isolation. Perceived family environment may explain different levels of participation of patients with myelomeningocele in employment, community mobility, and social activity as an adult, even beyond what can be explained by lesion level and intelligence. A positive correlation exists between perceived family encouragement of independence and outcomes in young adults with myelomeningocele.

○   **What is the lifetime prognosis for patients with myelomeningocele?**

For a child who is born with a myelomeningocele and who is treated aggressively, the mortality rate is approximately 10–15%, and most deaths occur before age 4 yr. At least 70% of survivors have normal intelligence, but learning problems and seizure disorders are more common than in the general population. Previous episodes of meningitis or ventriculitis adversely affect the ultimate intelligence quotient. Because myelomeningocele is a chronic handicapping condition, periodic multidisciplinary follow-up is required for life.

MOTOR NEURON DISORDERS

AMYOTROPHIC LATERAL SCLEROSIS (ALS)

O   **What is the basic classification scheme and definition of Amyotrophic Lateral Sclerosis (ALS)?**

Amyotrophic lateral sclerosis (ALS), which is also called motor neuron disease, Charcot's disease, or Lou Gehrig's disease, is an age dependent and generally fatal paralytic disorder caused by the degeneration of motor neurons in the motor cortex, brain stem, and spinal cord. About 10 percent of cases are familial (FALS) and the rest are sporadic (SALS). Broadly, there are three types of ALS usually considered in epidemiological studies: SALS, FALS, and a variant of ALS, sometimes called Guamanian ALS, found in the Western Pacific and characterized by the occurrence of parkinsonism, dementia, or both.

O   **What are the pathological findings in ALS?**

ALS is a primary disorder of motor cells and their axons. The hallmark of ALS is atrophy, degeneration, and loss of motor neurons in the lower brain stem and anterior horn of the spinal cord, followed by glial replacement. There is loss of pyramidal cells from the motor cortex of the prefrontal gyrus and large myelinated fibers of the anterior and lateral columns of the spinal cord, the brain stem, and the cerebrum. The posterior columns are usually spared in SALS. Lower brain stem nuclei are more often and more extensively involved than upper nuclei. Therefore, oculomotor nuclei loss is modest and rarely demonstrable clinically, whereas the hypoglossal nuclei are prominently degenerated.

O   **What pathophysiological processes have been described in ALS?**

A number of abnormalities in metabolism of the excitatory neurotransmitter glutamate have been identified in ALS, including alterations in tissue glutamate levels, transporter proteins, postsynaptic receptors, and indications of possible toxic agonists. Whether these are primary or secondary events and how they relate to the genesis of ALS is unclear but is under intense investigation.

O   **What is the incidence of Amyotrophic Lateral Sclerosis (ALS)?**

SALS has a worldwide incidence of 1 to 2 in 100,000 persons, with fairly uniform distribution worldwide and equal representation among racial groups. The occurrence of ALS before the age of 40 years is uncommon. The incidence is greatest between the ages of 50 and 70 years, and it seems to decline thereafter. The male to female ratio is about 1.3:1.

O   **Are there risk factors associated with SALS?**

The only indisputable risk factor other than age and gender is genetic susceptibility, with familial cases occurring in about 10 percent of most case series. Many isolated potential etiologies have been proposed for SALS, with the only consistent associations thus far being long term exposure to heavy metals, particularly lead, and a family history of parkinsonism and dementia. There is recent evidence of association between increased dietary fat and cigarette smoking.

O   **What are the diagnostic criteria for ALS?**

Summary of El Escorial Criteria for the Diagnosis of Amyotrophic Lateral Sclerosis
The diagnosis of ALS requires the *presence* of signs of lower motor neuron (LMN) degeneration by clinical, electrophysiological, or neuropathological examination and signs of upper motor neuron (UMN) degeneration by clinical examination, and the progressive spread of these signs within a region or to other regions, together with the *absence* of electrophysiological or neuroimaging evidence of other disease processes that might explain these signs.
Suspected ALS
LMN signs only in at least two regions
Possible ALS
UMN and LMN signs in only one region, or UMN signs only in at least two regions, or LMN signs rostral to UMN signs

Special cases: monomelic ALS, progressive bulbar palsy without spinal UMN and/or LMN signs, primary lateral sclerosis without spinal LMN signs
Probable ALS
UMN signs in at least two regions, with some UMN signs above LMN signs
Definite ALS
UMN signs and LMN signs in bulbar region and at least two spinal regions, or UMN and LMN signs in three spinal regions

○   **What other variants of ALS have been described?**

Other diseases classified as adult onset motor neuron diseases have more restricted presentations and can evolve into idiopathic ALS if the patient is tracked for a long period. These diseases include the following:
Progressive bulbar palsy - Pure bulbar involvement
Progressive muscular atrophy - Pure lower motor neuron degeneration
Primary lateral sclerosis - Pure upper motor neuron degeneration
Adult onset spinal muscular atrophy - Includes a broad range of primary motor neuron diseases classified by pattern of inheritance, distribution of weakness, or age of onset

○   **What is the clinical presentation of ALS?**

Although the disease may present in many different ways and in different parts of the body, generally the patient seeks attention because of symptomatic weakness. Alternatively, there may be a history of fasciculations, muscle cramping, and atrophy before weakness is apparent. A frequent diagnostic feature is the presence of hyperreflexia in segmental regions where muscles are starting to atrophy and an absence of sensory disturbance in the same distribution.

○   **What patterns of weakness have been described in ALS?**

Limb involvement occurs more often than bulbar involvement, and upper limbs are more often affected than lower limbs in SALS; this pattern is reversed in FALS. However, the pattern of involvement is frequently asymmetrical or focal.

○   **What symptoms are more salient with upper motor neuron involvement?**

If more upper motor neurons are affected, the symptoms will be primarily clumsiness, stiffness, and fatigue, whereas lower motor neuron degeneration will present as weakness or atrophy and occasionally fasciculations. Bulbar symptoms include hoarseness, slurring of speech, choking on liquids, and difficulty initiating swallowing. Paresthesias and sensory symptoms affect up to 25 percent of patients, but if present, these complaints are mild.

○   **What are the characteristics of disease progression in ALS?**

There is wide variation in disease progression and duration, neither of which can be accurately predicted from age or site of onset, although generally elderly patients have a shorter survival. Although fasciculations, especially of the tongue, are considered by some to be specifically associated with ALS, they may actually be seen in any disorder affecting the motor neuron or their axons.

○   **Are bladder and bowel function affected in ALS?**

Bowel, bladder, and sexual functioning are usually spared, with about 4 percent of patients experiencing loss of sphincter control.

○   **What do ancillary diagnostic tests reveal in ALS?**

Electromyographic (EMG) features commonly seen include fibrillation, positive sharp waves, and complex repetitive discharges that indicate denervation. Simultaneously, reduced numbers and increased amplitude and duration of motor unit potentials indicate reinnervation. Multifocal fasciculations are also characteristic of the disease. Increased jitter on single fiber EMG reflects immature endplates and inefficient reinnervation. Cerebrospinal fluid examination either is normal or shows mildly elevated protein (<100 mg/dL). There may be a moderate increase in creatine kinase (CK) of the muscle enzyme type.

O   **What protocol should be followed during EMG needle examination?**

Examine at least 3 levels—cervical/thoracic/lumbar paraspinal muscles and bulbar muscles.
1.   Most involved limb first—2 or more weak muscles with different innervation
2.   Distal muscles of other possibly abnormal extremities.
3.   If other levels are not abnormal then check bulbar muscles.
4.   If necessary, for respiratory involvement, check intercostal and respiratory diaphragm.
5.   Somatosensory evoked potentials to rule out a demyelinating process or primary spinal cord disease.

O   **What is the most common cause of death in ALS patients?**

ALS remains a fatal disease, with a mean survival of 3 years after the onset of symptoms. The cause of death is respiratory failure and aspiration.

O   **What pattern of weakness is common in patients with ALS?**

In the upper extremity, the wrist extensor, finger extensor, and hand intrinsic muscles tend to be weakest, with relative sparing of the wrist and finger flexors and elbow extensors. Other commonly affected muscles are the neck extensors, arm abductors, external rotators, and elbow flexors. In the lower extremities, the ankle dorsiflexor, invertor, and evertor muscles are weakest, with relative sparing of the ankle plantarflexors. Later, the knee extensors and hip girdle musculature become weak. Bulbar weakness tends to involve muscles innervated by cranial nerves X, XI, and XII more than V and VII and usually sparing the extraocular muscles.

O   **What is the exercise response often reported in ALS patients?**

In general, ALS patients show an abnormal response to exercise at the muscle level and systemic metabolic level, which decreases the tolerance to exercise. This is more pronounced in more severely involved patients. The recommendation that exercise above and beyond that provided by ADLs is warranted only in patients with mild difficulties and for slowly progressive disease appears to have support from metabolic studies.

O   **What is the time frame for loss of ambulation in ALS patients?**

ALS patients become wheelchair bound in 12 to 18 months on average. Whether patients require an electric or manual wheelchair depends on the distribution and degree of muscle weakness.

O   **What contractures are often encountered in ALS patients?**

The most commonly involved are the finger and wrist flexors, shoulder internal rotators and adductors, as well as ankle plantar flexors. Intrinsic hand muscle weakness may cause a "claw hand" type of deformity. Twice daily prolonged stretch to the affected muscles is primary treatment. Splinting with a static wrist hand orthosis or AFO may be necessary. Management of underlying spasticity, if present, will also be of benefit.

O   **What upper extremity orthosis may be of benefit in the symptomatic ALS patient?**

Patients with poor grasp can be provided with a universal cuff, and patients with hand weakness can be braced in 20-25° of extension to improve grip strength. For patients with proximal upper extremity weakness, a balanced forearm orthosis (i.e., deltoid aid) may be beneficial to enhance upper extremity movement by eliminating the effects of gravity.

O   **What assistive devices may aid the patient with advanced ALS?**

For patients with severe limb involvement, introduce environmental control units (ECUs) that utilize oral motor movements. In patients with severe bulbar involvement, extraocular movements are usually preserved so ECUs incorporating eye gaze technology can be used.

O   **What considerations should be taken to address restrictive airway disease in ALS patients?**

Patients should be educated early in the disease process, so informed decisions can be made further down the line. Routine pulmonary function tests (PFTs), including forced vital capacity (FVC) and maximal inspiratory and expiratory pressures (MIP/MEP) should be monitored closely. The MIP reflects diaphragmatic strength and the ability to ventilate. The MEP reflects chest wall and abdominal muscle strength and the ability to cough and clear secretions.

O   **What other monitoring is indicated to assess hypoventilation ?**

End tidal CO_2 levels or arterial blood gases (ABGs) should be measured periodically, depending on the clinical condition of the patient?

O   **What respiratory aids are appropriate for the ALS patient with symptomatic hypoventilation?**

Intermittent positive pressure ventilation (IPPV) by mouth avoids the need for tracheostomy and maintains reasonable QOL. Bimodal positive airway pressure (BiPAP) is the best initial form. This technique can be performed in the home and should be considered the preferred modality of assisted ventilation in ALS

O   **What role does glossopharyngeal breathing play in advanced ALS?**

A respiratory therapist can teach patients glossopharyngeal breathing. This involves gulping boluses of air into the lungs to add to the user's deep breath and can be useful in those with nonbulbar ALS who do not have a tracheostomy. One glossopharyngeal breath contains 6-9 gulps and can provide the patient with weak inspiratory muscles and no vital capacity a safe way to breathe if, for any reason, a ventilator cannot be used or there is sudden ventilator failure.

O   **What diagnostic and therapeutic strategies should be considered for ALS patients with dysphagia?**

Patients should be evaluated with videofluoroscopic swallowing studies if symptoms such as coughing after meals or food sticking in the back of the throat occur. Dietary modifications of food and liquid consistency as well as use of compensatory techniques may be helpful. For patients with pharyngeal constrictor weakness, clearing leafy vegetables may be particularly difficult. Severe cases may require gastrostomy tube feeding to prevent aspiration. Patients who aspirate their secretions may require surgical intervention.

O   **What communication disturbances are encountered in ALS patients?**

Communication problems may result from dysarthria. Vocal quality may be harsh and strangled (spastic dysarthria) or breathy with audible inspirations (flaccid dysarthria), or may be a combination. Patients with bulbar ALS rarely have normal speech, progress to a more severe dysarthria, and may require an augmentative communication device (ACD). The rate of progression is quite variable, with some patients requiring an ACD within a year after diagnosis while others barely change over several years.

O   **Are there any pharmacotherapeutic agents advantageous to the ALS patient?**

Thus far, only the benzothiazole riluzole has been shown to extend life span, although in double blind studies, the extension averages only 3 months and mortality rates are unaffected. In larger follow up studies, the increase in life may be as long as 12 months. Riluzole acts to block voltage activated sodium channels and to protect against glutamate toxicity.

POST POLIO SYNDROME (PPS)

O   **What is the incidence of PPS?**

The percentage of polio survivors in the United States experiencing new symptoms that may be related to their previous polio illness is unknown, but estimates have ranged from 25% to 60%. Thus, one might estimate that there are between 160,000 and 380,000 individuals in the United States at the present time that may be experiencing the late effects of polio. In all likelihood, this number will increase as polio survivors' age.

O   **What are the clinical manifestations of acute poliomyelitis?**

Paralysis is usually asymmetric and the legs are more commonly involved than the arms. Severe bulbar weakness occurs in 10% to 15% of paralytic patients.

O   **What factors govern motor recovery in poliomyelitis?**

The amount of recovery of strength and endurance following the acute poliomyelitis illness was determined by four major factors: 1) the number of motor neurons that recover and resume normal function, 2) the number of "orphaned" muscle fibers that are reinnervated by the surviving motor units through terminal axonal sprouting, 3) muscle hypertrophy resulting from increasing activity after the acute illness, and 4) improvement in muscle endurance capacity resulting from increasing activity after the acute illness.

O   **How does the pathological findings in the anterior horn compare to MMT?**

Manual muscle testing showed normal results in several muscle groups in a polio patient during his lifetime, although more than half of those muscle's anterior horn cells were shown to be destroyed at the time of a detailed postmortem study.

O   **What findings have been reported regarding loss of strength in PPS?**

It has been reported that the average postpolio patient, deemed to have normal strength of the quadriceps muscles by manual muscle testing, had a 50% reduction in strength when muscle strength was measured quantitatively. It is certainly plausible that a chronic deficit in strength in some muscle groups may be one contributing factor to the development of postpolio syndrome in some polio survivors at the present time.

O   **What other factors may be responsible for weakness and fatigue in PPS patients?**

Disuse muscle atrophy, overuse muscle injury, weight gain, chronic muscle weakness.

O   **What cascade of events may produce decreased activity in PPS?**

Simple muscle overuse may result in pain, which may lead to the individual decreasing his or her level of activity. This may then result in disuse weakness and the decreasing level of activity may result in weight gain. With decreased activity, joint contracture may develop, leading to increasing joint or muscle pain, which may result in yet a further decrease in activity and further deterioration.

O   **What are the complaints typically reported by PPS patients?**

The complaints are varied but generally can be divided into complaints of pain, fatigue, weakness, and other problems. Most prevalent of these complaints are complaints of musculoskeletal pain from muscle overuse or myofascial origin; pain from a progressive increase in skeletal deformity; pain in biomechanically disadvantaged, deformed, or marginally stable joints; fatigue; new muscle weakness or atrophy; respiratory impairment; cold intolerance; and a decline in activity of daily living (ADL) function.

O   **What ventilation and respiratory problems occur in PPS patients?**

A number of reports documented respiratory insufficiency in some polio survivors many years after the onset of acute illness. These problems included chronic hypoventilation, nocturnal rapid eye movement (REM) sleep–induced hypoxemia, and sleep apnea syndrome.

○ **What other problems have been reported in the PPS patient?**

Dysphagia with an impaired pharyngeal phase of swallowing.

○ **Which categories of ADL's are more problematic for PPS patients?**

Instrumental ADLs rather than basic ADLs.

○ **What psychosocial problems are encountered in the PPS patient population?**

In men, elevated scores on subscales of the Symptom Check List 90 Revised (SCL-90R) were found for somatization, depression, anxiety, hostility, and phobia, while in women elevations were found for somatization, depression, anxiety, and psychoticism. Elevated scores were found in the subscales of the Psychosocial Adjustment to Illness Scale (PAIS-SR) (pooling men and women) on health care orientation, social environment, and extended family relationships.

○ **What are the difference between asymptomatic vs. symptomatic patients with PPS?**

1. Unstable postpolio individuals had evidence of more widespread initial poliomyelitis illness in unstable postpolio individuals.
2. Unstable postpolio individuals had their acute illness at an older age.
3. Unstable postpolio individuals hospitalized longer at the time of their acute polio illness.
4. Unstable postpolio individuals acknowledge higher level of recent activity.
5. Unstable postpolio individuals have weaker muscles.
6. Unstable postpolio individuals have reduced capacity for muscular work.
7. Unstable postpolio individuals have a deficit in strength recovery after fatiguing exercise.

○ **What technique can be used to reduce muscle fatigue in PPS patients?**

Pacing (interspersing rest breaks during activity) can significantly reduce local muscle fatigue even when similar or greater amounts of total activities are actually performed.

○ **What criteria are recommended to establish a diagnosis of PPS?**

1. A prior episode of paralytic polio confirmed by history and physical examination.
2. A period of neurologic recovery followed by an extended interval of neurologic and functional stability preceding the onset of new problems. The interval of stability usually lasts 20 years or more.
3. A gradual or abrupt onset of new weakness that may or may not be accompanied by other new health problems such as excessive fatigue, muscle pain, joint pain, decreased endurance, decreased function, and atrophy.
4. Exclusion of other medical or neurologic conditions other than polio related conditions that might cause the health problems just listed.

○ **What role can an orthosis play in the management of gait associated pain in PPS patients?**

Proper orthotic use may definitely reduce pain at multiple sites by altering the lurching gait pattern that is often used by the individual in the absence of a properly fitted orthosis. Common examples of orthotically correctable gait patterns are the forward weight shift to move the center of gravity anterior to the axis of the knee joint to assist with knee extension, and the side to side pattern, to circumduct the leg, in patients with footdrop.

○ **What lifestyle adjustments and energy conservation techniques may be utilized by PPS patients?**

Lifestyle adjustments and energy conservation techniques can also be useful in the reduction and control of fatigue. Some of the simple energy conservation techniques include using a handicap license plate (when appropriate), planning one's day and reducing the number of trips, balancing activity and rest, learning and then using techniques of work simplification as well as appropriate assistive devices in occupational therapy, and using a motorized scooter for long distance mobility when appropriate.

○ **What role do non fatiguing exercise program play in PPS management?**

Patients should exercise for short intervals and then rest to recover between the bouts of exercise. Exercise may be performed on alternate days to allow for full recovery and to avoid overuse. Patients with PPS who were able to exercise at a level that avoided overuse (excessive muscle fatigue or increasing muscle or joint pain) have experienced positive results. Muscle fatigue, similar to the treatment of generalized fatigue, can be improved by interspersing bouts of activity with rest breaks (pacing) to avoid excessive fatigue. Non fatiguing exercise programs have used both submaximal and maximal strength combined with short duration repetitions. This simple procedure significantly improved strength recovery after activity. Improvements in cardiopulmonary reserve and mobility may also occur.

○ **What interventions may be considered for PPS patients with ventilatory deficits?**

Both sleep disorder breathing and chronic hypoventilation can be reversed and symptoms markedly improved with the utilization of ventilatory assistance. Inspiratory positive pressure ventilation (IPPV) can be delivered in a number of different ways including by continuous positive airway pressure (CPAP) or bilevel positive airway pressure (Bi-PAP). Bi-PAP independently varies the inspiratory and expiratory pressures. Both CPAP and Bi-PAP can be delivered by an oral, nasal, or oral nasal ventilator hose. Treatment for respiratory difficulties in postpolio patients is not different from that for patients with other neuromuscular disorders.

○ **What clinical interventions are appropriate for a PPS patient with dysphagia?**

Dysphagia results from involvement of the bulbar musculature. For patients who present with dysphagia, videofluoroscopy supervised by a speech and language pathologist can oftentimes determine the causative factors for the problem and whether compensatory techniques may be helpful for the patient. Such compensatory techniques include 1) changing the consistency of the food or liquid, 2) turning the head to one side or leaning to one side so that the food travels down the patient's stronger side, 3) tucking the chin, 4) alternating food and liquid, 5) swallowing twice for each bolus and 6) avoiding ingestion when fatigued.

○ **Are there pharmacotherapeutic options for symptomatic PPS patients?**

Currently, there are no medications that significantly improve strength in polio survivors. Pyridostigmine, which is generally gradually increased to a dose of 60 mg tid, has been used with mixed results to improve strength. In patients with chronic debilitating fatigue, methylphenidate hydrochloride and bromocriptine have been tried with mixed results. More recently, modafinil has been used for treating fatigue pharmacologically. The starting dose is usually 200 mg po every morning and may be increased to 400 mg.

○ **Summarize rehabilitative and palliative interventions for the patient with MND**

SYMPTOM	TREATMENT
Muscle weakness and Fatigue	Physiotherapy to prevent muscle contractures and joint stiffness
	Devices to maintain mobility and independence such as ankle-foot orthoses, head supports, mobile arm supports, bathroom aids etc.
	Acetylcholinesterase inhibitors (pyridostigmine) can cause a short term improvement in fatigue in some patients
Fasciculations	Antispasticity agents (Baclofen, Tizanidine): Dose must be carefully titrated as loss of tone can worsen mobility
Painful muscle cramps	Quinine sulphate for cramps
Spasticity	Low dose diazepam for cramps or fasciculations
Sialorrhea	Hyoscine transdermal patches, amitriptyline or atropine
	Portable suction devices.
	Low dose parotid irradiation may be considered if drug treatment is not successful.

	B-blockers or carbocysteine reduce viscosity of secretions.
Pseudobulbar Affect :	Responds well to amitriptyline or selective serotonin reuptake inhibitors (SSRIs)
Psychological Problems:	A grief reaction is a normal response to a devastating diagnosis.
	Clinical depression is also common and under diagnosed.
Depression and Anxiety	It can be treated with tricyclic antidepressants or SSRIs.
Sleep Disorders	Treatment should be directed at the cause of insomnia. Common causes in MND are respiratory insufficiency, anxiety depression, muscle cramps, and inability to change position.
	Use of sedatives should be avoided unless other options fail.
Constipation	Review medications (Analgesics and anticholinergics worsen constipation) and ensure adequate fluid intake.
	Bulk-forming or osmotic laxatives, glycerol suppositories
Musculoskeletal Pain	Non-steroidal anti-inflammatories and physiotherapy are most effective
Dysarthria	Simple strategies to improve communication can be taught by a speech therapist. When these become ineffective, a variety of communication aids are available, such as a light-writer
Dysphagia	See text
Dyspnea	See text

NEUROMUSCULAR DISORDERS

NEUROPATHIES

○   **Classify the peripheral neuropathy syndromes**

Peripheral Neuropathy Syndromes
I. Acute-Subacute Generalized Polyneuropathies
A. Sensorimotor

1. Acute motor and sensory axonal neuropathy syndrome
   2. Alcohol/nutritional
   3. Toxins (metals)

B. Motor > sensory

1. Guillain-Barre syndrome
   2. Acute motor axonal neuropathy syndrome
   3. Porphyria
   4. Diphtheria
   5. Toxins (dapsone, vincristine)

C. Sensory

1. Paraneoplastic/autoimmune (anti-Hu associated)
   2. Vitamin B_6 toxicity
   3. Toxins (cisplatin)
   4. Human immunodeficiency virus

II. Chronic Generalized Symmetric Polyneuropathies
A. Sensorimotor

1. Diabetes
   2. Uremia
   3. Alcohol/nutritional
   4. Dysproteinemias
   5. Connective tissue diseases

B. Motor > sensory

1. Chronic inflammatory demyelinating polyradiculoneuropathy
   2. Dysproteinemias
   3. Hypothyroidism
   4. Toxins (amiodarone, cytosine arabinoside, metals, tacrolimus)

C. Sensory

1. Paraneoplastic/autoimmune (anti-Hu associated)
   2. Vitamin B_6 toxicity
   3. Sjögren's syndrome
   4. Vitamin E deficiency

III. Inherited Generalized Symmetric Sensory and Motor Polyneuropathies
A. Charcot-Marie-Tooth disease types 1,2,3 and X B. Familial amyloidosis C. Hereditary predisposition to pressure palsies (focal and symmetric)
IV. Asymmetric Generalized Sensory and Motor Polyneuropathies
A. Vasculitis B. Sarcoidosis C. Diabetes D. Lyme disease
V. Mononeuropathies
A. Compression and entrapment neuropathies B. Vasculitis C. Diabetes

VI. Autonomic Neuropathies and Polyneuropathies with Prominent Autonomic Features

A. Acute

1. Acute pandysautonomia (paraneoplastic and idiopathic)
2. Guillain-Barre syndrome
3. Botulism
4. Porphyria
5. Toxins (vincristine, amiodarone, cisplatin, organic solvents, metals)

B. Chronic

1. Diabetes
2. Chronic pandysautonomia (paraneoplastic and idiopathic)
3. Amyloidosis
4. Riley-Day syndrome

○ **What drugs may induce polyneuropathies?**

Drugs that May Induce Polyneuropathies	
Drug	**Clinical Features of Polyneuropathy**
Antibiotic	
Chloramphenicol	Sensory, optic neuropathy
Chloroquine	Sensory
Dapsone	Motor
Didanosine	Sensory
Ethambutol	Sensorimotor
Ethionamide	Sensory
Isoniazid	Sensory (vitamin B_6 deficiency)
Metronidazole	Sensory
Nitrofurantoin	Sensorimotor
Savudine	Sensory
Suramin	Sensorimotor
Zalcitabine	Sensory
Chemotherapeutic	
Cisplatin	Sensorimotor, ototoxicity
Cytarabine	Sensory
Docetaxel	Sensorimotor
Paclitaxel	Sensorimotor
Procarbazine	Sensorimotor
Vinblastine	Sensorimotor
Vincristine	Sensorimotor
Cardiovascular	
Amiodarone	Sensorimotor, ototoxicity
Captopril	Sensorimotor
Enalapril	Sensorimotor
Flecainide	Sensory
Hydralazine	Sensory (vitamin B_6 deficiency)
Perhexiline	Sensorimotor
Rheumatologic	
Allopurinol	Sensorimotor
Colchicine	Sensory
Gold	Sensorimotor
Indomethacin	Sensorimotor

Miscellaneous	
Disulfiram	Sensory
Interferon alfa	Sensorimotor
Lithium	Sensorimotor
Lovastatin	Sensorimotor
Phenytoin	Sensorimotor
Pyridoxine	Sensory
Simvastatin	Sensorimotor
Thalidomide	Sensorimotor

O   **What are the environmental and industrial toxins that cause polyneuropathy?**

Environmental and Industrial Toxins that Cause Polyneuropathy	
Toxin	**Clinical Features of the Polyneuropathy**
Acrylamide	Sensorimotor, ataxia
Allyl chloride	Sensory
Arsenic	Sensorimotor
Carbon disulfide	Sensorimotor
Ethylene oxide	Sensorimotor, ataxia
Hexacarbons	Sensorimotor
Lead	Sensorimotor, motor > sensory
Mercury	Sensorimotor, motor > sensory
Organophosphorus esters	Sensorimotor, autonomic (cholinergic)
Thallium	Sensorimotor

O   **What is the classification of the heredofamilial polyneuropathies?**

Heredofamilial Polyneuropathies			
Disorder	**Inheritance**	**Clinical**	**Pathology**
CMT type 1	AD	Common, childhood onset, S/M	D
CMT type 2	AD	Rare, later onset than type 1, S/M	A
CMT type 3 (Dejerine-Sottas Disease)	AD	Rare, infantile onset, severe S/M	D
CMT, X-linked	XR	Second-most common, S/M, earlier onset, more severe	D
HNNP	AD	Variable onset, compression neuropathies, S/M	D
Familial amyloidosis	AD	Variable onset, autonomic and S/M	A
Refsum's disease	AR	Variable onset, ataxia, retinitis pigmentosa	D
Tangier disease	AR	Very rare, variable onset, splenomegaly, orange tonsils	A
Fabry's disease	XR	Childhood onset, SFN	A
CMT = Charcot-Marie-Tooth disease, HNPP = hereditary neuropathy with liability to pressure palsies, AD =autosomal dominant, XR = X-linked recessive, AR = autosomal recessive, A = axon loss, D = demyelinating, S/M = sensorimotor, SFN = small-fiber neuropathy			

○   **What are the small fiber neuropathies?**

Small-Fiber Neuropathies
Diabetes mellitus
Alcohol/nutritional deficiency
Amyloidosis (familial and primary)
Drugs/toxins
Cisplatin
Disulfiram
Isoniazid
Metals (gold, arsenic, thallium)
Metronidazole
Primary biliary cirrhosis
Hypothyroidism
Heredofamilial
Hereditary sensory and autonomic neuropathy types I, III, IV
Fabry's disease
Tangier disease
Dominantly inherited burning foot neuropathy
Sjögren's syndrome
Human immunodeficiency virus
Hyperlipidemia
Monoclonal gammopathy of uncertain significance
Idiopathic

○   **What is the differential diagnosis of neuropathies by clinical course?**

Differential Diagnosis of Neuropathies by Clinical Course

Acute onset (within days)	Subacute onset (weeks to months)	Chronic course/ insidious onset	Relapsing/ remitting course
Guillain-Barré Syndrome	Maintained exposure to toxic agents/medications	Hereditary motor sensory neuropathies	Guillain-Barré syndrome
Acute intermittent Porphyria	Persisting nutritional deficiency	Dominantly inherited sensory neuropathy	CIDP
Critical illness Polyneuropathy	Abnormal metabolic state	CIDP	HIV/AIDS
Diphtheric neuropathy	Paraneoplastic syndrome		Toxic
Thallium toxicity	CIDP		Porphyria

CIDP=chronic inflammatory demyelinating polyradiculoneuropathy; HIV=human immunodeficiency virus; AIDS=acquired immunodeficiency syndrome.

○   **What is the classification of neurophysiological findings in peripheral neuropathy?**

Neurophysiologic Classification of Generalized Neuropathies

Pathophysiology	Acute/Subacute	Chronic
Demyelinating	GBS	CIDP
	Diphtheria	MMN
	CMT1a with vincristine	HNPP
	Toxic (arsenic)	IgM (MAG and non-MAG)
		OSM
		CMT (demyelinating forms)
Axonal	GBS (axonal forms)	Chemotherapy induced
	Porphyria	CMT (axonal forms)
	SNS	Paraneoplastic
	Toxins	SNS

		(vasculitis)	HSN
			Toxins
			AIDS (late)
			Vasculitis (late)
			Toxic/metabolic like uremia
			Amyloidosis
Mixed		Diabetes	Diabetes
		CIDP (late forms with	CIDP
		axonal damage)	Some toxic

GBS, Guillain-Barré syndrome; CMT1a, Charcot-Marie-Tooth type 1a; SNS, subacute neuronopathy syndrome, either autoimmune or paraneoplastic; CIDP, chronic inflammatory demyelinating polyneuropathy; MMN, multifocal motor neuropathy; HNPP, hereditary neuropathy with pressure palsies; IgM, monoclonal IgM protein in blood; MAG, neuropathy associated with antibody against myelin-associated glycoprotein; OSM, osteosclerotic myeloma; HSN, hereditary sensory neuropathy AIDS, acquired immunodeficiency syndrome

○ **What are the electromyogram parameters of demyelination and axonal degeneration?**

Electromyogram Parameters of Demyelination and Axonal Degeneration

Pathophysiology	Distal Latency	Conduction Velocity	Amplitude	F-wave Latency	Needle EMG
Demyelinating	Prolonged DL-est	< 80% LLN	N or slightly low, CB and dispersion	Prolonged vs. CV	Variable acute changes, mild in most
Axonal	N or slightly prolonged if CMAP low; not > DL-est	80% LLN, decreased when CMAP low (< 50% LLN)	Decreased, often < 50% LLN in feet	Not > F-est	Marked active and chronic denervation changes distally

EMG, electromyogram; DL, distal latency; DL-est, the expected distal latency prolongation based on proximal CV; LLN, lower limit of normal for that nerve; N, normal; CV, conduction velocity; CMAP, maximal compound muscle potential amplitude obtained after nerve stimulation; F-est, the expected F-wave latency based on the conduction velocity.

○ **What is the diagnostic testing for idiopathic peripheral neuropathy?**

Diagnostic Testing for Idiopathic Neuropathy

1. **Routine**—almost all patients
   • CBC
   • Sedimentation rate
   • Chemistries: FBS, BUN, creatinine, calcium, phosphorus, albumin, liver function tests, electrolytes, serum lipids suspected
   • Fasting blood sugar and hemoglobin A1C if diabetes or glucose intolerance
   • Thyrotropin, vitamin B12, folate, serum protein electrophoresis, immunoglobulin levels, serum immunofixation electrophoresis
   • Chest x-ray
2. **Selective patients**—if above not diagnostic
   • 24-hour urine for heavy metals if history of exposure or clinical picture fits
   • Porphyrin levels if picture fits
   • Urine protein electrophoresis and immunofixation electrophoresis for free light chains in selected cases
   • Special immunologic and genetic tests in special cases
   • VDRL, Lyme disease, West Nile virus, and HIV titers
   • Skin, fat pad, and/or rectal biopsy if amyloid suspected
   • 2-hour GTT
   • CSF exam if GBS, CIDP, malignant infiltration or infection possible
   • Clinical and NCV examination of blood relatives if gene tests negative and inherited neuropathy a possibility
   • X-ray skeletal survey of OSM suggested
3. **If all negative**
   • Consider nerve biopsy in selected cases.

CBC, complete blood cell count; FBS, fasting blood sugar; BUN, serum urea nitrogen; VDRL, venereal disease research laboratory slide test; HIV, human immunodeficiency virus; GTT, glucose tolerance test; CSF, cerebrospinal fluid; GBS, Guillain-Barré syndrome; CIDP, chronic inflammatory demyelinating polyneuropathy; NCV, nerve conduction velocity; OSM, osteosclerotic myeloma.

○   **What are the available drug therapies for neuropathic pain?**

Drug Therapy for Neuropathic Pain		
I. Antidepressants		
Drug	**Daily Dosage, Range**	**Comments**
Amitriptyline	10-150 mg	Sedation, anticholinergic side effects, weight gain, arrhythmia
Nortriptyline	10-150 mg	Similar to amitriptyline but less sedating
Imipramine	10-300 mg	Similar to amitriptyline but less sedating
Desipramine	10-300 mg	Similar to amitriptyline but less sedating
Venlafaxine XR	37.5-225 mg	Asthenia, nausea sweating, ejaculatory dysfunction
II. Antiepileptics		
Gabapentin	300-3600 mg	Sedation, dizziness
Carbamazepine	200-1200 mg	Sedation, dizziness, nausea, bone marrow suppression
Oxcarbazepine	600-2400 mg	Fatigue, nausea, dizziness, leukopenia
Lamotrigine	50-500 mg	Serious rash, dizziness, nausea sedation
Topiramate	25-400 mg	Sedation, weight loss, nephrolithiasis, myopia, angle closure glaucoma
III. Miscellaneous		
Mexiletine	150-750 mg	Dyspepsia, dizziness, tremor, arrhythmia
Tramadol	50-400 mg	Dizziness, nausea, constipation, seizures
Capsaicin 0.75%	Topical tid-qid	Burning, erythema

○   **Are patients with diabetes mellitus (DM) at risk for peripheral neuropathy (PN)?**

Peripheral neuropathies have been described in patients with primary (types 1 and 2) and secondary diabetes of diverse causes, suggesting a common etiologic mechanism based on chronic hyperglycemia. The undoubted contribution of hyperglycemia has received strong support from the Diabetes Control and Complications Trial (DCCT). Neuropathies are characterized by a progressive loss of nerve fibers that can be assessed noninvasively by several tests of nerve function, including electrophysiology, quantitative sensory testing, and autonomic function tests. Pathologically, numerous changes have been demonstrated in both myelinated and unmyelinated fibers, although Schwann cell changes may be the primary pathologic change.

○   **Summarize the pathophysiology of diabetic neuropathy**

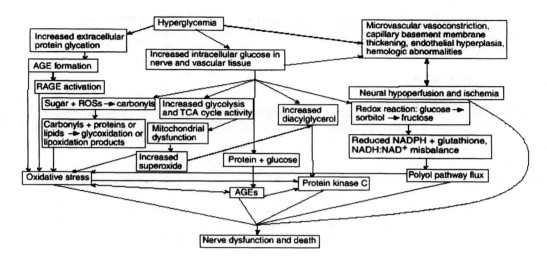

What is the pathogenesis of (PN) in patients with DM?

The pathophysiologic basis leading to the development of peripheral neuropathy in diabetes is not understood completely, and multiple hypotheses have been advanced. It generally is accepted as a multifactorial process.

What is the Diabetic Neuropathy Classification and Staging?

I. **Subclinical neuropathy**
  A. Abnormal electrodiagnostic tests
    1. Decreased nerve conduction velocity
    2. Decreased amplitude of evoked muscle or nerve action potentials
  B. Abnormal neurologic examination
    1. Vibratory and tactile tests
    2. Thermal warming and cooling tests
    3. Other
  C. Abnormal autonomic function tests
    1. Abnormal cardiovascular reflexes
    2. Altered cardiovascular reflexes
    3. Abnormal biochemical responses to hypoglycemia
II. **Clinical neuropathy**
  A. Diffuse somatic neuropathy
    1. Sensorimotor or distal symmetrical sensorimotor polyneuropathy
      a. Primarily small-fiber neuropathy
      b. Primarily large-fiber neuropathy
      c. Mixed
  B. Autonomic neuropathy
    1. Cardiovascular autonomic
    2. Abnormal pupillary function
    3. Gastrointestinal autonomic neuropathy
      a. Gastroparesis
      b. Constipation
      c. Diabetic diarrhea
      d. Anorectal incontinence
    4. Genitourinary autonomic neuropathy
      a. Bladder dysfunction
      b. Sexual dysfunction
  C. Focal Neuropathy
    1. Mononeuropathy
    2. Mononeuropathy multiplex
    3. Amyotrophy

What is the prevalence of diabetes Mellitus?

Estimates of the prevalence of diabetic polyneuropathy vary widely in literature, largely because of discrepancies in diagnostic criteria, methods of patient selection, and assessment. An estimated 10-65% of patients with diabetes have some form of peripheral neuropathy. It is estimated to be present in 7.5% of patients at the diagnosis of diabetes. Wide variability is due to lack of consistent criteria for the diagnosis of peripheral neuropathy and because most patients with diabetic polyneuropathy are initially asymptomatic, making detection extremely dependent on careful neurologic examination by the primary care giver. One half of patients have distal symmetric polyneuropathy, and one fourth have compression or entrapment neuropathies (mainly carpal tunnel syndrome).

❍   **What is the clinical time course of PN in DM?**

Typically in type I diabetes mellitus, distal polyneuropathy occurs after many years of chronic prolonged hyperglycemia. Conversely, in type II, it presents after few years of poor glycemic control. Occasionally in type II, diabetic neuropathy is found at the time of diagnosis.

❍   **What sensory symptoms may occur in patients with diabetic neuropathy?**

Sensory symptoms may be negative or positive, diffuse or focal. Negative sensory symptoms include numbness; deadness; feeling of wearing gloves or walking on stilts; loss of balance, especially with the eyes closed; and painless injuries. Positive symptoms include burning, pricking pain, electric shocklike feelings, tightness, and hypersensitivity to touch.

❍   **What motor symptoms occur?**

Motor symptoms can cause distal, proximal, or focal weakness. Distal motor symptoms include impaired fine coordination of the hand, inability to open jars or turn keys, foot slapping, and toe scuffing. Symptoms of proximal weakness include difficulty with stairs, difficulty in getting up from a sitting or lying position, falls due to the knee giving way, and difficulty raising arms above the shoulders.

❍   **What autonomic symptoms occur?**

Autonomic symptoms may be sudomotor (dry skin, lack of sweating, excessive sweating in defined areas), pupillary (poor dark adaptation, sensitivity to bright lights), cardiovascular (postural light headedness, fainting), urinary (urgency, incontinence, dribbling), gastrointestinal (nocturnal diarrhea, constipation, vomiting of retained food), and sexual (erectile impotence and ejaculatory failure in men, loss of ability to reach sexual climax in women).

❍   **What is the distal symmetric polyneuropathy?**

It is the most common diabetic neuropathy. It is chronic symmetric symptoms involving the distal extremities .The peripheral nerves affected in a length dependent pattern with the longest nerves affected first. Sensory, motor, and autonomic functions are affected in varying degrees, with sensory dysfunction predominating.

❍   **How do the sensory symptoms present with regard to symptoms and signs?**

Commonly it presents as nighttime painful paresthesias and numbness that begin in the toes and ascend proximally in a stocking like distribution over months. When the sensory symptoms reach the knees, the hands develop similar symptoms progressing proximally in a glove like distribution. There is pain and temperature loss with involvement of small fibers, predisposing to development of foot ulcers. There is impaired proprioception, vibratory perception, and gait (sensory ataxia) with involvement of large fibers.

❍   **What features may occur later in the disease process?**

The anterior aspect of the trunk and the vertex of the head possibly affected at a late stage. Weakness of foot muscles and decreased ankle and knee reflexes develop later in the disease process.. Anhidrosis, bladder atony, and unreactive pupils are possible from autonomic dysfunction.

❍   **What is the Small fiber neuropathy?**

It is less common distal symmetric neuropathy involving predominantly small diameter sensory fibers (A delta and C fibers). It presents as painful paresthesias that are burning, stabbing, crushing, aching, or cramplike, with increased severity at night. There is loss of pain and temperature sensation present, with sparing of distal reflexes and proprioception.

○   **What is the Large fiber neuropathy?**

It is less common distal symmetric neuropathy involving mainly the large diameter sensory fibers.
There is a painless electric tingling or a snug bandlike sensation around ankles and feet; prominent ataxia.
There are absent ankle jerk reflexes, prominent proprioceptive sensory impairment, and gait instability with eyes closed.

○   **What is Diabetic autonomic neuropathy?**

It is a pure autonomic neuropathy (rare). There is some degree of autonomic involvement present in most patients with diabetic polyneuropathy. The signs including orthostatic hypotension, resting tachycardia, loss of sinus arrhythmia, and small pupils with sluggish light reflex.

○   **What is Diabetic neuropathic cachexia?**

It usually occurs in older men with a history of significant weight loss. The symptoms begin with severe aching or stabbing pain in feet, worse at night. There is impotence (common). There is sensory loss and muscle weakness (uncommon).

○   **What is diabetic cranial mononeuropathy?**

Common nerves involved are the oculomotor (III, IV, VI), facial (VII), and optic (causing anterior ischemic optic neuropathy). Diabetic oculomotor cranial mononeuropathies primarily involve cranial nerve (CN) III, followed by CN VI; CN IV rarely affected alone. It often presents as acute or subacute periorbital pain or headache followed by diplopia. Muscle weakness typically is in a distribution of a single oculomotor nerve with sparing of pupillary reflex. Complete spontaneous recovery usually occurs within 3 months. Facial neuropathy presents with acute or subacute facial weakness (often taste is not involved); can be recurrent or bilateral; most recover spontaneously in 3-6 months. Anterior ischemic optic neuropathy presenting with acute visual loss or visual field defects (usually inferior altitudinal). The optic disk is often pale and swollen, accompanied by flame shaped hemorrhages.

○   **What are examples of diabetic somatic mononeuropathies?**

Focal neuropathies in the extremities are caused by either entrapment or compression of the nerve where it crosses common pressure points or by ischemia and subsequent infarction of the nerve. Entrapment and compression tends to occur in the same nerves and at the same sites as in individuals without diabetes. Common sites include the median nerve at the wrist (carpal tunnel syndrome), ulnar nerve at the elbow, and common peroneal nerve at the fibular head; often bilateral. Neuropathy secondary to nerve infarction presents acutely with focal pain associated with weakness and variable sensory loss in the distribution of the affected nerve. Multiple nerves are possibly affected at random, one after the other (mononeuritis multiplex).

○   **What is Diabetic Polyradiculopathy?**

It is single or more commonly multiple contiguous spinal roots involved. It Includes 2 syndromes, thoracoabdominal neuropathy and lumbosacral radiculoplexopathy.

○   **What is diabetic Thoracoabdominal neuropathy?**

It occurs in patients older than 50 years; more common in diabetes mellitus type II; often associated with significant weight loss. It presents with chest and/or abdominal pain in the distribution of thoracic and/or upper lumbar roots. There is burning, stabbing, boring, beltlike, or deep aching pain that is more intense at night .The onset of pain is usually unilateral; then may become bilateral. Touch possibly hypersensitive; contact with clothing may be unpleasant. Sensory deficits are usually with a dermatomal distribution; most prominent in distal distribution of intercostal nerves. Weakness presents as bulging of the abdominal wall from abdominal muscle paresis or weakness of quadriceps in L3-L4 involvement. Territorial extension of symptoms often occur in the cephalad, caudal, or contralateral side. Coexisting diabetic distal symmetric polyneuropathy is often present.

○   **What is diabetic lumbosacral radiculoplexopathy?**

Synonyms include asymmetric proximal motor neuropathy, diabetic amyotrophy, diabetic femoral neuropathy, femorosciatic neuropathy, and diabetic myelopathy (Bruhn-Garland syndrome). It often occurs in patients older than 50 years, in patients with poorly controlled diabetes, and predominantly in men rather than women. There is significant weight loss in 50% of patients. Symptoms begin unilaterally; later may spread to the opposite limb. It starts as sudden, severe, unilateral pain in the lower back or hips and spreads to the anterior thigh. Weakness develops days to weeks later in the hip and thigh muscles; can lead to profound atrophy of the proximal lower limb musculature. Usually there is an absent knee reflex; the ankle reflex may be depressed. Numbness and paresthesias are uncommon..

O   What is acute painful neuropathy (diabetic cachexia)?

It is a less common diabetic neuropathy syndrome characterized by precipitous and profound weight loss followed by severe and unremitting cutaneous pain, typically worse at night, and by small fiber neuropathy characterized by distal burning pain, hypesthesia, and autonomic dysfunction. Symptoms usually improve with prolonged hyperglycemia control. Pharmacologic treatment is usually not effective. Nonpharmacologic treatments that have been tried with limited success include sympathectomy, spinal cord blockade, and electrical spinal cord stimulation.

O   What are some of the clinical findings in patients with diabetic PN?

Diabetic polyneuropathy typically develops as generalized asymptomatic dysfunction of peripheral nerve fibers. The most common early dysfunction is abnormal nerve conduction studies or a reduction of the heart beat response to deep breathing or to Valsalva maneuver. The first clinical sign that usually develops with abnormal nerve conductions is decrease or loss of ankle jerks or decrease or loss of vibratory sensation over the great toes. With more severe involvement, the patient develops varying degrees and modalities of pain; sensory loss of the toes, feet, and distal legs; deep tendon reflex abnormalities; and weakness of small foot muscles.

O   Is there a role for electrodiagnostic studies in the patient with presumed diabetic polyneuropathy?

Electrophysiologic studies of peripheral nerve function are the most sensitive, reliable, and reproducible measures of nerve function, which also correlate with the morphologic findings on nerve biopsy. Although they can define and quantitate nerve dysfunction, the abnormalities found are not specific to diabetes.

O   What do motor nerve conduction studies reveal?

Motor nerve conduction is monitored by the amplitude of compound muscle action potentials or measured motor conduction velocities. Conduction abnormalities reflect losses of large diameter myelinated nerve fibers and usually are more pronounced in the legs than the arms. These effects reflect the length dependent degeneration of large diameter nerve fibers. Motor nerve conduction velocities should not be less than 50% of the normal mean; if so, seek another cause. Neither should conduction block be present. Abnormalities of sensorimotor conduction testing may be found in patients with diabetes even without clinical evidence of distal symmetric polyneuropathy. The initial abnormality may be found in the sensory nerves (sural, superficial peroneal, median nerves).

O   What do SNAPs reveal in diabetic polyneuropathy?

The sensory nerve action potentials (SNAP) show reduced, poorly formed amplitude or absent responses and slow conduction velocities. Low amplitude motor responses and slight reduction of the amplitudes may be seen in the common peroneal nerves. The late responses (common peroneal and tibial F waves, tibial H reflexes) are prolonged or absent. Overall, these reflect the primary pathologic changes of axonal degeneration.

O   What does EMG reveal in diabetic polyneuropathy?

Electromyographic sampling of distal muscles of the lower extremities reveals evidence of denervation in the form of positive sharp waves and fibrillations (spontaneous discharges). Reinnervation changes such as high amplitude, long duration, and polyphasic motor unit potentials reflect chronicity. Abnormalities in the paraspinal muscles by needle examination (spontaneous discharges) are found bilaterally and may reflect polyradiculopathy.

O   What is the most effective treatment for diabetic polyneuropathy?

Of all the treatments, tight and stable glycemic control is probably the only one that may provide symptomatic relief as well as slow the relentless progression of the neuropathic state. Because blood glucose flux, with rapid swings from hypoglycemia to hyperglycemia, has been suggested to aggravate and induce neuropathic pain, the stability rather than the actual level of glycemic control may be more important in relieving neuropathic pain. The DCCT demonstrated that tight blood sugar control decreased the risk of neuropathy by 60% in 5 years.

O   **What is uremic neuropathy?**

Uremic neuropathy is a distal sensorimotor polyneuropathy caused by uremic toxins. A strong correlation exists between the severity of neuropathy and severity of the renal insufficiency. Uremic neuropathy is considered a dying back neuropathy or central-peripheral axonopathy associated with secondary demyelination. However, uremia and its treatment also can be associated with mononeuropathy at compression sites.

O   **How common is uremic neuropathy?**

Peripheral neuropathy associated with end stage renal disease is common, affecting as many as 65% of patients at the time of initiation of dialysis.

O   **What symptoms are present?**

Typical uremic neuropathy symptoms are insidious in onset and consist of a tingling and prickling sensation in the lower extremities. Paresthesia is most common and is usually the earliest symptom. Increased pain sensation is a prominent complaint. Weakness of lower extremities and atrophy follow the sensory symptoms. As disease progresses, symptoms move proximally and involve the upper extremities. Muscle cramps and restless legs syndrome were reported by 67% of uremic patients. The symptoms can also be seen in uremic patients without neuropathy. Patients report that crawling, prickling, and itching sensations in their lower extremities are relieved partially by movement of the affected limb.

O   **What physical findings are encountered?**

Impaired vibratory perception and absent deep tendon reflexes are the most common clinical signs in 93% of patients. Sensory loss to pinprick in a glove and stocking distribution occurred in 16%. Paradoxic heat sensation was found in the foot in 42% of patients with chronic renal failure compared to less than 10% of healthy controls. Paradoxic heat sensation probably results from lowering of heat pain threshold. Muscular weakness and wasting were observed in 14%. Cranial nerve involvement is rare; transient nystagmus, miosis, impairment of extraocular movement, and facial asymmetry may be rarely found on physical examination. Focal weakness, sensory loss, and positive Tinel sign at compression sites can be found in the median, ulnar, or peroneal nerve distribution if compressive mononeuropathy is present. Abnormal Valsalva maneuver and orthostatic hypotension may be found in the patients with autonomic neuropathy.

O   **What abnormalities are evident on NCS/EMG?**

Nerve conduction study is a sensitive test for diagnosis of neuropathy in patients with uremia. Both sensory and motor nerve conduction velocities are reduced. Prolonged distal latencies are due to involvement of distal nerve segments; reduced compound action potential amplitudes are due mainly to reduced density of large myelinated motor and sensory fibers. .

O   **What effect does renal transplantation have on uremic neuropathy?**

Numerous case reports exist on the beneficial effect of renal transplantation. Nielsen reported that all successful transplantation patients showed definite improvement. Paresthesia disappeared within 1-3 months in mild uremic neuropathy. The remission after transplantation had 2 phases, with an early rapid and a late slow phase in moderate to severe neuropathy. Rapid improvement in nerve conduction velocity shortly after successful transplantation was noted. Renal transplantation reverses the sympathetic and parasympathetic autonomic dysfunction in as early as 3-6 months.

O   **What are the manifestations of thyroid neuropathy?**

Polyneuropathy is usually subacute, sensory, and occurs in 31-65% of patients. Subclinical hypothyroidism also may present with peripheral nerve involvement. Sensory complaints include painful dysesthesias in the hands and feet and radiating lancinating pains, occasionally suggesting nerve root compression. Examination findings may reveal distal glove and stocking sensory loss and ataxia. Weakness is a common complaint, but it usually is related to myopathic involvement. Hyporeflexia and delayed relaxation phase of the ankle jerk are common. Transient swelling on percussion of the skin (mounding phenomenon) may be observed. Occasionally, hyperthyroidism may be associated with polyneuropathy.

O   **What are the clinical features of Monoclonal gammopathies, such as cryoglobulinemia, monoclonal gammopathy of undetermined significance (MGUS), and myelin associated glycoprotein (MAG)–associated gammopathy?**

It is associated with the presence of monoclonal proteins in the serum. Amyloidosis, osteosclerotic myeloma, or related disorders are absent. MGUS presents as a symmetric sensorimotor polyneuropathy that begins insidiously and progresses slowly over months or years. It occurs especially in the fifth, sixth, and seventh decades of life. Males are affected more commonly than females. Paresthesias, ataxia, and pain may be prominent. Cranial nerves are not affected.

O   **What are the clinical features of amyloid neuropathy (nonfamilial?)**

Progressive involvement of small diameter fibers with loss of pain and temperature sensation is typical of amyloid neuropathy, but occasionally patients can develop large fiber neuropathy as well. It presents commonly as CTS or as a painful peripheral neuropathy. Initial symptoms of neuropathy are sensory, with more extensive involvement of the lower extremities. With time, motor symptoms develop and are more prominent in the lower limbs. Occasionally, amyloid neuropathy may manifest as autonomic dysfunction with severe orthostatic hypotension, syncopal episodes, or sexual impotence. In patients whose amyloidosis begins with neuropathy, the clue to the diagnosis may be involvement of the heart, bowel, or kidneys.

O   **What are the clinical features of porphyric neuropathy?**

Disorders of porphyrin metabolism are a rare cause of peripheral neuropathy. Only hepatic porphyrias are associated with neurologic disease. Acute intermittent porphyria may be associated with attacks of acute motor neuropathy with mild sensory symptoms very similar to Guillain-Barré syndrome. Attacks are precipitated by drugs like phenytoin and phenobarbital and may be accompanied by abdominal pain, confusion, and seizures.

O   **What is the pathogenesis of ethanol polyneuropathy?**

The precise pathogenesis of alcohol neuropathy remains unclear. Nutritional deficiency (frequently associated with alcohol neuropathy) and/or the direct toxic effect of alcohol or both have been implicated and studied. Most studies of peripheral neuropathy in humans and animals implicate nutritional deficiency as an etiology as opposed to the direct toxic effect of alcohol.

O   **What does NCS/EMG reveal?**

Electrophysiologic findings primarily reveal evidence of primary axonal polyneuropathy.

O   **What are the sensory electrophysiological findings?**

Sensory conduction studies may be abnormal even before the advent of clinical symptoms. Sural nerve sensory action potentials (SNAP) are reduced slightly to moderately in conduction velocity and SNAP amplitudes also are reduced. As the condition worsens, the sensory potentials may become unobtainable. The median, radial, and ulnar nerves show the same response as the disease progresses.

O   **What do the motor electrophysiological findings reveal?**

Motor conduction studies of the lower extremities (tibial and peroneal nerves) may reveal a slight reduction in conduction velocity (not to exceed 70-80% of the lower limit of normal), with diminution of the compound muscle action potential (CMAP) amplitude with a slight prolongation in distal latency. The upper extremity nerves follow the same pattern as time progresses.

O   **What is observed with regard to the late responses?**

The tibial H reflex latency is prolonged and becomes unobtainable if the condition continues to progress. The F waves are obtained more easily but reveal slight to moderate prolongation of latency.

O **What does needle electromyography reveal?**

Needle electromyography (EMG) examination of the distal muscles of the lower extremities shows active denervation as well as chronic changes in the form of reinnervation patterns. Spontaneous activity (positive sharp waves and fibrillation) is seen in the tibialis anterior and gastrocnemius. The motor unit action potentials are reduced in recruitment pattern, with high amplitude, long duration, and polyphasic motor units.

O **What is the basic definition of the Acute inflammatory demyelinating polyneuropathy (AIDP)?**

It is an autoimmune process that is characterized by progressive weakness and mild sensory changes. Many variants exist. In the West, the most common presentation is a subacute ascending paralysis. This is associated with distal paresthesias and loss of deep tendon reflexes. The condition usually plateaus after about 2-3 weeks before slowly improving. Clinically it is commonly referred to as Guillain-Barré syndrome.

O **Summarize the Acquired Demyelinating Disorders of the Peripheral Nervous System.**

Acquired Demyelinating Disorders of the Peripheral Nervous System
Acute
Guillain-Barré syndrome
Acute inflammatory demyelinating polyradiculoneuropathy (AIDP)
Acute axon loss ("axonal") polyradiculopathy
Acute motor axonal neuropathy
Acute motor-sensory axonal neuropathy
Chronic
Chronic inflammatory demyelinating polyradiculopathy (CIDP)
Monoclonal gammopathies of undetermined significance (MGUS)
MGUS IgM neuropathy with anti-MAG antibody
MGUS IgG, IgA, IgM neuropathy without anti-MAG antibody
CIDP with multiple myeloma
CIDP with osteosclerotic myeloma
CIDP with Waldenström's macroglobulinemia
Motor neuropathy with multifocal conduction block

O **What is the basic pathophysiology of AIDP?**

AIDP is believed to be caused by an immunologic attack that is directed against myelin components. This results in a demyelinating polyneuropathy. Both cellular and humoral immune mechanisms appear to play a role. Early inflammatory lesions consist of a lymphocytic infiltrate that is adjacent to segmental demyelination. Macrophages are more prominent several days later. Immune responses are directed against the antigen components associated with antecedent entities. These components produce antibodies that cross react with myelin to cause demyelination. This process has been termed molecular mimicry.

O **What is the incidence of GBS?**

In a recent epidemiological survey in the United States, the average annual incidence was 3.0 cases per 100,000 population. In comparing age groups, the annual mean rate of hospitalizations related to GBS increased with age with a rate of 1.5 cases per 100,000 population in persons aged less than 15 years to a peak of 8.6 cases per 100,000 in persons aged 70-79 years.

O **What morbidity and mortality associated with GBS?**

In epidemiologic surveys, the overall death rates range from 2-12% of patients. GBS associated mortality rates increase markedly with age. In the United States, the case fatality ratio ranges from 0.7% among persons aged less than 15 years to 8.6% among persons aged more than 65 years.

○ **Is there a gender associated disparity in mortality with GBS?**

Though the death rate increases with age in both males and females, males have a death rate 1.3 times greater than females after the age of 40 years.

○ **What is the usual causes of death in GBS patients?**

GBS related deaths usually occur in ventilator dependent patients due to complications such as pneumonia, sepsis, adult respiratory distress syndrome, or, less frequently, autonomic dysfunction. Underlying pulmonary disease and the need for mechanical ventilation increase the risk of death, especially in elderly patients. Length of hospital stays also increases with advancing age, due to disease severity and associated medical complications.

○ **What antecedent history is significant in patients with GBS?**

Up to two thirds of patients with GBS report an antecedent illness or event 1-3 weeks prior to the onset of weakness.

○ **Summarize the Antecedent Events Associated with Guillain-Barré Syndrome**

Antecedent Events Associated with Guillain-Barré Syndrome
Viral
Influenza
Herpes
Cytomegalovirus
Epstein-Barr virus
Hepatitis
Human immunodeficiency virus
Surgery
Bacterial
Campylobacter jejuni
Mycoplasma pneumoniae
Spirochetal
Borrelia burgdorferi
Vaccination
Rabies (some strains)
Vaccinia

○ **What is the differential diagnosis of AIDP?**

Differential Diagnosis of Guillain-Barré Syndrome
Hysteria/conversion reaction
Malingering
Brain stem infarction (Locked-in syndrome)
Acute myelopathies
Poliomyelitis

Rabies
Enteroviruses
Necrotic
Transverse
Focal compression
Cauda equina lesions
Peripheral neuropathies
Heavy metals; arsenic, thallium, gold
Alcohol
Organophosphates
Hexacarbons
Diphtheria
Drugs
Lyme disease
Critical illness
Vasculitis
Neuromuscular transmission disorders
Botulism
Tick-bite paralysis
Myasthenic syndrome
Myasthenia gravis
Snake venom
Sea urchin venom
Hypermagnesemia
Muscle disorders
Hypokalemia
Hyperkalemia

❍   **What characterizes the history of weakness in the GBS patient?**

The hallmark of classic AIDP is progressive weakness that usually begins in the feet before involving all 4 limbs. At presentation, 60% of patients have weakness in all 4 limbs. Weakness plateaus at 2 weeks after onset in 50% of patients and by 4 weeks in over 90%. It is usually symmetric, although mild asymmetry is not uncommon early in the disease course. In the arms, weakness may be worse proximally than distally. At presentation, half of patients have some facial weakness, although only 5% have varying degrees of ophthalmoplegia. Oropharyngeal or respiratory weakness is a presenting symptom in 40% of patients. Improvement in strength usually begins 1-4 weeks after the plateau. About one third of patients require mechanical ventilation because of respiratory failure.

❍   **What sensory symptoms occur in the patient with GBS?**

Most patients complain of paresthesias, numbness, or similar sensory changes. Sensory symptoms often precede the weakness. Sensory symptoms frequently are ascending in nature and are more pronounced in a distal distribution. Sensory symptoms are usually mild. Objective findings of sensory loss tend to be minimal and variable in most cases. On nerve conduction studies (NCS), 58-76% of patients exhibit sensory abnormalities.

❍   **What cranial nerve deficits occur in GBS?**

Cranial nerve involvement is observed in 45-75% of patients with GBS. Common complaints may include the following: Facial droop, Diplopias, Dysarthria, and Dysphagia.

O   **Is pain a concomitant symptom in the presentation of GBS?**

In a prospective, longitudinal study of pain in patients with GBS, 89% of patients reported pain attributable to GBS at some time during their illness. On initial presentation, almost 50% of patients described the pain as severe and distressing. The mechanism of pain is thought to be inflamed nerve roots. Dysesthetic symptoms are observed in approximately 50% of patients during the course of their illness. Other pain syndromes in GBS can include myalgic complaints with cramping and local muscle tenderness, visceral pain, and pain associated with conditions of immobility (eg, pressure nerve palsies, decubitus ulcers). Intensity of pain on admission correlates poorly with neurologic disability on admission and end outcome.

O   **What are the characteristics of the neuropathic pain associated with GBS?**

Dysesthesias frequently are described as burning, tingling, or shocklike sensations and are often more prevalent in the lower extremities than in the upper extremities. Dysesthesias may persist indefinitely in 5-10% of patients.

O   **What autonomic symptoms occur in the GBS patient?**

Autonomic nervous system involvement with dysfunction in the sympathetic and parasympathetic systems can be observed in patients with GBS. Autonomic changes can include the following: Tachycardia, Bradycardia, Facial flushing, Paroxysmal hypertension, orthostatic hypotension, Anhidrosis and/or diaphoresis. Urinary retention and paralytic ileus also can be observed. Bowel and bladder dysfunction rarely presents as an early symptom or persists for a significant period of time. Dysautonomia is more frequent in patients with severe weakness and respiratory failure. Autonomic changes rarely persist in the patient with GBS.

O   **What respiratory symptoms may be reported in the GBS patient?**

Upon presentation, 40% of patients have respiratory or oropharyngeal weakness and typical complaints may include the following: Dyspnea on exertion, Shortness of breath, Difficulty swallowing, slurred speech. Ventilatory failure with required respiratory support is observed in up to one third of patients at some time during the course of their disease.

O   **What vital sign disturbances may be encountered in the GBS patient?**

Cardiac arrhythmias, including tachycardias and bradycardias, can be observed due to autonomic nervous system involvement. Tachypnea may be a sign of ongoing dyspnea and progressive respiratory failure. Blood pressure lability is also a common feature with alterations between hypertension and hypotension.

O   **What Cranial nerve abnormalities may occur in the GBS patient?**

Facial weakness (cranial nerve VII) is observed most frequently, followed by symptoms associated with cranial nerves VI, III, XII, V, IX, and X. Involvement of facial, oropharyngeal, and ocular muscles results in facial droop, dysphagia, dysarthria, and findings associated with disorders of the eye. Ophthalmoparesis may be observed in up to 25% of patients with GBS. The most common limitation of eye movement is from a symmetric palsy associated with cranial nerve VI. Ptosis from cranial nerve III (oculomotor) palsy often is associated with limited eye movements. Pupillary abnormalities also are relatively common, especially accompanying ophthalmoparesis.

O   **What abnormal findings are encountered in the Motor examination?**

Lower extremity weakness usually begins first and ascends symmetrically and progressively over the first several days. Upper extremity, trunk, facial, and oropharyngeal weakness is observed to a variable extent. Marked asymmetric weakness calls the diagnosis of GBS into question.

O   **What abnormal findings may manifest in the sensory examination?**

Despite frequent complaints of paresthesias, objective sensory changes are minimal. A well demarcated sensory level should not be observed in patients with GBS, and such a finding calls the diagnosis of GBS into question.

○ **What Reflex changes occur in the GBS patient?**

Reflexes are absent or hyporeflexic early in the disease course and represent a major clinical finding on examination of the patient with GBS. Pathologic reflexes, such as Babinski, are absent. Hypotonia can be observed with significant weakness.

○ **What do CSF studies reveal in GBS?**

During the acute phase of GBS, the characteristic findings include albuminocytologic dissociation, which is an elevation in CSF protein (>0.55 g/L) without an elevation of white blood cells (<10lymphocytes/mm^3). The increase in CSF protein is thought to reflect the widespread inflammatory disease of the nerve roots. However, this finding is not specific to AIDP.

○ **What is the diagnostic role of NCS/EMG in GBS?**

Abnormalities in the NCS consistent with demyelination are sensitive and represent specific findings for classic GBS. Though NCS results classically show a picture of demyelinating neuropathy in most patients, other electrophysiologic subgroups include axonal and inexcitable groups. The inexcitable studies may represent either axonopathy or severe demyelination with distal conduction block. Though most patients' exhibit sensory abnormalities on NCS, these findings are much less marked than in motor nerves.

○ **What are the typical NCS findings in GBS?**

On NCS, demyelination is characterized by nerve conduction slowing, prolongation of the distal latencies, prolongation of the F waves, conduction block, and/or temporal dispersion. Changes on NCS should be present in at least 2 nerves in regions not typical for compressive mononeuropathies, preferentially in anatomically distinct areas (eg, an arm and a leg, a limb and the face).

○ **What does EMG reveal in GBS?**

The needle examination is of limited value in GBS. Reduced motor unit recruitment and absent denervation help support suggestion of a demyelinating mechanism, though the same changes can be observed in early axonal damage with pending Wallerian degeneration. Denervation changes may be observed later in the disease course with severe cases .In the axonal variant of the disease, absent or markedly reduced distal compound muscle action potentials (CMAP) are observed on NCS. On needle examination, profuse and early denervation potentials also support the conclusion that there has been axonal injury.

○ **What do PFTs reveal in GBS?**

Maximal inspiratory pressures and vital capacities are measurements of neuromuscular respiratory function and predict diaphragmatic strength. Maximal expiratory pressures also reflect abdominal muscle strength. Frequent evaluations of these parameters should be performed at bedside to monitor respiratory status and the need for ventilatory assistance. Respiratory assistance should be considered when the expiratory vital capacity decreases to <18 mL/kg or there is a decrease in oxygen saturation (arterial PO$_2$ <70 mm Hg).

○ **What is the role of physical therapy in the rehabilitation of the GBS patient?**

Early in the acute phase of the disease course, patients may not be able to participate fully in an active therapy program. At that stage, patients benefit from daily range of motion (ROM) exercises and proper positioning to prevent muscle shortening and joint contractures. Addressing upright tolerance and endurance also may be a significant issue during the early part of rehabilitation. Active muscle strengthening then can be introduced slowly and may include isometric, isotonic, isokinetic, or progressive resistive exercises. Mobility skills, such as bed mobility, transfers, and ambulation, are targeted functions. Patients should be monitored for hemodynamic instability and cardiac arrhythmias, especially upon initiation of the rehabilitation program. The intensity of the exercise program also should be monitored, as overworking the muscles, paradoxically, may lead to worsening weakness.

○   **What is the role of occupational therapy in the rehabilitation of the GBS patient?**

Occupational therapy professionals should be involved early in the rehabilitation program to promote upper body strengthening, ROM, and activities to promote functional self care. Both restorative and compensatory strategies can be used to promote functional improvements. Energy conservation techniques and work simplification also may be helpful, especially if the patient demonstrates poor strength and endurance.

○   **What is the role of speech therapy in the GBS patient?**

Speech therapy is involved to work on safe swallowing and speech skills for patients with significant oropharyngeal weakness, with resultant dysphagia and dysarthria. In ventilator dependent patients, alternative communication strategies also may need to be implemented. Once weaned from the ventilator, patients with tracheostomies can learn voicing strategies and eventually can be weaned from the tracheostomy tube. Cognitive screening also can be performed conjointly with neuropsychology to assess for deficits, as cognitive problems have been reported in some patients with GBS, especially patients after an extended stay in the intensive care unit (ICU).

○   **What is the role of immunomodulatory therapy?**

Immunomodulatory therapy, such as plasmapheresis or intravenous immunoglobulin (IVIG), frequently is used in GBS patients. The efficacy of plasmapheresis and IVIG appears about equal in shortening the average duration of disease. The efficacy of IVIG in GBS patients has been shown to equal that of plasma exchange in well controlled clinical trials. IVIG is easier to implement and potentially safer, and use of IVIG versus plasma exchange may be a choice of availability and convenience. The decision to use immunomodulatory therapy is based on the severity of the disease, rate of progression, and length of time between the first symptom and presentation. Patients with rapidly progressive severe disease are most likely to benefit from treatment, with improvements in the rate of functional recovery.

○   **Is there any therapeutic efficacy associated with the administration of corticosteroids in AIDP?**

Oral and intravenous steroids have been tried in GBS without any clinical benefit and are not used currently in the treatment of GBS.

○   **What is the outcome for GBS patients?**

Though most patients with GBS make good recovery, 2-12% die from complications related to GBS, and a significant percentage of survivors have persistent motor sequelae. Estimates indicate that 75-85% of patients experience good recoveries, 15-20% have moderate residual deficits, and 1-10% are left severely disabled. Though the exact prevalence is uncertain, up to 25,000-50,000 persons in the United States may have long term functional deficits from GBS. The speed of recovery varies. Recovery often takes place within a few weeks or months; however, if axonal degeneration has occurred, recovery can be expected to progress slowly over many months as regeneration may require 6-18 months. In general, slower and less complete recovery is observed in older patients.

○   **What patient related factors impact prognosis in GBS?**

Older age, poor upper extremity (UE) muscle strength, the need for mechanical ventilation, Medical Research Council (MRC) scores of <40, and preceding gastrointestinal infections all have been found to have an adverse effect on outcomes associated with GBS. A rapidly progressive onset of weakness also has been associated with less favorable outcomes in many studies, though delayed time to peak disability has been shown to be an independent predictor of poor outcome at 1 year in other studies. Low mean CMAP amplitudes of less than 20% of the lower limit of normal or the presence of inexcitable nerves on initial electrophysiologic studies are other predictors of poorer functional outcomes. Persistence of a low mean CMAP on later testing (more than 1 month after onset) results in an even higher sensitivity and specificity of testing than the initial test after onset. The sex of the patient, the presence of underlying pulmonary disease, or manifestation of dysautonomia has no prognostic significance.

○   **What is Charcot Marie tooth Disease?**

Also known as hereditary motor and sensory neuropathy (HMSN), Charcot-Marie-Tooth (CMT) syndromes are among the most common hereditary NMDs, with prevalence ranging from 14-282 cases per million population. At least 8 forms of HMSN exist. Types I, II, and III represent the Charcot-Marie-Tooth syndrome. HMSN I (hypertrophic nerve), the most common HMSN, is characterized by markedly reduced conduction velocities in peripheral motor and sensory nerves. HMSN II (neuronal form) exhibits predominant axonal loss, while conduction velocities remain relatively normal. CMT1 has four subtypes (CMT1 A, B, C and D), which have the same clinical presentations but different genetic causes. HMSN II usually is a less severe disease than HMSN I, although clinically it may not be distinguished easily from type I. CMT2 has five subtypes (CMT2 A, B, C, D and E). HMSN III is a congenital hypomyelinating neuropathy, with symptoms beginning in infancy.

O   **What are the clinical features of HMSN type I?**

In all CMT1 genotypes, 50-75% of affected individuals present with pes cavus and hammertoes. Approximately 65% of the cases have distal upper limb involvement. Distal sensory impairment is present, but is usually asymptomatic; vibratory sensation is typically diminished.

O   **What are the clinical features of CMT2?**

It is an axonal form of CMT that is characterized by chronic axonal loss and normal or near normal NCVs. CMT2A and CMT2B have similar clinical presentations as CMT1, but symptoms usually develop in the second decade. Individuals with CMT2 tend to be less disabled and have less sensory loss, as well.

O   **What are the features associated with Déjérine-Sottas Neuropathy (DSN)?**

DSN is a severe demyelinating neuropathy with onset in infancy or early childhood. The disorder is characterized by very slow (<6 m/s) NCVs.

O   **What is CMT4?**

CMT4 is a rare form of demyelinating CMT characterized by progressive motor/sensory neuropathies with autosomal recessive inheritance. Affected individuals have the typical CMT phenotype of distal muscle weakness and atrophy associated with sensory loss and, frequently, pes cavus, although it is usually more severe and the onset is earlier. CMT4 comprises six subtypes (CMT4 A, B, C, D, E and F) and is usually marked by slow (15-30 m/s) NCVs.

O   **What are the CMT1X Clinical Presentations?**

CMT1X is an X-linked form of CMT that may be inherited dominantly or, rarely, recessively. CMT1X clinical features overlap with those of CMT1. Males are more severely affected than females. Affected males have childhood or adolescent onset of a slowly progressive motor/sensory neuropathy associated with foot drop, pes cavus and distal limb atrophy. Affected females exhibit milder symptoms or may be asymptomatic.

O   **What are the pathological features associated with CMT1X?**

Pathologically, there is primary axonopathy with secondary demyelination, although a mixed picture (myelinopathy/axonopathy) may be identified by electrodiagnostic studies. NCVs of affected males are typically faster (20-30 m/s) than those of individuals affected by CMT1, but there is an overlap in NCV ranges between the two types. Mild slowing of NCVs is typical in affected females.

O   **How do the Charcot-Marie-Tooth Disorders compare genetically and electrophysiologically?**

Type	Mode of inheritance	Nerve conduction velocities	Proportion of HMSN cases
CMT1	Autosomal dominant	Slow (10-30 m/s)	50%
CMT1X	X-linked dominant (recessive in rare instances)	Faster than CMT1 NCVs (10-30 m/s), but some overlap between the two types	10-15%
CMT2	Autosomal dominant	Normal or near normal, occasionally	20-40%

	(recessive in rare instances) [10]	mildly slow (35-50 m/s)	
Déjérine-Sottas Neuropathy	Autosomal dominant and autosomal recessive	Very slow (<6 m/s) [10]	Unknown
CMT4	Autosomal recessive	Slow (15-30 m/s) [10]	Rare
HNPP	Autosomal dominant	Mildly slowed, conduction blocks	Unknown

MONONEUROPATHIES

○   **What are the clinical sequelae of an axillary nerve injury?**

Paresis of the deltoid muscle leads to a paresis of abduction of the arm (acromial part of the muscle), a paresis of elevation (clavicular part), and a paresis of backward movement of the horizontally elevated arm (spinal part). Cause of a lesion may be a trauma to the shoulder, repositioning after shoulder luxation, or proximal fracture of the upper arm. A true compression of the nerve in the lateral axillary gap (quadrilateral space) is very rare. It is characterized by pain and paresthesia in the shoulder and upper arm with irradiation down to the hand.

○   **What therapeutic intervention is recommended?**

The rare compression of the nerve in the posterior axillary gap is best cured by operative dorsal decompression. With other types of lesion, stretching the shoulder joint and painful pericapsular adhesions of this joint have to be avoided by carrying the arm in a sling and by passive movement. If there is no spontaneous reinnervation after 6-8 weeks after a traumatic lesion, an operative revision is advisable, including if necessary neurolysis, nerve suture, or nerve transplantation. Surrogate operations frequently proposed for irreversible palsies usually show indifferent results, so that in the presence of isolated axillary nerve lesions training should be used to strengthen the supraspinatus muscle for arm abduction, the clavicular part of the pectoralis major muscle, the coracobrachialis muscle, and the long head of the biceps. If the result of physical training is insufficient, arthrodesis of the shoulder joint may be considered, but only if the motion of the scapula is unrestricted.

○   **Summarize the Compression Syndromes of Proximal Arm & Shoulder Girdle Nerves: (may need polishing up via formatting)**

Nerve	Clinical signs	Etiology	Therapy
Dorsal scapular nerve (dorsal branch of the plexus from root C3-C5), innervating the levator scapulae and rhomboid muscles	Slight dislocation of the scapula (medial rim and inferior angle slightly rotated outward, medial rim slightly sticking out, bad fixation of the scapula, pain medial to the scapula)	Gunshot and stab lesions; because of its covered position compressions are rare; rarely seen with hypertrophy of the scalenus medius muscle	Usually not necessary, with stab wounds nerve suture, surgery for substitute of rhomboid function: connection of the lower scapular angle to the latissimus dorsi muscle
Suprascapular nerve (from roots C4-C6 via the upper primary bundle), innervates supra- and infraspinatus muscles, branches to the scalenus medius muscle	Paresis of lateral rotation and abduction, especially within above the scapula, especially during pull forward and to the opposite side of the body	Chronic compression at the incisura scapulae, especially by frequent pull of the shoulder forward; fractures of the collum scapulae	Incision of the ligamentum transversum scapulae, if necessary, neurolysis; surrogate operation for paresis of lateral rotation: transposition of the teres major muscle to the dorsal side of the humerus
Subscapular nerve (from roots C5-C8 from the upper primary bundle and posterior fascicle), innervates subscapular and teres major muscle	Atrophy invisible because of deep anatomical position of the muscle; inward rotation of upper arm hardly involved if the function of other inward rotators (pectoralis major muscle, latissimus dorsi, and anterior part of the deltoid muscle) is intact	Isolated lesion very rare because of the deep protected position	Usually not necessary in an isolated lesion of the nerve
Long thoracic nerve (from	Sticking out of the scapula,	Compression by bandages,	Immobilization to avoid pull

roots C5-C7 before the formation of the primary bundle), innervates the serratus anterior muscle	especially during arm elevation (scapula alata) displacement of the scapula rostrally and of the lower scapula angle medially, lateral tilt of the acromion	carrying of loads (rucksack paresis), iatrogenic tear during thoracotomy, extirpation of lymph nodes in the axilla, paresis as a part of neuralgic shoulder amyotrophy, parainfectious neuritis	of the muscle by the weight of the arm; if necessary, fixation of the lower scapula angle at the scapula of the opposite side or at the ninth rib or by the latissimus dorsi and pectoralis major muscle
Thoracodorsal nerve (from roots C6-C8 and the medium primary bundle), innervates latissimus dorsi muscle and partly also teres major muscle	Weakness of adduction, inward rotation and lowering of the upper arm	Isolated lesions rare	Usually not necessary, loss of function is compensated for by the pectoralis major and teres major muscles
Nerve pectorales mediales and laterales (from C5-Tl), innervate pectoralis major and minor muscle	Weakness of upper arm adduction and anteversion, atrophy visible (differential diagnosis congenital aplasia, muscular dystrophy)	Isolated lesions rare	Usually not necessary

O **What are the circumstances under which the musculocutaneous nerve may be injured?**

Two sites are predisposed to compression of the musculocutaneous nerve, proximally where it pierces the coracobrachialis muscle and distally at the upper arm where it pierces the fascia brachii at the elbow. Proximal lesions lead to a paresis of elbow flexion and supination, very high lesions also to a weakness of arm elevation by paresis of the coracobrachialis muscle. Flexion of the elbow can, however, still be accomplished by the brachioradialis and pronator teres muscles, supination by the supinator muscle. Except for very rare traumatic lesions, proximal lesions may occur during anesthesia when the arm is in abduction. Occasionally after hard muscle effort (i.e. weight lifting), either a proximal or distal type of paresis may be seen, depending on the type of movement.

O **What treatments are recommended?**

With compression syndromes, especially after hard muscle work, immobilization and the use of nonsteroidal anti inflammatory drugs and, if this is insufficient, the use of oral steroids and local anesthetics is advisable. Acute lesions have a good prognosis. If conservative treatment fails, especially in distal compression syndromes, a surgical revision of the nerve in the cubital fossa with a resection of fibrous tissue and incision of the biceps tendon may be successful. With an isolated traumatic lesion, surgery is the treatment of choice. With irreversible lesions surrogate operations may be considered.

O **What is the clinical presentation for proximal radial nerve lesions?**

Proximal lesions of the nerve, for example in the axilla provoked by using crutches, are relatively uncommon. They can be recognized clinically by the presence of triceps paresis and sensory loss posteriorly in the upper arm. The relatively frequent lesions of the nerve at the site of the bony sulcus of the upper arm, caused by upper arm fractures and compression of the nerve against the bone under the influence of alcohol or drugs (Saturday night palsy) or occasionally by pressure of the edge of the operation table during anesthesia, go along with an intact function of the triceps. The same is the case with lesions at the lateral intermuscular septum (mid portion of the upper arm) provoked by strong contraction of the triceps or chronic strain of the triceps.

O **What treatments are recommended?**

The acute pressure injury and the acute and chronic occupational palsy have a good spontaneous prognosis, if traumatization of the nerve is discontinued. If conservative treatment or if the initial surgical repair is not successful within 2 months, a revision and neurolysis of the nerve may be advisable after previous precise localization of the lesion by means of neurophysiological methods. Lesions of the nerve by upper arm fracture may also initially be treated conservatively as the trauma usually leads to contusion of the nerve but only rarely to a complete disruption of the nerve. If signs of reinnervation are missing after 5-6 months, an operative exploration and repair is suggested. The nerve is usually found compressed by scar tissue and not by callus. If the palsy is irreversible, a transposition of the latissimus dorsi muscle may be considered to compensate for the missing function of the triceps.

O   **Describe the Posterior Interosseous Nerve syndrome**

Posterior Interosseous Nerve syndrome (pain and paresis)
Causes (FREAS)
Fibrous tendinous band at origin of supinator (30% of people)
Radial recurrent vessels (the **leash of Henry**) (less convincing evidence)
Extensor carpi radialis brevis
Arcade of Frohse
Supinator (the distal border).
RA. of elbow
dislocation of elbow, Monteggia fracture
surgical resection of radial head
mass lesions
Symptoms
pain in 50%
weakness of extension of wrist and MCP joints
Signs
Radial deviation of wrist with dorsiflexion (ECRL supplied by Radial nerve)
If partial, pseudo clawed hand
Able to extend IP joints due to interossei
no loss of sensation
Investigations
NCS -decreased latency across arcade of Frohse
EMG denervation fibrillations of affected muscles
Treatment
Conservative observe for 8-12 wks if no evidence of mass lesion
Surgical decompression

O   **Describe the radial tunnel syndrome**

Radial tunnel syndrome (pain but no paresis)
Mild compression of post interosseous nerve *without paresis*
Causes
As for posterior interosseus syndrome but not usually any mass lesions
Symptoms
dull aching in extensor muscle mass
worse at end of day
Signs
local tenderness 5 cm distal to lateral epicondyle
pain elicited by resisted active supination
middle finger test.
Each finger is tested under resisted extension. Testing the middle finger increases the pain. Due to **ECRB inserting into base of 3rd metacarpal.**
Performed with the elbow and middle finger completely extended with the wrist in neutral position.
Firm pressure is applied by the examiner to the dorsum of the proximal phalanx of the middle finger.
The test is positive if it produces pain at the edge of the ECRB in the proximal forearm.
Differential diagnosis
Tennis elbow
Investigation
NCS
Increased motor latency in active forceful supination
Injection of local anesthetic into radial tunnel
Management
Conservative, anti inflammatories, avoidance of repetitive provoking activities
Surgical, decompression. Internervous plane between ECRB and E Digitorum developed. PIN found just proximal to arcade of Frohse.

O   **What outcomes are expected for surgical intervention?**

In operative revision at the arcade of Frohse frequently fibrous tissue, rarely a lipoma, neurinoma or ganglion may be found. In the painful variant, operation usually leads to improvement or even complete relief shortly after the operation in more than 80% of the patients. With the paretic form, improvement is much slower (3-18 months). With permanent paresis, surrogate operation with transposition of the flexor carpi ulnaris and palmaris muscles and, if necessary, the pronator teres muscle to the tendons of the extensor muscles may be performed.

O   **What is the pathogenesis of injury to the superficial radial nerve?**

A lesion of the sensory superficial branch of the radial nerve is usually the consequence of a trauma at the forearm, rarely the consequence of repetitive pronation and supination of the forearm or chronic pressure (operating gloves, bracelet, hand cuffs!) and has good prognosis of spontaneous recovery.

O   **What proximal injuries to the median nerve can occur?**

Lesions at the upper arm are rare and may be caused by trauma, sleep paresis, pressure of crutches in the axilla, and pressure of cuffs used for a blood free field during operation. Of the population, 1-3% has a supracondylar process 5 cm proximal to the medial epicondyle at the humerus, sometimes accompanied by a fibrous band from the medial epicondyle to the supracondylar process (Struther's ligament).

O   **What is the clinical presentation?**

The nerve and the brachial artery, which run behind and below the process and the ligament and cross them, may be irritated here, leading to pain at the elbow, in the volar forearm, and in the sensory innervation territory of the median nerve of the hand and fingers during flexion and pronation of the arm. Tinel's sign may be provoked by pressure 3-5 cm proximal to the medial epicondyle. The degree of sensory loss in the median territory at the hand is very variable. Marked paresis caused by a supracondylar process and Struther's ligament are rare. The lesions at the upper arm just mentioned may cause marked tenderness often associated with a paresis of pronation (pronation is partly carried out by the brachioradialis muscle) and of hand and finger flexion. Flexor carpi ulnaris muscle and the ulnar part of the flexor digitorum profundus muscle are, of course, unaffected. During innervation of the hand flexors the predominance of the flexor carpi ulnaris muscle may lead to an ulnar deviation of the hand.

O   **What is the prognosis?**

The prognosis for the spontaneous course of pressure injury at the upper arm is favorable, so that only in rare cases with long lasting deficit is an operative revision indicated. Compression of the nerve at the distal upper arm by a supracondylar process or Struther's ligament has a good prognosis with operative treatment.

O   **What is the pronator teres syndrome?**

Pronator Teres Syndrome
Compression at
Lacertus fibrosus
Pronator teres muscle
Fibrous arcade of FDS
Ligament of Struthers (present in 1.5 % of people)
Causes
Repeated minor trauma/ repetitive use of elbow
Fracture / fracture dislocation of elbow
Tight/scarred lacertus fibrosus
Tendinous bands in pronator teres
Abnormal anatomy of pronator teres
Tight fibrous arch at prox FDS
Symptoms
Aching / fatigue of forearm after heavy use
Clumsiness
Vague, intermittent paresthesia, but rarely numbness
Signs
Local tenderness to deep pressure and reproduction of symptoms

Tinel's test
Pain on resisted pronation of forearm with elbow extended = Pronator teres
Pain on resisted elbow flexion and supination= lacertus fibrosus
pain on resisted flexion of PIP joint middle finger = FDS arch
Investigations
NCS not much use, intermittent symptoms
EMG may show evidence of reduced innervation of muscles and thus may differentiate from CTS
Management
Conservative-avoidance of repetitive elbow movements, NSAIDS, Splintage with elbow flexed with pronation
Surgical- Decompress all the structures

O   **What is the Anterior Interosseous Syndrome**

Anterior Interosseous Syndrome
Compression under **humeral part of pronator teres**
Anterior interosseous nerve motor to FPL, radial side of FDP and pronator quadratus
Does not supply skin sensation
Afferent sensory fibers from **capsular ligament structures** of wrist and DRUJ
Clinical diagnosis
Spontaneous vague forearm pain
Reduced dexterity
Weakness of pinch
Unable to make 'OK sign' due to weakness of FPL & FDP index finger (makes square instead of circle)
Weak pronation with elbow in full extension (isolates PQ)
Direct pressure over nerve can elicit symptoms
Tinel's sign usually negative
Investigations
NCS unhelpful
Management
Conservative- NSAIDS, avoiding aggravating movements
Surgical exploration- most common compressing structure deep head of pronator teres

O   **What are the demographics of carpal tunnel syndrome (CTS)?**

The carpal tunnel syndrome (CTS) is by far the most frequent peripheral nerve compression syndrome. It causes about 20% of all compression syndromes and about 50% of all cases of brachialgia. It occurs twice as frequently in women as in men, usually at ages above 50. The dominant side is affected more frequently, and if the compression is bilateral (40-50% of the cases); the dominant side is usually more affected.

O   **What is the incidence of CTS?**

The incidence is 1-3 cases per 1000 subjects per year; prevalence is approximately 50 cases per 1000 subjects in the general population. Incidence may rise as high as 150 cases per 1000 subjects per year, with prevalence rates greater than 500 cases per 1000 subjects in certain high risk groups.

O   **What is the clinical presentation?**

Frequently, carpal tunnel syndrome announces its presence with brachialgia paraesthetica nocturna. The patient is awakened from sleep by paresthesia and a feeling of swelling of the fingers without objective signs of edema. The pain may radiate to the upper arm or even to the shoulder. Massages, changes of arm position, or shaking of the hand may bring relief. Morning stiffness with diminished dexterity and numbness in the finger will decrease in the morning hours.

O   **What provocation tests may be used to aid in the diagnosis of CTS?**

Tinel's sign -74% sensitivity, 91 % specificity
Gentle tapping over median nerve at the wrist in a neutral position. Positive if this produces paraesthesia or dysesthesia in the distribution of the median nerve
Phalen's sign –61% sensitivity, 83% specificity

Elbows on the table allowing the wrists to passively flex. If symptoms provoked within 60 secs then positive
Median nerve compression test – 86% sensitivity, 95% specificity
Elbow extended, forearm in supination, wrist flexed to 60 degrees, ,even digital pressure applied with one thumb over the carpal tunnel. Test positive if paresthesia or numbness within 30 secs
Elbows on the table allowing the wrists to passively flex. If symptoms provoked within 60 secs then positive

○ **What is the pathogenesis of CTS?**

The syndrome is caused by compression of the median nerve in the carpal tunnel, which is enclosed by the carpal bones and the transverse carpal ligament and contains, in addition to the nerve, the tendons of the flexor muscles. Frequent anatomical variations may play a role in eliciting the syndrome. Pressure in the carpal tunnel is least in the mid-position and increases with flexion and even more with extension of the wrist. In patients with CTS resting pressure is increased even in the mid-position. The provocation of paresthesia by full flexion or extension of the wrist for 30-40 sec is of diagnostic significance.

○ **What is the clinical etiology of CTS?**

1. Frequent flexion and extension of the hand or vibrating machines;
2. Tendosynovitis;
3. Infectious diseases like tuberculosis or histoplasmosis;
4. Rheumatic inflammation;
5. Bleeding, thrombosis, neoplasms;
6. Disorders of water and lipid contents (obesity, pregnancy, menopause, oral contraceptives, myxedema, acromegaly);
7. Rare hereditary diseases (amyloidosis, mucopolysaccharidosis, mucolipidosis).

All may lead to a relative increase of the contents of the carpal tunnel and thereby to CTS.

○ **What factors may predispose to idiopathic CTS?**

In idiopathic CTS, the carpal tunnel may be narrow (measured by computerized tomography), or there may be other anatomical variations of muscles, tendons, and blood vessels. Apart from a history, the diagnosis is made on the basis of the typical sensory deficit, paresis, or atrophy of thenar muscles; a positive Phalen test (flexion of the wrist by gravity for 60 sec while keeping the forearm vertical and the elbow supported on the surface of a table); or by a positive dorsal extension test of the wrist. Nerve conduction testing and electromyographic examination may strongly support the diagnosis, which, like all diagnoses, must be clinical.

○ **What are the range of sensitivities for electrodiagnostic procedures utilized in the assessment of CTS?**

Relative sensitivity of electrodiagnostic tests for carpal tunnel syndrome

Most Sensitive
- Serial motor studies
- Serial sensory studies
- Repetitive sensory stimulation
- Transcarpal motor conduction
- Transcarpal sensory conduction ipsilateral nerve comparisons
- Threshold distal motor latency
- Distal sensory latency

Less Sensitive
- Residual motor latency
- Terminal latency index
- Distal motor latency

Insensitive

- Electromyographic evidence of axonal interruption

Rare

- Electromyographic evidence of spontaneous repetitive discharges

○   **What are the reported pooled sensitivities and specificities according to the Practice parameter: Electrodiagnostic studies in carpal tunnel syndrome Report of the American Association of Electrodiagnostic Medicine, American Academy of Neurology, and the American Academy of Physical Medicine and Rehabilitation ?**

	Technique	Pooled sensitivity*	Pooled specificity*
A.	Median sensory and mixed nerve conduction: wrist and palm segment compared with forearm or digit segment	0.85† (0.83, 0.88)	0.98† (0.94, 1.00)
B.	Comparison of median and ulnar sensory conduction between wrist and ring finger	0.85 (0.80, 0.90)	0.97 (0.91, 0.99)
C.	Median sensory and mixed nerve conduction between wrist and palm	0.74† (0.71, 0.76)	0.97† (0.95, 0.99)
D.	Comparison of median and ulnar mixed nerve conduction between wrist and palm	0.71 (0.65, 0.77)	0.97 (0.91, 0.99)
E.	Median motor nerve conduction between wrist and palm	0.69† (0.64, 0.74)	0.98† (0.93, 0.99)
F.	Comparison of median and radial sensory conduction between wrist and thumb	0.65 (0.60, 0.71)	0.99 (0.96, 1.00)
G.	Median sensory nerve conduction between wrist and digit	0.65† (0.63, 0.67)	0.98† (0.97, 0.99)
H.	Median motor nerve distal latency	0.63† (0.61, 0.65)	0.98† (0.96, 0.99)
I.	Median motor nerve terminal latency index	0.62† (0.54, 0.70)	0.94† (0.87, 0.97)
J.	Comparison of median motor nerve distal latency (second lumbrical) to the ulnar motor nerve distal latency (second interossei)	0.56‡ (0.46, 0.66)	0.98‡ (0.90, 1.00)
K.	Sympathetic skin response	0.04 (0.00, 0.08)	0.52 (0.44, 0.61)

○   **What are the guidelines according to the Practice parameter: Electrodiagnostic studies in carpal tunnel syndrome Report of the American Association of Electrodiagnostic Medicine, American Academy of Neurology, and the American Academy of Physical Medicine and Rehabilitation ?**

In patients with suspected CTS, the following EDX studies are recommended

1. Perform a median sensory NCS across the wrist with a conduction distance of 13 to 14 cm
If the result is abnormal, comparison of the result of the median sensory NCS to the result of a sensory NCS of one other adjacent sensory nerve in the symptomatic limb
2. If the initial median sensory NCS across the wrist has a conduction distance greater than 8 cm and the result is normal, one of the following additional studies is recommended:
a. Comparison of median sensory or mixed nerve conduction across the wrist over a short (7 to 8 cm) conduction distance with ulnar sensory nerve conduction across the wrist over the same short (7 to 8 cm) conduction distance
OR
b. Comparison of median sensory conduction
across the wrist with radial or ulnar sensory conduction across the wrist in the same limb

OR
 Comparison of median sensory or mixed nerve conduction through the carpal tunnel to sensory or mixed NCSs of proximal (forearm) or distal (digit) segments of the median nerve in the same limb

3. Motor conduction study of the median nerve recording from the thenar muscle (Technique H) and of one other nerve in the symptomatic limb to include measurement of distal latency
4. Supplementary NCS: Comparison of the median motor nerve distal latency (second lumbrical) to the

ulnar motor nerve distal latency (second interossei)
median motor terminal latency index
median motor nerve conduction between wrist and palm, median motor nerve compound muscle action
potential (CMAP)
wrist to palm amplitude ratio to detect conduction block
median sensory nerve action potential (SNAP)
wrist to palm amplitude ratio to detect conduction block, short segment (1 cm) incremental median sensory
nerve conduction across the carpal tunnel
5. Needle electromyography of a sample of muscles innervated by the C5 to T1 spinal roots, including a
thenar muscle innervated by the median nerve of the symptomatic limb

O   **What is the initial treatment recommended for CTS?**

In the presence of painful paresthesias without objective neurological deficits, volar splinting of the wrist in mid-position
during the night is the treatment of choice (initial improvement in 50% of all cases, long lasting relief of complaints,
however, only in 1-14% of the patients), nonsteroidal inflammatory drugs may be used at this stage although not during
pregnancy. If rapid improvement is expected after trauma or heavy use of the wrist, even in the presence of neurological
deficits, nonsteroidal may be useful.

O   **What is the role of injection therapy for CTS?**

In the presence of incomplete remission of complaints in chronic compression syndromes, especially near the end of
pregnancy, the injection of 25 mg of prednisolone or 1 mg of depot methyl prednisolone into the carpal tunnel after previous
injection of 2-3 ml of 1% lidocaine may be tried. This treatment may be repeated after 3 to 8 days (however, maximally two
to three times because the risk of infection increases with increasing frequency). This treatment almost regularly leads to
initial improvement; however, long term results are less favorable (after 1-2 years only 20-50% of the patients are free of
pain).

O   **What is the role of surgery in CTS?**

In cases with definite sensory or motor defects surgery to release the transverse carpal ligament is the treatment of choice, as
well as in all cases with incomplete success of conservative treatment. Many variations of surgical procedure have been
described. Most frequently, the operation is done after plexus or local anesthesia in a blood free field, complete section of the
retinaculum is carried out to the tendon of the flexor palmaris longus muscle. Visualization of the motor branch is advisable
as it may be subject to isolated compression. In addition to freeing the nerve from compressing fibrous tissue, some authors,
when there is strangulation of the nerve by the epineurium and by interfascicular scar tissue, recommend a microsurgical
epineural and endoneural neurolysis. The resection of the palmaris longus tendon is occasionally done.

O   **What is the prognosis after surgical release of the carpal ligament?**

After a correct diagnosis, completely cutting the ligament almost regularly leads to instantaneous relief from pain. Sensory
deficits show good improvement within about 18 months in most (90%) cases. Improvement of motor function depends
mainly on the preoperative function loss and the duration of the compression; atrophy rarely improves if duration is longer
than 12 months.

O   **What are the outcomes for endoscopically released carpal ligaments?**

Using a two portal technique in over 1000 procedures, only 2% were considered failures (longest follow up was 30 months),
and patients could return to work after 2 weeks. Complications included injury to the superficial palmar arch, wound
hematoma, and severe paresthesias lasting up to 3 months. The technique has also been suggested to be safe and reliable. A
multicenter randomized study of endoscopic surgery reported comparable results ' and patients returned to work 3 weeks
earlier than with the standard operation. Many report similar good results in carefully selected patients. Complications
include tendon laceration, infection, bleeding, neurapraxias, median nerve laceration, and wound dehiscence. Choice of
surgical technique is highly dependent upon surgical experience and cost. In most cases in which patients had conventional
surgery on one hand and endoscopic release on the other, the latter was preferred.

O   **What is the post-operative rehabilitation for transverse ligament release?**

The wrist is usually immobilized for 2 weeks after surgery. After suture removal, soft tissue massage around the suture line helps to soften the maturing scar. Ice or cold towels can be used to control edema. The patient begins active motions of the digits. To prevent adhesions, gentle selective tendon gliding can be achieved by selected FDS and FDP exercises. Light ADL are allowed around PO Weeks 2 to 3, but no forceful activities or exercises are permitted until PO Weeks 4 to 6. Strength returns slowly (over 6 months) and sometimes without reversal of thenar muscle atrophy.

○   **How frequent is the Martin Gruber anastomosis?**

The frequency of the Martin-Gruber anastomosis, in which motor fibers from the median nerve pass to and travel with the ulnar nerve to the small hand muscles, is estimated to be 10-44%.

○   **What is the etiology of cubital tunnel syndrome?**

Cubital tunnel syndrome may be caused by constricting fascial bands, cubitus valgus, bony spurs, hypertrophied synovium, tumors, ganglia, or direct compression. Work may aggravate cubital tunnel syndrome secondary to repetitive elbow flexion and extension. Certain occupations are associated with the development of cubital tunnel syndrome; however, a definite relationship with occupational activities is not well defined. Habitual luxation of the nerve because of a flat cubital sulcus (according to the literature in 2-36% of the operated patients) may cause injury.

○   **What is the pathophysiology associated with the cubital tunnel syndrome?**

As the elbow moves from extension to flexion, the distance between the medial epicondyle and the olecranon increases 5 mm for every 45 degrees of elbow flexion. Elbow flexion places stress on the medial collateral ligament (MCL) and the overlying retinaculum. The shape of the cubital tunnel changes from a round to an oval tunnel with a 2.5-mm loss of height because the cubital tunnel rises during elbow flexion and the retrocondylar groove on the inferior aspect of the medial epicondyle is not as deep as the groove is posteriorly. The cubital tunnel's loss in height with flexion results in a 55% volume decrease in the canal, which further results in the mean ulnar intraneural pressure increasing from 7 mm Hg to 14 mm Hg. A combination of shoulder abduction, elbow flexion, and wrist extension results in the greatest increase in cubital tunnel pressures, with an increase in intraneural pressure 6 times normal.

○   **What are the presenting symptoms and signs of cubital tunnel syndrome?**

Patients who are affected with cubital tunnel syndrome often experience numbness and tingling along the little finger and ulnar half of the ring finger, often accompanied by weakness of grip. Frequently, this occurs when the patient rests upon or flexes the elbow. Patients may experience pain and tenderness at the level of the cubital tunnel, and this discomfort may radiate proximally or distally. Symptoms vary from a vague discomfort to hypersensitivity at the elbow. Symptoms may be intermittent at first and then become more constant. Nocturnal symptoms, especially with elbow flexion, may be quite disturbing. Patients with chronic ulnar neuropathy may complain of loss of grip and pinch strength and loss of fine dexterity. Rare patients with severe prolonged compression present with intrinsic muscle wasting and clawing or abduction of the little finger.

○   **What does the physical examination address first?**

Check elbow ROM and examine the carrying angle, examine for areas of tenderness or ulnar nerve subluxation. Palpate the cubital tunnel region to exclude mass lesions.

○   **What is the significance of a Tinel's sign?**

A positive Tinel sign finding is typically present in cubital tunnel syndrome. However, a positive Tinel sign finding is found in up to 24% of the asymptomatic population.

○   **What is the elbow flexion test?**

The elbow flexion test is the most diagnostic test for cubital tunnel syndrome. The test involves the patient flexing the elbow past 90 degrees, supinating the forearm, and extending the wrist. Results are positive if discomfort is reproduced or paresthesia occurs within 60 seconds. The addition of shoulder abduction may enhance the diagnostic capacity of this test. Examine for intrinsic muscle weakness.

O   **What sensory modalities are tested?**

Check vibratory perception and light tough with Semmes-Weinstein monofilaments. This is more important than static and moving 2 point discrimination tests, which reflect innervation density, as the initial changes in nerve compression affect threshold. Check 2 point discrimination. Further evaluate sensation, especially the area on the ulnar dorsum of the hand supplied by the dorsal ulnar sensory nerve; hypesthesia in this area suggests a lesion proximal to the Guyon canal.

O   **What pathological causes should be entertained in the differential?**

Exclude other causes of dysesthesias and weakness along the C8-T1 distribution, such as cervical disk disease or arthritis, thoracic outlet syndrome, or ulnar nerve impingement at the Guyon canal.

O   **What general conservative treatment plan is utilized?**

With nonoperative treatment, strengthening the elbow flexors/extensors isometrically and isotonically within 0-45 degrees ROM is helpful. Limit the arc of elbow motion to a more extended range to avoid ulnar nerve impingement in the cubital tunnel. Recommend decreasing activities of repetition that may exacerbate the patient's symptoms. Administer nonsteroidal anti inflammatory drugs (NSAIDs) in an attempt to decrease inflammation around the nerve. Protect the ulnar nerve from prolonged elbow flexion during sleep, and protect the nerve during the day by avoiding direct pressure or trauma.

O   **What are the recommendations for initial conservative treatment for cubital tunnel?**

Recommendations are to use an elbow pad and/or night splinting for a 3 month trial period. Consider daytime immobilization for 3 weeks if symptoms do not improve with splinting. Consider surgical release if the symptoms do not improve with conservative treatment. If the symptoms do improve, continue conservative treatment for at least 6 weeks beyond the resolution of symptoms to prevent recurrence.

O   **What interventions are considered for mild cubital tunnel syndrome?**

For mild cubital tunnel symptoms, a reversed elbow pad that covers the antecubital fossa, rather than the olecranon, serves as a reminder to the patient to maintain the elbow in an extended position and to avoid pressure on the nerve. At night, position a pillow or folded towel in the antecubital fossa to keep the elbow in an extended position. Another option is to apply a commercial soft elbow splint, with a thermoplastic insert, for persistent symptoms.

O   **What orthosis may be considered in highly symptomatic cases?**

For constant pain and paresthesia, consider a rigid thermoplastic splint positioned in 45 degrees of flexion to decrease pressure on the ulnar nerve. Initially, patients should wear this splint at all times. As symptoms subside, patients can wear the splint just at night.

O   **What surgical techniques may be utilized?**

The following *surgical meth*ods are recommended:
1.   Decompression of the nerve by cutting the tendinous arcade crossing the nerve at the insertion point of the flexor carpi ulnaris muscle.
2.   Ventral transposition of the nerve, either into the subcutaneous tissue or into the ulnar flexor muscles. The latter procedure has the advantage of better protecting the nerve. The ventral transposition includes cutting the tendinous insertion of the flexor carpi ulnaris muscle at the medial epicondyle.
3.   Medial epicondylectomy is carried out, removing most of the bony prominence with an osteotome, which allows the nerve to ride freely into this new area.

O   **What are the postoperative rehabilitation guidelines for these patients?**

With medial epicondylectomy, no postoperative immobilization is necessary, and active motion is started immediately according to patient tolerance. Within 1-2 months, normal activities should be resumed. With subcutaneous transposition, postoperative immobilization of the elbow in 45 degrees of flexion for 2 weeks is necessary. Then, active mobilization with muscle stretching and strengthening is carried out for 2-3 months. Submuscular transposition requires immobilization for 3-4 weeks in a sugar tong splint with slight pronation and the wrist in neutral position. Active range of motion, stretching, and strengthening are then carried out for 3-4 months. Intramuscular transposition requires 3 weeks of immobilization at 90 degrees of elbow flexion with the forearm in full pronation. This is followed by gradual active range of motion exercises, stretching, and muscle strengthening.

O   **What are the surgical outcomes for ulnar nerve transposition?**

The results after submuscular transposition of the nerve show rates of improvement of 80-90% the same is the case for subcutaneous transposition.

O   **What is the most common site of distal ulnar entrapment?**

The Guyon canal is the second most common site of entrapment and is located at the wrist. Entrapment may cause purely motor, purely sensory, or a mixed lesion, depending on the site of compression.

O   **What are the anatomical features of Guyon's canal that account for variability in its clinical presentation?**

Anatomically, the canal is divided into 3 zones. Zone 1 is the area proximal to the bifurcation of the ulnar nerve. Compression in zone 1 causes combined motor and sensory loss. It is most commonly caused by a fracture of the hook of the hamate or a ganglion. Zone 2 encompasses the motor branch of the nerve after it has bifurcated. Compression causes pure loss of motor function to all of the ulnar innervated muscles in the hand. Ganglion and fracture of the hook of the hamate are the most common etiological factors. Zone 3 encompasses the superficial or sensory branch of the bifurcated nerve. Compression here causes sensory loss to the hypothenar eminence, the small finger, and part of the ring finger, but it does not cause motor deficits. Common causes are an aneurysm of the ulnar artery, thrombosis, and synovial inflammation.

O   **What is the presentation of distal ulnar nerve injury?**

A complete lesion of the ulnar nerve near the wrist, including superficial and deep branch may lead to combined motor and sensory (volar side only) deficits. Compression of the deep branch leads to motor deficits only; with more distal compressions of the deep branch the hypothenar muscles may be spared. Now and then a compression in the canal of Guyon may lead to pure sensory deficits on the volar side of the hand. Pure motor paresis is usually painless; with sensory deficits pain is usually located at the wrist and may radiate into the fingers and the forearm. Pain may increase during the night and with movement of the wrist.

O   **What treatment approaches are considered for distal ulnar nerve compression syndromes?**

Treatment of ulnar nerve compression in this location depends on the origin and duration of the condition. For mild compressions associated either with a single traumatic event or with chronic trauma, conservative treatment should be initially prescribed. Avoidance of the trauma, with or without splinting, often results in complete return of function. In cases not responding to nonsurgical care, surgical exploration, decompression, and neurolysis should be done. If the hook of the hamate bone is fractured, it should be excised along with decompression and neurolysis of the nerve. Ganglia and other soft tissue masses should be removed.

O   **Describe a protocol for postsurgical distal ulnar nerve decompression:**

Ulnar Tunnel Syndrome, Surgical Decompression
0 to 7 days: Fit the patient with a soft splint and encourage wrist flexion and extension exercises.
7 days: Remove the splint and increase wrist extension and flexion exercises to full motion,
7 to 14 days: Emphasize light grip activities and finger motion (marble hunt in corn or rice or soft putty exercises). Remove
                 sutures at 2 weeks.
2 to 4 weeks: Treat the scar with deep friction massage and a silicone based scar pad.
                 Begin resistive exercises (hand-helper, clothes pin pinch, forearm and wrist curls),
4 to 6 weeks: Encourage normal activity.

Allow the patient to begin work related activities.
Desensitization techniques may be necessary for palmar scar tenderness, and a padded glove may allow the patient an early return to moderate to heavy work activities.

O **What are the clinical categories of TOS?**

Neurogenic, vascular and 'functional'.

O **Where are the putative sites of neural compression in the thoracic outlet syndrome (TOS)?**

Depending on the site of the compression, the thoracic outlet syndrome (TOS) was separated into different entities such as scalenus syndrome (compression between the scalenus anterior and medius muscle and the first rib), costoclavicular syndrome (compression between the first rib and the clavicle), and the hyperabduction syndrome (compression of the plexus below the origin of the pectoralis minor muscle at the coracoid).

O **What is the incidence of TOS?**

The prevalence of TOS was estimated to be 1 case per 1 million population.

O **Is there a gender predilection for TOS?**

Females are diagnosed more commonly with TOS than males, with some reports of a 9:1 female-to-male ratio. The shape of the chest wall is believed to predispose women by encouraging closure of the thoracic outlet. Large pendulous breasts have been particularly implicated, adding to the anterior forces on the chest, which leads to drooped shoulder posturing and further closing the outlet.

O **What possible pathological origins of neurogenic TOS have been espoused?**

Anomalies leading to a TOS is a cervical rib or a prolonged transverse process of the seventh cervical vertebra or a ligament between C7 and the first rib. These structures may compress the inferior trunk of the plexus from below, accompanied by pressure of the plexus against the rim of the scalenus anterior or medius muscle, especially if the gap between the muscles is narrow as a result of closely located origins of the muscles. Additional sources of pathology include congenital cervical connective tissue bands, scalene and subclavius muscles.

O **What surgical anatomical pathogenies has been described for TOS?**

Roos observed that 98% of his patients with TOS had anomalous fibrous muscular bands that probably irritated or compressed the brachial plexus. Nine different bands were described. The most frequent one is type 3, which is a fibromuscular structure originating on the neck of the first rib and passing horizontally across the thoracic outlet to lie between the T1 root of the plexus and the subclavian artery.

O **What symptoms occur when the upper plexus is involved?**

The patient clinically presents with symptoms of median nerve compression. The most frequent upper plexus anomaly is type 3, in which the anterior scalene muscle passes between the roots and trunks of the plexus.

O **What is the most common contributing dysfunctional phenomena to TOS?**

Postural and muscle imbalance of the shoulder girdle muscle groups.

O **What are the typical symptoms a TOS patient presents with?**

The typical TOS patient complains about brachialgia of the ulnar side of the hand and forearm; especially in uncommon arm positions (elevation of the arm, working, and also sleeping with an elevated arm) or carrying loads with the arm hanging down. Therefore, pulling the arm downward may be a diagnostic maneuver provoking pain. With time, signs of a lower plexus lesion with sensory and motor deficits and disturbances of control of finger movements may develop.

O   **What are the sensitivities of the TOS provocation maneuvers?**

Of normal asymptomatic persons, 38% have a positive Adson's test, 68% have a positive costoclavicular maneuver, and 54% have a positive hyperabduction maneuver. But used in conjunction with other findings and history, these tests serve to bolster the benign nature of the symptoms.

O   **What is an appropriate diagnostic workup for TOS?**

DIAGNOSTIC WORKUP FOR THORACIC OUTLET SYNDROME

History
1.   Intermittent pain, paresthesia, and swelling of part or all of an upper extremity
2.   Aggravating factors, such as hyperabducting arms, at work or during sleep
3.   Absence of specific features of carpal tunnel syndrome, cervical disc disease, or other systemic disease

Physical Examination
1.   Observation for structural disorders (e.g., drooping shoulders, heavy pendulous breasts)
2.   Check for masses in supraclavicular fossa
3.   Perform special tests and maneuvers (e.g., Roos test, cervical rotation-lateral flexion test, Adson's test, hyperabduction, costoclavicular maneuvers
4.   Absence of objective swelling or atrophy in most patients

Routine Tests
1.   Cervical spine and chest roentgenograms
2.   Serological tests for inflammatory disorders
3.   Electrocardiogram if chest pain coexists

Special Tests
1.   Electrodiagnostic studies especially static and dynamic (positional NCS+SSEP)
2.   Vascular studies, including venography, venous flow rates, angiography, or magnetic resonance angiography
3.   MRI of the brachial plexus

O   **What is the differential diagnosis for TOS?**

Differential Diagnoses for Thoracic Outlet Syndrome
Bursitis
Cervical arthritis
Glenohumeral joint instability
Myositis
Fibrositis
Brachial plexus neuritis
Raynaud's disease
Thromboangiitis
Neoplasm of the spinal canal
Neoplasm of the peripheral nerve
Apical pulmonary neoplasm
Cervical disk disease
Peripheral nerve compression (cubital and carpal tunnels)

O   **Describe the conservative approach to TOS rehabilitation**

Evaluation

Nerve entrapment sites
Posture
Range of motion and movement patterns: cervical, scapula, shoulder, arm
Exclude or identify other pathologic conditions: cervical disc disease, nerve root impingement, shoulder tendinitis
Education

Pathophysiologic process of single and multiple level nerve compression
Positions of most risk and least risk for nerve compression
Posture and position correction
Integration of corrected postures in activities of daily living at work, home, and sleep
Impact of obesity, breast hypertrophy, and general physical condition
Treatment

Postural and positional correction
Neutral wrist splint at night, elbow pad, soft neck support for night use, lumbar support in sitting
Physiotherapy

Pain control and range of motion
Stretching exercises for upper trapezius, levator scapulae, scalenes, sternocleidomastoid, pectorals and chin retraction exercises (begin in supine with pillow support)
Strengthening exercises for middle/lower trapezius, serratus anterior, lower rhomboids(begin in gravity-assisted positions)
Aerobic conditioning program
Diaphragmatic and lateral costal breathing exercises
Progressive walking program and other aerobic conditioning exercises
Patient education and encouragement with compliance to home exercise program and behavior modification

O   **What invasive techniques may be considered for refractory cases of TOS?**

Trigger point injections to the periscapular muscle groups and scalene motor blocks may have a role in the therapeutic plan. Surgery is indicated when conservative treatment does not relieve symptoms. Cervical rib resection, thoracic rib resection, scalenectomy, scalenotomy, and fibromuscular band excision may be used individually or in combinations.

O   **What are the intrinsic etiologies of sciatic nerve injury?**

Sciatic nerve lesions usually lead to partial damage, more likely and more severe in the peroneal division. Masses within the pelvis can compress the sciatic nerve. Endometriosis leads to pain in the hip and buttock radiating into the leg and foot, sometimes varying with the menstrual circle (cyclical sciatica). Other tumors in the gluteal region include schwannomas, neurofibromas, lipomas, and lymphomas. Hematomas may occur as a complication of anticoagulation or hip surgery. During childbirth pressure on the nerve may occur due to the fetal head.

O   **What entrapment syndrome may involve the sciatic nerve?**

Entrapment syndromes of the sciatic nerve are rare. Some authors believe that compression of the nerve by the piriform muscle may occur due to an anatomical variation of the course of the nerve during its passage through the sciatic notch *(piriformis syndrome)*. Usually the peroneal trunk deviates and runs above or between the parts of the piriform muscle. Rarely, nerve entrapments by fibrosis or fibrovascular bands are found. Complete palsy of the sciatic nerve is extremely rare and not expected from an entrapment disorder.

O   **What are the symptoms associated with piriformis syndrome?**

Patients usually present with a history of blunt trauma to the gluteal or sacroiliac region with complaints of pain in the lower region of the sacroiliac joint, the greater sciatic notch, and the piriformis muscle occasionally radiating down the posterior aspect of the lower extremity. The pain may also be described as a cramping or a feeling of tightness in the hamstring muscles. Stooping or lifting exacerbates the symptoms.

O   **How is the diagnosis of piriformis syndrome established?**

Diagnosis of piriformis syndrome can be difficult and somewhat controversial. On examination, patients may be noted to have a palpable mass over the piriformis muscle during an exacerbation of symptoms. This mass is markedly tender has been called the pathognomonic sign. Buttocks pain may be exacerbated by hip flexion and passive internal rotation. Results of the straight leg raising test are occasionally positive. Electrodiagnostic studies usually demonstrate normal long latency signals at rest but become abnormal with hip flexion and internal rotation maneuvers.

O   What are the extrinsic causes of sciatic nerve injury?

External compression occurs mainly by prolonged pressure against the buttock or posterior thigh during coma or surgery with the patient in a sitting position. In severe cases a compartment syndrome with pressure induced swelling and necrosis of muscles within the posterior compartment of the thigh can occur.

O   What are the treatment approaches to sciatic nerve injury?

Patients with piriformis syndrome may have pain relief from injections of local anesthetics or corticosteroids or both into the piriformis and sciatic nerve area. Surgical dissection of a portion of the muscle or tenotomy produces mostly pain relief and is rarely carried out because the surgical success rate is low. Entrapment by other deeply located structures may require surgical intervention with dissection of fibrous bands or resection of a tumor or hematoma. Endometriosis should be treated with synthetic hormones or surgical resection of the tissue or both, according to gynecological principles. Postoperative sciatic neuropathies without hematoma, resulting from patient positioning, do not need to be surgically explored. Spontaneous recovery is frequent.

O   What are the therapeutic options are practiced in the conservative management of piriformis syndrome?

Consider the use of ultrasound and other heat modalities prior to physical therapy sessions. Prior to performing piriformis stretches, the hip joint capsule should be mobilized anteriorly and posteriorly to allow for more effective stretching. Soft tissue therapies of the piriformis muscle can be helpful, including longitudinal gliding with passive internal hip rotation, as well as transverse gliding and sustained longitudinal release with the patient lying on his/her side. Addressing sacroiliac joint and low back dysfunction also is important.

O   What is the clinical presentation of femoral nerve injury?

Lesions of the femoral nerve produce weakness of the quadriceps muscle, a diminished or absent knee reflex, and sensory disturbances over the anteromedial side of the thigh and the medial side of the lower leg. The most common compressive cause of femoral palsy is retroperitoneal hemorrhage due to hemophilia or anticoagulant therapy, rarely to rupture of an arterial aneurysm or traumatic avulsion of the iliacus muscle. The main symptom is severe pain that begins below the inguinal ligament and spreads to the distribution of the saphenous nerve, and local tenderness in the groin. Examination reveals signs of femoral palsy. Extension of the hip increases pain and occasionally ecchymoses are present in the upper thigh.

O   What other disorders may give rise to femoral nerve injury?

Other disorders leading to less acute compression of the femoral nerve are iliac abscesses, aneurysms of the internal iliac artery, or tumors arising from the iliopsoas muscle or the ileum. Iatrogenic causes include various surgical procedures (e.g., lithotomy position), leading to kinking and compression of the nerve under the inguinal ligament during hip flexion. CT scanning will demonstrate acute hemorrhage very well. MRI may give better visualization of nonhemorrhagic lesions such as abscess or tumor.

O   How are femoral nerve injuries managed?

The early management of iliacus hematomas depends on the severity of the injury and the patient's condition. Analgesic treatment and correction of bleeding disorders are necessary. Indications for surgery are controversial because conservative treatment may give satisfactory results and no controlled trials are available. In severe cases most authorities would agree that prompt surgical evacuation of the hematoma may be required. Percutaneous drainage may be a useful alternative. Compression by malignant tumors should be treated by surgical excision, radiotherapy, or chemotherapy. Retroperitoneal abscesses require drainage and antimicrobial treatment, and aneurysms should be removed surgically.

○   **What rehabilitation interventions are warranted?**

Regardless of cause, every femoral nerve lesion with weakness of the quadriceps muscle requires stretching and strengthening exercises to maintain joint mobility and enhance stability. If genu recurvatum is severe a Swedish knee cage orthosis may be provided, otherwise patients often rely on compensatory strategies to overcome quadriceps weakness.

○   **What is the etiology of saphenous nerve injury?**

The saphenous nerve is the terminal sensory branch of the femoral nerve. It descends through the adductor canal and penetrates the fascia above the level of the knee, supplying the medial calf, the medial malleolus and the medial portion of the arch of the foot. Compression of the nerve may occur anywhere in its long course, in the thigh, at the knee, or in the lower leg. In the thigh, compression results from fibrous bands and from anomalous branches of the femoral artery, rarely from schwannomas of the nerve.

○   **What are the clinical manifestations of saphenous nerve injury?**

The symptoms are radiating pain and sensory disturbances over the distribution of the nerve. Often Tinel's sign is elicit able along the nerve. Entrapment may occur at the exit of the nerve from Hunter's canal leading to pain near the knee and the medial lower leg that may be increased by walking. Entrapment of the nerve where it pierces the sartorius tendon results in pain and paresthesias in the distribution of the infrapatellar branch of the saphenous nerve. External compression of the saphenous nerve may occur due to patient positioning, leg holders during gynecological surgery, plaster casts, or braces.

○   **What treatment is appropriate?**

The treatment of the saphenous nerve entrapment syndromes is that of neuropathic pain. A TENS trial may be warranted initially. Systemic or topical pharmacological agents may be considered. If a series of injections of local anesthetic agents or corticoids or both is not successful, a surgical decompression should be performed. Compression of the infrapatellar ramus may be treated by displacement of the nerve into subcutaneous fatty tissue or by neurectomy.

○   **What is the prognosis for femoral nerve injury?**

In femoral nerve compression due to positioning, spontaneous recovery is frequent within a few weeks.

○   **What is meralgia paresthetica?**

Meralgia paresthetica is a painful condition attributed to entrapment or injury to the lateral femoral cutaneous nerve at the site where the nerve leaves the pelvis.

○   **What is the incidence of meralgia paresthetica?**

The incidence rate of MP is 4.3 per 10,000 person years.

○   **Is there a gender predilection?**

Meralgia paresthetica affects men more than women due to possible occupational considerations and may be bilateral in approximately 25 percent of cases.

○   **What patient related factors may be responsible for meralgia paresthetica?**

Numerous factors may contribute to mechanical damage of the lateral femoral cutaneous nerve as it exits under the inguinal ligament, such as obesity, constricting garments or girdles, direct pressure on the thigh in the region of the nerve, postural alterations, or increased demands placed on the abdominal muscles secondary to pregnancy or marching.

○   **What anatomical factors may be responsible for meralgia paresthetica?**

Various hypotheses have been formulated for the cause of this condition based on the anatomical relationship between the lateral femoral cutaneous nerve and the structures associated with the inguinal region:
The nerve may be angulated or compressed against a sharp edge of fascia as it pierces the iliac fascia prior to exiting the pelvis beneath the inguinal ligament. The nerve may be subjected to friction where it is wedged between the attachment of the inguinal ligament with the ASIS. The nerve may pass through the tendinous fibers of the inguinal ligament and be pinched at this site. The nerve may be compressed as it crosses the iliac crest or may be compressed within the substance of the sartorius muscle or tensor fascia lata muscle.

O   **What symptoms are often attributed to meralgia paresthetica?**

The patient with meralgia paresthetica may complain of a dull ache, itching, numbness, tingling, or burning sensation over the lateral and anterolateral thigh. The pain associated with this condition may vary in intensity from mild to very severe and frequently occurs following activity with relief following rest. Clinically, the history may reveal that the pain is potentiated by extension and relieved by flexion, as well as being aggravated by long periods of standing or walking.

O   **What findings may be encountered on clinical examination?**

Physical examination may reveal a sensory loss taking the form of a reduction of tactile sensation in the distribution of the lateral femoral cutaneous nerve. These findings may be accompanied in three fourths of cases by a tender spot over the inguinal ligament that is two finger widths medial to the anterior superior iliac spine.

O   **What is the differential diagnosis?**

In diagnosing meralgia paresthetica, care should be taken to rule out intraspinal, retroperitoneal, abdominal, or pelvic pathologies, diabetes mellitus, and L3 disc prolapses. Clinically, the L3 disc prolapse may produce alteration of the patellar reflex. In contrast, the reflex will not be altered in meralgia paresthetica.

O   **What is the prognosis of meralgia paresthetica?**

In meralgia paresthetica symptoms usually disappear spontaneously in a few weeks or months.

O   **What are the treatment choices?**

Drugs(local anesthetics corticoids or both)should be injected under the fascia lata medial and below the anterior superior iliac crest to relieve the pain. Constricting belts and binders should be avoided; in adipose patients weight reduction may help.

O   **What physical rehabilitation interventions are appropriate?**

Physical therapy may be recommended as an adjunct to analgesic medications for pain control in patients with MP. In addition to moist heat, other modalities that may be recommended by the physical therapist include transcutaneous electrical nerve stimulation (TENS), interferential current, or low intensity phonophoresis. These modalities are used to help alleviate pain and enable the patient to perform gentle stretching exercises with greater ease. Soft tissue techniques (eg, trigger point therapy) also may be beneficial for pain and tightness in the hip and thigh muscles. The physical therapist also may instruct the patient in a general fitness program to assist with weight reduction, as well as proper biomechanics and postural re-education.

O   **What considerations may be given to the patient with refractory meralgia paresthetica?**

In a minority of patients the symptoms persist or become severe so that surgical intervention is required. The nerve should be decompressed by neurolysis with incision of the iliac fascia and the inguinal ligament *which* is highly effective. Sectioning of the nerve is effective in pain relief but may lead to numbness of the thigh and recurrence of symptoms due to neuroma formation.

O   **What rehabilitation interventions may be appropriate?**

Weakness and gait abnormalities often occur secondary to the peroneal and tibial nerve divisions involved in the injury patients are often able to compensate for incomplete sciatic nerve injury. If it is complete a DMU or SAFO may be required.

○ **What are the symptoms of peroneal nerve injury?**

The symptoms of common peroneal nerve palsy include foot drop and partial sensory loss and vary according to the etiology of the lesion. In many peroneal neuropathies the muscles supplied by the deep branch are more severely affected and sensory loss is variable or lacking.

○ **What are the etiologies for peroneal nerve injury?**

The most common of the causes for damage of the peroneal nerve is external compression in its course around the head and neck of the fibula during sleep, anesthesia, coma, prolonged bed rest, or by plaster casts. Habitual crossing of legs or prolonged squatting are frequent causes of common peroneal neuropathy. In some patients there is a history of excessive weight loss due to cancer or diet, leading to changes in behavior and increased vulnerability to compression. Entrapment of the nerve rarely occurs at the head of the fibula (fibular tunnel), resulting in a slowly progressive and painful peroneal neuropathy. Other conditions for compression of the nerve are ganglia and cysts arising from the knee joint, lipomas, callus, or tumors of the fibula.

○ **What is the anterior compartment syndrome?**

The anterior compartment syndrome (anterior tibial syndrome) is caused by compression of the deep peroneal nerve by acute muscle swelling within the anterior fascial compartment. The syndrome includes severe anterior lower leg pain, swelling and redness, with motor and sensory dysfunction of the deep peroneal nerve. It results from excessive exercise, soft tissue trauma, fractures, hemorrhage, occlusion of the anterior tibial artery, or restoration of blood flow after acute arterial insufficiency in the leg. The acute compartment syndrome of the lower leg is a surgical emergency and requires prompt fasciotomy.

○ **What is the anterior tarsal tunnel syndrome?**

Compression of the distal part of the deep peroneal nerve can occur where it crosses the anterior ankle (anterior tarsal tunnel syndrome) due to tight shoes or trauma. Symptoms are painful paresthesias. The distal part of the superficial peroneal nerve can be compressed where it pierces the deep fascia of the lower leg. This leads to local tenderness and painful paresthesias in the distribution of the nerve. Compression of the distal parts of the deep and superficial peroneal nerve should be followed conservatively; pressure from tight shoes should be avoided. Orthosis to change foot position or local steroid injections may help. If there is no improvement, surgical decompression by incision of constricting fascial bands should be performed.

○ **What is the treatment approach to peroneal nerve injury?**

Peroneal neuropathies due to external compression do not require surgical treatment. Patients with conduction block due to a demyelinative lesion recover in a few weeks, whereas recovery of axonal damage lesions will take much longer, at least several months. Patients with mixed axonal and conduction block lesions may show a biphasic recovery. Treatment consists of avoidance of further compression, stretching and strengthening exercises to the ankle muscle groups, and a posterior leaf spring or semisolid AFO to provide stability of the foot. Tendon transfers are rarely needed in complete injury.

○ **What are the etiologies for tibial nerve injury?**

Compression of the proximal tibial nerve is infrequent and may be due to a ganglion, Baker's cyst, or nerve tumor, sometimes to positioning or plaster casts.

○ **What are the presenting symptoms?**

Symptoms include weakness of the plantar flexors, long toe flexors, and the intrinsic foot muscles and sensory loss in the sole of the foot.

○ **What is the prognosis of tibial nerve injuries?**

Lesions due to external compression usually recover spontaneously. Chronic lesions from masses in the popliteal fossa require surgical exploration and decompression of the nerve and have a more guarded prognosis for recovery..

○   **What is the tarsal tunnel syndrome?**

The tarsal tunnel syndrome in its basic form is an entrapment of the posterior tibial nerve within the tarsal canal. It may involve only one of the terminal branches distal to the tarsal canal. The tarsal canal is located behind the medial malleolus and becomes the tarsal tunnel as the flexor retinaculum passes over the structures, creating a closed compartment. Distally, at about the level of the medial malleolus, the posterior tibial nerve divides into its terminal branches, giving rise to the medial plantar nerve, the lateral plantar nerve, and the medial calcaneal branches.

○   **What is the etiology associated with tarsal tunnel syndrome?**

The cause of tarsal tunnel syndrome is idiopathic in about 50% of cases, and in the other 50% a specific cause can be identified. The most commonly identified cause is a space occupying lesion such as a synovial cyst, ganglion protruding from a tendon sheath, a lipoma, neurilemoma, venous varicosities, tenosynovitis, severe pronation or valgus hindfoot deformity, trauma resulting in a fracture of the distal tibia or calcaneus, or occasionally after a severe ankle sprain.

○   **What are the symptoms associated with tarsal tunnel syndrome?**

Most patients with tarsal tunnel syndrome complain of a poorly defined burning, tingling, or numb feeling on the plantar aspect of the foot. At times, this pattern of pain may be localized to one of the three terminal branches of the posterior tibial nerve rather than the entire nerve. Generally, the pain is aggravated by activity and relieved by rest, but sometimes patients note that the symptoms are most bothersome in bed at night; this type of pain can be relieved by getting up, moving around, and massaging the foot.

○   **What are the findings on exam suggestive of tarsal tunnel syndrome?**

Initially, the patient is examined in the standing position to evaluate the overall posture of the foot and the presence of edema, venous varicosities, or thickening around the medial aspect of the ankle or heel. The range of motion of the ankle and of the subtalar and transverse tarsal joints is evaluated. The physician then gently taps along the course of the posterior tibial nerve starting above the malleolus and passing distally below the malleolus along each terminal branch of the nerve. As this area is percussed, an attempt is made to elicit tingling along the course of the posterior tibial nerve or its terminal branches to identify the site of possible pathology. Careful palpation along the tendon sheaths is important because at times a cyst or ganglion may arise, placing pressure on the posterior tibial nerve or one of its terminal branches. A sensory examination on the plantar aspect of the foot is made, and the motor function to the toes is evaluated.

○   **What elements of electrodiagnostic testing for tarsal tunnel syndrome?**

The terminal latencies of the medial plantar nerve to the abductor hallucis and the lateral plantar nerve to the abductor digiti quinti are determined. The terminal latency of the medial plantar nerve to the abductor hallucis should be less than 6.2 msec, and that of the lateral plantar nerve to the abductor digiti quinti should be less than 7.0 msec. Needle examination of the abductor hallucis and/or abductor digiti quinti may show denervation, active and/or chronic changes.

○   **What is the treatment for tarsal tunnel syndrome?**

Nonoperative treatment includes use of proper shoes, arch supports when indicated, ensuring proper gait and stride, orthoses if significant pronation is present, and NSAIDs. Perhaps the best diagnostic test is response to a corticosteroid-local anesthetic injection into the region of the tarsal tunnel, with relief confirming the presence of the syndrome. In most persistent cases a corticosteroid-local anesthetic mixture injected once or twice into the region inferior and posterior to the medial malleolus and injected in a fan-like pattern provides relief. Injection of 20 mg methylprednisolone mixed with 1% procaine or lidocaine hydrochloride, take care not to inject the nerve.

○   **What are the surgical considerations?**

Some practitioners report only a 30% response and recommend decompression surgery. However, the value of decompression surgery itself has been questioned; in one large study only 44% benefited from surgery. Thus it has been suggested that surgery be restricted to patients who have an associated lesion near or within the tarsal tunnel. It may be that surgical intervention is most often required when the tarsal tunnel syndrome follows fracture or dislocation or when imaging reveals a space occupying lesion. Surgeons often recommend surgery no later than 10 months after onset of symptoms; results were poor in those with longer symptom duration.

○   **What is Morton's neuralgia?**

Morton neuroma is a perineural fibrosis and nerve degeneration of the common digital nerve occurring most frequently between the third and fourth metatarsal heads. Morton neuroma is not a true neuroma but, rather, fibrosis due to repetitive irritation of the nerve.

○   **What are the demographics for Morton's neuroma?**

Forefoot neuromas tend to occur most commonly between the ages of 18 to 60 years. They are more frequent in women than in men. More than one nerve in the same foot can be effected. Morton neuromas are more common in women, with a female-to-male ratio of 4:1.

○   **What factors are proposed to account for Morton's neuroma?**

1.   The junction of the medial and lateral plantar nerves near the muscle belly of the flexor digitorum brevis is subject to increased tensile forces on the nerve fiber during digital dorsiflexion, causing greater risk of neuroma formation.
2.   Compression of digital nerves by the metatarsal heads and the transverse intermetatarsal ligament appears to be a major cause of Morton's neuroma. This conclusion is supported by histologic evidence and the anatomic distribution of the lesion.
3.   Further, the second and third intermetatarsal spaces, recognized as the most common places for neuroma formation are also the most probable sites of nerve compression. Intermetatarsal head distances here are significantly less than those at the first and fourth intermetatarsal. The smaller zone through which the nerve passes is likely to increase the risk of nerve compression, accounting for the prevalence of intermetatarsal neuroma at these sites.

○   **What are the symptoms associated with Morton's neuroma?**

Symptoms of intermetatarsal neuroma are localized to the forefoot and toes. The condition may initially present as a dull ache or cramping sensation, with associated numbness. Tingling or burning radiating to the toes along with intermittent symptoms of sharp, shooting pain are reported with neuroma formation. Progression results in increased intensity and duration of symptoms, possibly radiating proximally. In chronic cases, patients may describe sensations of a hardened mass within the foot at the site of discomfort. Digital dorsiflexion may cause pain during propulsive phases of walking or during forefoot weight bearing activity, such as sprinting, jumping, squatting, or repeated hopping. Narrow fitting footwear usually induces symptoms; relief is often reported with shoe removal or massage of the foot.

○   **What findings on clinical examination are suggestive of Morton's Neuroma?**

Clinically, dorsoplantar compression of the intermetatarsal space often reveals a palpable mass and usually reproduces pain that may radiate to the toes or proximally along the course of the affected nerve. The patient may display relative paresthesia at the web space supplied by the injured nerve; this may be assessed through tests of light touch perception at the web spaces of both feet. Dynamic assessment may reveal excessive foot pronation, contributing to increased mobility of the metatarsals and increased risk of neural compression.

○   **What provocative test has been cited in the diagnosis of Morton's Neuroma?**

Mulder's sign has been reported as a useful diagnostic aid. By applying manual pressure to the medial and lateral aspects of the forefoot, the neuroma may be compressed between two metatarsals. On subsequent palpation of the area plantar and distal to the transverse intermetatarsal ligament, a "click" may or may not be heard. This sound is said to result from the neuroma mass crossing the ligament.

○   **Can ultrasound be used to further assess the diagnosis of Morton's neuroma?**

Sonographic imaging has been shown to accurately portray the location and magnitude of intermetatarsal neuroma. Given the definitive nature of clinical diagnosis and the expense of imaging, ultrasound is often reserved for cases in which diagnosis of forefoot pain is unconfirmed or for use in a presurgery workup. Suspicion of a second neuroma within the same foot may be confirmed through sonographic evaluation. Magnetic resonance imaging may also demonstrate the presence of Morton's neuroma, particularly if lesions are multiple or recur following neuroma surgery.

O   **What is the differential diagnosis of Morton's neuroma?**

A range of conditions may mimic Morton's neuroma, including metatarsal stress fracture, metatarsophalangeal joint synovitis, intermetatarsal bursitis, extensor tendon tenosynovitis, tumor, and nerve injury more proximally. Metatarsal stress fracture will present with bony tenderness and pain upon palpation of the metatarsal shaft, rather than the common digital nerve. Metatarsophalangeal joint synovitis will often prove painful during active or passive joint motion. Competing diagnoses may be definitively excluded through plain film radiography, bone scan, computed tomography, or magnetic resonance imaging.

O   **What treatments are appropriate for Morton's neuroma?**

Conservative therapy of Morton's metatarsalgia consists of padding the appropriate metatarsal heads. . Wearing athletic shoes that offer suitable motion control and using foot orthoses may serve as ongoing methods of addressing foot function. The use of footwear that exacerbates symptoms should be discouraged. Local injections of anesthetics and corticosteroids are often successful.

O   **Describe the injection procedure for Morton's neuroma?**

Perform injection into the dorsal aspect of the foot, 1-2 cm proximal to the web space, in line with the MTP joints. Advance the needle through the mid web space into the plantar aspect of the foot until the needle gently tents the skin. Then withdraw it about 1 cm to where the tip of the neuroma is located. Inject a corticosteroid/anesthetic mix. A reasonable volume is 1 mL of corticosteroid and 2 mL of anesthetic. The anesthetic used should not contain epinephrine, as necrosis may result. Care also should be taken not to inject into the plantar pad. Adverse outcomes include plantar fat pad necrosis.

O   **What options are considered for the patient with refractory symptoms?**

If these measures fall, surgical intervention with excision of the nerve or incision of the deep intermetatarsal ligament is required. Both approaches have good results.

BRACHIAL PLEXOPATHY

O   **What is the incidence of neonatal brachial plexus injuries?**

Brachial plexus injury is a common problem, with an incidence of 0.6–4.6 per 1,000 live births.

O   **Is there a lateralizing pattern in neonatal brachial plexus injuries?**

The right side is injured more commonly, comprising 51% of cases. Left BPP occurs in 45% of patients and bilateral injuries in 4%.

O   **Which infants are at risk?**

These injuries occur in macrosomic infants and when lateral traction is exerted on the head and neck during delivery of the shoulder in a vertex presentation, when the arms are extended over the head in a breech presentation, or when excessive traction is placed on the shoulders. Approximately 45% are associated with shoulder dystocia.

O   **What are the specific risk factors associated with neonatal brachial plexopathy?**

Most neonatal BPP occurs in the birthing process. Risk factors for this type of injury, also referred to as obstetrical brachial plexus palsy (OBPP), include the following:
Large birth weight (average vertex BPP 3.8-5.0 kg; average breech BPP 1.8-3.7 kg; average unaffected 2.8-4.5 kg), breech presentation maternal diabetes, multiparity, second stage of labor that lasts more than 60 minutes, assisted delivery (eg, use of mid/low forceps, vacuum extraction), previous child with obstetric brachial plexopathy, intrauterine torticollis, shoulder dystocia.

O   **Describe the Erb-Duchenne paralysis in the infant.**

In **Erb-Duchenne paralysis,** the injury is limited to the 5th and 6th cervical nerves. The infant loses the power to abduct the arm from the shoulder, rotate the arm externally, and supinate the forearm. The characteristic position consists of adduction and internal rotation of the arm with pronation of the forearm. Power to extend the forearm is retained, but the biceps reflex is absent; the Moro reflex is absent on the affected side. The outer aspect of the arm may have some sensory impairment. Power in the forearm and hand grasp are preserved unless the lower part of the plexus is also injured; the presence of hand grasp is a favorable prognostic sign.

O   **Describe the Klumpke paralysis presentation in the infant.**

Klumpke paralysis is a rarer form of brachial palsy; injury to the 7th and 8th cervical nerves and the 1st thoracic nerve produces a paralyzed hand and ipsilateral ptosis and miosis (Horner syndrome) if the sympathetic fibers of the 1st thoracic root are also injured. Mild cases may not be detected immediately after birth. Differentiation must be made from cerebral injury; from fracture, dislocation, or epiphyseal separation of the humerus; and from fracture of the clavicle. MRI demonstrates nerve root rupture or avulsion.

O   **What is the prognosis in neonatal brachial plexopathy?**

Full recovery occurs in most patients, the prognosis depending on whether the nerve was merely injured or was lacerated. If the paralysis was due to edema and hemorrhage about the nerve fibers, function should return within a few months; if due to laceration, permanent damage may result. Involvement of the deltoid is usually the most serious problem and may result in shoulder drop secondary to muscle atrophy. In general, paralysis of the upper part of the arm has a better prognosis than paralysis of the lower part does.

O   **What is the incidence of permanent disability?**

The incidence of permanent impairment is 3-25%.

O   **What treatment is initiated after diagnosis of neonatal brachial plexopathy?**

The rehabilitation of children with BPP must begin in infancy to achieve optimal functional returns.

O   **What rehabilitation interventions are carried out during the first two weeks?**

For the first 2 weeks, the child may have some pain in the affected shoulder and limb, either from the injury or from an associated clavicular or humeral fracture. The arm can be fixed across the child's chest by pinning of his or her clothing to provide more comfort. Recently, some authors have discouraged this pinning in favor of immediate institution of gentle ROM exercises. Parents should be instructed in techniques for dressing the child to avoid further traction on the arm. Often a wrist extension splint is necessary to maintain proper wrist alignment and reduce the risk of progressive contractures.

O   **What are the goals in promoting an optimal rehabilitation outcome?**

A comprehensive therapy program should consist of ROM exercises, facilitation of active movement, strengthening, promotion of sensory awareness, and provision of instructions for home activities. Overall goals should focus on minimizing bony deformities and joint contractures associated with BPP, while optimizing functional outcomes.

O   **What specific guidelines and special consideration should be given to the shoulder and elbow in any program of ROM exercises?**

In children with BPP and persistent peripheral neurologic deficits, internal rotation and adduction contractures develop because of muscular imbalance around the glenohumeral joint. Early and consistent stretching of internal rotators should minimize the risk of this problem. External rotation, performed with the shoulder adducted alongside the chest and the elbow flexed to 90°, provides maximum stretch of internal rotators (specifically, the subscapularis) and the anterior shoulder capsule. The scapula should be stabilized while stretching shoulder girdle muscles to maintain mobility and preserve some scapulohumeral rhythm. Early development of flexion contractures at the elbow is common and can be exacerbated by radial head dislocation caused by forced supination. Aggressive forearm supination, therefore, should be avoided.

O   **What role does static and dynamic splinting of the arm play in neonatal brachial plexopathy?**

It is useful to reduce contractures, prevent further deformity, and, in some cases, assist movement. Commonly prescribed splints include resting hand and wrist splints, elbow extension splints, dynamic elbow flexion and supinator splints. Careful selection and timing of splint use is essential to optimize the desired effect.

O   **What role do sensory awareness activities play in the rehabilitation program?**

Sensory awareness activities are useful to enhance active motor performance, as well as to minimize neglect of the affected limb. Use of infant massage and drawing visual attention to the affected arm can be incorporated easily into play and daily activities. Weight bearing activities with the affected arm in all positions not only provide necessary proprioceptive input but also can contribute to skeletal growth.

O   **What parental teaching is implemented for the infant with brachial palsy?**

A comprehensive program including stretching exercises, safe handling and early positioning techniques, developmental and strengthening activities, and sensory awareness should be developed and updated as needed. In older children with persistent disability, the focus on home instruction shifts to independence with self stretching and strengthening exercises and instruction on strategies to achieve specific life skills. The focus of therapy often is directed to more recreational activities, such as swimming or basketball.

O   **What is the most frequent etiology of brachial plexus injury in adults?**

Brachial plexus injuries are estimated to account for 5% of peripheral nerve injuries. In military combat penetrating wounds cause most brachial plexus injuries. In civilian life, in addition to injuries related to birth, the plexus may be injured by missiles, stab wounds, traction applied to the plexus during falls, vehicular accidents, or sports activities, as well as radiation. Closed injury to the brachial plexus most commonly occurs in young adult males and the cause is frequently a motorcycle accident. Previous studies have noted that 70-80% of the complete brachial plexus injuries were related to motorcycle accidents.

O   **What associated injuries occur in conjunction with brachial plexus injury?**

Common associated injuries include fractures of the proximal humerus, the scapula, the ribs, the clavicle, and the transverse processes of the cervical vertebrae and dislocation of the shoulder, the acromioclavicular, and the sternoclavicular joints. A torn rotator cuff also has been described in conjunction with brachial plexus injury.

O   **What are the classification schemes cited most often in brachial plexus injury?**

Many classifications of brachial plexus injuries exist with the most familiar distinguishing between upper plexus injuries (Erb) and lower plexus injuries (Klumpke). Leffert has classified brachial plexus injuries according to mechanism and level of injury.

O   **What are the characteristics of an upper plexus (Erb's Palsy)?**

C5 and C6 +/- C7, waiters tip deformity, limb extended at elbow, flaccid at side of trunk, adducted, internally rotated. Abduction of the shoulder is impossible due to paralysis of deltoid, supraspinatus. External rotation of shoulder impossible due to paralysis of infraspinatus and teres minor muscle. Active flexion at elbow is impossible due to paralysis of biceps, brachialis, and brachioradialis. Supination of forearm is impossible due to paralysis of supinator. Sensation is absent over deltoid, lateral aspect of forearm and hand.

○   **What are the characteristics of a lower brachial plexus (Klumpke's palsy)?**

C8 and T1 +/- C7 deficits are the defining features; It is often caused by penetrating wounds, difficult births, falls onto the outstretched arm, or trauma from crutches Weak intrinsics of hand, paralysis of wrist and finger flexors are evident. There is a sensory deficit over medial aspect of arm forearm and hand.

○   **What is the Leffert classification?**

Open injuries
Closed (traction) injuries
A. supraclavicular
1.Supraganglionic
2.Infraganglionic
B. Infraclavicular
C. Postanesthetic palsy
Radiation injury to the brachial plexus

○   **What is the most common mechanism of injury?**

The mechanisms of injury are usually related to stretching, compression, or penetration of the plexus components. In a motorcycle injury to the plexus, the biomechanical forces that result in stretch or avulsion injuries are produced with the arm down at the side or in the abducted position, with the head and neck tilted away from the side of the stretched plexus.

○   **How are brachial plexus injuries anatomically defined?**

A plexus injury can occur at any point from the takeoff of the spinal roots at the spinal cord level distally to the peripheral nerves as they arise from the cords of the plexus. The level of closed plexus injury can be classified as supraclavicular or infraclavicular. Supraclavicular injuries have poorer prognostic outcomes when it comes to neurologic recovery with the return of function in the arm and hand.

○   **What is the anatomical representation of brachial plexus injury?**

The supraclavicular portion of the brachial plexus includes the plexus elements from the intradural spinal roots distally to the divisions. The infraclavicular portion includes the cords and terminal branches that are the individual peripheral nerves. The supraclavicular portion of the plexus is most consistently and severely damaged by the traction injuries described earlier. Supraclavicular lesions account for about 75% of brachial plexus injuries. In general, a neurapraxic injury is not as common in the setting of a supraclavicular plexus injury as in the setting of an infraclavicular injury.

○   **What are the neuropathological characteristics of complete brachial plexus injury?**

If there is a complete nerve injury, the distal neurons are disassociated from their cell bodies and undergo wallerian degeneration. The portions of the neuron proximal to the lesion will attempt to regenerate and scar tissue forms around the regenerating axons forming a neuroma.

○   **What are the different categories of incomplete brachial plexus injury?**

Neurapraxia, axonotmesis, and neurotmesis can be seen with brachial plexus injuries. Neurapraxia presents the best prognosis, and complete recovery should be anticipated within a short time (days to a few weeks) after injury. With axonotmesis, where the axonal sheath is intact, neural recovery is incomplete. Proximal muscles and sensation are more likely to recover than distal sensation and motor function. With neurotmesis, spontaneous recovery is unlikely and surgery will be required for the best opportunity of functional return.

○   **What are the subdivisions of supraclavicular nerve injuries?**

Supraclavicular root injuries (75%) can be subdivided into upper, middle, lower, and total plexus palsies.
The upper plexus (C5, C6, and C7) is involved in 20% to 25% of patients while lower plexus involvement (C8, T1) represents only 2% to 3%. Involvement of the middle plexus (C7) is associated with upper or lower plexus paralysis. Involvement of all plexus elements (C5–C8, T1) is most frequent, representing 75% to 80% of all plexus injuries.

○   **What clinical findings suggest a supraclavicular brachial plexus injury?**

1. Fracture of the clavicle or cervical transverse process
2. Evidence of injury to nerves arising from the supra-clavicular portion (i.e., long thoracic or dorsal scapular nerves)
3. Horner syndrome
4. Swelling, induration, or tenderness in the supraclavicular fossa

○   **What are the distinguishing characteristics of infraclavicular brachial plexus injuries?**

Infraclavicular plexus lesions of the distal cords or peripheral nerves arising from the cords account for 25% of all brachial plexus injuries. These lesions usually involve the posterior cord (axillary and radial nerves), or with specific shoulder or humeral trauma, there may be individual radial or axillary damage.

○   **What associated diagnoses accompany infraclavicular brachial plexus injury?**

Common associated diagnoses include shoulder dislocation and humeral fracture. A common infraclavicular injury to the axillary nerve occurs with shoulder dislocation. The nerve is rendered taut as it is stretched across the humeral head.

○   **What is the prognosis of infraclavicular brachial plexus injuries in the clinical context given above?**

Most of these lesions recover spontaneously, but more slowly than expected. Signs of recovery may be delayed for 3 to 6 months or longer. The milder nature of the infraclavicular injury is due to the restricted excursion of the fractured or dislocated humerus. Also, since the traction occurs laterally at a point far removed from an anatomic point of anchorage, the normal elasticity of the nerve roots protects them from damage. The branch of the plexus nearest its anchorage is the axillary nerve.

○   **What value does the Tinel sign have in the evaluation of a patient with a brachial plexus injury?**

In the case of distal rupture of a trunk, a positive Tinel sign gives strong evidence of the availability of proximal axons from which to graft. With axonotmesis and the nerve in continuity, repeated examinations over time will demonstrate distal migration along the nerves of the point from which the Tinel sign arises. A Tinel sign can be present before any testable muscle has been reinnervated.

○   **What patterns of electrodiagnostic findings occur in brachial plexus lesions?**

Since serious traumatic injuries of the plexus produce axonal change, signs of denervation should be present on the EMG recording. In addition, small or absent M-waves and sensory nerve action potentials (SNAP) should occur. Little, if any, slowing in conduction velocity should be found. Persistence of SNAP implies a lesion proximal to the dorsal root ganglion (i.e., root avulsion). A combined lesion may also lead to small or absent SNAP, and concomitant pathology at the root level can be hard to recognize unless needle EMG indicates involvement of the paraspinal or other muscles innervated by proximal plexus elements. Loss of functional continuity of components of the plexus may be confirmed by F-wave responses or somatosensory-evoked potential (SEP) studies.

O **What is the current axiom regarding the timing of surgical therapeutics?**

The current axiom for brachial plexus surgery is that surgery should be performed in closed injuries if there is no recovery by 3 months or if the recovery has plateaued before 6 months following the injury. If surgery is performed more than 6 months following the injury, the chance for maximal recovery is reduced. Exploration of the plexus and neurorrhaphy, autogenous interfascicular nerve grafting, or neurolysis are indicated 3 to 6 weeks after open injury.

O **What electrodiagnostic findings occur in a supraclavicular brachial plexus injury?**

In patients with supraclavicular injuries, special EMG studies can answer how far proximally or medially the roots or spinal nerves are injured. A sampling of paravertebral muscles will help to establish if the posterior primary nerve has been involved, indicating a nerve root avulsion. In this case, signs of denervation will be present in paraspinal muscles as early as 10 days following the injury. Other proximal muscles may show spontaneous motor activity at 14 days and distal muscles should show positive signs by 21 days.

O **What rehabilitation interventions are pursued initially after brachial plexus injury?**

1. If there is extensive anesthesia in the hand and forearm, protective care is taught.
2. An understanding of osteoporosis in the presence of paralysis should help prevent long bone trauma.
3. Additionally, passive range of motion exercises performed within the normal range are taught to patients and families so they can be accomplished at home at least twice daily.
4. The paralyzed limb should be positioned so as to prevent edema and to provide support for the glenohumeral joint in an attempt to reduce subluxation.

O **If the dominant arm is compromised by brachial plexus injury what rehabilitation interventions are considered?**

If the affected limb is the dominant arm, then the teaching of one handed activities of daily living and change of dominance activities should be instituted immediately after the injury. Special activities to concentrate on include: writing (penmanship), food cutting (rocker knife), buttoning (button hook), and using one handed methods to tie bows or knots. Other adaptive equipment may be useful based on the person's functional needs. Electrical stimulation of the muscles that show weak but volitional control may assist in strengthening them more quickly than do active assistive range of motion exercises alone.

O **What orthosis may be considered for a patient with loss of C 5, 6 myotomal function?**

An orthosis with a shoulder piece and joint can assist to stabilize the shoulder, but it is quite bulky. The shoulder piece and joint can be attached to an elbow locking mechanism that is manually activated. Alternatively, an axilla loop with a control cable can actively lock and unlock the elbow joint.

O **What orthosis may be considered for a patient with loss of C 8, T1 myotomal function?**

In the plexus injured person with a C8–T1 injury, the hand is usually flail and assumes an intrinsic minus
Deformity in the claw position. A long opponens orthosis that positions the hand in a functional attitude can be worn to protect the hand from injury and to attempt to prevent a claw deformity.

O **What hand function is preserved in C7 myotomal loss?**

If C7 function is present, then the hand can provide gross grasp and release, which can be helpful in assisting the opposite hand in bimanual tasks. However, power grasp cannot be provided with orthotic or surgical interventions.

O **What orthosis may be considered for a patient who has sustained C7 myotomal loss in addition to C 8, T1?**

The radial wrist extensors will provide wrist dorsiflexion and a weak key pinch through a tenodesis effect. A stronger tenodesis pinch can be achieved orthotically with a wrist driven flexor tenodesis orthosis. Surgically, improved pinch may be obtained using a variety of reconstructive procedures about the wrist and hand.

O **What are the surgeons goals in operative repair of a brachial plexus injury?**

The surgeon should have clear and reasonable surgical goals, which are in order of priority: (1) restoration of elbow flexion, (2) restoration of shoulder abduction, and (3) restoration of sensation to the medial border of the forearm and hand.

○   **What surgical reconstructive techniques are utilized in the patient with brachial plexopathy?**

The surgical techniques for reconstruction of plexus elements include neurolysis, primary nerve repair, cable grafting, interfascicular grafting, neurotization (nerve transfers), and a combination of these procedures.

○   **What role does direct intraoperative nerve stimulation and recording play in surgical repair?**

Direct intraoperative nerve stimulation and recording are required across damaged elements; if nerve action potentials are obtained, simple neurolysis is indicated. If neural integrity is completely lost or if no nerve action potentials are recorded across a damaged element, excision and nerve grafting are required.

○   **What is neurolysis?**

Neurolysis is performed to remove the scar tissue from an injured nerve in continuity. Removal of the scar tissue is done to facilitate axon growth.

○   **What is the most commonly utilized technique of nerve repair in the patient with brachial plexopathy?**

The most commonly used technique for plexus repair is nerve grafting. These grafts are placed to facilitate return of muscle function in the shoulder girdle and across the elbow. Return of innervation to the distal region of the forearm and hand is much less likely to occur.

○   **What are interfascicular grafts?**

Interfascicular grafts are used to repair the cords and branches and cable grafts are used for the repair of nerve roots and trunks.

○   **What are nerve transfers?**

Nerve transfers are most commonly performed using the intercostal nerves, the cervical plexus nerves, the spinal accessory nerve or a combination of these.

○   **What surgical options are appropriate for root avulsions at the cervicobrachial level?**

In root avulsions of the upper plexus in which no proximal neural stump is available for nerve grafting, neurotization between the intercostal nerves and the musculocutaneous nerve to restore elbow flexion may be considered.

○   **What is the most common nerve grafting method to close gaps in brachial plexus reconstruction?**

Currently, interfascicular nerve grafting using the sural nerve from one or both legs is the most common method used to close nerve gaps in brachial plexus reconstruction. This allows earlier mobilization, since tension at the site of repair is minimal.

○   **What does the post operative management consist of?**

When an interfascicular grafting technique is used, a Velpeau bandage is applied for immobilization. Any drains left in the wound are removed at 36 to 48 hours. The sutures are removed at 10 to 14 days, and the Velpeau dressing is removed at 3 to 4 weeks. Active pendulum exercises are started at 4 weeks and gentle abduction exercises at 6. Significant return of function may require 3 to 5 years. During this time physical therapy to prevent contractures of joints and muscles is essential. Vocational rehabilitation is equally important. Whether electrical stimulation of denervated muscles is beneficial is not known for certain.

○   **What is the prognosis of surgically repaired brachial plexopathy?**

In general, surgical repair of the infraclavicular injury carries a better prognosis than that of the supraclavicular injury.

○ **What is the role of orthopedic reconstruction of the patient with brachial plexopathy?**

Upper extremity reconstructive surgery in the individual with an incomplete brachial plexus injury may provide useful arm function, especially if the scapula and glenohumeral joints are stable and forearm flexion can be restored.

○ **What is the surgical time table for additional reconstructive surgery after brachial plexus surgery?**

After brachial plexus repair and reconstruction, 12 to 18 months are required to determine the extent of neural regeneration. Then if recovery is considered inadequate, peripheral reconstruction should be considered. Tendon transfers about the shoulder that may be considered include trapezius to deltoid transfer to improve abduction and latissimus dorsi transfer to improve external rotation.

○ **What is the recommended timing for tendon transfer procedures?**

Tendon transfers should be performed no sooner than 1 year after the injury occurred, to permit time for evidence of spontaneous return. An exception to this would be if there is documented evidence of neurotmesis, as seen at the time of surgical exploration. If the shoulder is flail and arthrodesis is to be performed, it has been suggested that the humerus be placed in 30 degrees of flexion and 30 degrees of internal rotation. Abduction at the shoulder should be in the 20- to 30-degree range.

○ **What techniques are utilized in operative transfers?**

Operations to restore elbow flexion include transfers of the latissimus dorsi, the pectoralis major, the triceps, the sternocleidomastoid, and the flexor-pronator mass. Restoration of elbow flexion is helpful to the patient even if the hand is functionless.

○ **What considerations are given prior to planning reconstructive surgery?**

If the serratus anterior is of normal strength, thereby stabilizing the scapula on the thorax, but there is significant weakness in the C5–C6 innervated muscles creating glenohumeral instability, a glenohumeral arthrodesis should be considered. If no active elbow flexion is present but there is residual C7–C8 muscle function, a tendon transfer to produce elbow flexion can be accomplished. Any muscle that has well to normal strength can be transferred; the pectoralis major, the triceps, or the latissimus dorsi muscles are used most frequently.

○ **What is the recommended timing for tendon transfer procedures?**

Tendon transfers should be performed no sooner than 1 year after the injury occurred, to permit time for evidence of spontaneous return. An exception to this would be if there is documented evidence of neurotmesis, as seen at the time of surgical exploration. If the shoulder is flail and arthrodesis is to be performed, it has been suggested that the humerus be placed in 30 degrees of flexion and 30 degrees of internal rotation. Abduction at the shoulder should be in the 20- to 30-degree range.

○ **What residual function is required when considering trans humeral amputation of the flail upper extremity?**

Proximal scapular and glenohumeral stability is essential if useful prosthetic function is to be an expected outcome. The glenohumeral joint must be stabilized if there is insufficient intrinsic shoulder muscle strength. Glenohumeral stabilization can be performed at the time of the amputation. A distal trans humeral level of amputation should be chosen to provide the optimal lever arm to transmit forces to the prosthesis.

○ **What prosthetic prescription is appropriate for the plexus injured patient upper extremity amputee?**

The plexus patient who has had a transradial amputation should be fitted with a body powered transradial prosthesis. If there is insufficient residual elbow flexion strength to lift the terminal device, a forearm flexion lift assist can be added to the elbow hinge. This assist will counterbalance the weight of the residual forearm and prosthesis, making elbow flexion easier.

O   What considerations are taken into consideration in the prosthetic prescription for the brachial plexus injured amputee?

The body powered prosthesis for the plexus injured patient who has had an amputation at a trans humeral level should contain the lightest weight terminal device and wrist joint. Generally, there is not sufficient muscle signal remaining in the affected limb for an externally powered or myoelectric prosthesis to work in the brachial plexus–injured amputee. Proximal axial muscles may produce excellent EMG signals but their signals are difficult to isolate for prosthetic motor activation of the prosthesis.

O   Describe the differential diagnosis for hypotonia children

Hypotonia
Hereditary motor and sensory neuropathies
Neuromuscular transmission defects
Transient neonatal myasthenia
Congenital myasthenic   syndromes
Infantile botulism
Congenital myopathies with distinguishing structural abnormalities
Central core disease
Nemaline myopathy
Centronuclear myopathy
Muscular dystrophies
Metabolic myopathies
Glycogen storage diseases
Lipid storage myopathies
Mitochondrial myopathies
Inflammatory myopathies
Dermatomyositis/polymyositis
Connective tissue disorders
Osteogenesis imperfecta
Marfan disease
Ehlers-Danlos syndrome
Metabolic diseases
Aminoacidopathies
Organic acidurias
Renal reabsorption defects
Endocrinopathies
Prader-Willi syndrome
Nutritional disorders

O   Outline the differential diagnosis for the child presenting with progressive weakness

Progressive Muscle Weakness
Peripheral neuropathies

Subacute inflammatory polyradiculoneuropathy
Hereditary motor neuropathies
Muscular dystrophies
Metabolic myopathies
Glycogen storage diseases
Lipid storage myopathies
Inflammatory myopathies
Dermatomyositis/polymyositis

O   **What is arthrogryposis multiplex congenita?**

Arthrogryposis multiplex congenita (AMC) is not a specific diagnosis but rather a general descriptive term for infants born with multiple joint contractures.

O   **What is the incidence?**

The incidence is 1 in 3000 to 4000 live births.

O   **What is the etiology?**

An exact etiology is unknown, but it is speculated that a congenital or acquired defect occurs in utero during the first trimester. This leads to the common pathogenesis of decreased intrauterine fetal movements that result in the abnormal development of joints and the formation of contractures. Various etiologic agents including chromosomal defects, viral or bacterial infection, chemical or drug agents, and environmental factors have been implicated.

O   **How is it classified?**

AMC may be classified into either neuropathic or myopathic forms, based on pathologic and muscle biopsy data. The neurogenic type accounts for more than 90% of cases, the majority being related to CNS disorders and degeneration of the anterior horn cells, although more distal components of the peripheral
nervous system may be responsible. The resultant syndromes associated with these neuropathic lesions are
nonhereditary.

O   **What are the typical clinical features of AMC?**

The description of AMC is applied based on the typical clinical features. In addition to three or more, usually symmetric, joint contractures at birth, there is decreased or absent joint motion actively and passively; absent or atrophic muscle with shapeless, cylindrical limbs; absence of normal skin creases with dimpling of the skin; and normal sensation.

O   **What is most common clinical presentation of AMC?**

The most common syndrome affects the limbs only and is referred to as "classic arthrogryposis" or amyoplasia. These infants are born with a typical positioning of the limbs giving them a "wooden doll"–like appearance. In the upper extremities, there is internal rotation of the shoulders, fixed extended elbows, and flexed wrists in ulnar deviation. In the lower extremities, the hips are flexed, externally rotated, and abducted, and there are severe equinovarus deformities of the feet.

O   **What is the prognosis of AMC?**

AMC is non progressive, and the prognosis is good. AMC is non progressive, and the prognosis is good
for those who survive the first 2 years of life. Pulmonary hypoplasia is the most common cause of death in children with AMC. In general, those with limb involvement only do well and those with extra-axial or
CNS involvement tend to do worse.

SPINAL MUSCULAR ATROPHIES (SMAs)

○   **Briefly describe the conceptual grouping of the SMAs**

The spinal muscular atrophies (SMAs) are a clinically and genetically heterogeneous group of disorders. They are characterized by primary degeneration of the anterior horn cells of the spinal cord and often of the bulbar motor nuclei without evidence of primary peripheral nerve or long tract involvement. Because bulbar features are often present, the term SMA does not technically describe the disorder. The SMAs present with a diversity of symptoms and differ in age of onset, mode of inheritance, distribution of muscle weakness, and progression of symptoms. Additionally, atypical forms of the disease have been described, including those with associated sensory deficits, hearing loss, or arthrogryposis.

○   **What is the genetic origin of the spinal muscular atrophies (SMAs)?**

The SMAs are transmitted via an autosomal recessive trait that has been specifically mapped to chromosome 5q.

○   **Have advances in genetics aided the classification of SMAs?**

The classification of the SMAs by phenotypic variation has undergone revision as the underlying molecular and genetic information has become available. Identifying the linkages between markers in the chromosome region 5q11.2-13.3 for SMA types I-III and discovering neighboring candidate genes (i.e., the survival motor neuron [*SMN*] and neuronal apoptosis inhibitor protein genes) have been significant advances toward classification by genetic variation.

○   **What is the overall incidence of the SMA's?**

SMAs as a group comprise the second most common autosomal recessive inherited disorder after cystic fibrosis. The acute infantile-onset SMA (type I) affects approximately 1 per 10,000 live births; the chronic forms (types II and III), 1 per 24,000 births. The autosomal dominant form is rare, accounting for fewer than 2% of all childhood onset SMAs. The adult onset form is less frequent, accounting for 0.32 per 100,000 births in the general population.

○   **What is the overall distribution of the SMAs?**

Overall, SMA type I accounts for about one fourth of cases. SMA type II represents the largest group at one half of all cases, while SMA type III accounts for one fourth of cases.

○   **What current classification system is recommended?**

The most recent clinical classification system was proposed by an international consortium and retains the three types of SMA, described by age at onset and two other criteria: course or maximal functional status, and age at death.

Designation	Symptom (MU)	Course	Death
I (severe)	0-6	Never sit	<2
II (intermediate)	<18	Never stand	>2
III (mild)	>18	Stands alone	Adult

○   **Describe an alternate classification for the SMAs**

Types of Spinal Muscular Atrophy					
Type	Inheritance Pattern	Age of Onset	Presenting Symptoms	Hallmark	Prognosis
SMA type I (severe infantile SMA, acute or fatal SMA, Werdnig-Hoffman, Oppenheim disease, amyotonia	AR	In utero to 6 months	Hypotonia and weakness; problems with sucking, swallowing, and breathing	Never able to sit	Average life months, expectancy is 8 months, 95 percent dead before age 1

Types of Spinal Muscular Atrophy					
Type	Inheritance Pattern	Age of Onset	Presenting Symptoms	Hallmark	Prognosis
congenita)					
SMA type II (intermediate)	AR	Generally between 3 and 15 months	Proximal leg weakness, fasciculations, fine hand tremor	Never able to stand; facial muscles spared	Dependent on extent of timing of respiratory complications
SMA type III (chronic SMA, Kugelberg-Welander)	AR, AD	15 months to teen years	Proximal leg weakness, delayed motor milestones		Dependent on extent and timing of respiratory complications
SMA type IV (adult-onset SMA)	AD, AR, or very rarely X-linked recessive	Median age of onset, 37 years	Proximal weakness; variable within families; more severe in AD form		Life expectancy not markedly reduced
Distal SMA (progressive SMA, Charcot-Marie-Tooth-type SMA)	AR, AD	AR: birth or infancy; AD: adulthood	Distal weakness		Very slow clinical progression; does not alter life span
AD, Autosomal dominant; AR, autosomal recessive.					

O **What are the main characteristics of Type I - Acute infantile, severe form (Werdnig-Hoffmann disease) ?**

Thirty five percent of all SMA cases are this type. It presents between birth and age 6 months, although 95% of patients show signs of the disease by age 3 months. It is inherited with an AR pattern. Infants appear hypotonic; fetal movements are impaired in 30% and 60% are "floppy babies." Cyanosis may be prolonged at birth. Muscle weakness is progressive with symptoms cumulating in total immobility. Bulbar dysfunction results in a mean life expectancy of 5.9 months; 95% of patients are dead by age 18 months. With few exceptions, most patients are never able to sit without support. This acute form may be differentiated from early onset chronic forms (type II) by its relative rapid progression of symptoms. Serum creatine kinase (CK) level is usually normal.

O **What are the laboratory findings of patients with SMA type I?**

Normal serum levels of muscle enzymes differentiate SMA from the primary myopathies. Examination of muscle biopsy specimens demonstrates groups of small, rounded, atrophic type I and II fibers intermingled with groups of hypertrophied, mainly type I fibers. There are no degenerative muscle fiber changes and the nuclei are usually in the normal, peripheral position. Diminished muscle bulk and occasional "myopathic" features can make both the electromyographic (EMG) and muscle biopsy findings difficult to interpret.

O **What is the main focus of care in patients with SMA type I?**

Pulmonary toilet is a main focus of care in infants with SMA type I. They often require assisted ventilation, supplemental oxygen or tracheostomy. Frequent suctioning, assisted coughing, and postural drainage can improve secretion management. This is especially important prior to and after feeding, as bulbar weakness increases the risk of aspiration of food and upper airway secretions. Supported sitting can help with postural drainage, but external supports are poorly tolerated. Respiratory infections require aggressive antibiotic treatment and supplemental oxygenation.

O **What is the major role of rehabilitation for children with SMA type I?**

The major role of rehabilitation for children with SMA type I has been to maximize the parent child relationship and minimize physical discomfort. In addition, rehabilitation of these infants can potentially enhance the outcome of those who go on to have a less severe course. However, while there are reports of SMA type I children surviving long term, the prognosis should not be unrealistically optimistic, given the more typical trend for limited function and survival.

○ **What are the clinical findings for patients with SMA type I?**

All of these infants are born floppy and on examination have profound weakness of the more proximal muscles of the extremities and the trunk. The lower limbs tend to be affected earlier and more severely than the upper limbs. These infants have a characteristic, gravity dependent posture in a supine position, with the lower extremities externally rotated, abducted, and flexed at the hips and knees in a "frog leg" position, and the upper extremities partially abducted at the shoulders with flexion at the elbows in a "jug handle" position.

○ **What mechanical ventilation deficits are evident?**

There may be a pectus excavatum deformity of the chest because of intercostal muscle weakness. During inspiration, the unaffected diaphragm descends, and the abdomen protrudes, with paradoxical thoracic depression and intercostal space retraction. The infants may make some whimpering sounds, but do not develop speech.

○ **What methods of feeding are advised in the patient with SMA type I?**

Most infants with SMA type I require total or supplemental feeding via a nasogastric tube or gastrostomy. Tube feedings should be continuous rather than by bolus to prevent gastric distention, which can limit diaphragmatic excursion. A feeding program can be pursued if safe swallowing can be documented by a modified barium swallow study and if the infant's pulmonary status is stable. The airway should be suctioned prior to feeding. Frequent, small feedings and jaw support with the infant in the semi reclined position are recommended, along with the use of nipples with large openings that do not emit food without a suck.

○ **What are the recommendations for positioning patients with SMA type I?**

Infants with SMA type I are limp and immobile and have no head control. These infants should be positioned supine or on their side, with their heads elevated with foam wedges, in an appropriate seating device fashioned from various plastics, foam rubber, or urethane foam.

○ **Are spinal orthoses advisable in patients with SMA type I?**

Spinal orthoses for sitting are not well tolerated because of increased abdominal pressure causing elevation of the diaphragm and skin problems due to decreased muscle bulk.

○ **What other guidelines are recommended for patients with SMA type I regarding positioning?**

Positioning with rolled towels or bolsters can be used to allow the hands to come together in the midline and to reach from the body. This gives infants the opportunity for exploration of and stimulation by lightweight toys or rattles that can be placed close to the hands or attached to the wrists with Velcro straps.

○ **What are the characteristics of intermediate SMA?**

Intermediate SMA is also known as SMA type II or chronic Werdnig-Hoffmann disease. In this group of patients, signs can be present as early as the age of 3 months, but are definitely apparent by 18 months. The creatine kinase (CK) level is normal to mildly elevated. Most children achieve the ability to sit unaided but then are unable to take weight on the legs and stand or ambulate independently. There is variable progression and survival is into adolescence or adulthood.

○ **What ventilatory problems develop in these patients?**

The majority of these patients develop restrictive lung disease, and this is the most important factor determining prognosis. Respiratory muscle weakness may be out of proportion to extremity weakness and result in chronic, alveolar hypoventilation and impaired secretion clearance. Such pulmonary compromise may be exacerbated by scoliosis. An aggressive maintenance program of chest physiotherapy (CPT), postural drainage, and deep breathing exercises is indicated. The children with more severe weakness often require tracheostomy or negative or positive pressure ventilation. However, some may be able to be weaned once they survive into adolescence. SMA type II patients who required definitive ventilatory support later in childhood or as adults were found to benefit, with greatly prolonged survival and function in society.

O   **What pattern of clinical weakness is evident in SMA type II patients?**

Clinical weakness is similar to that seen with SMA type I, with symmetric involvement, more proximally than distally, and more pronounced in the lower than the upper extremities with associated atrophy. There is generalized hypotonia and joint extensibility, often striking in the hands. Tremors of the hands and fasciculations and atrophy of the tongue are often seen. The progression of weakness is static to slowly progressive. Weakness may be exacerbated by obesity and in situations that result in immobilization such as acute illness, fractures, and surgeries.

O   **What is the pattern of motor milestone development in patients with SMA type II?**

Some children will attain, but then lose some of their early motor milestones such as independent sitting and standing. Some achieve limited ambulation, usually with orthoses.

O   **Do patients with SMA type II benefit from strength training exercises?**

Several studies that included limited numbers of SMA patients showed increases in strength with moderate resistance training, suggesting such exercise programs may be indicated for all SMA patients except those with the most severe and progressive weakness.

O   **How can independence in self care skills be achieved?**

Independence with self care can be facilitated with the use of adaptive clothing with Velcro fasteners, lightweight eating and writing utensils with built up handles, balanced forearm orthoses, and toileting and bathing equipment. The ability to produce a measurable force for pinch or gross grasp was associated with independence in mobility, hand function, and ADLs in one study of this population.

O   **How common are contractures in the SMA type II patients?**

In the child who is nonambulatory, prevention of postural deformities is an essential aspect of care. In children who ambulate, prevention of contractures may prolong ambulation. Contractures are common in SMA type II patients and occur most frequently at the shoulders, related to shoulder girdle weakness, and hips, knees, and feet, corresponding to prolonged sitting.

O   **How can mobility be optimized in the SMA type II patient?**

Transportation of the infant or toddler can be accomplished with an adapted stroller that provides adequate back and neck support. The child should be seated in a wheelchair when he or she outgrows or is not age appropriate for a stroller. The wheelchair should also have a firm seat and back and be able to grow with the child. However, the weaker child who does not sit or stand may require a spinal orthosis for support. Floor mobility devices such as scooters can help these children enjoy a variety of typical developmental motor experiences. Parents should be taught to move the children as much as possible to give them motor experiences they cannot gain on their own. In the child with adequate strength and respiratory reserve, mobility can be facilitated with the use of HKAFOs or reciprocating gait orthoses.

O   **What gait deviations are noted in the patient with SMA type II?**

Ambulatory children often show a hyperlordotic, Trendelenburg gait with shuffling feet.

O   **What is the mobility prognosis for SMA type II patients?**

In a 10 year retrospective review SMA patients were classified by maximal motor function achieved. This study found that children who never walked became power chair dependent by age 14. In those who achieved ambulation with gait aids, walking ceased by age 14 and power mobility was needed by age 18.

O   **What interventions are recommended in the type II SMA patients to reduce the impact of contractures?**

Range of motion exercises must be performed at least daily. Torticollis and hip tightness are best controlled by proper positioning in supine and side lying positions, often with the use of wedges and bolsters with attention to neutral spine and joint alignment. The feet should be plantigrade while seated, and this can be achieved with the footplate and straps or with a molded AFO. Night splints can also help to prevent contractures. Children with adequate head control can be stretched in the prone stander or parapodium, but may need external trunk support.

○ **What is the incidence of scoliosis in SMA type II patients?**

In studies of combined SMA type II and III patients, the incidence of scoliosis was very common, estimated to be around 60% to 90% for SMA type II children who are wheelchair dependent. Both ambulators and nonambulators can develop scoliosis, but the curves appear much earlier and are more severe in the latter, weaker group. A rigid, straight spine may result in loss of ambulation and decreased upper extremity reach in some children, so the risks and benefits must be carefully considered prior to scoliosis surgery.

○ **How does the scoliosis progress in the SMA type II patients?**

The deformity is a paralytic curve with early onset and continuous progression, even after spinal growth is completed, which may relate to the underlying joint hypermobility. The curve is typically thoracolumbar and C shaped, progresses by 8 degrees per year from 4 to 21 years, and is often associated with marked kyphosis and pelvic obliquity. The literature does not support the use of spinal orthoses for the prevention of scoliosis or its progression.

○ **What psychosocial issues needs the SMA type II patients present with?**

These children have normal intelligence and from an early age, they should be encouraged to strive for social, emotional, and financial independence. Even if on a ventilator, they should be able to attend a regular school program with the appropriate accommodations and lack of barriers. If they are not healthy enough to attend school, either for short or long periods, a home program is necessary to provide early stimulation for the toddler and preschooler and quality educational programs for the school age child. Computer skills are important to develop during the school years and can be incorporated into vocational planning. These children also benefit from participation in recreational activities such as wheelchair sports, swimming, and horseback riding to improve their endurance and self-esteem.

○ **What family support interventions are recommended?**

Families of these children will benefit from ongoing support and counseling with regard to parenting a child with a disability, and anticipation of medical needs. Families need to be prepared for any major changes in the child's status, such as need for gastrostomy placement, spine surgery, or ventilatory support.

○ **What are the presenting features of SMA type III?**

Mild SMA is also known as SMA type III or Kugelberg-Welander disease. In contrast to SMA types I and II in which there is significant morbidity and mortality, the impairments seen with SMA type III are relatively mild. Typical onset is late in the first decade or early adolescence, although weakness can be obvious in the early years of life. Children affected with SMA type III achieve early developmental milestones, although they may walk somewhat late and then begin to show evidence of mild proximal weakness. They may present with a complaint of difficulty keeping up with their peers, climbing stairs, and rising from the floor, which may require use of the Gower maneuver. As seen in SMA type II, patients also may demonstrate fasciculations and hand tremors. Pseudohypertrophy of the lower extremities can be seen.

○ **Can bulbar findings manifest in SMA type III?**

Dysphagia and dysarthria may occur as late findings.

○ **What are the diagnostic findings in SMA type III?**

The diagnosis may need to be supported with special investigations. CK levels may be elevated slightly to markedly. Examination of muscle biopsy specimens shows a histologic pattern of small group atrophy versus the large group atrophy seen in types I and II. In addition, a number of more "myopathic" changes have been described, such as central cores, target fibers, and internal nuclei, thought to be related to the chronicity of this type of SMA.

○ **Is scoliosis and restrictive lung disease common in SMA type III?**

No they are both uncommon.

○ **What are the basic features of the dystrophinopathies?**

The muscular dystrophies are degenerative hereditary disorders, with the most common being the dystrophinopathies and disorders of dystrophin associated proteins. In 1987, with the identification of a defect in the dystrophin gene as the cause of Duchenne muscular dystrophy (DMD), Monaco and Kunkel opened the door for research into the role of dystrophin and functionally related proteins in muscle function and maintenance.

Muscular Dystrophinopathies

○ **What are the two most significant dystrophinopathies?**

Different mutations in the dystrophin gene produce different allelic disorders, most commonly either the lethal DMD or Becker muscular dystrophy (BMD), a milder myopathy. Very rarely, patients with cardiomyopathy with mild weakness, dilated cardiomyopathy without weakness, exercise intolerance associated with myalgias, muscle cramps, or myoglobinuria and asymptomatic elevation of serum CK have also been identified.

○ **What is the genetic pathogenesis of Duchenne's muscular dystrophy (DMD)?**

DMD is inherited as an X-linked recessive gene that is passed to boys by mothers who are asymptomatic, except for a small percentage that are very mildly symptomatic. The prevalence is 63 per million, and the incidence is approximately 1 per 3500 live male births, of which one third of cases are from spontaneous mutations. The DMD gene locus is responsible for this high mutation rate, as it includes over 2.5 million base pairs of human X chromosome, localized to the short arm of chromosome 21. The gene codes for the dystrophin protein, which is a component of normal skeletal muscle sarcolemma and is involved in maintaining its structural integrity.

○ **How does the genetic anomaly translate into clinical pathophysiology?**

Because of gene deletions (55%–65% of cases), duplications (5%–10% of cases), or point mutations (30%–40%), dystrophin and its associated sarcolemmal glycoproteins are absent in the skeletal muscle fibers of DMD patients.. Dystrophin is integral to the structural stability of the myofiber, as is evinced by the widespread destruction that occurs when it is defective or absent. The functional loss of dystrophin initiates a cascade of events, including loss of other components of the dystrophin associated glycoprotein complex, sarcolemmal breakdown with attendant calcium ion influx, phospholipase activation, oxidative cellular injury, and, ultimately, myonecrosis.

○ **What is dystrophin?**

Dystrophin is 427 kDa in size and consists of 2 apposed globular heads with a flexible rod shaped center. Its amino terminal end insinuates with the subsarcolemmal actin filaments of myofibrils, while cysteine rich domains of the carboxy terminal end associate with beta-dystroglycan as well as elements of the sarcoglycan complex, all of which are contained within the sarcolemmal membrane. Beta-dystroglycan in turn anchors the entire complex to the basal lamina via laminin.

○ **How is the diagnosis of DMD made?**

A diagnosis of DMD is strongly suggested by the family history or clinical examination, or both, along with elevation of serum CK levels. Any male toddler who is not ambulating by 18 months should have serum CK levels measured. In DMD, the serum CK value is 50 to 100 times normal around the ages of 3 to 6 years and thereafter decreases approximately by 20%

per year, reflecting a loss of muscle bulk. Confirmation of the diagnosis is made by muscle biopsy and histologic examination. Chromosome and dystrophin analysis may be necessary to confirm the diagnosis if the clinical and laboratory data are not conclusive.

○   **What pathological findings are evident on histopathological analysis in DMD?**

Similar pathological changes are present in BMD and DMD, particularly necrotic and regenerating fibers, branching fibers, abnormal fiber size, and endomysial fibrosis. Generally there are more necrotic, hypercontracted, and regenerating fibers with a more severe phenotype. Additionally, inflammatory cells are evident at perivascular, endomysial, and perimysial sites in DMD. Plasma membrane defects that lead to segmental fiber necrosis and eventual regeneration are observed with electron microscopy.

○   **Are genetic analysis tests available to aid in the diagnosis of DMD?**

Several advances in molecular genetics over the last 15 years have revolutionized the diagnosis of DMD. Gene amplification through the PCR technique detects gene deletions in two thirds of patients affected with DMD. This can be performed on a blood sample using DNA gleaned from lymphocytes. Immunoblot analysis of muscle homogenates with dystrophin antibodies confirms abnormalities in at least 95 percent of DMD patients and differentiates DMD from BMD.

○   **How is dystrophin assayed in a muscle biopsy sample?**

Immunostaining of the muscle using antibodies directed against the rod domain and carboxy and amino terminals of dystrophin shows absence of the usual sarcolemmal staining in boys with DMD. Patients with BMD show more fragmented and patchy staining of sarcolemmal regions.

○   **What are the clinical manifestations of DMD through the age of 6 ?**

Usually, the child is asymptomatic in the neonatal period, with the earliest problems perceived by caregivers being developmental delays, particularly in walking and climbing, and the appearance of enlarged calf muscles. Between the ages of 3 and 6, the gait becomes waddling and lordotic.
Gowers' sign appears, in which the child stands from a prone position by a process of climbing up the legs, using the hands first on the knees and then on the thighs to support her or himself .

○   **What are the characteristic patterns of muscle dysfunction occurs from the age of 6?**

Usually by the age of 6 years, there is enlargement of calf, gluteal, lateral vastus, deltoid, and infraspinatus muscles, and weakness is readily apparent, with the proximal extremities more severely affected than the distal extremities, and lower extremities and torso more severely affected than the upper extremities. Weakness of the arms may be present but is not obvious without careful examination.

○   **What are the characteristic patterns of muscle dysfunction occurs after the age of 6?**

The strength of limb and torso muscles continues to decline steadily from ages 6 though 11 years. Proximal muscles continue to be more severely affected than distal muscles, with neck flexors becoming more involved than extensors, wrist extensors more than flexors, biceps and triceps more than deltoid, quadriceps more than hamstrings, and the tibialis posterior and peroni more than the gastrocnemius, soleus, and tibialis anterior. Tendon reflexes decrease and disappear as muscle weakness progresses.

○   **What is the pattern of muscle dysfunction observed by age 10?**

By the age of 10 years, 50 percent of patients have lost biceps, triceps, and knee reflexes, in contrast with the ankle reflex, which remains in one third of patients even in end stage disease. Significant contractures of the iliotibial bands, hip flexors, and heel cords are present in 70 percent of the children by the age of 10 years.

○   **What clinical changes are observed during the second decade?**

The second decade brings progressive kyphoscoliosis from weakened paraspinal muscles and decreased vital and total lung capacities and maximal inspiratory and expiratory pressures from weakened respiratory muscles. These problems first appear between the ages of 8 and 9 years and progress as functional status deteriorates.

○ **What other systems are affected in DMD?**

Degeneration of smooth muscle also occurs in DMD. There may be dystrophic and fibrotic changes in the myocardium and 90% of ECGs are abnormal but most patients do not have cardiac symptomatology. Similar muscle pathology can occur in the gastrointestinal tract, commonly causing esophageal and intestinal hypomotility, symptoms of reflux, and constipation, and in rare and potentially fatal cases, acute gastric dilatation.

○ **What are the electrodiagnostic findings in DMD?**

Electromyography (EMG), even though not diagnostic, narrows the differential diagnosis by effectively excluding primarily neurogenic processes such as spinal muscular atrophy. In general, the proximal muscles of the lower extremities may exhibit the more prominent EMG findings. A sufficient number of muscles need to be sampled to establish the presence of a diffuse process such as a dystrophy. The more revealing findings will be obtained in muscles of intermediate involvement with respect to weakness.

○ **What are the motor unit action potentials (MUAPs) findings in DMD?**

The motor unit action potentials (MUAPs) in DMD or BMD patients are typically of short duration, particularly the simple (i.e. non polyphasic) MUAPs. MUAP amplitudes are variable (normal to reduced) and they are typically polyphasic from the variability in muscle fiber diameters, resulting in longer MUAP durations. Early recruitment of MUAPs may be seen. If muscle fiber loss is severe, then what appears to be a loss of motor units may be seen with fast firing individual spikes. The latter are distinguished from neurogenic processes by the generally lower than normal amplitudes and reduced area of the spikes.

○ **What pattern of spontaneous activity is observed?**

Fibrillation potentials and positive sharp waves, which represent spontaneously depolarizing muscle fibers bereft of nervous innervation, are encountered in active disease as necrosis engulfs the motor endplate or separates the endplate from other portions of the muscle fiber. These may be difficult to see in some muscles, requiring higher than usual sensitivity settings on the amplifier.

○ **What are the pulmonary complications of DMD?**

The pulmonary complications of DMD are the result of the severe, progressive restrictive lung disease
present in all DMD boys, usually beginning in the second decade. Death from DMD usually occurs in the late teens and in approximately 70% of patients is related to the pulmonary complications associated with restrictive lung disease. Clinically, there may be no symptoms in younger boys, but changes in the mechanical properties of the thorax can be documented by early decreases in maximal static airway pressures. Decreased static airway pressures, particularly maximal inspiratory pressure, are considered more sensitive than vital capacity in the early stages of disease, since vital capacity increases with growth. Vital capacity, which reflects both thoracic wall compliance and respiratory muscle weakness, becomes a better indicator of pulmonary impairment later in the disease when mobility is lost.

○ **What are the characteristic features of progression in pulmonary dysfunction in DMD patients?**

The course of restrictive lung disease is directly correlated with the progression of weakness with age. Deterioration in pulmonary function was found to occur around the time a DMD boy cannot rise from a chair until the time when assistance is needed for walking. The survival time for those with 35% or less of normal forced vital capacity was 3.2 years in one study. Early intervention is recommended to limit cardiopulmonary morbidity and to delay early death from respiratory failure. Several studies showed that advanced DMD patients on noninvasive or invasive ventilatory assistance have a longer life expectancy as well as a meaningful quality of life.

○ **Is obesity a health problem among DMD patients?**

Obesity may be seen in up to one third of patients. This tendency is usually obvious in childhood and persists into adolescence. Loss of ambulation in early adolescence is not correlated with acute weight gain. In fact, in late adolescence, there is frequently weight loss, due to a state of relative hypercatabolism along with the influences of worsening restrictive lung disease, dysphagia, and impaired self feeding.

O   **What therapeutic options are available to patients with DMD?**

Prednisone is the only medication that has demonstrated even a modest benefit in modifying the course of the disease. Alternate day dosing of prednisone (0.75-1.5 mg/kg/d) retards muscle wasting; clinical improvement is seen as early as 1 month after starting treatment and lasts as long as 3 years. This benefit is tempered by the frequently encountered adverse sequelae of steroid use. Children who discontinue steroids for these reasons soon revert to the natural downward progression of the disease. Because of the potential risks of high dose steroids, it is currently recommended as a short term intervention while patients are still in the ambulatory phase. Other immunosuppressive therapies have been studied, but overall medical therapies do not appear to be effective.

O   **What future therapeutic interventions show promise for patients with DMD?**

Advancements in molecular genetics, such as cell and gene therapy, are more promising, but still experimental. Gene therapy involves the direct implantation of a normal, cloned dystrophin gene, either directly or via some transfer agent such as a virus vector, liposome, or myoblast. Human myoblasts are donated from close male relatives, cultured, and injected into the affected boy's muscle. Success has been limited thus far by the low efficiency of transfer of the normal genetic material o the abnormal skeletal muscle cells. A carefully controlled study determined that injecting normal myoblasts into affected muscle did not increase muscle force generation or the amount of dystrophin in muscle.

O   **How does the progression of weakness correlate with the loss of function in DMD?**

The course of loss of function is quite variable and progression of the disease in general as opposed to weakness per se may correspond better to time when function is lost than to chronologic age.   A number of studies timed the duration of functional activities to document progression of weakness. The findings in these studies suggest that the variability in function over time relates to both the progression of muscle weakness and the ability of DMD boys to use compensatory postures.

O   **What factors influence the ability to compensate in DMD?**

The ability to compensate in order to maintain function may be influenced by many factors such as preservation of range of motion, scoliosis, obesity, medical illness, and psychological and emotional issues. Differences in the ability to compensate may explain some of the variability in function between DMD boys of similar age or extent of weakness, or both.

O   **What is the pathophysiologic basis for the limitation of therapeutic exercise in DMD patients?**

Dystrophin-deficient muscle is very susceptible to exercise induced muscle injury. Studies have been completed using voluntary running protocols, looking at the effects of exercise on skeletal muscle from both normal mice and MDX mice (mice lacking dystrophin), a genetically homologous murine model of DMD. In contrast to normal mice, the MDX mice show considerable avoidance behavior for exercise, which may be an intuitive survival strategy. After exercise on a mouse wheel ad libitum, the extensor digitorum longus (EDL) and soleus muscles of adult MDX mice became significantly weaker and showed histochemical signs of further damage compared to control MDX muscles.

O   **What therapeutic exercise rationale and recommendations are appropriate for patients with DMD?**

Based on animal studies with dystrophic mice, the recommendations for strengthening in neuromuscular disease in general includes initiation of resistance training early in the disease course, and increasing resistance gradually. Avoidance of eccentric contractions and overexertion is also suggested, based on the concern for overwork weakness and the potential for increased muscle damage. If initiated early in the progression of DMD, the key muscles for strength training include the hip extensors and abductors, abdominals, and quadriceps.

O   **What gait deviations manifest early in the course of DMD?**

The affected child first develops a waddling type gait and increased lumbar lordosis due to hip extensor weakness, representing the first postural compensation in DMD gait. A balanced stance in the setting of increasing weakness of the hips and knee extensors requires knee hyperextension and ankle plantarflexion, as well as further lumbar lordosis.

○   **What adaptive equipment may be indicated to assist ADL's in a patient with DMD?**

Dressing usually requires some physical assistance at this stage of the disease. A balanced forearm orthosis can allow hand-to-mouth function when hand function is intact, but there is poor proximal strength. Robotic arms mounted on the wheelchair tray can be used with only finger movements for wheelchair operation, feeding devices, and environmental controls. Mouth sticks can be used for turning pages, painting, buttoning, and maneuvering smaller objects. Voice-, eye-, and blink-operated environmental controls are available to give patients access to all appliances, computers, and telecommunication equipment. Bathroom equipment, such as raised toilet seats, grab bars, bath seats, and roll in showers, can assist in promoting safety and independence.

○   **What changes in gait occur with disease progression?**

DMD boys experience a decrease in gait cadence and velocity as they progress from the early through the transitional to the late stages of gait. The early stage is characterized by progression of weakness and worsening contractures, resulting in a more vertical alignment of the centers of the hip, knee, and ankle joints. In the late stage, the gait of DMD boys requires significant energy expenditure and effort to maintain stability at the hips and knees.

○   **What factors are responsible for the loss of ambulatory ability in DMD patients?**

Impairments in mobility and the termination of ambulation have been related to muscle strength, contractures, specific gait abnormalities, and loss of other mobility functions. A number of studies found that ambulation is discontinued specifically when the quadriceps and gluteal muscles lose more than 50% strength. Loss of ambulation occurred with an increased double support phase in gait analysis. The average interval between assisted ambulation and wheelchair reliance was 3.3 years.

○   **What is the role of musculoskeletal surgery in patients with DMD ?**

Several investigators advocated earlier surgery, reporting increased time of brace free ambulation by 1 to 2 years. Lower extremity soft tissue surgery for prolongation of reambulation in DMD typically involves a combination of releases at the iliotibial band, hip flexors, Achilles tendon, or hamstrings.

○   **What are the criteria for reambulation after orthopedic surgery?**

The criteria for re ambulation after orthopedic surgery include a non ambulatory period of no longer than 3 to 4 weeks.

○   **What wheelchair adaptations may be warranted in DMD patients who come nonambulatory?**

Adaptations for the wheelchair, such as lateral trunk supports, adductor pads, seat belt, chest strap, lap tray, and head support, should be added when indicated. A reclining back will allow for position changes and pressure relief. Pressure relief can also be accomplished with lateral weight shifts, with manual assistance if necessary.

○   **What pattern of contractures occurs in the lower extremity of the DMD patient?**

Early tightness of the iliotibial band, tensor fasciae latae, and gastrocnemius muscles occurs without significant muscle strength loss. Contractures gradually develop in these muscles as well as in the hip flexors and hamstrings.

○   **What pattern of contractures develops in the upper extremities?**

In the upper extremities, contractures tend to develop from static positioning and the effects of gravity, and usually occur in the wrist and elbow flexors and ulnar deviators. Tightness in the fingers with various distal interphalangeal deformities also occurs.

○   **What are the benefits of a standing program in the DMD patient?**

A standing program with knee ankle foot orthoses, or standing frames or tilt tables or even swivel walkers provides prolonged stretching as well as opportunities to participate in school and home activities in the upright position.

○   **Does bracing alter the progression of scoliosis?**

Orthotic management of scoliosis in DMD with thoracolumbar supports does not prevent progression or decrease the rate of progression.

○   **What is the current treatment approach to scoliosis in patients with DMD?**

The current treatment approach is aggressive, with most authors recommending fusion when the curve is 25 to 30 degrees with segmental type instrumentation and fusion to the sacrum. Early correction of spinal deformity is done to avoid unacceptable operative risks due to restrictive lung disease, and permit maximal correction and balance of the spine. The major benefits of scoliosis correction are ease and comfort of seating and positioning. It does not necessarily improve pulmonary function parameters of restrictive airway disease.

○   **Does mental retardation occur in DMD?**

There is a relative mental retardation in the DMD population. Various studies have indicated an average IQ of around 85 or one standard deviation below normal for DMD boys, with approximately one third of DMD boys having an IQ less than 75. This subgroup is classified as mentally retarded and will need special classroom placements or tutoring. Neuropsychological testing revealed mild impairments of a global nature, but several studies detected specific problems in language abilities, reading, and memory.

○   **What is the etiology of DMD mental retardation?**

Dystrophin is found in the brain and has been localized to the neocortex, cerebellum, and hippocampus. It is not the same as muscle dystrophin. A general malfunction of the dystrophin gene as opposed to a specific deletion pattern is believed to be responsible for the variable reduction in intellectual function seen across the spectrum of Xp21 dystrophies.

○   **How does Becker muscular dystrophy compare to DMD?**

Becker muscular dystrophy (BMD) is a more benign phenotype of DMD. There is involvement of both skeletal and cardiac muscle, but the course is more slowly progressive and the associated impairments and disabilities are less severe. BMD is less common than DMD, with an estimated incidence of 1 per 20,000 births. BMD is also inherited through an X-linked mechanism and is related to a mutation, typically a deletion, on the same gene as in DMD. This results in dystrophin of abnormal size or reduced amounts of normal dystrophin.

○   **What is typical developmental history of a patient with BMD?**

Delayed gross motor milestones (eg, late walking, running, jumping, and difficulty with stair climbing) may be reported. Initially, some children later diagnosed with BMD may be called clumsy. Increasing numbers of falls, toe walking, and difficulty rising from the floor may be later features. Proximal muscle weakness is reported.

○   **What are the temporal features of BMD?**

Age of onset ranges from 1 to 70 years of age, with a mean of 12 years. Ninety percent of patients are affected by age 20. Lower extremity weakness appears on average by age 11, with upper extremity weakness by age 20. Loss of ambulation generally occurs around 40 but can occur as early as age 12. Age at death ranges from 23 to 89 years of age, with the average being 42.

○   **What cardiac pathology occurs in BMD?**

Cardiac problems similar to those associated with DMD are present in about half of the patients with BMD. The extent of cardiac involvement does not correlate with degree of myopathy. Myocardial pathology includes degeneration of cardiac muscle and fibrous replacement of myocardiocytes, particularly in the posterobasal region and the adjacent lateral wall of the left ventricle.

O   **What specific diagnostic test may help differentiate BMD form DMD?**

Immunoblot analysis of muscle homogenates with dystrophin antibodies confirms abnormalities in at least 95 percent of DMD patients and differentiates DMD from BMD.

O   **What is Myotonic muscular dystrophy (MMD)?**

Myotonic muscular dystrophy is an autosomal dominant multisystem hereditary muscular dystrophy with an incidence of 1 case per 8000 population, is characterized clinically by progressive predominantly distal muscle weakness and myotonia. Associated findings include frontal baldness, gonadal atrophy, cataracts, and cardiac dysrhythmias.

O   **What are the two types of myotonic dystrophy?**

The two types of MMD are recognized, noncongenital (NC-MMD) and congenital (C-MMD).

O   **What are the temporal features of myotonic dystrophy?**

The adult form of this disease has a median onset at 21.2 years and a mean of 23 ± 13 years. The 10 year mortality in one study was 21%, with the mean age at death 55 ± 12 years.

O   **What pattern of weakness is most common among patients with myotonic dystrophy?**

The classic presentation of noncongenital myotonic dystrophy includes marked weakness in the face, jaw, and neck muscles and milder distal extremity weakness. Weakness of the extremities is often the first problem perceived by the patient, even when a careful evaluation may reveal a clear history of myotonia (sometimes termed muscle stiffness or cramping by patients), facial weakness, and nasal speech.

O   **What neurological maneuver is used in the examination of the patient with MMD?**

Using a percussion hammer, myotonia can be elicited in patients with MMD with a brisk tap on the thenar muscle, causing flexion-opposition of the thumb with slow relaxation.

O   **What changes occur in the appearance of patients with advanced MMD?**

The person with advanced DM has a characteristic appearance: a long, thin face with sunken cheeks due to temporal and masseter wasting, a so called "swan neck" because of sternocleidomastoid wasting, and ptosis, with relatively strong muscles in the posterior neck and shoulder girdle.

O   **What is the presentation in congenital MMD?**

Congenital DM presents a distinctive picture that is different from other disorders. Facial diplegia and jaw weakness without concomitant extremity weakness are hallmarks. Weakness of the respiratory muscles with respiratory distress is present in at least 50 percent of patients and is the most common cause of death in these infants. Hypotonia is present in severely affected neonates, but it may disappear within weeks. Clinical myotonia is generally absent and is usually detectable only by EMG.

O   **What treatments are available for symptomatic management of myotonia?**

100 mg of phenytoin taken three times daily is effective in reducing myotonia and does not produce the cardiosuppressive complications of either quinine or procainamide.

O   **Outline Symptoms of myotonic dystrophy and potential treatment options.**

Symptom	Treatment
Myotonia	Drug therapy, if severe
Neck weakness	Neck brace, head support in car seats and chairs
Ptosis (drooping eyelids)	Special glasses to lift lids Surgery
Foot drop due to lower limb weakness	Ankle foot orthosis, ankle splints Wheelchair if severe
General weakness	Wheelchair, especially for outdoor use
Digestive problems	Diet Medication
Excessive sleeping	Exclude poor respiration as a cause Medication Establish regular sleeping pattern
Cardiac abnormalities	Monitor with regular ECGs
Cataracts	Surgery

O   **What is Facioscapulohumeral muscular dystrophy (FSH):**

Fascioscapulohumeral dystrophy (FSHD) is a slowly progressive myopathy with autosomal dominant inheritance and prominent involvement of facial musculature. Exact prevalence is difficult to ascertain due to undiagnosed mild cases but has been estimated at 10-20 cases per million population. The abnormal gene is on the end of chromosome 4, and DNA testing for diagnostic purposes is now commercially available. FSHD can be quite heterogeneous in its clinical presentation and course, which leads to questions regarding genetic homogeneity. Sporadic forms may be referred to as FSH syndrome (FSHS).

O   **What are the symptoms associated with FSH?**

Symptoms of FSH are vary greatly. They most commonly begin in the teens or early twenties, but infant or childhood onset has been documented. Symptoms usually begin with difficulty lifting objects above the shoulders. The weakness in the shoulders causes scapular winging, where the shoulder blades stick out sharply from the back. Muscles in the upper arm often lose bulk sooner than the forearm. Symptoms related to facial weakness include loss of facial expression, difficulty closing the eyes completely, and the inability to drink with a straw, blow up a balloon, or whistle. Contracture of the calf muscles may cause frequent tripping over curbs or uneven areas. The earlier the onset of symptoms, the more likely the patient is to need a wheelchair for mobility. Children with FSH often develop partial or complete deafness.

O   **What is Limb girdle syndrome (LGS)?**

It is a very heterogeneous group of myopathies that share some clinical features, has been classified into at least 5 types:
1. Autosomal recessive muscular dystrophy of childhood (ARMDC)
2. Autosomal dominant late onset (ADLO)
3. Pelvifemoral (PF)
4. Scapulohumeral (SH)
5. Myopathy limited to quadriceps

Expression of any of these conditions may be observed in either sex, with primary involvement of the shoulder and/or pelvic girdle muscles and a variable rate of progression. LGS is no longer considered to be a distinct nosological entity and is thought to be a wide variety of muscle disorders predominantly affecting the limb girdle muscles.

O   **What is late onset limb girdle muscular dystrophy?**

Late onset limb girdle muscular dystrophy with autosomal dominant inheritance has been linked to chromosome 5 but also may be present in childhood; this condition is referred to as Bethlem myopathy. Pelvifemoral LGS is so heterogeneous that its existence as a discrete disorder remains controversial. Due to the substantial heterogeneity, prevalence rates for these syndromes have not been reported.

○   **What are the characteristic symptoms of late onset limb girdle muscular dystrophy?**

Symptoms include progressive weakness and loss of the muscles closest to the trunk. Leg contractures may occur. The patient usually loses the ability to walk about 20 years after the onset of symptoms. Some people with LGMD need to use a ventilator because of respiratory weakness. Lifespan may be slightly shortened.

○   **What is Oculopharyngeal Muscular Dystrophy (OMD)?**

Oculopharyngeal muscular dystrophy is a disorder of late adult onset characterized by progressive ptosis and dysphagia.

○   **What are the clinical characteristics of OMD?**

Asymmetrical weakness of the levator palpebrae and pharyngeal muscles is the initial presentation, generally after the age of 50. Eventually all extraocular muscles may become involved. There is no cardiac involvement.

○   **What are the EMG findings?**

The EMG shows myopathic changes.

○   **What are the muscle biopsy findings?**

Muscle biopsy reveals changes found in other muscular dystrophies: loss of muscle fibers, variation in fiber size, increased numbers of nuclei and internal nuclei, and increased fibrous and fatty connective tissue. On histochemistry, there are small angulated fibers that react strongly for oxidative enzymes and "rimmed" vacuoles, particularly in type I fibers from extremity muscles rather than extraocular muscles. On electron microscopy, there are unique intranuclear tubular filaments.

○   **What rehabilitation interventions are options in OMD?**

Interventions, such as eyelid crutches to alleviate the ptosis and a feeding tube to provide adequate nutrition, are palliative. If the patient does not receive a feeding tube, the dysphagia will lead to early death by malnutrition and starvation.

○   **What is Emery-Dreifuss muscular dystrophy?**

Generally it is X-linked recessive, although there are very rare autosomal dominant and recessive forms. The incidence of the X-linked type is estimated to be about 1 in 100,000. The classic symptoms of ED MD include (1) contractures of elbows, Achilles' tendon, and postcervical muscles before weakness is present; (2) slowly progressive weakness and muscle wasting, generally starting in the humeroperoneal muscles; and (3) a cardiomyopathy that frequently presents as heart block.

○   **What care plan is indicated in EDMD patients?**

The care provided to the patient is similar to that for the other muscular dystrophies, with the notable exception of cardiac intervention. Merlini documented that up to 40 percent of patients with ED MD die suddenly, many of them without any preceding cardiac symptoms. Therefore, a thorough cardiac evaluation and insertion of a pacemaker when indicated is essential.

○   **Summarize the proximal inherited myopathies**

PROXIMAL INHERITED MYOPATHIES	CHARACTERISTIC MUSCLE INVOLVEMENT	INHERITANCE *age at onset*	MOLECULAR DIAGNOSIS
DMD Duchenne's muscular dystrophy	toe-walking calf hypertrophy Gower's maneuver cardiomyopathy	X-linked *3-5y*	mutations in dystrophin gene absent staining

BMD Becker's muscular dystrophy	as for DMD but much milder post-exercise cramps cardiomyopathy	X-linked *3-20+y*	mutations in dystrophin gene	
LGMD Limb-girdle muscular dystrophies	pelvic>>shoulder girdle can look like DMD, BMD or humeroperoneal weakness sparing face no cardiac involvement	AR (AD) *3-20+y*	various mutations incl. calpain-3, _ -, ̄ -,α -,β -sarcoglycans	
PROMM Proximal myotonic myopathy (DM2)	limb-girdle stiffness, pain myotonia cardiac conduction defects can be similar to DM1	AD *20-60y*	quadruplet expansions in ZNF9	

O   **Summarize the distal inherited myopathies**

DISTAL **INHERITED** **MYOPATHIES**	CHARACTERISTIC MUSCLE INVOLVEMENT	INHERITANCE	MOLECULAR DIAGNOSIS	*age at* *onset*
Myotonic dystrophy	myotonia bilateral ptosis masseter/temporalis sternocleidomastoid bulbar muscles cardiomyopathy	AD	triplet expansions in DM-PK	*any age*
Distal myopathies • Welander	no cardiac involvement forearm extensors	AD	few identified genes	*>40y*
• Nonaka	anterior compartment leg	AR		*<30y*
• Miyoshi/LGMD 2B	posterior compartment leg	AR	with decreased/absent dysferlin	*<30y*

O   **Summarize the distinctive inherited myopathies**

DISTINCTIVE **INHERITED** **MYOPATHIES**	CHARACTERISTIC MUSCLE INVOLVEMENT	INHERITANCE *age at onset*	MOLECULAR DIAGNOSIS	
FSH Facioscapulohumeral muscular dystrophy	asymmetric weakness facial onset shoulder>>pelvic girdle humeroperoneal weakness no cardiac involvement	AD *10-30y*	deletions in 4qter	
OPMD Oculopharyngeal muscular dystrophy	ptosis dysphagia ± limb-girdle weakness late onset no cardiac involvement	AD *40-60y*	triplet expansions in PABP2 DNA studies	
EDMD Emery-Dreifuss muscular dystrophy	elbow, neck contractures humeroperoneal weakness cardiac conduction defects	X-linked (AD) *3-20y*	mutations in STA gene absent emerin staining	
Bethlem myopathy	finger, elbow contractures limb-girdle weakness no cardiac involvement	AD *0-50y*	mutations in collagen VI gene	

INFLAMMATORY MYOPATHIES

O   **What is the incidence of Polymyositis (PM) ?**

The overall incidence is reported as 0.2 to 0.9 per 100,000. PM affects women more frequently than men (2:1 ratio); it is most common in black females. PM usually affects adults older than 20 years, and especially people aged 45-60 years. PM rarely affects children, unlike DM. The age of onset of PM with another collagen vascular disease is related to the associated condition

○ **What are the mortality rates of PM?**

Five year survival rates have been estimated at more than 80%. Causes of death include severe muscle weakness, pulmonary involvement, cardiac involvement, associated malignancy, and complications of immunosuppressive therapy, especially infection.

○ **How are dermatomyositis and polymyositis (DM & PM) related?**

Polymyositis (PM) and dermatomyositis (DM) are usually considered together as idiopathic inflammatory myopathies, owing to the similar clinical manifestations, except for the dermatologic findings seen in DM.   While DM has both childhood and adult forms, PM presents almost exclusively in patients over 18 years
old.

○ **How is PM classified by Walton and Adams ?**

Dermatomyositis and polymyositis have been classified into the following clinical groups as originally proposed by Walton and Adams:
   Primary polymyositis (idiopathic, adult)
   Dermatomyositis (idiopathic, adult)
   Childhood dermatomyositis or myositis with necrotizing vasculitis
   Polymyositis associated with connective tissue disorder (i.e., overlap syndrome)
   Polymyositis or dermatomyositis associated with neoplasia

○ **What is the classification by Bohan and Peter?**

Bohan and Peter classify the idiopathic inflammatory myopathies as follows:
   I - Primary idiopathic PM
   II - Primary idiopathic DM
   III - PM or DM associated with malignancy
   IV - Childhood PM or DM
   V - PM or DM associated with another connective tissue disease
   VI - IBM
   VII - Miscellaneous (eg, eosinophilic myositis, myositis ossificans, focal myositis, giant cell myositis)

○ **What is the pathogenesis of PM?**

Polymyositis is presumed to be an autoimmune mediated disease secondary to defective cellular immunity, which may be due to diverse causes that may occur either alone or in association with viral infections, malignancies, or connective tissue disorders. Evidence exists for a T cell–mediated cytotoxic process directed against unidentified muscle antigens. This conclusion is supported by the presence of CD 8 T cells, which, along with macrophages, initially surround healthy non-necrotic muscle fibers and eventually invade and destroy them.

○ **Characterize the autoimmune response assays for PM?**

Autoimmune response to nuclear and cytoplasmic autoantigens is detected in about 60-80% of patients affected with polymyositis and dermatomyositis. Some of the serum autoantibodies are shared with other autoimmune diseases (i.e., myositis-associated antibodies [MAA]) and some of them are unique to myositis (i.e., myositis-specific antibodies [MSA]). The MSA are found in approximately 40% of patients with polymyositis and dermatomyositis, whereas the MAA are found in 20-50% of the patients.

○ **What are the Myositis-specific antibodies?**

The identified MSA targets include 3 distinct groups of proteins: the aminoacyl–transfer RNA (tRNA) synthetases (anti-Jo-1), the nuclear Mi-2 protein, and components of the signal recognition particle (SRP).

○ **What are the Myositis-associated antibodies?**

The MAA are found in 20-50% of patients' sera; they are commonly encountered in other connective tissue diseases. The most important antigenic targets of the MAA are the PM/Scl nucleolar antigen, the nuclear Ku antigen, the small nuclear ribonucleoproteins (snRNP), and the cytoplasmic ribonucleoproteins (RoRNP). The anti-PM/Scl autoantibodies are generally found in patients affected by polymyositis overlapping with scleroderma. Anti-Ku antibodies are found in patients with myositis overlapping with other connective tissue diseases.

○ **What is the pathogenesis of Dermatomyositis?**

Dermatomyositis is likely the result of a humoral attack on the muscle capillaries and small arterioles. Complement c5b-9 membrane attack complex is deposited, which is needed in preparing the cell for destruction in antibody mediated disease. B cells and CD4 (helper) cells are also present in abundance in the inflammatory reaction associated with the blood vessels. As the disease progresses, the capillaries are destroyed and the muscles undergo microinfarction. Perifascicular atrophy occurs in the beginning, but, as the disease advances, necrotic and degenerative fibers are present throughout the muscle.

○ **What is the age distribution for DM?**

Dermatomyositis affects children and adults equally. Peak incidence is observed in individuals aged 45-64 years, with a smaller peak in children aged 5-14 years.

○ **Does the morbidity and mortality vary between DM and PM?**

The active period of the disease is approximately 2-3 years in both children and adults. The duration is greater for patients with cardiac or pulmonary complications; approximately 20% of the patients recover completely. The mortality rate after several years of the disease is approximately 15%; it is higher for patients with dermatomyositis with connective tissue diseases and malignancy.

○ **What are the symptoms and history suggestive of PM?**

The weakness is painless in two thirds of the patients. A rash is not present. Eye muscles are not involved, and facial muscles are involved only with severe disease. Family history of neuromuscular disease, endocrinopathy, or exposure to myotoxic drugs or toxins is absent. The disease may exist for several months before the patient seeks medical advice, and all the muscles of the thighs, trunk, shoulders, hips, and upper arms are usually involved. Symptoms include difficulty getting up from a chair, climbing steps, stepping onto a curb, lifting objects, and combing hair. Fatigue, myalgias, and muscle cramps may also be present. In contrast, fine motor movements that depend on the strength of distal muscles, such as buttoning a shirt, sewing, knitting, or writing are affected only late in the disease.

○ **What are the physical findings encountered in PM?**

Nothing is characteristic about the muscle weakness. It is not painful, although a minority of patients report aches or cramps. The weakness may fluctuate from week to week and month to month. Ocular muscles remain normal even in advanced untreated cases. Facial muscles remain normal except in rare advanced cases. The pharyngeal and neck flexor muscles are often involved, causing dysphagia and difficulty in holding up the head. In advanced cases and rarely in acute cases, respiratory muscles may also be affected. Severe weakness is almost always associated with muscular wasting. Sensation remains normal. Occasionally, the muscle may be sore to palpation and may have a nodular grainy feel. The tendon reflexes are preserved, but they may be absent in severely weakened or atrophied muscles.

○ **How do patients with DM present?**

Patients often present with skin disease as one of the initial manifestations. Sometimes, perhaps in as many as 40% of the patients, the skin disease may be the sole manifestation at the onset. Muscle disease may occur concurrently, may precede the skin disease, or may follow the skin disease by weeks to years.

O   **What integumentary symptoms occur?**

Patients often notice an eruption on exposed surfaces. The rash is often pruritic, and intense pruritus may disturb sleep patterns. Patients may also report a scaly scalp or diffuse hair loss.

O   **What muscular symptoms occur?**

Muscle involvement is manifested by proximal muscle weakness. Patients often begin to note fatigue of their muscles or weakness when climbing stairs, walking, rising from a sitting position, combing their hair, or reaching for items in cabinets that are above their shoulders. Muscle tenderness may occur, but tenderness is not a regular feature of the disease.

O   **What other systemic symptoms may occur?**

Systemic manifestations may occur; therefore, the review of systems should assess for the presence of arthralgia, arthritis, dyspnea, dysphagia, arrhythmia, and dysphonia.

O   **What is the association of malignancy with DM?**

Malignancy is possible in any patient with DM, but it occurs more frequently in adults older than 60 years. Only a few children with DM and malignancy have been reported. The history should include a thorough review of systems and an assessment for previous malignancy.

O   **What are the clinical symptoms that a child may present with?**

Children with DM may have an insidious onset that defies diagnosis until the dermatologic disease is clearly observed and diagnosed. Calcinosis is a complication of juvenile DM but is rarely observed at the onset of disease. Ask questions about hard nodules of the skin during the initial examination.

O   **What are the characteristic cutaneous features of DM?**

The characteristic, and possibly pathognomonic, cutaneous features of DM are heliotrope rash and Gottron papules. Several other cutaneous features, including malar erythema, poikiloderma (i.e., variegated telangiectasia, hyperpigmentation) in a photosensitive distribution, violaceous erythema on the extensor surfaces, and periungual and cuticular changes, are characteristic of the disease even though they are not pathognomonic.

O   **What are the characteristics of the heliotrope rash?**

The heliotrope rash consists of a violaceous to dusky erythematous rash with or without edema in a symmetrical distribution involving periorbital skin. Sometimes, this sign is quite subtle and may involve only a mild discoloration along the eyelid margin. A heliotrope rash is rarely observed in other disorders; thus, its presence is highly suggestive of DM.

O   **What are Gottron Papules?**

The Gottron papules are found over bony prominences, particularly the metacarpophalangeal joints, the proximal interphalangeal joints, and/or the distal interphalangeal joints. Papules may also be found overlying the elbows, knees, and/or feet. The lesions consist of slightly elevated violaceous papules and plaques. A slight scale and, occasionally, a thick psoriasiform scale may be present. These lesions may resemble lesions of lupus erythematosus (LE), psoriasis, or lichen planus (LP).

O   **How is the diagnosis of PM established?**

Diagnosis of polymyositis is established by serum enzyme levels and electromyography (EMG) studies and is confirmed by obtaining a diagnostic muscle biopsy.

O   **What is the most sensitive enzyme assay in PM?**

The most sensitive enzyme is creatine kinase, which, in the presence of disease, can be elevated as much as 50 times the reference level. The creatine kinase level usually parallels disease activity. It is only rarely within the reference range in active polymyositis. The creatine kinase level may also be within the reference range in some patients with polymyositis associated with a connective tissue disease.

○   **Are the Anti-Jo-1 antibodies relevant in the diagnosis of PM?**

Anti-Jo-1 antibodies are present in one fifth of the patients.

○   **What EMG findings are encountered in PM?**

EMG may be helpful in diagnosis, although findings can be normal in 15% of patients. It shows a typical myopathic pattern with irritability, although it is not specific for the condition. These findings are most consistently observed in weak proximal muscles. EMG also is helpful in selecting a muscle for biopsy. Needle EMG shows myopathic potentials characterized by short duration, low amplitude polyphasic units on voluntary activation and increased spontaneous activity with fibrillations, complex repetitive discharges, and positive sharp waves along with early recruitment.

○   **What is the role of muscle biopsy in PM?**

Muscle biopsy is the definitive test not only for establishing the diagnosis of polymyositis but also for excluding other neuromuscular diseases. In polymyositis, the presence of inflammation is the histological hallmark of the disease. The diagnosis of polymyositis is definite when a patient has subacute elevated levels of serum creatine kinase and findings on muscle biopsy consistent with the histological features of polymyositis

○   **What are the histological findings?**

The endomysial infiltrates mostly are in foci within the fascicles, initially surrounding healthy muscle fibers and finally invading these cells and resulting in phagocytosis and necrosis. Because the inflammatory infiltrates can be small and multifocal, they can be missed in a small size muscle biopsy specimen. Perifascicular atrophy or prominent perivascular infiltrates are not present and the blood vessels are normal. When the disease becomes chronic, the connective tissue increases.

○   **What pulmonary dysfunction may be encountered in patients with DM/PM?**

Pulmonary function test results are abnormal in 50% of patients and show a restrictive pattern. Interstitial lung disease occurs in 5% to 10% of patients and may be fatal.

○   **What cardiac disorders may be encountered in patients with PM/DM?**

Arrhythmia and cardiomyopathy were seen in 33 of 55 patients with PM or DM studied retrospectively.
Cardiac arrhythmias include atrioventricular block, premature ventricular contractions, and ventricular and supraventricular tachycardias. Congestive heart failure may result from myocardial inflammation.

○   **How common is dysphagia among patients with DM/PM?**

Dysphagia occurs in 20% to 50% of patients with PM or DM. Striated muscle weakness in the hypopharynx and upper esophagus causes decreased propulsion of the food bolus into the esophagus. Pressures generated in the hypopharynx may not be able to overcome a fibrotic cricopharyngeal muscle or the prolonged pharyngeal transit time may miss the relaxation of the cricopharyngeal muscle. There is evidence of smooth muscle involvement in the lower esophagus and delayed gastric emptying.

○   **What does videofluoroscopic examination reveal in patients with DM/PM?**

Videofluoroscopic examination may show pharyngeal pooling and decreased contrast below the cricopharyngeal muscle.

○   **What therapeutic interventions may be pursued in DM/PM patients with dysphagia?**

Solid dysphagia exceeds liquid dysphagia, and frequent small feedings, softer solid consistencies, frequent sips of liquids, and a slow feeding rate can improve symptoms. Upright positioning during and after meals can improve reflux symptoms. Cricopharyngeal myotomy may alleviate dysphagia in patients who fail to respond to conservative measures. Patients with very severe disease may require gastrostomy feedings to maintain nutrition. Unless they have more distal muscle involvement, most patients can feed themselves.

O **What is the role of prednisone in the treatment of PM?**

Prednisone is the first line treatment of choice for PM. Typically, the dose is 1 mg/kg/d, either as a single dose or divided. This high dose is usually continued for 4-8 weeks, until the CK level returns to reference ranges. Taper prednisone on a monthly basis by 5-10 mg until the lowest dose that controls the disease is reached.

O **What effect do corticosteroids have on DM/PM?**

High dose prednisone results in complete improvement in 25% of patients and partial improvement in 61%, with DM showing a better response than PM. On the other hand, avascular necrosis and osteoporotic compression fractures resulting from steroid use contribute significantly to disability. PM and DM are truly systemic diseases.

O **When are Immunosuppressive agents indicated?**

Immunosuppressive agents indicated are indicated if patients do not show improvement with steroids within a reasonable period of time (i.e., 4 wk) or if adverse effects from corticosteroids develop. Patients with poor prognostic indicators, such as dysphagia or dysphonia, are likely to require immunosuppressive agents. Under these circumstances, methotrexate is the second line agent. Patients with IBM usually respond poorly to corticosteroids and immunosuppressive agents.

O **What poor prognostic factors are associated with PM/DM?**

Poor prognostic factors include the following: older age, female sex, African American race, interstitial lung disease, Presence of anti-Jo-1 (lung disease) and anti-SRP antibodies (severe muscle disease, cardiac involvement),associated malignancy, delayed or inadequate treatment, dysphagia, dysphonia, cardiac and pulmonary involvement.

O **What are appropriate guidelines for initiating and progressing a physical rehabilitation in the PM patient?**

When muscle strength is 2/5 or less (an inability to resist gravity) all range of motion stretching should be done by the therapist, but as muscle strength approaches 3/5 an active, assisted program should be instituted. This involves a combination of isotonic and isometric exercises with elastic straps of varying resistance. As muscle strength improves to 4-/5 (near normal strength) a more aggressive approach with free weights or resistive machines should be used. Patients with acute and chronic myopathy often have tightness of tendons and capsules as well as muscle around their joints. In this circumstance, heat should be applied to increase mobility prior to instituting a range of motion and strengthening program in patients without acute arthritis. As patients improve with pharmacologic treatment and a resistive exercise program, an aerobic conditioning regimen to address fatigue should be implemented.

O **What benefits can be achieved through therapeutic exercise during an active episode of PM?**

In a study by Cecília Varjú et al, during the acute phase of inflammatory myopathies the proximal muscles of the body were far more seriously affected; consequently the average strength improvement of the proximal muscles was not significant in the early recovery group patients. Yet the physical training was helpful in preventing or at least reducing muscle atrophy caused by inactivation and corticosteroids. Meanwhile, the distal muscles that are less seriously affected may become significantly stronger, contributing to an overall improvement in activities of daily living.

O **What functional gains can be achieved with therapeutic exercise in PM?**

In this study the functional independence scales, HAQ scores indicated some improvement in almost all cases. The improvement was greater in the early recovery group than in their chronic stage group.

O **Can a home exercise program be safely administered to patients with PM?**

In a study by Alexanderson, H et al The group showed significantly improved function and quality of life compared to the start of study. It seems that this exercise program safely can be employed in patients with active PM or DM, and we suggest that physical exercise should be included in the rehabilitation of these patients.

O   **What is sporadic Inclusion Body Myositis (s-IBM)?**

Sporadic inclusion body myositis (s-IBM) and inherited inclusion body myopathies (i-IBM) encompass a group of disorders that have the common pathological finding of "inclusion bodies" on muscle biopsy (MBx). They collectively demonstrate a wide variation in clinical expression, age of onset, associated diseases, and prognosis. The specific hallmarks of inclusion body myositis (IBM) are inflammation, vacuolated muscle fibers, intracellular amyloid deposits, and 15- to 18-nm tubulofilamentous inclusions.

O   **What is the pathogenesis of s-IBM?**

1.   The inflammatory cells that are present in affected muscle are mostly CD 8^+ lymphocytes or macrophages expressing MHC II surface markers. These findings suggest a directed response against specific antigens and a role of immune mediated cytotoxicity.
2.   In addition, there are changes in the mitochondria and the nuclei of the myofibers, amyloid protein, and abnormally present filaments that suggest a possible "neurodegenerative" pathogenic mechanism.
3.   It is also suggested that the expression of an abnormal gene product may lead to a cytodestructive process and help explain the inflammatory and neurodegenerative evidence.

O   **What is the epidemiology of s-IBM?**

IBM is the most common inflammatory muscle disease occurring over the age of 50. Patients are greater than 30 years of age and usually greater than 50 at the time of onset of symptoms. Men are more often affected than women, in contrast with other autoimmune and inflammatory diseases. There are no known risk factors other than genetic risk in those families with a history of IBM.

O   **What is the incidence of s-IBM?**

In series of inflammatory myopathies from the United States and Canada, s-IBM is reported to account for approximately 15-28% of cases.

O   **What is the clinical presentation of s-IBM?**

The clinical weakness of IBM may resemble that of PM or DM but more typically evolves over years and resembles a limb girdle dystrophy. Distal weakness is common, and dysphagia occurs in as many as 60 percent of patients. The weakness and atrophy may be asymmetrical and involve solitary muscles such as the quadriceps, iliopsoas, biceps, or triceps. Over years, there is more symmetry and weakness of the involved muscles. Unlike other inflammatory myopathies, patients with IBM do not have an increased risk of malignancy.

O   **When is s-IBM suspected?**

IBM is suspected when a patient with the diagnosis of PM does not respond to corticosteroid therapy, has early involvement of distal muscles such as long finger flexors of the hand and wrist and extensors of the foot, or has dysphagia.

O   **What is the distribution of weakness in s- IBM?**

The distribution of weakness in s-IBM is variable, but both proximal and distal weakness can be present. Characteristic changes are predominant knee extensor weakness in the legs and wrist/finger flexor weakness in the arms .A common and distinct characteristic of s-IBM is its severe involvement of the wrist and finger flexors, out of proportion to their extensor counterparts. Hence, loss of finger dexterity and grip strength may be a presenting or prominent symptom; whereas in polymyositis the distribution of weakness is typically symmetric, in s-IBM it is often asymmetric.

O   **What other symptoms may be present in s-IBM?**

Fatigue and reduced tolerance of exertion are common, particularly in ambulatory individuals. Dysphagia is also common; patients should be questioned about difficulties in chewing/swallowing. Myalgias and cramping are relatively uncommon. Sensory and autonomic dysfunctions are not present except in patients having a concurrent polyneuropathy. Cardiac disease is common; it is most likely due to the older age of most patients. Direct cardiac muscle involvement by the disease has not been demonstrated.

O   **Tabulate the Characteristic Features and Diagnostic Criteria for Inclusion Body Myositis**

Characteristic Features and Diagnostic Criteria for Inclusion Body Myositis
Characteristic Features
Clinical
Duration of illness >6 months
Age of onset >30 years old
Weakness of proximal and distal arm and leg muscles; must include at least one of the following features:
Finger flexor weakness
Wrist flexor > wrist extensor weakness
Quadriceps muscle weakness (≤ grade 4 MRC)
Laboratory
Serum creatine kinase <12 times normal
Muscle biopsy:
Inflammatory myopathy characterized by mononuclear cell invasion of non necrotic muscle fibers
Vacuolated muscle fibers
Intracellular amyloid deposits or 15- to 18-nm tubulofilaments by electron microscopy
Electromyography consistent with inflammatory myopathy
Diagnostic Criteria
Definite *inclusion body myositis*
Patients must exhibit all of the muscle biopsy features including invasion of non necrotic fibers by mononuclear cells, vacuolated muscle fibers, and intracellular (within muscle fibers) amyloid deposits or 15- to 18-nm tubulofilaments
None of the other clinical or laboratory features are mandatory if the muscle biopsy features are diagnostic
Possible *inclusion body myositis*
If the muscle shows only inflammation (invasion of non necrotic muscle fibers by mononuclear cells) *without* other pathological features of inclusion body myositis, *then* a diagnosis of possible inclusion body myositis can be given if the patient exhibits the characteristic clinical and laboratory features

O   **Tabulate the differential diagnosis of s-IBM**

Disease	Points of Differentiation
i-IBM	Positive family history with confirmatory MBx
Polymyositis*	MBx shows inflammation; no other morphologic criteria present for s-IBM
Dermatomyositis	Presence of skin lesions plus appropriate MBx findings
Oculopharyngeal dystrophy	Predominant involvement of oculopharyngeal musculature; no ocular muscle involvement shown with s-IBM; MBx shows similarities to s-IBM, but muscle fiber inclusions are smaller and no inflammation seen; positive family history and genetic testing; rare oculopharyngodistal variant (one type described in Japan)
Other late-onset distal myopathies	Positive family history unless sporadic case; MBx may show rimmed vacuoles and inclusions in Swedish (Welander) type and Japanese (Nonaka) type
Sarcoid (chronic atrophic sarcoid myopathy)	Progressive generalized weakness may occur in sarcoid rarely, independent of presence of polyneuropathy; MBx shows scattered MF atrophy and degeneration; does not respond to

	immunosuppressive therapy
Myasthenia gravis	In s-IBM, extraocular muscles not involved; motor unit action potential (MUAP) instability (i.e., jitter) on EMG rare, repetitive nerve stimulation should not show any decrement; negative for antibodies to acetylcholine receptors
Motor neuron disease	Upper motor neuron signs such as hyperreflexia and extensor plantar responses not present in s-IBM; EMG in s-IBM may show "neurogenic" changes (i.e., enlarged MUAPs), but these changes are relatively minor compared to predominance of smaller MUAPs, suggesting myopathy; in s-IBM, fibrillation potentials relatively infrequent except in early, severe cases, and fasciculation potentials have not been reported
Acid maltase deficiency	EMG is "myopathic," similar to that of s-IBM; in acid maltase deficiency, however, insertional activity (complex repetitive discharges and myotonia) increased prominently; myotonia not seen in s-IBM and complex repetitive discharges uncommon; MBx positive for glycogen storage products
Chronic inflammatory demyelinating polyradiculoneuropathy	Weakness usually greater distally but may be asymmetric; abnormal nerve conductions consistent with demyelination; chronic reinnervating changes present on needle electrode examination; serum creatine kinase (CK) typically normal

O   **What are the electrodiagnostic findings in IBM?**

The MUAPs typically show normal to reduced amplitude. There is reduced duration for simple (non polyphasic) MUAPs and variable increase in complexity (phases and turns). When assessing duration, only simple MUAPs should be measured so as to increase diagnostic sensitivity. Increase in complexity (eg, increases in phases, turns, or the presence of late components or satellites) is a nonspecific finding and may be seen as an early abnormal finding in neurogenic or myopathic processes. Occasional MUAPs in s-IBM may appear "enlarged" or high amplitude. Careful assessment shows that these are narrow spikes with minimal area. In s-IBM, MUAPs are generally stable. In other words, jitter typically is not increased. If at least 4 MUAPs in a muscle are considered to be abnormal and have changes consistent with myopathy, examining the muscle further is not necessary unless other issues need be addressed (eg, polyneuropathy, radiculopathy).

O   **What other pathological conditions are encountered in s-IBM patients?**

Polyneuropathy is present in 15% to 20% of patients with s- IBM. IBM is associated with other immune mediated diseases such as systemic lupus erythematosus, Sjögren syndrome, interstitial lung disease, idiopathic thrombocytopenic purpura, and diabetes mellitus. Patients with s IBM may have distal lower extremity paresthesias that may or may not be associated with concomitant diabetic neuropathy.

NEUROMUSCULAR JUNCTION DISORDERS

O   **What is the estimated annual incidence of myasthenia gravis (MG)?**

The estimated annual incidence of MG is 2 per 1,000,000.

O   **What is the Mortality/Morbidity associated with MG?**

Recent advances in treatment and care of critically ill patients have resulted in marked decrease in the mortality rate. The rate is now 3-4%, with principal risk factors being age older than 40 years, short history of severe disease, and thymoma. Previously, the mortality rate was as high as 30-40%.

O   **What is the female-to-male ratio in MG?**

It is said classically to be 6:4, but as the population has aged, the incidence is now equal in males and females.

O   **What is the association of age and MG?**

MG presents at any age. Female incidence peaks in the third decade of life, whereas male incidence peaks in the sixth or seventh decade. Mean age of onset is 28 years in females and 42 years in males.

O **What are the clinical characteristics of MG?**

MG is characterized by fluctuating weakness increased by exertion. Weakness increases during the day and improves with rest. Presentation and progression vary.

O **What patterns of muscle weakness are most common?**

Extraocular muscle (EOM) weakness or ptosis is present initially in 50% of patients and occurs during the course of illness in 90%. Bulbar muscle weakness is also common, along with weakness of head extension and flexion.

O **What variations in weakness pattern may present?**

Weakness may involve limb musculature with myopathic like proximal weakness greater than distal muscle weakness. Isolated limb muscle weakness as the presenting symptom is rare and occurs in fewer than 10% of patients.

O **What is the temporal pattern of progression in MG patients?**

Patients progress from mild to more severe disease over weeks to months. Weakness tends to spread from the ocular to facial to bulbar muscles and then to truncal and limb muscles. The disease remains ocular in only 16% of patients. About 87% of patients generalize within 13 months after onset. In patients with generalized disease, the interval from onset to maximal weakness is less than 36 months in 83% of patients.

O **What neurological findings are encountered on examination?**

Weakness can be present in a variety of different muscles and is usually proximal and symmetric. Sensory examination and deep tendon reflexes are normal.

O **What are the characteristics of facial muscle weakness?**

Weakness of the facial muscles is almost always present. Bilateral facial muscle weakness produces a masklike face with ptosis and a horizontal smile. The eyebrows are furrowed to compensate for ptosis, and the sclerae below the limbi may be exposed secondary to weak lower lids. Mild proptosis due to EOM weakness also may be present.

O **What are the bulbar findings associated with MG?**

Weakness of palatal muscles can result in a nasal twang to the voice and nasal regurgitation of food and especially liquids. Chewing may become difficult. Severe jaw weakness may cause the jaw to hang open (the patient may sit with a hand on the chin for support). Swallowing may become difficult and aspiration may occur with fluids, giving rise to coughing or choking while drinking. Weakness of neck muscles is common and neck flexors usually are affected more severely than neck extensors.

O **What are the characteristics of limb muscle weakness**

Certain limb muscles are involved more commonly than others (eg, upper limb muscles are more likely to be involved than lower limb muscles). In the upper limbs, deltoids and extensors of the wrist and fingers are affected most. Triceps are more likely to be affected than biceps. In the lower extremities, commonly involved muscles include hip flexors, quadriceps, and hamstrings, with involvement of foot dorsiflexors or plantar flexors less common.

O **What patterns of ocular muscle weakness occur in MG?**

Typically, EOM weakness is asymmetric. The weakness usually affects more than 1 EOM and is not limited to muscles innervated by a single cranial nerve. This is an important diagnostic clue. The weakness of lateral and medial recti may produce a pseudointernuclear ophthalmoplegia, described as limited adduction of 1 eye, with nystagmus of the abducting eye on attempted lateral gaze. The nystagmus becomes coarser on sustained lateral gaze as the medial rectus of the abducting eye fatigues. Eyelid weakness results in ptosis.

○   **What serological test is utilized in the diagnosis of MG?**

The Anti-acetylcholine receptor antibody test is reliable for diagnosing autoimmune MG. The result of the test for the anti-AChR antibody (Ab) is positive in 74% of patients. Results are positive in about 80% of patients with generalized myasthenia and in 50% of those with pure ocular myasthenia. Thus, the anti-AChR Ab test result is frequently negative in patients with only ocular MG.

○   **What treatments are available for MG?**

AChE inhibitors and immunomodulating therapies are the mainstays of treatment. In the mild form of the disease, AChE inhibitors are used initially. Most patients with generalized MG require additional immunomodulating therapy. Plasmapheresis and thymectomy are important modalities for treating MG. They are not traditional medical immunomodulating therapies, but they function by modifying the immune system.

○   **What are the most important different characteristics of the two diseases?**

	Myasthenia gravis	**Lambert-Eaton Syndrome**
muscle strength	decreasing during ongoing exercise	maximum contraction delayed
ocular muscles paresis	typical	Rare
autonomic nervous system	normal	anticholinergic syndrome
tendon reflexes	normal	reduced with posttetanic facilitation
single nerve stimulation	normal amplitude	reduced amplitude
repetitive stimulation	decrement at 3-Hz stimulation	additional increment at 20-Hz stimulation
acetylcholine receptor autoantibodies	positive	Negative
calcium channel autoantibodies	negative	Positive

○   **Is therapeutic exercise safe in patients with MG?**

Lohi EL. Et al established that moderate resistance exercise therapy was safe in patients with MG without causing exacerbation of the disease. Improvements in exercise tolerance and quality of life were also cite

REHABILITATION PROBLEM FOCUSED ISSUES

SPASTICITY

○ **What is a definition of spasticity?**

Spasticity (meaning to draw or tug) is involuntary velocity-dependent increased muscle tone resulting in resistance to movement that may occur secondary to spinal cord injury (SCI), brain injury, tumor, stroke, multiple sclerosis (MS), or a peripheral nerve injury. A lag time may exist between injury and spasticity onset, and severity may wax and wane over time. Spasticity may be static or dynamic in nature.

○ **What are some advantages of spasticity?**

Substitutes for strength, allowing standing, walking, gripping.
May improve circulation and prevent deep venous thrombosis (DVT) and edema.
May reduce the risk of osteoporosis.

○ **What are disadvantages of spasticity?**

Orthopedic deformity such as hip dislocation, contractures, or scoliosis.
Impairment of activities of daily living (ADL) (eg, dressing, bathing, toileting).
Impairment of mobility (eg, inability to walk, roll, sit).
Skin breakdown secondary to positioning difficulties and shearing pressure.
Pain or abnormal sensory feedback.
Poor weight gain secondary to high caloric expenditure.
Sleep disturbance.
Depression secondary to lack of functional independence.

○ **What patterns of spasticity are encountered in the upper extremity?**

Adduction and internal rotation of the shoulder.
Flexion of the elbow and wrist.
Pronation of the forearm.
Flexion of the fingers and adduction of the thumb.

○ **What upper extremity muscle groups are targeted for therapy?**

Pectoralis major.
Latissimus dorsi.
Teres major.
Biceps.
Brachioradialis.
Brachialis.
Pronator teres and quadratus.
Flexor carpi radialis and ulnaris.
Flexor digitorum profundus and superficialis.
Adductor pollicis.

○ **What patterns of lower extremity spasticity are encountered?**

Hip adduction and flexion.
Knee flexion.

Ankle plantar flexion or equinovarus positioning.

○   **What lower extremity muscle groups are targeted for therapy?**

Adductor magnus.
Iliopsoas.
Hamstrings (medial more often than lateral).
Tibialis posterior.
Soleus.
Gastrocnemius.

○   **What factors may influence the degree of spasticity?**

Infection (eg, otitis, urinary tract, pneumonia).
Pressure sore.
Noxious stimulus (eg, ingrown toenail, ill-fitting orthotics, occult fracture).
Deep venous thrombosis.
Bladder distention.
Bowel impaction.
Fatigue.
Seizure activity.
Cold temperature.
Malpositioning.

○   **What is the Spasm Frequency Scale?**

How many spasms has the patient had in the last 24 hours in affected muscles or extremity?

Definitions of Spasms: (1) Spasm is a jumping or twitching of the muscle or limb without control; **(2)** A spasm can be a "shooting" of the body part into a position without control; **(3)** A rapid series of "spasms" without significant pausing/resting is defined as one spasm.

0=No spasms
1=One spasm or fewer per day
2=Between one and five spasms per day
3=Between five and nine spasms per day
4=Ten or more spasms per day

○   **What is the Medical Research Council Scale (motor testing)?**

As far as possible, the action of each muscle should be observed separately.
0=No contraction
1=Flicker or trace of contraction
2=Active movement, with gravity eliminated
3=Active movement against gravity
4=Active movement against gravity and resistance
5=Normal power

○   **What is the Modified Ashworth Scale?**

0=No increase in muscle tone
1=Slight increase in muscle tone, manifested by a catch and release or by minimal resistance at the end range of motion when the part is moved in flexion or extension/abduction or adduction, etc.
1+=Slight increase in muscle tone, manifested by a catch, followed by minimal resistance throughout the remainder (less than half) of the ROM

2=More marked increase in muscle tone through most of the ROM, but the affected part is easily moved
3=Considerable increase in muscle tone, passive movement is difficult
4=Affected part is rigid in flexion or extension (abduction or adduction, etc.)

O **What are the goals of spasticity management?**

| To improve function with activities of daily living (ADL), mobility, ease of care for caregivers, sleep, cosmesis, and overall functional independence. |
| To prevent pressure areas from developing, orthopedic deformity, and the need for corrective surgery |
| To reduce pain. |
| To allow stretch of shortened muscles, strengthening of antagonistic muscle, and appropriate orthotic fit. |

O **What considerations are there in managing spasticity?**

| Duration of spasticity and likely duration of therapy. |
| Severity of spasticity. |
| Location of spasticity. |
| Success of prior interventions. |
| Current functional status and future goals. |
| Underlying diagnosis and comorbidities. |
| Ability to comply with treatment. |
| Availability of support/caregivers and follow-up therapy. |

O **What is the progression of therapy for plasticity?**

A step ladder approach from conservative to aggressive measures often is used, sometimes combining therapies from various levels.

1. Preventative measures.
2. Therapeutic interventions and physical modalities.
3. Positioning/orthotics.
4. Oral medications.
5. Injectable medications.
6. Surgical interventions.

O **What preventative measures consist of?**

Prevention consists of alleviation or treatment of precipitating factors, such as the following:

| Pressure areas. |
| Infections (eg, bladder, toenail, ear, skin). |
| Deep venous thrombosis. |
| Constipation. |
| Bladder distention. |
| Fatigue. |
| Cold. |

O **What physical agents/modalities are used to treat spasticity?**

| Sustained stretching. |
| Massage. |
| Vibration. |
| Heat modalities. |
| Cryotherapy. |
| Functional electrical stimulation (FES)/biofeedback. |
| Strengthening of antagonistic muscle groups. |

Hydrotherapy.

O   **What roles do orthotics/positioning play in the management of spasticity?**

Serial or inhibitive casting of the ankles, knees, fingers, wrists, and elbows
Splinting &orthotics: Upper and lower extremities, soft or hard, custom or prefabricated orthosis may help hold a limb in a functional position, reduce pain, and prevent deformity.
Positioning to reduce synergy patterns (eg, wheelchair seating, bed positioning)
Children may require a new orthosis every few months due to growth.
When newly casting, splinting, or positioning, monitor the skin closely for signs of breakdown.

O   **What are the characteristics and properties of injectable phenol in spasticity management?**

Usually in a 5% concentration, phenol is injected near motor points in the affected muscle. A neurostimulator with a Teflon-coated needle electrode is used for guidance. Gamma fibers are demyelinated for about 6 months, resulting in a less irritable, weakened muscle that can be stretched more easily. Because phenol injections do not cause permanent reduction in spasticity, a focus on obtaining functional improvements after injections is important. Injections can be uncomfortable for some patients, and children may need to be sedated before injection. Phenol is inexpensive, easily compounded, and has an immediate onset of action.

O   **What are possible adverse effects associated with phenol injections for spasticity management?**

Possible adverse effects include pain and swelling at the site of injection. In a very small number of patients, dysesthesias may occur if injections are done near sensory-rich nerve branches. If lengthening of a shortened muscle is desired, serial casting following injections may enhance effectiveness.

O   **What is the rationale for Botulinum toxin type A or B use in spasticity?**

Botulinum toxin injections can be used for regional or focal management of spasticity. The toxin inhibits the release of acetylcholine at the neuromuscular junction by cleaving one or more members of the complex that fuse acetylcholine vesicles to the plasma membrane at the nerve terminal. Botulinum toxin A and B provide chemical denervation and muscle paralysis on a temporary basis in selective muscle groups that are injected. With dosage limits of approximately 10 to 12 U/kg up to approximately 400 U, multiple muscle groups cannot be simultaneously injected. Additionally, because of its reversibility it requires reinjection approximately every 3 months.

O   **What are the characteristic therapeutic effects of botulinum toxin injection for spasticity?**

Botulinum toxin effects are dose dependent. The main action is localized to a 4- to 5-cm area with the clinical effect apparent in 48 hours and peak action in 2 to 4 weeks. Duration is 3 to 4 months, although improvements may outlast the direct effect on the nerve terminal. Possible explanations for these prolonged effects include improved balance of the muscle groups with the over-stretched antagonists shortening and muscle lengthening in the agonists at the injection site

O   **Which patients are best suited for botulinum toxin injection therapy?**

Patients best suited for botulinum toxin injections demonstrate muscle imbalance with stronger spastic agonist muscles. Sufficient power in the antagonist muscles is necessary to offset weakened agonists. Fixed contractures and bony deformities do not adequately benefit from the relaxation of muscle and are only amenable to orthopedic intervention, such as casting or surgery. Patients in the acute rehabilitation phase of an injury, such as traumatic brain injury, also may benefit. If the increased tone is adequately addressed, then the orthopedic abnormalities are not magnified.

O   **What are the clinical outcomes of botulinum toxin injection?**

Botulinum toxin provides decreased tone and functional improvement in the injected muscle groups with efficacy in upper and lower extremities. The side effect profile is good, with a 6% incidence primarily related to the discomfort of local injections

O **What role is there for tenotomy/tendon transfer/osteotomy in spasticity management?**

Orthopedic interventions release muscle contractures, lengthen shortened tendons, protect against or reduce bony deformities, and may reduce the strength of a spastic muscle group. The timing of procedures is critical. If performed too early, repetitive procedures may be necessary or developmental milestones may be delayed. If delayed too long, future pain or irreversible bone deformity may occur. Orthopedic interventions do not alter the spasticity of muscle groups inherently; they only alter the effects of spasticity.

O **What role is there for myelotomy/cordectomy in spasticity management?**

Transection or resection of portions of the spinal cord result in reduced spasticity but potentially cause loss of bowel and bladder function, as well as a loss of strength, pain, and temperature sensation. These procedures rarely are performed.

O **What is the role of selective dorsal rhizotomy in managing spasticity?**

Selective transection of the posterior spinal nerve roots from L2-S1 results in reduced lower extremity spasticity. Nerve roots are selected for ablation by evaluating the peripheral muscle and EMG activity that occurs during intraoperative stimulation. Trunk and upper extremity function as well as sensation also may be altered. The procedure appears to be most effective in a select group of young children with CP, who have strength underlying their spasticity. Physical and occupational therapy are important postsurgical interventions to achieve the best outcome.

O **What caution is needed in children?**

Children with spasticity should be monitored regularly for onset of orthopedic or other abnormalities, as rapid growth may result in permanent contractures or loss of function.

O **What problems may caregivers encounter during patient spasticity management?**

If spasticity worsens, caregivers may have difficulty transferring patients safely or providing adequate hygiene and general care. Recognizing caregiver difficulties and intervening to educate and help ensures that patients are cared for properly. Monitoring skin integrity is essential, as pressure ulcers can lead to sepsis and death.

O **Are there caveats to spasticity management?**

Overly aggressive surgical lengthening of severe contractures should be avoided, as compression or over stretch injuries to the nerves and arteries of the limb may occur. The ability of muscles to function after spasticity reduction varies. Treating spasticity does not guarantee acquisition of previously undeveloped skills. The importance of physical and occupational therapy intervention for achieving functional goals cannot be overemphasized.

O **What role do the benzodiazepines play in the management of spasticity?**

The benzodiazepines are centrally acting agents that increase the affinity of GABA to its receptor. They have been shown to bind in the brain stem and at the spinal cord level.

O **What are the key features of diazepam in the management of spasticity?**

Diazepam is the oldest and most frequently used benzodiazepine for managing spasticity related to spinal cord injury, cerebral palsy, and cerebral vascular accident. The clinical effects of diazepam include improved passive range of motion and reduction in hyperreflexia as well as painful spasms. Diazepam also causes sedation and improves anxiety. Diazepam has a half-life of 20-80 hours and active metabolites that prolong its effectiveness.

O **What other benzodiazepine is used in the management of spasticity?**

Clonazepam which has a half-life ranges from 18-28 hours.

O **What are the limitations to benzodiazepine use in spasticity management?**

Sedation, weakness, hypotension, GI symptoms, memory impairment, incoordination, confusion, depression, and ataxia are possible side effects of benzodiazepine treatment. Tolerance and dependency from these agents may occur and withdrawal phenomena have been associated with abrupt cessation of therapy. Tolerance may also lead to unacceptable dosage escalation to continue obtaining good clinical response. Benzodiazepines should be carefully monitored when used with similar agents, such as baclofen or tizanidine that may potentiate sedation and other central depressant properties.

O   **What is baclofen?**

Baclofen has been widely used for spasticity since 1967. It is a GABA agonist that has presynaptic and postsynaptic effects on monosynaptic and polysynaptic pathways. The primary site of action is the spinal cord where baclofen reduces the release of excitatory neurotransmitters.

O   **What are the benefits of baclofen in the management of spasticity?**

Most studies indicate that baclofen improves clonus, spasm frequency and joint range of motion resulting in improved functional status for the patient.

O   **What is the dosing recommendation for baclofen?**

The dose ranges from 30-100 mg/day in divided amounts.

O   **What precautions are needed in monitoring and adjusting the dosage of baclofen?**

Tolerance to the medication may develop. Baclofen must be slowly weaned to prevent withdrawal effects such as seizures, hallucinations and increased spasticity. It must be used with care in patients with renal insufficiency as its clearance is primarily renal. Side effects are predominantly from central depressant properties including sedation, ataxia, weakness and fatigue. These side effects may be minimized by direct intrathecal infusion of baclofen because the concentration gradient favors higher levels at the spinal cord versus the brain. When baclofen is used in combination with tizanidine or benzodiazepines the patient should be monitored for unwanted depressant effects.

O   **What is the rationale for intrathecal baclofen in spasticity management?**

For patients who have multisegmental or more extensive spasticity, and for whom oral medications are not effective or appropriate, intrathecal baclofen (ITB) is a strong consideration. Baclofen is a presynaptic inhibitor that activates the $GABA_B$ receptors. The Food and Drug Administration (FDA) has approved intrathecal use for spasticity of cerebral and spinal origin. A continuous supply of medication is delivered by an infusion system that uses a catheter in the intrathecal space, a pump in the abdomen, and telemetry programming.

O   **What are the administration and dosing guidelines?**

The intrathecal dose required is (often or frequently) 0.3% to 0.5% of the oral route and is better tolerated in patients who have systemic side effects from oral baclofen. The rate, mode, and pattern of infusion may be modified noninvasively to meet the patient's needs. The patient may receive a 24-hour simple continuous infusion dose.

O   **What clinical caveats may need to be addressed with ITB therapy?**

If there are variable needs throughout the day, however, then the infusion rate can be adjusted up to 10 distinct rates in a more complex infusion pattern. A common pattern is to increase the dose in the evening to aid sleep and reduce it in the morning to facilitate transfers. The catheter can be placed in the high thoracic or lower cervical area to better address upper extremity spasticity and dystonia.

O   **What criteria are utilized to help establish appropriateness for ITB therapy?**

Appropriate candidates for intrathecal infusion should have an Ashworth score of 3 or higher in the lower extremity and must have enough body mass at a minimum age to support the pump. Before placement, the patient should have a positive response to a trial bolus dose of ITB. An adequate response is a 1-point decline in the Ashworth scale for cerebral origin and a 2-point drop in patients who have spinal cord origin.

O   **Which patients benefit from ITB therapy?**

Patients who benefit from ITB include those who have poor underlying strength whose extremity movements are impeded by spasticity, nonambulatory spastic quadriparetics whose spasticity interferes with daily living skills, nonfunctional patients for whom the goal is to enhance quality of caregiving, and patients who have dystonia or other movement disorders.

O   **What is the efficacy of ITB therapy for spasticity?**

Studies have demonstrated improvement in tone, spasm, pain and quality of life. Compared with oral therapies, ITB reduces intolerable side effects. ITB can be used in conjunction with other therapies.

O   **What are the drawbacks to ITB therapy?**

There is potential for side effects from **baclofen** and the indwelling technology, including hypotonia, weakness, nausea and vomiting, and changes in urinary or bowel function. The frequency of seizures in patients previously diagnosed with epilepsy does not seem to be influenced by the ITB. Device related and surgery-related events include seroma, infection, and catheter related problems, including kinking, breakage, and dislodging. Serious medical issues are related to overdose and acute withdrawal of the medication:

O   **What are the physiological effects of ITB therapy?**

Long-term ITB infusion causes down-regulation of $GABA_B$ receptors in the CNS and spinal cord. Down regulation of $GABA_B$ receptors accounts for the decreased sensitivity to the baclofen over time. Although $GABA_B$ receptors are down-regulated, it is the baclofen itself that causes increased inhibitory tone in the CNS and spinal cord.

O   **What is the effect of abrupt discontinuation of ITB therapy?**

Abrupt ITB withdrawal results in a predominance of excitatory effects and simulates other conditions that are associated with CNS hyperexcitability and severe spasticity. Sudden cessation of ITB administration can cause mild symptoms like reappearance of baseline level of spasticity associated with pruritus, anxiety and disorientation. These mild symptoms represent "loss of drug effect". All patients experience "loss of drug effect" when ITB is discontinued.

O   **What is the most dangerous effect of abrupt ITB therapy withdrawal?**

Severe symptoms like hyperthermia (109.4°F), myoclonus, seizures, rhabdomyolysis, disseminated intravascular coagulation, multisystem organ failure, cardiac arrest, coma and death have been well reported, and represents a full-blown life-threatening ITB withdrawal syndrome. Food and drug administration (FDA) of USA has included a drug label warning for baclofen withdrawal syndrome in April 2002. Most reported episodes of ITB withdrawal were caused by preventable human errors or oversights. However, catheter dislodgement, catheter migration and kinks, and other catheter related issues might be more common than pump-related malfunctions. Close attention to pump refilling and programming procedures may reduce the incidence of ITB withdrawal syndrome.

O   **What therapeutic options are available to attenuate the ITB withdrawal syndrome?**

Benzodiazepines are helpful in controlling spasticity and seizures during ITB withdrawal syndrome. Benzodiazepines activate central receptors and $GABA_A$ receptors of spinal cord by different mechanisms. Therefore, ITB induced down-regulation of $GABA_B$ receptors do not interfere with benzodiazepine's mechanism of action. Benzodiazepines could be an initial life saving strategy even before analysis and restoration of ITB pump is achieved, or in cases, where resumption of ITB administration is not as simple as correcting a programming error.

O   **How is the implant baclofen dose adjusted and monitored?**

After the implant, the dosage of baclofen gradually is titrated until the desired effect is obtained. The pump reservoir is refilled every 1-3 months via injection into a refill port. Potential problems include catheter kinks or disconnection, which are diagnosed by clinical symptoms and injection of dye into an access port. Batteries within the pump need replacement every 5-7 years. Patients as small as 18 lb (8.2 kg) have undergone this implant procedure successfully. The procedure is reversible.

O   **What considerations are there for the continuum of care of the patient with spasticity undergoing treatment?**

Because tolerance can occur with medications, drug dosages should be regularly reviewed and implantable devices (pumps, stimulators) should be checked. Ongoing documentation of compliance with therapeutic interventions and evaluation of orthotic or positioning devices is important.

O   **What is the role of dantrolene in the management of spasticity?**

Unlike all other oral agents for spasticity, dantrolene sodium acts peripherally at the level of the muscle fiber. It affects the release of calcium from the sarcoplasmic reticulum of skeletal muscle and thus reduces muscle contraction. Dantrolene sodium is generally indicated for spasticity of supraspinal origin. The medication has peak effect at 4-6 hours with a half-life of 6-9 hours. There is a linear correlation between blood levels and spasmolytic effect. The dose range is between 25-400 mg/day in divided doses (children, dose range between 0.5 mg/kg/day - 3.0 mg/kg/day). It is less likely than the other agents to cause drowsiness, confusion and other central effects because of its mechanism of action. Dantrolene sodium has been shown to decrease muscle tone, clonus and muscle spasm.

O   **What are the drawbacks to dantrolene in the management of spasticity?**

The action of dantrolene sodium is not selective for spastic muscles and it may cause generalized weakness, including weakness of the respiratory muscles. The side effects include drowsiness, dizziness, weakness, fatigue and diarrhea. In addition, there is potential hepatotoxicity that occurs in < 1% of patients who take dantrolene sodium. This increase in liver function tests is seen particularly in adolescents and women who have duration of treatment for greater than sixty days and dosages greater than 300 mg/day. This agent should not be used in combination with other agents known to cause hepatotoxicity, including tizanidine. If no benefit is seen after forty five days of treatment with dantrolene sodium at maximal therapeutic doses, then it should be discontinued.

O   **What is tizanidine?**

Approved in the United States in 1996, tizanidine has been available in other countries since 1977 for the treatment of spasticity caused by multiple sclerosis and spinal cord injury. As a central alpha 2 noradrenergic agonist, tizanidine facilitates short-term vibratory inhibition of the H-reflex, associated with anti spasticity effects without muscle weakness. Although the exact mechanism of action is not yet known, it does differ from other anti spasticity agents, enabling the avoidance of certain drug dependence, intolerance and interactions. Objective measures of muscle strength demonstrate no adverse effects from tizanidine. Patients report less muscle weakness from tizanidine than baclofen or diazepam.

O   **What is the proposed mechanism of action of tizanidine?**

Tizanidine is an alpha-adrenergic agonist. It acts by increasing presynaptic inhibition of motor neurons at the alpha $_2$-adrenergic receptor sites, possibly by reducing the release of excitatory amino acids and inhibiting facilitory coerulospinal pathways, resulting in a reduction in spasticity. Some studies suggest a possible postsynaptic action at the excitatory amino acid receptors. In addition, tizanidine may have some activity at the imidazoline receptors. A study in animals found that tizanidine acts mainly on the polysynaptic pathways, thereby reducing facilitation of spinal motor neurons. Tizanidine may also have minor effects on monosynaptic reflexes, which are associated with the facilitory effect of the coerulospinal pathways. The exact mechanism of action of tizanidine is unknown.

O   **What is the efficacy of tizanidine in the management of spasticity?**

The efficacy of tizanidine in reducing muscle tone based on various placebo controlled studies is comparable to baclofen and better than diazepam. While spasms and clonus are reduced in patients using tizanidine, the Ashworth Scale does not reveal significant differences from placebo groups. However, the long term impact of tizanidine on spasms and clonus does show anti spasticity value.

○ **What are the administration and dosing concerns associated with tizanidine?**

The anti spasticity effects of tizanidine, using traditional tests, demonstrate a striking relationship to the plasma concentration, which peaks at 1-2 hours and dissipates between 3 to 6 hours after oral use. Since there is broad patient variability in titrating the optimal therapeutic dosage of tizanidine, an initial treatment dosage regimen of 2 to 4 weeks is required. Global tolerability scores were significantly higher among patients taking tizanidine than patients using baclofen, dantrolene or diazepam—the most commonly used anti spasticity agents. The usual starting dose 2 mg by mouth once daily, titrated over 2 to 4 weeks to the maximum tolerated dose, usually 8 mg three times daily. The maximum dose is 36 mg daily in three or four divided doses.

○ **What adverse effects are encountered with tizanidine?**

Dry mouth, somnolence, asthenia and dizziness are the most common adverse events associated with tizanidine. Liver function problems and hallucinations are rare tizanidine-related serious adverse events. From a review of 50 clinical trials, tizanidine appears to be an effective therapeutic option in the limited number of approaches to managing spasticity due to cerebral or spinal damage.

CONTRACTURES

○ **What are the clinical ramifications of joint contracture?**

Clinically, depending on location, the limb or body part with a joint contracture is less likely to participate in or perform functional tasks. Ankle, knee, or hip contractures commonly interfere with normal ambulation and mobility patterns and result in high energy costs when the patient adapts by using postural substitutions to compensate.

○ **What are the clinical consequences of ankle plantarflexion contracture?**

An ankle plantarflexion contracture of at least 15 degrees, for example, prevents normal progression of loading over the supporting foot during the stance phase. This results in premature heel off during the mid-stance phase and excessive weight bearing by the metatarsal heads. To compensate, the patient will often attempt to lean the trunk forward during the stance phase or hyperextend the knee, which can result in genu recurvatum. This compensatory motion results in increased energy expenditure by the trunk muscles to maintain trunk control.

○ **What are the clinical consequences of a knee flexion contracture?**

Knee flexion contractures between 15 and 30 degrees will increase demand on the quadriceps to support the body weight during the stance phase by increasing tension from 20% to 50% of normal strength. It has been demonstrated that a linear increase in electromyographic activity of the vastus lateralis during standing with simulated knee flexion contractures of increasing magnitude (0–40 degrees). This increased muscle activity greatly increases energy cost and reduces endurance during standing and walking. Knee flexion contractures also impair standing balance by altering the center of pressure.

○ **What are the clinical consequences of a hip flexion contracture?**

A hip flexion contracture of 30 degrees reduces hip extension and is accommodated by increasing the lumbar lordosis, by walking in increased plantarflexion with excessive weight bearing on the metatarsal heads, and by standing with the unaffected knee in flexion to equalize limb height. These substitutions also increase energy cost during standing and walking. Because the hamstring muscles cross both the hip and the knee joints, patients with a hip flexion contracture shorten their hamstring muscles and may also develop a secondary knee flexion contracture.

○ **What are the clinical consequences of a hip adduction contracture?**

A hip adduction contracture may occur in isolation or in association with a hip flexion contracture. If the abnormal adduction is unilateral, scissoring during the swing phase of gait may impair ambulation. Bilateral hip adduction contractures will have a more pronounced effect on ambulation and may compromise perineal hygiene in the non-ambulating patient.

○ **How are stretching techniques used in the management of spasticity?**

For contractures that are relatively mild (limited to approximately 80%–95% of functional ROM), sustained stretching for 20 to 30 minutes twice a day has been suggested. For more severe contractures (<80% of the functional ROM), stretching for a duration of 30 to 45 minutes or longer may be necessary. Several methods for applying prolonged stretch, using a variety of limb weighting and mechanical pulley systems, have been described. These techniques are used most often on large joints, such as the hip, knee, and shoulder. Although literature support for these techniques is scant and has methodologic limitations, low-load, prolonged stretching can reduce contractures and may be superior to manual stretching techniques.

○ **How does the application of heat facilitate contracture management?**

For severe contractures, application of therapeutic heat to the affected joint capsule or musculotendinous junction can enhance the effectiveness of stretching the elasticity of connective tissue increases when heated in the therapeutic range (40°–43°C). Ultrasound is established as a popular method of heating contractures of large joints or joints covered by abundant layers of tissue. However, depending on the size and location of the involved joint, other heating modalities may accomplish similar objectives. For example, contractures of small, relatively superficial joints, such as metacarpophalangeal or interphalangeal joints may be more easily heated with a paraffin bath immersion.

○ **What are dynamic splints?**

Dynamic splints, also called low-load prolonged stretch (LLPS) orthoses, are used to reduce contractures by applying prolonged, low-intensity stretching across the joint. Dynamic splints employ a static-base orthosis, usually on the dorsal or ventral aspect of a limb. The static supporting part of the orthosis extends just proximal to the joint with the contracture. The joint itself is usually left unencumbered to allow movement in the direction of contracture reduction. A separate part of the dynamic splint supports part of the limb or digit immediately distal to the involved joint.

○ **How is tension applied in a dynamic splint?**

Tension is applied to this distal part of the limb or digit and across the involved joint, through the use of an elastic band, wire, or spring device, opposing the direction of the contracture shortening. For example, extension is applied for a flexion contracture. This allows persistent tension that is adjustable during the course of treatment. Some dynamic splints are "homemade" out of thermoplastic materials. Commercial prefabricated dynamic splints are available and have been used for reduction of contractures at hand, wrist, knee, and ankle joints.

○ **How is a patient positioned for pulley in order to manage contractures?**

The patient is positioned on a table or bed for stabilization. A stretch force (against the direction of the contracture shortening) is applied across the joint by pulling the free part of the limb (leg or thigh) into extension with a weighted traction apparatus. Similar forces can be generated either by having the patient lie supine with the hip joint supported (and padded) but most of the thigh and leg extending off the table unsupported, or by lying prone with the knee joint supported but the leg partially extending past the table. The weight of the unsupported limb and added weight to the distal limb (thigh or ankle) from a weighted traction and pulley apparatus produce extension force to help reduce the contracture.

○ **What are the parameters for this method of treatment?**

Weights of 2 to 5 kg or 5% to 10% of body weight have been used. Clinicians have suggested a treatment time of 20 to 30 minutes or more for 3 to 5 days, depending on patient tolerance. This method of contracture reduction reportedly is better tolerated than high-intensity, brief duration, manually applied stretching. Contracture reductions in the 20- to 70-degree range and greater have been reported.

○ **What is serial casting?**

In serial casting, the joint contracture is measured and cast padding is applied to protect nerves and bony prominences on the part of the limb to be enclosed in the cast. The affected joint is then manually stretched to reduce the contracture, and held in a position of maximally tolerated stretch while a plaster or fiberglass cast is applied. Serial casting has been used to reduce adult and pediatric contractures in a variety of upper- and lower limb joints, including elbow flexion, wrist extension, knee flexion, and ankle plantarflexion contractures.

○ **How is serial casting used in the management of contractures?**

After the initial cast is worn for several days, the process is repeated as a series of casts are applied at weekly intervals. Between cast changes, the limb is inspected for pressure areas (subsequent cast modifications or padding adjustments are made as necessary). The joint ROM is remeasured, and the limb is taken through its maximum possible range prior to reapplication of the cast.

○ **What is a drop out cast?**

 Some protocols call for cutting and removing half of the cast (bivalving). This leaves half of the cast to maintain the joint in stretch and converts the cast into a splint, which can be removed to facilitate better hygiene and allow the skin to be checked for pressure areas. This type of cast is called a drop-out cast.

PRESSURE ULCERS

○ **What is the epidemiology of pressure ulcers?**

The estimated prevalence among patients in acute care hospitals ranges from 3.5 to 29.5% but is higher in quadriplegic (60%); elderly post-hip fracture (66%), and critical care (41%) patients. The estimated prevalence among nursing home residents is as high as 23%; among home care patients, as high as 12.9%. The prevalence of pressure ulcers in the United States has been estimated to be between 1.5 million and 3 million.

○ **How are pressure ulcers defined?**

Pressure ulcers are localized areas of tissue necrosis that tend to occur when soft tissue is compressed between a bony prominence and an external surface for a prolonged period of time. Pressure ulcers commonly occur over the sacrum, greater trochanter, ischial tuberosity, malleolus, heel, fibular head, and scapula.

○ **What are the intrinsic risk factors associated with pressure sore formation?**

Immobility
Limited functional ability
Fecal incontinence
Impaired sensation
Diminished level of consciousness
Poor nutritional status
Age, especially >75 yr.
Comorbid conditions, including stroke, Parkinson's disease, fracture, sepsis, prior ulcers

○ **What are the extrinsic risk factors associated with pressure sore formation?**

Pressure
Friction
Shearing
Moisture

○ **What are the stages of pressure sores according to the National Pressure Ulcer Advisory Panel?**

Stage I   Non-blanchable erythema of intact skin, considered to be the heralding lesion of skin ulceration.

Stage II   Partial thickness skin loss involving the epidermis and/or dermis. The ulcer is superficial and presents clinically as an abrasion, blister, or shallow crater.

Stage III   Full thickness skin loss involving damage or necrosis of subcutaneous tissue, which may extend down to, but not through, underlying fascia. The ulcer presents clinically as a deep crater with or without undermining of adjacent tissue.

Stage IV   Full thickness skin loss with extensive destruction, tissue necrosis, or damage to muscle, bone, or supporting structures, such as tendons or joint capsules.

O   **Compare the different classification schemes for pressure ulcers**

Stage or grade	Shea	Yarkony-Kirk	NPUAP
		A comparison of different classification systems of pressure ulcers	
1	Erythema +/- epidermis	Erythema:	Nonblanchable erythema of intact skin
		A. 30 min-24 hr	
		B. >24 hr	
2	Epidermis +/- dermis	Epidermis +/- dermis	Epidermis +/- dermis
3	Subcutis	Subcutis	Subcutis
4	Muscle, bone, joints	Muscle/Fascia	Muscle, bone, joints
5	Closed; large cavity draining through sinus; +/- muscle and bone involvement	Bone	--
6		Joint	

O   **What is the pathogenesis of pressure sores?**

Four key factors are thought to be involved in causing skin breakdown: pressure, shearing forces, friction, and moisture.

O   **How does pressure contribute to ulcer formation?**

Pressure beneath bony prominences can impede blood flow to the skin and underlying tissues, resulting in ischemic injury. Since muscle and subcutaneous tissues are more susceptible to pressure-induced injury than the epidermis, pressure ulcers are frequently worse than they initially appear. The visibly damaged tissue that one sees on the surface of a pressure ulcer may merely represent the "tip of the iceberg".

O   **How does shearing contribute to ulcer formation?**

Shearing forces result from the sliding of adjacent structures, causing a relative displacement. This commonly occurs when patients are propped up in bed more than 30 degrees, or are seated, and then slide down. Under these circumstances, subcutaneous tissues are stretched and angulated, while the sacral skin remains stationary. This causes angulation and occlusion of subcutaneous blood vessels, resulting in tissue ischemia.

O   **How do friction and moisture contribute to ulcer formation?**

Friction and shearing forces can occur when skin is moved across bed sheets, during transfers in and out of bed, or with frequent limb movements in patients with restlessness, agitation, or spasticity. Moisture, often resulting from incontinence or perspiration, can lead to tissue maceration and facilitate skin breakdown when any of the other factors listed are present.

O   **Why is aged skin more vulnerable to pressure sore formation?**

A number of changes occur in normal skin with aging which may predispose older individuals to the development of pressure sores: Epidermal turnover decreases, the dermal epidermal junction flattens, and there are fewer dermal blood vessels. In addition, there is an increase in dermal collagen, a decrease in elastic fibers, a loss of cells that synthesize vessel basement membrane, and an increase in skin permeability. Older individuals may also experience a decrease in the perception of pain.

O **Diagram the pathophysiology of the fundamental factors role in pressure sore formation**

☐ Pressure
  - Exceed normal capillary filling pressure of 32 mmHg
  - Hypoxia → acidosis → hemorrhage into interstitium → accumulation of toxic cellular wastes → cell death → tissue necrosis
  - Pressure highest in tissue nearest to the bone
  - 100-150 mmHg: sacral pressure in patient lying in standard hospital bed
  - 300 mmHg: sacral pressure in seated patient
  - Pressure greater than 70 mmHg for 2 hours = irreversible damages

☐ Shearing Forces
  - Occur in patient placed on incline
  - Deeper tissue (muscle and fat) pulled down by gravity while epidermis and dermis remain fixed
  - Alone, do not cause ulceration, rather have an additive effect

☐ Friction
  - Occur in patient dragged across an external surface
  - Result in abrasion leading to Stage 2 lesions

☐ Moisture
  - i.e., perspiration, feces, urine
  - Lead to skin maceration and predispose to superficial ulceration

---

O **What is the Norton scale?**

In the Norton scale, general physical condition as well as mental state, activity, mobility, and incontinence are assessed with a 4 grade scale. A total score of 14 or below indicates risk. Several modifications to the Norton scale have been suggested, including a category for nutrition and clarification of the terms good, fair, poor, and very bad in describing physical condition. This scale has been used in numerous studies; however, it is reported to have limited predictive accuracy.

O **What is the Braden scale?**

The Braden scale consists of six items including sensory perception, moisture, activity, mobility, nutrition, friction and shear. Each is graded with a score of 1, 2, 3, or 4. A total score of 16 or less indicates a risk for the development of pressure ulcers. The Braden scale is reported to have good interrater reliability.

O **Compare the two scales**

- Norton Scale
  - Uses 1-4 scoring system in 5 subscales
    - Physical condition
    - Mental condition
    - Activity
    - Motility
    - Incontinence
  - Score < 14 = high risk
- Braden Scale
  - Scores range from 1 to 3 or 4 in 6 subscales
    - Sensory perception
    - Moisture
    - Activity
    - Motility
    - Nutrition
    - Friction/Shear
  - Score less than or equal to 16 = high risk

O   How is cellulitis diagnosed?

Cellulitis can be difficult to diagnose because its appearance may be similar to the reactive hyperemia and erythema associated with normal healing. All pressure ulcers are colonized with bacteria, whether infection is present or not. Swab culturettes of the wound surface are virtually always positive; however they only identify surface organisms, and do not accurately identify causative organisms even when infection is present. When an ulcer does not heal, the possibility of infection should always be considered. Infection is typically caused by a mixture of organisms, which may include gram positive cocci (Staphylococcus and Streptococcus), gram negative bacilli, and anaerobes. Clinically infected ulcers and non healing wounds require further evaluation to rule out osteomyelitis.

O   Is osteomyelitis difficult to diagnose?

Osteomyelitis has been found to occur in the bone underlying 26% of non-healing ulcers. If an ulcer fails to show evidence of healing after pressure has been removed, or if purulent drainage visibly extends into bone, then osteomyelitis should be ruled out The diagnosis of osteomyelitis can be difficult. Even when infection is not present, soft tissue cultures, radiographs and nuclear imaging studies are often abnormal in areas surrounding a pressure ulcer. These tests have poor positive predictive value, but their negative predictive value is quite good.

O   What is the gold standard for diagnosing osteomyelitis?

The gold standard for diagnosing osteomyelitis still remains bone biopsy, with microscopic examination and quantitative culture for organisms. .Magnetic Resonance Imaging has become the test of choice among radiologic methods of evaluating suspected osteomyelitis. Alternatively, a bone scan, or a bone scan in conjunction with an indium leucocyte scan may be used. A negative bone scan rules out osteomyelitis. If the bone scan is positive, bone biopsies should then be considered.

O   What are the general principles of pressure ulcer treatment?

Relief of pressure
Removal of devitalized tissue
Optimization of the wound environment to promote granulation and reepithelialization
Avoidance of maceration, trauma, friction or shearing force
A search for reversible underlying conditions, which may predispose to ulcer development or impede wound healing.

O **What are air-fluidized beds?**

An air fluidized bed (e.g. Clinitron® bed) is an oval space in which up to 2000 pounds of glass beads are contained and covered with a polyester sheet. The beads are fluidized by a flow of warm, pressurized air, which floats the polyester cover upon which the patient is placed. These beds have been available since 1969. The patient's feces and body fluids are able to flow through the polyester sheet, keeping the skin dry. Bowel and bladder management is still necessary to minimize incontinence. In addition to being quite heavy, these beds are expensive. The circulating warm air tends to make the bed hot and may not be tolerated by patients with heat intolerance, as seen with multiple sclerosis.

O **How effective are air-fluidized beds?**

Most studies of air fluidized bed therapy have shown faster rates of wound healing compared to conventional treatment. Regardless of the method of treatment, however, severe pressure ulcers take a long time to heal. In one nursing home study, the median length of treatment was 119 days. In a study of patients with pressure ulcers who were being treated in their own homes, patients using air fluidized beds spent fewer days in the hospital, but there was no difference in clinical outcome or cost.

O **What are the indications for air fluidized bed use?**

Because of the need for prolonged treatment, and the high cost of air-fluidized beds, it has been recommended that air fluidized beds should be used primarily for medically stable patients whose prognosis is otherwise good. Air-fluidized beds should be used for at least sixty days before discontinuation for lack of therapeutic response. They can also be used to treat pressure sores successfully in debilitated patients who are not candidates for surgery.

O **What are low air loss beds?**

Low Air Loss Beds, such as the Kinair® bed, are made up of multiple inflatable fabric pillows, which are attached to a modified hospital bed frame. An electric fan maintains buoyancy of the pillows. The head and foot of the bed can be elevated, much like regular hospital beds. The low air loss bed is cooler, considerably lighter, and more portable than air-fluidized beds. Unlike air fluidized beds, Urine and feces do not pass through the fabric of low air loss beds.

O **How effective are low air loss beds?**

The use of low air loss beds in nursing home patients with pressure ulcers was associated with a threefold increase in the rate of wound healing, compared with patients in the same facility treated with foam mattresses... Similar beds were found to be useful for the prevention of pressure sores in critically ill intensive care unit (ICU) patients. Once ulcers appeared, however, there was no difference in ulcer resolution compared to ICU patients treated with conventional therapy.

O **Compare the different effects of pressure reducing surface beds**

Performance Characteristics	Selected characteristics for classes of support surfaces					
	Air-fluidized	Low-air-loss	Alternating-air	Static flotation	Foam	Standard
Increased support area	Yes	Yes	Yes	Yes	Yes	No
Low moisture retention	Yes	Yes	No	No	No	No
Reduced heat accumulation	Yes	Yes	No	No	No	No
Shear reduction	Yes	?	Yes	Yes	No	No
Pressure reduction	Yes	Yes	Yes	Yes	Yes	No
Dynamic	Yes	Yes	Yes	No	No	No
Cost per day	High	High	Moderate	Low	Low	Low

O **What role does debridement play in pressure sore management?**

Debridement of stage II ulcers with a small amount of superficial necrotic tissue can be accomplished by gentle mechanical debridement with coarse mesh gauze moistened with saline (removing and reapplying moist dressings every six-to-eight hours), hydrocolloid dressings, or enzymatic debriding agents.

○   **What are limitations of gauze and enzymatic dressings?**

If allowed to dry, gauze dressings can be painful to remove. The use of enzymatic agents can also be painful. They require a skin protectant such as petroleum jelly, zinc oxide, "Skin Prep" ® or "No Sting"® to prevent damage to adjacent normal tissues. Enzymatic agents cannot remove a hardened, black eschar or a large amount of necrotic tissue; however they can loosen the eschar to facilitate sharp debridement.

○   **What is the role of aquatic therapy?**

Whirlpool, shower cart, or pulsed-water (Waterpik)® debridement may be useful adjuncts for continued debridement of large ulcers.

○   **What treatment is considered for large stage III or stage IV ulcers?**

Stage IV ulcers and large stage III lesions are usually débrided surgically. Along with surgical debridement, a soft tissue flap may be needed in order to ensure adequate blood flow to large deep wounds and provide cushioning over bony prominences. Surgical consultation should also be considered for any wound greater than 10 centimeters in diameter.

○   **What is the role of film products in pressure sore management?**

Semipermeable polyurethane films allow gasses to pass through but are impermeable to water. They may enhance healing by sequestering wound fluids. Because they are transparent, the wound can be directly visualized with the dressing in place. They mimic the function of the skin. Such films are commonly used in the treatment of stage I or select stage II lesions. A skin sealant should be used to prevent maceration around the wound. A single dressing may remain in place up to 7 days.

○   **What is the role of foam products in pressure sore management?**

Semipermeable polyurethane foams are, like films, transparent and waterproof. Additionally, they provide cushioning to the wound, and absorb excess wound exudate. At the same time, a moist environment is maintained, and excessive autolysis or maceration avoided. Because they do not adhere to the wound, they must be secured with a cover dressing or tape, obscuring direct visualization of the ulcer. Foams should not be used for ulcers, which extend into underlying muscle, ulcers completely covered by eschar, clinically infected ulcers, or heavily exuding ulcers.

○   **What is the role for moist gauze dressings in pressure ulcer management?**

Moist gauze dressings are inexpensive. They must be changed at least two to three times a day, however, which requires additional nursing time and adds to overall costs. It may be difficult to maintain moisture, and when they dry out, they can adhere to the wound. Removing an adherent, dry dressing can cause pain and may remove healthy granulation tissue. Like foams, they must be secured with a cover dressing or wrap.

○   **What is the role of hydrocolloid dressings in pressure ulcer management?**

Hydrocolloid dressings (HCDs) contain an adhesive material that physically interacts with wound fluid. These occlusive or semi-occlusive dressings encourage wound cleansing and debridement through the process of autolysis, and promote the development of granulation tissue by stimulating angiogenesis.

○   **How effective are hydrocolloid dressings in pressure ulcer management?**

Several studies have found HCDs to be at least as efficacious as gauze dressings, and may require only one eighth as much nursing care...The dressing need not be changed for up to seven days, although one study found that the average lifespan of an HCD was only 3 and one-half days.

○   **What stage pressure ulcers are HCDs suitable for?**

HCDs are best for smaller, solitary stage II to III ulcers. The dressing should be checked 3 times a day and changed whenever there is any evidence of drainage or fluctuance.. The dressing itself must be removed carefully, to avoid desquamation of surrounding tissue. An adhesive remover such as acetone can facilitate removal.

O **What are the limitations of HCDs in pressure sore management?**

HCDs may not adhere well to highly exudative wounds, and should not be applied to clinically infected ulcers. Large or multiple lesions may not be covered by a single HCD, whereas a single moist gauze dressing may suffice. HCDs may macerate surrounding fragile skin. Skin Prep can be used before applying the HCD to protect the surrounding skin.

O **What are hydrogels?**

Hydrogels are three dimensional hydrophilic polymers that interact with aqueous solutions. They swell and maintain water in their structure. They are non-adhesive, many are transparent, and conform to the wound surface. Hydrogels are very absorbent, and dehydrate easily, especially when not covered properly with a dressing or wrap. Although they may be difficult to confine in large wounds, they can be used with stage IV ulcers.

O **What are alginate dressings?**

Alginate dressings, derived from seaweed, are highly absorbent. They have been used for ulcers with copious drainage. In one study supported by the manufacturer, alginates dried out and adhered to the wound in one fourth of the patients, and dissolved in another fourth. These nonadherent dressings must be secured with a cover dressing or wrap. They should not be used for dry wounds.

O **What is the role of topical disinfecting agents in pressure sore management?**

Irrigation with saline can retard bacterial growth in open pressure ulcers. Topical agents such as antibiotics or antiseptic solutions are not routinely recommended. The use of topical disinfecting agents may actually be counterproductive. Povidone® iodine, acetic acid, hydrogen peroxide, and sodium hypochlorite are all cytotoxic to fibroblasts, and may impair wound healing.

O **What are limitations of topical antimicrobials in pressure sore management?**

Topical antimicrobials such as mupirocin ointment and silver sulfadiazine can decrease bacterial counts; however use of such agents may result in selection of resistant organisms. Topical antibiotics generally do not penetrate deeply into the ulcer. Hypersensitivity, contact dermatitis, and systemic toxicity from drug absorption can all occur with topical antibiotic use. If topical antibiotics are used, the duration of therapy should be limited to seven to ten days, to prevent the selection of resistant organisms. With the exception of mupirocin, topical antibiotics do not seem to be superior to saline soaks with regard to prevention of bacterial growth.

O **Tabulate a comparison of dressing formulation to ulcer characteristics**

Dressing	Indication	Contraindication	Example
Transparent film	Stage I ulcer Protection from friction Autolytic debridement	Skin tears Draining ulcers Suspected skin infections	Tegaderm® Bioclusive Opsite®
Foam Island	Stage II and III Low to mod. Exudate	Excessive exudate Dry crusted wound	Alleyn® Lyofoam®
Hydrocolloids	Stage II, III Low to mod. Drainage Autolytic debridement Leave in place 3-5 days Can apply over alginate	Poor skin integrity Infected ulcers Wound needs packing	Restore® Duoderm® Tegasorb® Replicare®

Petroleum-based non-adherent	Stage II, III Graft sites		Vaseline gauze Xeroform®
Dressing	**Indication**	**Contraindication**	**Example**
Alginate	Stage II, III, IV Excessive drainage Requires secondary dressing	Dry or minimally draining wound Superficial wound	Sorbsan® Kaltostar® Algiderm®
Hydrogel (amorphous gel)	Stage II, III, IV Combine w/ gauze dressing Stays moist longer than saline gauze	Macerated areas Wounds w/ excess exudates	Curasol gel Solosite gel Intrasite gel
Hydrogel (gel sheet)	Stage II Skin tears Need topper dressing	Macerated areas Wounds w/ moderate to heavy exudate	Vigilon®
Gauze packing (moistened w/ saline)	Needs remoistening frequently		Iodophor gauze

O   **What are some of the conservative surgical options for pressure sore healing?**

The method of reconstruction depends mainly on the size of the tissue defect and its location. For clean wounds in patients for whom good nursing care is available, healing by second intention is an option. Primary closure with sutures is seldom used because it stretches the skin, creating tension that frequently leads to dehiscence. Because of the lack of padding and their inability to grow on exposed bone, skin grafts seem to have limited use in the treatment of pressure ulcers.

O   **What are the different types of flaps utilized in pressure sore management?**

In general, flaps with predictable blood supply are preferred to random flaps. These include axial flaps (a long, thin, vascularized segment of skin and subcutaneous tissue is developed and rotated into a defect), fasciocutaneous or musculocutaneous flaps (a fascial/muscle unit with its overlying skin receiving blood supply from a recognized pedicle is utilized), and microvascular flaps (a vascularized tissue unit on a single arteriovenous pedicle is dissected, the vessels are transected and anastomosed to recipient vessels adjacent to the defect).

O   **What is the most common type of flap utilized in pressure sore management?**

Muscle flaps are the most commonly used method of reconstruction for pressure ulcers, providing bulk, padding, hardiness, and durability. By providing a physiologic barrier to infection, eliminating dead space, and improving vascularity, they also provide an effective therapeutic modality for osteomyelitis.

O   **What are the healing rates for most ulcers?**

Stage 1→ one day to 1 week	
Stage 2→ 5 days to 3 months	
Stage 3→ 1 month to 6 months	
Stage 4→ 6 months to 1 year	

DECONDITIONING

O   **Summarize the adverse effects of immobilization on different organ systems**

Adverse effects of immobilization on different organ systems

Organ systems	Conditions
Muscles	Reduced strength, endurance, flexibility and bulk

Adverse effects of immobilization on different organ systems

Joints	Reduced flexibility; joint contractures
Bones	Osteopenia and osteoporosis
Heart	Reduced stroke volume, cardiac output, and exercise capacity tachycardia
Peripheral circulation	Reduced orthostatic tolerance and venous return; deep vein thrombosis
Lungs	Atelectasis and pneumonia; pulmonary embolism
Gastrointestinal tract	Reduced appetite and bowel motility; constipation
Urinary tract	Urolithiasis, infection
Skin	Pressure ulcers
Endocrine	Reduced endorphin production and insulin sensitivity; reduced lean body mass; obesity
Psychologic	Reduced self image and stress tolerance; anxiety and depression

O **What are the behavioral, affective and cognitive consequences of immobility?**

In studies with imposed sensory deprivation and bed rest, subjects experienced alterations in affect, perception, and cognition. Changes in affect included anxiety, fear, depression, and rapid mood changes. Changes in perception included disorientation to time and the perception that time was passing slowly, the appearance of hallucinations, a lowered pain threshold, and an increased auditory threshold. Changes in cognition that have been found include decreased concentration and impairments in judgment and problem solving.

O **What hemodynamic changes occur when moving from the supine to the erect position?**

In a normal healthy individual, moving from the supine to the erect position shifts 500 to 700 mL of fluid from the thorax into the legs, secondary to the force of gravity. The body adapts to this shift of fluid by several compensatory mechanisms, including the carotid and aortic mechanoreceptors (baroreceptors) and the cardiopulmonary mechanoreceptors. In the erect position, with less blood volume in the thorax, there is a decreased "stretch" in the mechanoreceptors, which produces pressor responses such as increased heart rate and contractility, vasoconstriction, venoconstriction, and antidiuresis. These responses combine to maintain adequate systolic blood pressure and cerebral perfusion.

O **What is orthostatic hypotension?**

After prolonged bed rest, a person loses this adaptation and develops an orthostatic intolerance. Blood pools in the legs, venous return decreases, stroke volume is diminished, heart rate rises, and the systolic blood pressure is not maintained in the erect position. This may be due to an altered carotid baroreflex and autonomic balance. Clinically, this is accompanied by the common signs and symptoms of orthostatic hypotension, that is, a feeling of light headedness, nausea, dizziness, sweating, pallor, tachycardia, and hypotension .

O **What is neurovascular deconditioning?**

Neurovascular deconditioning appears to occur mostly during the first 4 to 7 days of bed rest , and even more rapidly in the elderly and the medically frail. With resumption of physical activities, it may take twice as long to reverse these changes as it took for them to develop.

O **What changes fluid volume changes occur with prolonged bed rest?**

With prolonged bed rest, the relatively increased central blood volume is adapted to by depressed levels of aldosterone and antidiuretic hormone, with a resultant diuresis. Thus, the net effect is a decreased blood and plasma volume. From this decrease, it follows that the stroke volume is lower, the resting heart rate is higher (to maintain resting cardiac output), and the maximum oxygen consumption (VO$_2$max), which is a function of maximum cardiac output, is decreased.

O **What are the effects on red blood cell mass with deconditioning?**

Because red blood cell mass remains unchanged, hematocrit initially rises and blood viscosity increases. Over the course of 2 to 4 weeks, red blood cell mass decreases and hematocrit begins to fall. During this time period, the loss of plasma volume is proportionally greater than the loss of red blood cells. Later, red blood cell losses will exceed plasma losses.

O   **What happens to the heart rate with bed rest?**

Historical studies, typically in young healthy men, indicated that the heart rate at rest increases by one beat every 2 days during the first 4 weeks of immobilization. After 6 weeks of bed rest, the increase in heart rate in response to head up tilt from supine position may be as much as 89%, apparently related to imbalance of the autonomic nervous system .

O   **What changes occur with regard to plasma volume during bed rest?**

Plasma volume loss is approximately 10% after 1 week of bed rest and 15% by 4 weeks. The decrease in plasma and blood volume continues and most likely plateaus around 70% of normal plasma volume and 60% of normal blood volume. It is accompanied by a proportionate loss of plasma proteins. There also appears to be a loss of albumin, creatinine, chloride, phosphorus, calcium, potassium, and glucose. Urea nitrogen, globulin, sodium, and osmotic concentration are increased, while uric acid is decreased.

O   **What cardiac changes occur with bed rest?**

Stroke volume is decreased, left ventricular end-diastolic volume is decreased, and cardiac output is relatively unchanged or decreased. A decrease in left ventricular size occurs with bed rest or as a result of decreased activity, and atrophy of cardiac muscle develops with chronic disuse.

O   **What are the effects of deconditioning on Maximal oxygen uptake (VO_{2max})?**

Maximal oxygen uptake (VO_{2max}), an indicator of general aerobic fitness, is reduced by bed rest, as is the submaximal VO_2.

O   **What are the effects of deconditioning on the arteriovenous oxygen difference?**

Physical **deconditioning** produces an increase in the arteriovenous oxygen difference with submaximal, but not with maximal, exercise.

O   **What are the effects of deconditioning on the total peripheral resistance and mean arterial pressure?**

There is no significant change in the total peripheral resistance and mean arterial pressure at rest or during exercise after bed rest. In the deconditioned person, it takes longer for the heart rate to return to the resting state after a period of exercise than in an able bodied person

O   **What changes occur in the cardiovascular response to submaximal exercise in the deconditioned patient?**

At any level of submaximal exercise (in either the supine or the erect position) there is an abnormally large increase in heart rate in individuals after a period of bed rest compared with control subjects who have not been placed on bed rest. Stroke volume and cardiac output are reduced by about 25% and 15%, respectively, with submaximal exercise and by about 30% and 26% at maximal exercise. Similarly, VO2max, which is a measure of cardiovascular fitness and reserve, is reduced (by 15%–46%) after exercise in the upright position.

O   **What intrinsic changes occur in the vascular system, which increases the risk of thrombus formation?**

Increased blood viscosity may also occur with immobility, which increases the intrinsic predisposition of the blood to clot. Platelet aggregation may be stimulated and blood fibrinogen may be increased as well. Therefore, bed rest is a well-known and significant risk factor for developing venous thrombotic disease.

O   **What ventilatory changes occur with bed rest?**

Upon assumption of the supine position there are several immediate effects on the respiratory system. The diaphragm moves to a more cephalad position, with a resultant decrease in thoracic size. In addition, the central fluid shift results in increased blood in the thorax further reduce the available space for lung expansion and aeration. There is an increase in forced vital capacity and total lung capacity, whereas residual volume, functional residual capacity, maximal ventilatory volume, and maximal minute volume are relatively unchanged.

○   **What changes in ventilation occur during a change in position from upright to supine?**

A change in position from upright to supine results in a 2% reduction of vital capacity, a 7% reduction of total lung capacity, a 19% reduction in residual volume, and 30% reduction in functional residual capacity.

○   **Is there a ventilation perfusion dissociation with prolonged bed rest?**

Because of alterations in blood supply and aeration that occur in the supine position, a mismatch in lung ventilation and perfusion occurs and leads to decreased arterial oxygenation.

○   **What changes may impact chest wall and rib cage function during ventilation?**

Prolonged immobility and bed rest may lead to intercostal muscle and joint contractures, more shallow breathing, and an increased respiratory rate. These changes further impair the patient's oxygenation and thereby limit endurance and the ability to make functional gains.

○   **How is pulmonary clearance affected by bed rest?**

The ability to clear secretions is more difficult in a recumbent position. The dependent, usually posterior chest walls, accumulate more secretions, whereas the upper parts usually become dry, rendering the ciliary lining ineffective for clearing secretions and allowing the secretions to pool in the lower bronchial tree. The effectiveness of coughing is impaired both because of ciliary malfunction and respiratory muscle weakness.

○   **What affect does bed rest have on muscle strength?**

At bed rest there is a decrease in muscle strength (or torque around a joint) of approximately 1% per day (depending on the study, 0.7%–1.5% /day). The amount of strength that is lost plateaus at 20% to 50%. Loss of strength is consistently greatest in the postural muscles (such as the low back muscles) and weight-bearing lower extremity muscles (such as the quadriceps and gastrocnemius soleus muscle groups). pattern for loss of muscle strength. Upper extremity muscles are significantly less involved, as the finding of preserved handgrip strength in patients on bed rest illustrates. Paralleling this loss in strength of postural and lower-extremity muscles is loss of muscle mass and increased muscle atrophy.

○   **What muscle fiber changes occur with bed rest?**

On the anatomic and histologic level, many changes occur to the muscles, though many of these findings have been derived from animal studies. Animal studies (particularly rat studies) found that type I slow-twitch fiber muscles were predominantly affected by bed rest, compared with type II fast-twitch fibers. This finding is consistent with the relatively high cross-sectional area of type I fibers in the antigravity muscles most affected with disuse, and in humans it may be anatomic position and function rather than fiber type that is more important. In addition, the postural role of physiologic extensors explains their greater atrophy with immobility compared with flexors.

○   **What other muscle function characteristics change under conditions of immobilization?**

Additional changes with immobilization include a decrease in protein synthesis. The number of sarcomeres in the series decreases with muscles kept in a shortened position. A decrease in the strength of the myotendinous junction and changes in muscle electrical activity have been found. Furthermore, fatigability of the muscles increases, possibly because of decreased levels of adenosine triphosphate and glycogen stores, more rapid accumulation of lactic acid, and a decreased ability of muscles to utilize fatty acids after a period of immobility. The extent of atrophy is significantly increased if the muscle is kept in its contracted position, while stretching the muscle slows or prevents atrophy.

○ **What changes occur in synovial joints as a result of immobilization?**

Immobilization leads to changes in the collagen, ligaments, and muscles surrounding the joint, resulting in reduced range of motion and a decreased ability to withstand stress. There is fibrofatty proliferation of connective tissue within the joint cavity, with the development of atrophic synovium and deterioration of the subchondral bone. The articular cartilage can become necrotic in areas of contact and develop fissures in other areas. Typical contractures that develop with prolonged bed rest include the hips or knees in a flexed position and the ankles plantar flexed. Less common upper body contractures with bed rest include the fingers flexed, the elbows flexed, the shoulders internally rotated, and the thorax flexed.

○ **What is the affect of bed rest on the skeletal system?**

Bed rest and immobilization lead to disuse osteoporosis documented by both increased calcium excretion and decreased bone density. Bone loss occurs primarily in weight bearing bones such as the vertebral bodies, the long bones of the legs, the calcaneus, and the metacarpals. Bone mineral density of the vertebral bones decreases by about 1% per week of bed rest, which is nearly 50 times the predicted involutional bone loss.

○ **What metabolic changes occur with bed rest?**

Studies have demonstrated a decrease or no change in the basal metabolic rate. Total body weight remains unchanged with bed rest; however, lean body mass is decreased while body fat is increased. Body temperature remains normal during bed rest, but is minimally higher than expected during submaximal exercise after bed rest. Energy absorption from food is unchanged, but appetite and water intake is decreased.

○ **What additional effects on the endocrine system during bed rest?**

Additional effects on the endocrine system during bed rest are seen in the adrenocortical steroid pathways, with changes in circulating glucocorticoids. Examples of these changes include an increase in urinary hydrocortisone excretion, increased plasma renin activity, altered growth hormone production, and an alteration in the circadian rhythm

○ **What changes occur with regard to carbohydrate metabolism?**

Serum glucose levels usually remain normal; However, hyperglycemia may occur as a result of 50% decrease in peripheral muscle sensitivity to circulating insulin, occurring within 2 weeks of bed rest . Consequently, there is a rise in serum insulin levels, but it is not adequate to reduce the hyperglycemia. There is a progressive delay in the peak insulin concentration and an increase in the total insulin response after a glucose tolerance test, depending on the duration of the bed rest. Evidence also suggests increased secretion of insulin in response to glucose by beta cells of the pancreas.

○ **What changes occur with regard to nitrogen balance during bed rest?**

There is a daily net nitrogen loss with bed rest. The loss of nitrogen with bed rest in the young healthy individual is about 2 g/day via urinary excretion, and begins by day 5 or 6 of bed rest and persists throughout the period of inactivity. A reduction in muscle activity, muscle atrophy, and decreased protein synthesis leads to hypoproteinemia.

○ **What electrolyte disturbances occur during bed rest?**

There is increased excretion of electrolytes including potassium, sodium, and chloride during bed rest, although serum levels remain normal. The losses in sodium and potassium occur early during bed rest, paralleling the losses in plasma volume. There are losses in phosphorus that parallel calcium losses and in sulfur that follow nitrogen losses. There is also a loss of zinc during bed rest, likely secondary to bone loss and muscle atrophy.

○ **What happens to calcium metabolism during bed rest?**

Calcium is lost during bed rest via fecal and urinary routes, paralleling losses in bone mass. Within 2 to 3 days of bed rest, there is an increase in urinary calcium excretion, reaching maximum in 3 to 7 weeks. It is estimated that there is a 0.5% loss of total body calcium that occurs per month during immobilization . Absorption of 1, 25-dihydroxyvitamin D is also decreased during bed rest.

○ **What are the effects of immobility on genitourinary function?**

There are several effects of prolonged bed rest on the genitourinary system. These include increased diuresis, hypercalciuria, increased renal stone formation, urinary retention, bladder distention, urinary stasis, and increased urinary tract infections. With prolonged bed rest, hypercalciuria and hyperphosphaturia increase the propensity to form calcium-containing renal stones. Renal stones in turn increase the risk for, and make it more difficult to eradicate, urinary tract infections, by providing a nidus for bacterial growth.

○ **What affects occur in the gastrointestinal system in response to bed rest?**

Bed rest and immobility mechanically affect the gastrointestinal tract as the passage of food is slowed in the supine position. It has been shown that nonviscous, but not viscous materials, pass through the esophagus more rapidly in the upright position than supine , and the transit time through the stomach is 66% slower in the supine position than when standing. Bed rest also results in decrease of appetite, reduced peristalsis, slower rate of absorption, and an increase in symptoms of gastroesophageal reflux. Increased gastric acidity secondary to decreased bicarbonate secretion has been noted during bed rest.

HETEROTOPIC OSSIFICATION

○ **What heritable conditions are associated with heterotopic ossification?**

Fibrodysplasia ossificans progressiva (FOP), or Munchmeyer disease, is an autosomal dominant severely disabling disease resulting in progressive ossification of fascial planes, muscles, tendons, and ligaments. Congenital malformation of the great toes is associated with FOP. HO is a feature of several other diseases, including Albright hereditary osteodystrophy, progressive osseous heteroplasia, and primary osteoma cutis.

○ **What is the pathogenesis of heterotopic ossification (HO)?**

HO originates from osteoprogenitor stem cells lying dormant within the affected soft tissues. With the proper stimulus, the stem cells differentiate into osteoblasts and begin the process of osteoid formation, eventually leading to mature heterotopic bone. A variety of bone morphogenetic proteins (BMPs) can stimulate HO when experimentally deposited into soft tissues, suggesting that BMPs play a role in the initiation of HO. A degree of neurologic control is implied but is not well understood.

○ **Is there a genetic model to elucidate the pathogenesis of HO?**

Potentially causative mutations for FOP have been mapped to 2 sites, adding evidence of the BMP role in HO formation. The first site lies on the long arm of chromosome 17, in the region of the noggin gene (NOG). The noggin protein inhibits BMPs. The second genetic location is on the long arm of chromosome 4, in the region of a known BMP-signaling pathway gene. Bone morphogenetic protein 4 is overproduced in patients with FOP.

○ **What are the histological features of HO development?**

The typical histologic evolution of HO following trauma begins with spindle cell proliferation within the first week of the traumatic event. Primitive osteoid develops at the periphery of the lesion by 7-10 days. Primitive cartilage and woven bone can be seen in the second week, with trabecular bone forming at 2-5 weeks after the inciting trauma. After approximately 6 weeks, a zonal phenomenon can be seen with immature, undifferentiated, central tissues and mature lamellar bone peripherally.

□□ **What are the characteristics of mature HO?**

After approximately 6 months, the appearance of true bone is noted with trabeculae, marrow, and lamellar arrangements around abundant vascular channels. Predominantly adipose tissue is found in the marrow spaces, and hemopoiesis virtually is absent. The HO mass develops with mature bone intermixed with immature bone and eventually results in lamellar corticospongiosal bone with a thin cortex, tightly latticed spongiosa, and occasional Haversian systems.

○   **What is the incidence of HO in musculoskeletal disorders?**

Risk factors for HO include the presence of other bone-forming disorders such as diffuse idiopathic skeletal hyperostosis, ankylosing spondylitis, and Paget disease. A personal history of previous HO also increases the risk of future occurrences. Of total hip arthroplasty procedures, HO complicates 8-71%, with the higher incidence if the patient has had HO in a previous total arthroplasty site.

○   **What is the incidence of HO in SCI?**

The reported incidence of HO following SCI varies greatly from study to study. Incidence varies from a low of 3.4% to a high of 47% reported by Hassard, who found HO around the hips of 62 of 131 patients with SCI who were admitted to the Hot Springs Rehabilitation Center over a 2-year period. Most studies cite a range between these 2 extremes. Peak incidence is noted from 4-12 weeks post injury and can occur up to 5 months following trauma. Later onset has been reported, but it is very rare.

○   **What morbidity is associated with HO?**

Of patients with neurologic deficits, 8-10% has severe functional limitations resulting directly from HO. The extent of involvement is correlated positively with poorer outcome in rehabilitation patients recovering from traumatic brain injury. In patients with spinal cord injuries, large foci of HO can lead to skin breakdown and the inability to sit upright. Malignant degeneration to osteosarcoma has been reported but is extremely rare.

○   **What gender and age factors relate to HO?**

Male patients with spinal cord injury are twice as likely to develop HO as are female patients. No strong sex association exists in FOP. Isolated HO can occur at any age but is rare in very young children. Posttraumatic HO is, not surprisingly, most common in young athletic persons. In some studies, HO has been found to affect young patients with spinal cord injury more frequently (age 20-30 y). Other studies have found no correlation between age and HO formation. In contrast, FOP tends to manifest in patients by age 5 years, causing severe upper extremity restriction of movement in most patients by age 15 years.

○   **What is the clinical course of HO in SCI?**

Onset of HO usually is 1-4 months after injury in SCI patients, though it may occur as early as 19 days or as late as 1 year following injury. The condition may occur later with other precipitating circumstances (eg, fracture, surgery, severe systemic illness).Not uncommonly, incidental HO that was never noted clinically may be detected much later on x-ray. HO always occurs below the level of injury in SCI patients, and most authors agree there is no relation to presence or absence of spasticity in SCI patients. HO does tend to occur more frequently with complete injuries. In SCI patients with HO, the hips are involved most commonly. At the hip, the flexors and abductors tend to be involved more frequently than extensors or adductors. At the knee, the medial aspect most commonly is affected by HO. Shoulders and elbows are the joints affected most commonly in the upper extremities.

○   **What is the course of HO in TBI?**

 HO almost always occurs on the affected side, and most authors have noted that HO is more frequent in patients with spasticity than without. Garland and Blum studied 496 patients with severe head injuries. Clinically significant HO, causing pain and decreased ROM, was noted in 100 joints in 57 patients. Of the 100 involved joints, 89 were in spastic extremities. Frequency of involvement of different joints was slightly different than in patients with SCI; the hips were involved most commonly (44), then shoulders (27), and elbows (26). HO was detected in only 3 knee joints.

○   **What other factors may increase the risk of HO in TBI?**

Spielman also looked at occurrence of HO in patients with head injuries. In that study, inclusion criteria were (1) initial Glasgow Coma Scale score of 8 or less and (2) coma lasting more than 2 weeks. All patients had passive range of motion (PROM) of unknown frequency. Prolonged coma also appeared to increase the likelihood of development of HO. Once again, HO was more common in the limbs of patients with severe spasticity. In patients with neurologic deficits, increased limb spasticity, decreased joint ROM, and inflammatory signs near a joint strongly suggest the possibility of HO.

O **What laboratory findings may assist in the diagnosis of HO?**

Serial serum alkaline phosphatase (SAP) estimations can be useful. Elevation suggests bone growth, but the amount of increase is not proportional to the extent of HO. The alkaline phosphatase also may return to normal before maturity or may remain elevated for a prolonged period. SAP elevations always precede radiographic findings; however, alkaline phosphatase also can be elevated in patients with fractures or other skeletal or hepatic abnormalities. Elevation of SAP level from a previously abnormal level in a patient with an appropriate clinical presentation strongly suggests development of HO. One must exercise caution that coexisting fractures are not responsible for elevations of SAP.

O **What are the physical findings associated with HO?**

Diagnosis of HO can be made clinically if localized inflammatory reaction, palpable mass or limited ROM is observed. Clinically, onset of larger masses of HO is often characteristic of any inflammatory reaction. Fairly suddenly, a warm and swollen extremity becomes obvious, and associated low grade fever may be present. If sensation is intact, the area of swelling is painful. The swelling usually is localized more than in thrombophlebitis, and, within several days, a more circumscribed firmer mass is palpable within the edematous area. If the mass is adjacent to a joint, gradual loss of PROM may follow. With development of early HO at the hip or knee, effusion may be noted at the knee.

O **What are the limitations of plain x-ray in diagnosing HO?**

As soft tissue calcification must occur for radiographic evidence of HO to be present, x-rays are not helpful in the early stages. Radiologic examinations do not show evidence of HO until a flocculent patchy appearance develops, as calcium is deposited about 7-10 days after onset of clinical symptoms. This patchy appearance coalesces and enlarges on subsequent examinations, and, by 2-3 months, the boundaries of the HO demarcate with the appearance of mature bone. X-rays, however, are not reliable at assessing maturity of HO as more mature areas may hide immature areas.

O **What imaging modality is considered more useful for HO?**

Bone scan is the most useful investigation, as it can detect HO at onset of clinical symptoms. The 3-phase bone scan using technetium 99 is used in diagnosing and monitoring of HO. Images are obtained during dynamic blood flow phase, static phase immediately following injection, and 2-3 hours after injection, following bony uptake. The first 2 phases indicate hyperemia and blood pooling, precursors of ossification. These early phases are the most important for early diagnosis and monitoring of the ossification process.

O **How is HO maturity assessed clinically?**

Assessment of maturity of the HO is important because, if the lesion is significant enough for consideration of resection, the fact that resection prior to maturity almost always leads to recurrence of HO must be taken into account. Bone scans currently are considered to be the most reliable means of determining maturity of HO. Serial bone scans, performed weekly for 4-6 weeks, with decreasing uptake over time suggests maturation, although uptake can vary with serial examinations that make assessment of maturation less than 100% accurate.

O **What rehabilitation interventions are appropriate for HO?**

During the acute inflammatory stage, the patient should rest the involved joint in a functional position, and the physical therapist should initiate gentle PROM as soon as possible. The role of continuous PROM machines has not been studied in this situation. For patients with incomplete SCI or head injuries, maintaining ROM may be difficult because of pain from ROM exercises. Joint manipulation has been reported in cases of HO with functional limitations because of limited joint ROM, but it is controversial because of risks of formation of new hematoma and long-bone fracture risk in the patient population with secondary osteoporosis.

O **Is there a role for prophylactic treatment in HO?**

Successful prophylaxis of patients at high risk for HO has included external beam radiation and administration of nonsteroidal anti-inflammatory agents such as indomethacin and naproxen. The prophylactic use of medications to prevent HO has been studied in individuals with SCI, but the outcome has been mixed. Routine use of prophylactic etidronate sodium or nonsteroidal anti-inflammatory drugs (NSAIDs) probably is not justified for all patients with SCI or brain injuries, but NSAIDs do have a role in prevention of postoperative recurrence after excision of HO.

What is the rationale for radiation therapy?

Radiation therapy has been studied most in connection with prevention of HO in patients at high risk for recurrence following hip arthroplasty, but it also has been used in management of HO in SCI and TBI patients. Radiation may act on pluripotent mesenchymal stem cells, preventing differentiation into osteoblasts. The most common use in the rehabilitation setting is for prevention of postoperative recurrence, but the optimal dosage, frequency, and timing have not been established. A single irradiation of 7 Gy may be recommended for patients at high risk or who have developed HO after previous operations or in whom indomethacin is contraindicated .

What treatment is available for established HO?

Once HO has developed to the point that it interferes significantly with the functional capacity of the patient, the only treatment option remaining is surgery, which most commonly is required at the hip. Ensure that the HO has reached maturity before resection, as resection of immature HO leads to high recurrence rates. Hemorrhage may be a significant problem at the time of surgery with an average blood loss of 2100 cc reported. Postsurgical infection may lead to amputation; therefore, great care must be taken at the time of surgery. Initiate a pre surgery program to eliminate any possible nidus of bacteremia or infections (eg, decubitus ulcers, urinary tract infections).

What surgical technique is most often used for HO of the hip?

The usual surgical technique used on HO occurring anteriorly at the hip is anterior wedge resection.

What postoperative care is recommended?

Postoperatively, position the joint properly with foam wedges so that the surgical correction can be maintained and any strain on the incision or pressure sores can be prevented. Start gentle PROM about 72 hours post operation, and increase therapy intensity gradually to incorporate retraining in functional activities. Patient selection and careful identification of functional goals are critical for successful surgical intervention.

What is the role for bisphosphonates in HO?

The bisphosphonate group of compounds has properties similar to naturally occurring pyrophosphate, which may be a regulator of calcification. Etidronate disodium is the most extensively studied of this class of drugs for treatment of HO. Bisphosphonates act by (1) inhibiting precipitation of calcium phosphate from unsaturated solutions, (2) delaying aggregation of apatite crystals into layers, and (3) blocking conversion of calcium phosphate into hydroxyapatite. Bisphosphonates do not prevent the inflammatory process that initiates ossification, but they do inhibit mineralization and subsequent bone formation. The effectiveness of etidronate depends entirely on when and how long it is given, and it does not affect HO that has been formed already. There is limited of clinical evidence supporting the efficacy of HO prophylaxis and accretion.

What is the rationale for using NSAIDs in HO?

NSAIDs are presumed to have both direct and indirect effects on formation of HO. Direct effect refers to inhibiting differentiation of mesenchymal cells into osteogenic cells and indirect refers to inhibiting posttraumatic bone remodeling by suppression of the prostaglandin-mediated inflammatory response.

What is the proposed mechanism of action of NSAIDs in HO?

Nonsteroidal anti-inflammatory drugs (NSAIDs) that nonspecifically inhibit COX-1 and COX-2 can reduce bone resorption and inhibit osteoclast formation in vitro. Prostaglandins are potent local regulators of bone cell function and may play a critical role in both physiologic and pathologic changes in the skeleton. The major effects of PGs, particularly PGE_2, are to stimulate bone resorption by osteoclasts and bone formation by osteoblasts.

REHABILITATION TECHNOLOGY

PHYSICAL AGENTS

○ **What are the contraindications for heat therapy?**

Superficial heat modalities are contraindicated in the following situations:

Paraffin baths or fluidotherapy should not be used in open wounds that are either clean or infected.
Hydrotherapy is contraindicated in patients immediately following surgery, as a healing wound should be kept dry.
Special precautions should be used for therapy to be provided in a Hubbard tank for patients with either a tracheostomy or ostomy.

○ **When should radiant heat not be used in patients?**

Photosensitivity.
Acute inflammation or hemorrhage.
Bleeding disorder.

○ **What conditions should Hubbard tank therapy be contraindicated in patients?**

Hubbard tank therapy elevates core body temperature, patients with the following conditions that generate temperature-sensitivity should avoid this heating modality:

Multiple sclerosis.
Adrenal suppression or failure.
Systemic lupus erythematosus.
Pregnancy.

○ **What are hot packs?**

Hot packs or hydrocollator packs contain silicate gel in a cotton bag. These packs are placed in a hot water tank, which is thermostatically controlled at 71.1-79.4°C. The silicate gel absorbs a large quantity of water and has a high heat capacity.

○ **What is the duration of treatment?**

Hot packs are applied over layers of towels for 20-30 minutes. Most of the heat transfer from the hot pack to the patient is by conduction. Increasing the towel thickness reduces the heat flow and produces an intentional slowing in the temperature rise. Acceleration of heat transfer occurs if the hot pack leaks into the towel. The patient never should lie on the hot pack, as the body weight could squeeze hot water out of the pack into the towel and potentially cause a burn.

○ **What are the temporal properties of heat conduction?**

The maximum skin temperature is obtained after 8 minutes, followed by a reduction in temperature due to increased blood flow. Repeated application of hot packs may prolong the period of temperature elevation but does not alter the temperature distribution.

○ **What is a paraffin bath?**

Paraffin bath is another form of conductive heating. Paraffin baths are particularly useful for contractures due to rheumatoid arthritis, burns, and progressive systemic sclerosis (scleroderma). Paraffin usually is applied to the hands, arms, and feet.

Paraffin wax is melted and mixed with liquid paraffin. For therapeutic use, the paraffin bath is maintained at the melting point of 51.7-54.4°C in a thermostatically controlled insulated container.

O   What is the dip method?

The hand or foot is placed in the liquid paraffin bath and withdrawn when a thin layer of warm solid paraffin forms, becomes adherent, and covers the skin. The dipping procedure is repeated until a thick paraffin glove is formed. The heat can be retained by wrapping with towels for a period of 20 minutes; then, the cool solid paraffin glove is peeled away and the paraffin is recycled. The dip method is a mild heat application because only a limited amount of heat is available for transfer to the skin.

O   What is immersion?

Alternatively, the body part is immersed in the paraffin bath for 20-30 minutes. The immersion method transfers heat not only from the solid paraffin block but also from the liquid paraffin bath itself. The heat transfer rate from the liquid paraffin bath to the skin is slowed as the solid paraffin glove provides a poor thermal conductor. This modality represents a vigorous heat application, causing a significant increase in skin tissue temperature, up to 46°C, with a marked temperature decrease in the subcutaneous tissue. Water at the same temperature applied by the same method would be intolerable because of the high specific heat and thermal conductivity.

O   What is fluidotherapy?

Fluidotherapy is a form of convective heating that uses a bed of uniform finely divided round solids, such as glass beads, into which thermostatically controlled warm air is blown to generate a semifluid warm mixture. Part of the limb or hand/foot can be immersed for superficial heating. This technique applies dry heat, and the temperature is equivalent to the hot air that is blown into the bed of beads. The usual treatment temperature range is 45.6-47.8°C. Uses of fluidotherapy may include pain relief in arthritic conditions of small joints, joint mobilization following trauma/mobility, and analgesia/sedation in young patients undergoing exercise programs with painful and contracted joints due to sickle cell anemia.

O   What is hydrotherapy?

Hydrotherapy can include total immersion in a large hot tub or Hubbard tank. Partial immersion is available for upper or lower extremities by whirlpool baths. As hydrotherapy also may be used in treating infected draining wounds, the equipment must be sterilized between uses. The water is agitated, and the size of the tank determines the capacity (the entire body or just the upper or lower extremities).

O   What temperature settings are appropriate in hydrotherapy?

For total body immersion in water, the temperature should not exceed 40.6°C. Partial immersion of a limb should have a maximum temperature of 46.1°C.

O   What is the treatment time?

The treatment time is limited to 20-30 minutes each session.

O   What are the physiological characteristics of total body immersion?

As a precaution for total body immersion, oral temperature should be observed with water temperatures over 37.8°C to prevent a rise of body core temperature. With total body immersion, heat loss occurs primarily through the head and neck; therefore, the heat regulatory mechanism is impaired significantly. Total body immersion has a relaxing effect and may predispose the patient to hypotension due to peripheral blood pooling secondary to vasodilatation of all 4 limbs.

O   What are contrast baths?

Contrast baths provide a method of therapeutic hyperemia for management of rheumatoid arthritis or sympathetically mediated pain (eg, rheumatoid arthritis of distal joints, hands, feet; prolonged ankle swelling after an ankle sprain/strain in refractory joint effusions). A differential of approximately 25°C exists between the hot and cold water. The hot water is at a temperature of 40.6-43.3°C. The cold water temperature is maintained at 15-20°C.

○ **What does the contrast bath treatment regimen consists of?**

The greatest hyperemia response is produced by a 10-minute hot water immersion followed by cold water for 1 minute. The cycle continues with hot water immersion for 4 minutes and cold water for 1 minute; this 4:1 cycle is repeated for a total of 30 minutes at each physical therapy appointment or for each home-based self-treatment session.

○ **What is mechanism of radiant heat therapy?**

Radiant heat therapy is a type of conversion heating. The high-energy photons penetrate the tissues, and this energy is converted to heat. Because photons of longer wavelengths process less energy, penetration is more superficial; shorter wavelengths have a greater therapeutic benefit. The therapeutic radiant heat-producing temperature rise in tissues ranges from the spectrum of far infrared to visible yellow. Longer wavelengths of light from green to ultraviolet produce photochemical reactions that do not raise tissue temperature significantly.

○ **What types of devices are available?**

Most other commercially available radiant light sources produce infrared with some visible light. These lamps contain heating elements of Carborundum (silicon carbide), special quartz tubes, or metal alloys. The higher energy photons are produced by shorter wavelength radiant heat, resulting in a greater penetration of superficial tissue.

○ **How is the treatment carried out?**

A treatment time of 20-30 minutes is recommended, with the maximum effect occurring at a minimum of 20 minutes. The radiant energy source is positioned at 15-24 inches (38.1-61 cm) from the treatment site. The intensity is controlled by the light source, distance, type/quality of reflector, and air movement. With heat lamps, guidance concerning treatment time is given by the patient's subjective feeling of warmth. The conventional single heat cradle with an output of 300 watts is not likely to increase body temperature; however, a double cradle could. Patients also could receive increased radiation after an hour of treatment time.

○ **What are the physiological effects induced by cold?**

Decreased local metabolism.
Vasoconstriction.
Reactive hyperemia.
Reduced swelling/edema.
Decreased hemorrhage.
Reduced muscle efficiency.
Analgesia secondary to impaired neuromuscular transmission.

○ **What are the most common applications of cold therapy?**

The most common methods of cold application include cold packs, cold immersion, ice massage, and cooling during exercise (cryokinetics). Spray and stretch is an application of cryotherapy with a vapo-coolant spray, which then is followed by stretching of the involved muscles. This technique sometimes is used in the management of myofascial pain syndromes.

○ **What are the indications of cold therapy?**

To decrease swelling/edema following trauma (cooling in water at 8°C for 30 minutes decreases edema).
To treat burns.
To inhibit spasticity (in spasticity, the muscle must be cooled; this process takes 10 minutes in thin patients and up to 60 minutes in more obese persons).
To reduce muscle spasm.
To reduce acute inflammatory reaction.

To reduce pain.
To reduce limb metabolism (prior to amputation).
To produce reactive hyperemia.
To facilitate muscular contraction for various forms of neurogenic weakness and for muscle re-education.

O   What is the duration of treatment?

Therapeutic cold is applied for 5-20 minutes, followed by a rest period of 30 minutes. For treatment of acute sprains/strains and postoperative care, application of cold is recommended for the first 24-48 hours.

O   What are contraindications to cold therapy?

Hypertension (due to secondary vasoconstriction).
Raynaud disease.
Rheumatoid arthritis.
Local limb ischemia.
History of vascular impairment, such as frostbite or arteriosclerosis.
Cold allergy (cold urticaria).
Paroxysmal cold hemoglobinuria.
Cryoglobulinemia or any disease that produces a marked cold pressor response.

O   What are the salient physiological responses to heat and cold.

A longer time is necessary for cooled muscle to return to normal temperature. Because application of heat increases blood flow, a heated muscle returns to normal temperature after a few minutes.
The application of heat for relief of muscle spasm is secondary to muscle hyperemia, which decreases muscle spasm-induced ischemia/pain and interrupts this vicious cycle.
Increased tissue metabolism occurs with temperature elevation; reduced metabolism with cold modalities.
Heated muscle tissue can sustain a contraction for a shorter period of time; cooling to approximately 27°C increases the ability of muscle to sustain contraction.
Blood flow increases with heat and decreases with cold.
The tendency to bleed increases with heat and decreases with cold.
Formation of edema is facilitated by heat and decreased by cooling.
Immediate cooling of burns is beneficial; however, frostbite is treated by quick warming.
Joint stiffness is decreased with heating but increased with cold.
Due to blood pooling, orthostatic hypotension is produced by application of heat to large parts or all of the body. With cold treatment, hypotension is decreased secondary to vasoconstriction.

O   What is short wave diathermy (SWD)?

This deep heat modality is the therapeutic application of high radiofrequency electrical currents. The radiofrequency electromagnetic field usually is at a frequency of 27.12 MHz. Hyperemia, sedation, and analgesia are the basic physiologic effects. The reduction in muscle spasm due to muscle relaxation is a result of increased vascular supply to the treated area. A transverse technique is applied to treat a larger anatomic area with the primary concentration at the mid point between electrodes.

O   What are the treatment principles and techniques used in SWD application?

Proper application and tuning are required. The patient's electrical impedance becomes part of the impedance of the patient's own circuit. The patient's circuit must be set to resonance, so the patient's circuit frequency is equal to that of the machine. The patient should feel only a comfortable heat. The tissue temperature should be elevated to a range of 40-45°C for therapeutic benefit. Continuous supervision and observation of the patient is required. The treatment time is usually 20-30 minutes. At clinically relevant energies, shortwave diathermy can increase subcutaneous fat temperature 15°C and muscle 4-6°C at a depth of 4-5 cm. Application of this modality should be restricted to patients on either wooden tables or chairs.

○ **What is the condenser method?**

The technique of modality application includes the condenser method, which places the treatment site between 2 electrodes that function as capacitor plates. Monitoring of patient movement is required, as movement can affect the amplitude of the heat concentration applied. The condenser method of application should be used with felt or plastic spacers.

○ **What is the inductive coil method?**

The inductive coil method involves coil applicators that selectively heat superficial musculature unless applied to joints with minimal overlying soft tissue, resulting in selective heating of the joint. Inductively coupled units use induced eddy currents to heat tissue, especially in tissues with high water content such as muscle. Units joined to provide aggregate capacity use electrical fields to heat low water content tissues such as fat. Self-adjusting resonators minimize the positioning effect.

○ **What procedures are involved in utilization of SWD?**

A towel should be used to absorb perspiration with both the condenser and inductive methods to avoid localized heat concentration. The patient must be instructed to remain motionless. The output of the machine should be adjusted to a desired level so that movement does not change the impedance circuit and increase current flow, thereby increasing risk of an increased dose and resultant burns. The shortwave diathermy unit is tuned to low power as per patient tolerance, and the meter readings should be documented properly. Heating localization depends upon coupling of radio waves to the patient.

○ **What are indications for SWD?**

Localized musculoskeletal pain.
Inflammation (joint or tissue).
Pain/spasm.
Sprains/strains.
Tendinitis.
Tenosynovitis.
Bursitis.
Rheumatoid arthritis.
Periostitis.
Capsulitis.

○ **What are contraindications to SWD?**

Malignancy.
Sensory loss.
Tuberculosis.
Metallic implants or foreign bodies.
Pregnancy.
Application over moist dressings.
Ischemic areas or arteriosclerosis.
Thromboangiitis obliterans.
Phlebitis.
Use extreme care with pediatric and geriatric patients.
Cardiac pacemakers.
Contact lenses.
Metal-containing intrauterine contraceptive devices.
Metal in contact with skin (eg, watches, belt buckles, jewelry).
Use over epiphyseal areas of developing bones.
Active menses.

○ **What is microwave diathermy (MWD)?**

Microwave diathermy, a form of electromagnetic radiation, is another deep heat modality that selectively heats tissues with high water concentration. Hyperemia, sedation, and analgesia are the physiologic effects, similar to the results of shortwave diathermy. Secondary local vascular dilatation results in increased local metabolism.

○ **What frequencies are used in MWD?**

The 2 frequencies designated for microwave diathermy are 2,456 MHz and 915 MHz, the latter being the most commonly used. Since frequencies are higher than in shortwave diathermy and wavelengths are the same size as the applicator, microwave diathermy can be focused more easily than shortwave diathermy. The lower frequency is preferred because it provides selective heat deep into muscle, and less energy is converted to heat in the subcutaneous fat. Direct contact applicators with full aperture skin contact are optimal for improved coupling and reduced stray radiation.

○ **How is MWD carried out?**

A microwave director is used to aim the microwaves at the area of treatment, allowing observation of the treatment site. Heat can be reduced by increasing the distance of the microwave director from the treatment site. As with shortwave diathermy, hot spots and burns can occur secondary to localized perspiration associated with selective heating of the treatment zone. The microwave diathermy equipment is adjusted to provide comfortable heating with a treatment time of 20-30 minutes.

○ **What is ultrasound (US)?**

Ultrasound is a deep heating modality that uses high-frequency acoustic vibration above the human audible spectrum, defined as frequencies >17,000 Hz. Therapeutic ultrasound is in the frequency range of 0.8-1.0 MHz. Ultrasound energy is generated by the piezoelectric effect; electrical energy is applied to a crystal, causing it to vibrate at a high frequency and to produce ultrasound. Ultrasound is delivered by continuous or pulsed wave (the goal is to produce non-thermal affects such as streaming and cavitation) and provides a high heating intensity.

○ **What are the dosing parameters for US?**

Ultrasound energy is absorbed and transformed into heat energy as it propagates through tissue. The therapeutic dose is computed by the power output (total W) and the size of the ultrasound head. The usual initial dose is 1 W/cm^2 and is adjusted to patient tolerance, as well as to the goals of treatment. The practitioner must select the wave form (continuous or pulsed), intensity, and duration (usually 5-10 minutes). The patient should experience a comfortable heating or no sensation at all.

○ **What is the treatment period duration?**

The treatment time is 5-10 minutes, taking into account the patient's tolerance and comfort.

○ **What is a coupling agent?**

A coupling agent, such as ultrasound gel, is required after cleansing the skin, to provide effective conduction between the ultrasound head/transducer and the skin surface.

○ **What biological effects characterize ultrasound?**

Temporary analgesia.
Increased peripheral blood flow.
Increased vascularity with associated hyperemia/inflammatory response.
Increased cell membrane permeability.
Peripheral nerve conduction changes (reversible conduction block with high-intensity ultrasound exposure).
Relief of muscle spasms.

○ **What factors influence the propagation of ultrasound in biological tissue?**

Transmission.

Absorption.
Refraction.
Reflection.

○   **What are some indications for US?**

Joint contracture.
Joint adhesions.
Calcific bursitis.
Hematoma resolution.
Neuromas.
Fibrosis.
Phantom limb pain.
Myofascial pain.
Reflex vasodilatation.
Ulcer debridement.

○   **What are some contraindications to US treatment?**

Although the literature for physical therapy and for physical medicine has differing opinions, therapeutic ultrasound can be used over metal implants with caution and with constant motion of the ultrasound head. Additional contraindications of ultrasound include conditions in which application of deep heat would require direct exposure of the eye, pregnant uterus, spine, laminectomy sites, brain, heart, or known ischemic areas, which can result in detrimental cavitation and heating of those tissues.

○   **What is phonophoresis?**

Phonophoresis is a US technique in which medications such as corticosteroids, analgesics, and anesthetics are mixed in the coupling agent in the hope that they will be "driven" by the US through the skin into deeper tissues. Penetration to depths of several centimeters has been reported, but many find the concept arguable in that substances may not always pass through the skin and once past the epidermis, may be dispersed by the subcutaneous circulation. Whether phonophoresis is more beneficial than US alone is unclear. Both no and significant effects are reported, but the studies were small, blinding was ambiguous, and comparisons to local injection or oral administration of the same medication were lacking.

○   **What are some of the mechanisms underlying transcutaneous electric nerve stimulation (TENS)?**

Presynaptic inhibition in the dorsal horn of the spinal cord.
Endogenous pain control (via endorphins, enkephalins, and dynorphins).
Direct inhibition of an abnormally excited nerve.
Restoration of afferent input.

○   **What is the underlying mechanism, of TENS?**

The results of laboratory studies suggest that electrical stimulation delivered by a TENS unit reduces pain through nociceptive inhibition at the presynaptic level in the dorsal horn, thus limiting its central transmission. The electrical stimuli on the skin preferentially activate low- threshold myelinated nerve fibers. The afferent input from these fibers inhibits propagation of nociception carried in the small unmyelinated C fibers by blocking transmission along these fibers to the target cells located in the substantia gelatinosa (laminae 1, 2 and 5) of the dorsal horn.

○   **What are the components of a TENS unit?**

A TENS unit consists of one or more electric signal generators, a battery, and a set of electrodes. The units are small and programmable, and the generators can deliver trains of stimuli with variable current strengths, pulse rates, and pulse widths. The preferred waveform is biphasic, to avoid the electrolytic and iontophoretic effects of a unidirectional current.

○   **What parameters are utilized in TENS therapy?**

Amplitude Current at low intensity, comfortable level, just above threshold.
Pulse width (duration) 10-1000 microseconds.
Pulse rate (frequency) 80-100 impulses per second (Hz); 0.5-10 Hz when stimulus intensity is set high.

○   **What are the settings for conventions TENS?**

Conventional TENS has a high stimulation frequency (40-150 Hz) and low intensity, just above threshold, with the current set between 10-30 mA. The pulse duration is short (up to 50 microseconds). The onset of analgesia with this setup is virtually immediate. Pain relief lasts while the stimulus is turned on, but it usually abates when the stimulation stops. Patients customarily apply the electrodes and leave them in place all day, turning the stimulus on for approximately 30-minute intervals throughout the day. In individuals who respond well, analgesia persists for a variable time after the stimulation stops.

○   **What are the settings in acupuncture like TENS?**

In acupuncture-like settings, the TENS unit delivers low frequency stimulus trains at 1-10 Hz, at a high stimulus intensity, close to the tolerance limit of the patient. Although this method sometimes may be more effective than conventional TENS, it is uncomfortable, and not many patients can tolerate it. This method often is considered for patients who do not respond to conventional TENS.

○   **What is pulsed or burst TENS?**

Pulsed (burst) TENS uses low-intensity stimuli firing in high frequency bursts. The recurrent bursts discharge at 1-2 Hz, and the frequency of impulses within each burst is at 100 Hz. No particular advantage has been established for the pulsed method over the conventional TENS method.

○   **What considerations are given to the clinical application of TENS?**

The amount of output current depends on the combined impedance of the electrodes, skin, and tissues. With repetitive electrical stimuli applied to the same location on the skin, the skin impedance is reduced, which could result in greater current flow as stimulation continues. A constant current stimulator, therefore, is preferred to minimize sudden uncontrolled fluctuations of current intensity related to changes in impedance. An electro conductive gel applied between the electrode and skin serves to minimize the skin impedance. Patients need to be instructed in the use and care of TENS equipment, with particular attention to the electrodes.

○   **What are the precautions for TENS utilization?**

Medical complications arising from use of TENS are rare; however, skin irritation is a frequent problem and often is due partly to the drying out of the electrodes. Sometimes individuals react to the tape used to secure the electrodes. Skin irritation is minimized by using self-adhesive disposable electrodes and repositioning them slightly for repeated applications. The use of TENS is contraindicated in patients with demand-type pacemakers because their stimulus outputs may drive or inhibit the pacemaker.

○   **What is interferential current therapy?**

Interferential current therapy (IFC) is based on summation of 2 alternating current signals of slightly different frequency. The resultant current consists of cyclical modulation of amplitude, based on the difference in frequency between the 2 signals. When the signals are in phase, they summate to amplitude sufficient to stimulate, but no stimulation occurs when they are out of phase. The beat frequency of IFC is equal to the difference in the frequencies of the 2 signals. For example, the beat frequency and, hence, the stimulation rate of a dual channel IFC unit with signals set at 4200 and 4100 Hz is 100 Hz. IFC therapy can deliver higher currents than TENS. IFC can use 2, 4, or 6 applicators, arranged in either the same plane for use on regions such as the back or in different planes in complex regions (eg, the shoulder).

○   **What is high volt galvanic stimulation?**

High-voltage galvanic stimulation (HVGS) or high-voltage pulsed galvanic stimulation (HVPGS) was originally developed in the USA and given this name. The twin pulse waveform has almost instantaneous rises with exponential falls. The pair of pulses lasts for only 0.1 ms and each peak lasts for only a few microseconds; the shape and duration are normally fixed. The frequency of the double pulse can be varied, usually from 2 to 100 Hz. With such short peaks very high voltages are needed (hence the name) to provide high enough currents to stimulate nerve fibers. Peak currents of 2-2.5 A may be generated during the few microseconds of peak voltage but, of course, the total average current is very low, at around 1.2-1.5 mA. Such pulsed currents will pass easily through the tissues (in common with TENS) because they are so brief and will be relatively comfortable due to their wide discrimination between sensory, motor and nociceptor nerve fibers.

O   **What are other characteristics of HVGS?**

As well as the frequency the intensity can be varied (0-500 V) and the polarity altered. The pattern of current can be changed by a mode switch. In continuous mode the train of twin pulses is delivered continuously. Reciprocate mode refers to the alternate application of trains of pulses to one or other of two active pads and does not mean that the current direction is reversed. Surge mode gives a train of pulses whose intensity is gradually increased. A meter to indicate peak current may be provided. On some machines the interval between the two peaks may be altered; this is called the intrapulse interval. The current is applied by flexible electrodes and sponges. The electrodes are usually small and are sometimes mounted on a handle. Various special electrodes are available.

O   **What are the uses of HVPGS in wound healing?**

There seems to be evidence that low-intensity currents lead to tissue healing.

O   **What are the uses of HVPGS in pain modulation?**

Since both the frequency and intensity of HVPGS can be controlled it is possible to apply both high-frequency, low-intensity stimulation for pain gate control and low frequency, high intensity stimulation for enkephalin-type pain control. HVPGS has been recommended for controlling all kinds of pain -acute, chronic, and neurogenic and pain from many sources.

O   **What are the uses of HVPGS in muscle stimulation?**

HVPGS is used for the stimulation of innervated muscle and, due to the short pulses and hence good transmission in the tissues; it is an efficient way of doing so. Consider the strength duration curve which shows that short pulses at high intensities will be more selective in stimulating motor rather than pain nerves. HVPGS has therefore been used for muscle strengthening and the reduction of disuse atrophy of innervated muscle. A frequency of around 30 Hz has been suggested with long intervals between bouts of tetanic contraction as the optimum schedule.

O   **What is percutaneous electrical nerve stimulation (PENS)?**

Percutaneous electrical nerve stimulation (PENS) combines advantages of both electroacupuncture and TENS. Rather than using surface electrodes, PENS uses acupuncture like needle probes as electrodes, placed at dermatomal levels corresponding to local pathology. The main advantage of PENS over TENS is that it bypasses the local skin resistance and delivers electrical stimuli at the precisely desired   level in close proximity to the nerve endings located in soft tissue, muscle, or periosteum.

O   **What are the indications for iontophoresis?**

Iontophoresis is an accepted treatment of hyperhidrosis. The mechanism of action is unclear, but success rates of 90% are achieved with tap water alone and may persist for weeks. Typically the hands or feet are placed in water, and the circuit adjusted to deliver 10 to 30 mA. Iontophoretic antibiotic delivery is possible but has not become common. Other uses such as salicylates for postsurgical pain, iodine for scar tissue reduction, acetic acid for calcific tendinitis, zinc for ischemic ulcers, and lidocaine for local anesthesia are reported but effectiveness is not established.

O   **How often does skin irritation occur?**

Skin irritation can occur in as many as 33% of patients, at least in part, due to drying out of the electrode gel.

O   **What is iontophoresis?**

Iontophoresis uses electrical fields to drive charged or electrically polarized substances (e.g., salicylates, acetic acid) through the epidermis. Much of the penetration probably occurs at sweat glands and sites of skin breakdown. Penetration is variable and how much of a substance is actually delivered to the treated tissue rather than the blood remains contentious.

O   **Summarize the uses of electrical stimulation in innervated muscle**

Strengthening muscle in healthy subjects
Strengthening atrophied or potentially atrophied muscle due to disuse
Facilitation of motor control
Maintaining or increasing the range of joint motion
Functional electrical stimulation
To replace splinting and provoke motion
To control spasticity
Effect changes in muscle structure and properties with chronic electrical stimulation
Increase muscle metabolism and blood flow
Increase venous and lymphatic flow in adjacent tissues.

O   **Summarize the effects of pulsed currents:**

Sensory nerves prickling Sensation-
pain relief via pain gate mechanism
cutaneous vasodilation via axon reflex
Motor nerves skeletal muscle contraction-
reeducation of movement
increased strength and endurance
increased intramuscular blood flow
increased muscle metabolism
increased blood flow in adjacent tissues (pumping effect)
increased or maintained joint motion control *of* joint motion (FES)
Muscle fatigue
affect muscle fiber growth —trophic change
Nociceptors-   A-delta and C- fibers
pain sensation
modify pain perception
(due to release of endogenous opioids and other mechanisms)
Muscle tissue- muscle contraction
Autonomic nerves- possible effects on blood flow

O   **What does iontophoretic equipment consist of?**

Iontophoretic equipment consists of a direct-current power source, two electrodes, and moistened pads that are placed between the electrodes and the skin. The pads may be moistened with normal saline solution and a 1% solution of the chosen agent is placed on the pad under the electrode of the same polarity. Electrical fields, which are proportional to the voltage, provide the driving force. Currents are usually limited to produce intensities of 0.1 to 0.5 mA/cm $_2$ and are proportional to the active material delivered.

PROSTHETICS

O   **What are the goals of surgical amputation?**

The goals of surgical amputation are to 1) preserve functional length of the extremity, 2) preserve useful sensation, 3) prevent symptomatic neuromas or pain syndromes, 4) prevent adjacent joint contractures, 5) minimize recovery time, and 6) achieve early prosthetic fitting to facilitate return to work, activities of daily living (ADLs), recreation, and socialization.

○   **What is the most common type of upper extremity amputation?**

The most common type of upper extremity amputation is the fingertip amputation.

○   **Why are ray amputations done?**

Ray amputations are often done electively to minimize disability from a previous injury to a digit. This is usually not done at the time of trauma because the patient needs to determine if a digit stump is useful or not.

○   **What are the consequences of index finger amputation?**

If the index finger is very short and cannot be used for pinch, the remnant may interfere with the individual pinching between the thumb and the middle finger. Since the index finger provides stability to the power grip, significant effort is made to preserve the length and sensation of the index finger, particularly in manual laborers. Resection of the index ray can reduce grip strength by 20%, but can markedly improve cosmesis.

○   **What is the preferred length for a transradial amputation?**

For transradial or BE amputation, it is important to conserve all possible length of the limb, with a minimum of 10 cm below the lateral epicondyle of the humerus being preferred.

○   **What are the advantages to a long transradial residual limb?**

A longer residuum provides a greater lever arm and consequently greater forearm strength and power. Greater forearm rotation is preserved. An amputation at 2 cm or more proximal to the wrist allows more room for prosthetic components. At this level, approximately 70% to 80% of natural pronation and supination are preserved.

○   **What residual limb length is preferred for trans humeral amputations?**

A residual limb that is at least 10 cm long, measuring from the axillary fold, is preferred. The greater the upper limb loss, the less humeral rotation is preserved.

○   **Why is epiphyseal preservation important in children?**

In children, epiphyseal preservation is important. The growth potential of the distal epiphyses is greater than that of the proximal radial and ulnar epiphyses, while in the humerus, the proximal epiphysis has greater growth potential. Disarticulation allows for undisturbed epiphyseal bone growth, preserving longitudinal growth. Disarticulation also prevents the development of bony overgrowth at the terminal bone. Since bony prominences (e.g., condyles) become less prominent with age, disarticulation does not present the same cosmetic problems that are seen in adults.

○   **What is a body powered prosthesis?**

The body powered prosthesis uses a system of straps and cables to transfer energy of one body part to the prosthesis to perform a specific motion. For example, the AE amputee uses scapular and humeral motion to operate a prosthetic elbow and hand.

○   **What is an externally powered prosthesis?**

Externally powered systems rely on an external source of energy to operate the prosthesis. The most frequently used externally powered prosthesis employs the myoelectric control system, but other systems exist, including electric switch controls. Myoelectric prostheses use the electrical potential of a muscle to voluntarily operate components of the prosthesis, for example, to open and close a prosthetic hand.

O   **When should an upper extremity amputee be fitted with a prosthesis?**

Fitting a prosthesis within four weeks of upper extremity amputation dramatically improves the long term outcome. Some clinicians report success rates as high as 90%.

O   **For upper extremity amputees, which power system, is most commonly used?**

Estimates indicate that 90% of upper extremity amputees who use a prosthesis use a body powered system at least part time. Amputees prefer this system because it is relatively inexpensive, durable, reliable, and functional.

O   **What are some of the advantages of the body powered system?**

This system provides some sensory feedback via the cables and harness control systems. Many prefer the speed of operation and accuracy of body powered prostheses. Because they do not require external sources of power, there are no batteries to recharge or replace.

O   **What are some of the disadvantages of the body powered system?**

A body-powered prosthesis has a weaker grip than the myoelectric one, but it is more durable for manual work such as lifting.

O   **What are the basic operational features of a myoelectric powered system?**

It harnesses the electrical potential of a contracting muscle to operate the prosthesis. These prostheses require minimal proximal muscle control and can be used in all planes of motion (e.g., overhead reaching). Compared to body powered prostheses, myoelectric prostheses provide a stronger, graded grasp. Though more expensive than body powered prostheses, they are often more cosmetic since many do not require a harness for suspension.

O   **What are some of the disadvantages of myoelectrically powered prosthesis?**

Myoelectric prostheses are expensive. They are comparatively fragile devices and frequently break down.
Greater technical skill is needed to repair and maintain these systems. Unlike the body powered prostheses, myoelectric systems do not tolerate many environmental factors, such as dust and moisture. They are not as durable or as well suited as body-powered prostheses for manual labor. Because the weight of the prosthesis is not transferred to more proximal body parts, as in the body powered systems, myoelectric prostheses create more pressure at the point of suspension, the distal part of the limb. Additionally, they feel heavier to the user.

O   **What timing is characteristic for UE amputees in introduction and training with prosthesis?**

A typical prosthetic restoration and rehabilitation schedule has several stages. Initially, the amputee is fitted with prosthesis in the immediate or early postamputation period. Over the next 2 to 6 weeks, fitting and training with a preparatory body-powered prosthesis occur. Once trained, and after prosthetic needs are determined, the amputee is fitted with definitive body powered prosthesis. Typically, the amputee is ready for a definitive body powered prosthesis approximately 6 to 12 weeks after amputation. As a general rule, a person is fitted with a body powered prosthesis first. Once the individual is successfully using the body powered prosthesis, he or she is evaluated for the more expensive myoelectric system.

O   **What function does the harness serve?**

The harness provides suspension and a way to control the active parts of the prosthesis. The type of socket and the intimacy of the fit between the socket and the residual limb also provide suspension. The harness is composed of a collection of strategically placed straps around the shoulder or thorax to transmit the force of proximal body motion to the prosthetic components. The straps, which are typically made of Dacron, must be carefully placed and fitted so that body power is efficiently transmitted to the active prosthetic components. A cable system is secured proximally on the harness and terminates on the TD.

O   **What are the two basic types of control systems in the UE amputee?**

There are two basic types, the single control system, which typically operates the TD for the BE amputee; and the dual control system required by the AE amputee. The amputee transmits muscle tension along the stainless-steel cables of the prosthesis to perform the desired motion. For example, in the BE amputee, the cable terminates on the TD. The OT trains the patient to perform coordinated movements of arm flexion and shoulder abduction to operate the TD. The body powered AE prosthesis uses the same principles but requires a second cable to control the elbow unit.

○ **Under what circumstance dies a patient with a partial hand amputation not need prosthesis?**

Typically, prosthesis is not required to improve function if two or more digits remain. With two remaining digits, a person is able to adduct or oppose one finger to the other. If opposition is not possible with the remaining digits, a rotation osteotomy may be considered in an attempt to create opposition.

○ **What is the terminal device (TD)?**

The TD is the most distal component of upper extremity prosthesis. A TD is either active or passive. A passive TD is usually very light and has no moving parts. The typical active prehension TD is a hook, hand, or specialized device or tool with moveable parts. The opening width of the TD must be compatible with the ability to handle common objects. TDs can be voluntary opening (VO) or voluntary closing (VC). The hook TD has two "fingers," one stationary and one moveable. The amputee activates the hook using either a body powered or myoelectric control system.

○ **How is the grip force determined in a hook terminal device?**

In the conventional body-powered prosthesis, the number of rubber bands located at the base of the hook fingers determines the grip force of the TD. One rubber band is equivalent to approximately 1 lb (0.45 kg) of pinch between the two hook fingers. By producing tension on the cable, the amputee is able to open or close the hook.

○ **What wrist substitutes are available for the BE amputee?**

Three basic types of wrist units are available for conventional prostheses. The first two types provide pronation and supination but not wrist flexion and extension. The amputee must position the wrist unit in the desired position of pronation or supination. The variable friction wrist unit adjusts for variable rotation friction, that is, from loose to tight. Most individuals prefer the quick change wrist units because the amputee can change the TD quickly. The third type, the wrist flexion unit, provides not only variable friction for wrist rotation but also wrist flexion. This is an important option for the bilateral amputee, or the person with a nonfunctional contralateral limb, who is dependent on the prosthesis to do midline activities, such as dressing.

○ **What are the three basic types of elbow hinges for the BE amputee?**

There are three basic types of elbow hinges: the flexible hinges, the rigid hinges, and step up hinges. In the presence of a long residual forearm, flexible elbow hinges allow natural forearm rotation. Rigid hinges impede this motion. Rigid hinges are a better option for the shorter residual forearm because more forearm stability is needed.

○ **When are step up hinges advantageous for the BE amputee?**

The individual with a very short limb after transradial amputation can benefit from step up hinges since anatomic elbow flexion is usually limited to less than 90 degrees. These hinges amplify the range of motion (ROM) at the elbow in a ratio of 1 : 2. For instance, 50 degrees of elbow flexion results in approximately 100 degrees of prosthetic flexion. The step up hinge design requires that the socket be a separate unit from the prosthetic forearm (split socket design). This system is preferred for the amputee with a very short residual forearm with limited ROM for whom increased ROM is more important than strength.

○ **What is a drawback to the step up hinge?**

Unfortunately, though flexion is increased, the lever arm force is reduced approximately 50%. The force applied to the volar surface of the residual forearm is high and many patients do not tolerate the pressure.

O   What are the two harnesses available for the transradial amputee?

Two basic types of harnesses are available for the patient who underwent transradial amputation: the figure of eight harness and the shoulder harness with a chest strap. Because the figure of eight harness allows for the widest range of activities with the least restriction, it is the most common harness used by unilateral and bilateral upper extremity amputees.

O   What options are available for a trans humeral amputee?

Trans humeral amputation that is performed at least 5 cm proximal to the elbow leaves a limb that can accommodate an internal or inside locking elbow unit. The turntable multiple locking elbow unit, which is the most common unit used by the AE amputee, has 11 locking positions. It provides 5 to 135 degrees of flexion, whereas the elbow unit used in disarticulation prosthesis has only seven positions, or fewer if it is a heavy duty design. With a body-powered prosthesis, if the elbow is unlocked, pulling the cable flexes the elbow. If however the elbow is locked, a pull on the main cable operates the TD.

O   Are hybrid body systems considered in the AE amputee?

Hybrids of myoelectric and body-powered systems are very valuable for the AE amputee. A body powered elbow with a myoelectric hand is a common choice. The myoelectric hand, with its stronger grip and graded control, is valuable for the person whose work or avocation involves a lot of holding and stabilizing objects. The myoelectric elbow with a body powered TD affords more sensory feedback for the patient who needs feedback regarding TD function.

O   What does UE prosthesis training involves initially?

The patient first learns how to wear the prosthesis. Typically, the amputee learns to don and doff the prosthesis using either a pullover technique or a coat technique. The amputee initially wears the new prosthesis for periods of 30 to 60 minutes, and then gradually increases the wearing time. Within 1 or 2 weeks, the amputee should be comfortably wearing the prosthesis for an entire day. New amputees continue to wear shrinker socks or elasticized wraps when not wearing the prosthesis. This is required until the volume of the residual limb stabilizes, or indefinitely in patients with fluctuating limb volumes.

O   What does the UE amputee with a body powered system receives training in?

The wearer of a conventional, or body powered, prosthesis is taught how many socks to wear and the indications for changing the number of socks. The amputee must learn how many rubber bands to put on the VO hook. Typically, the individual begins with about 1 lb (0.5 kg) of pressure, as measured by the pinchometer. The number of rubber bands is gradually increased until sufficient pressure is provided to meet the amputee's functional needs, that is, 3 to 15 lb (1.35–6.75 kg) of pressure. Generally, BE amputees need approximately 8 lb (3.6 kg) of pinch force, while AE amputees develop about 5 lb (2.25 kg) of pinch force with the VO hook.

O   What training occurs for the upper extremity amputee who will use a myoelectric body powered system?

Control of muscle site signals is the basis of successful myoelectric prosthesis use. Dual site control is preferred over the more difficult single-site control. With dual site control, two muscles must be able to generate independently a sufficient electrical potential to operate the prosthesis without interfering with each other. Typically, the patient is taught to isolate antagonist muscles. For example, BE amputees learn to isolate the wrist flexors and extensors, while AE amputees learn to isolate the biceps and triceps.

O   What pinch force is needed for the basic ADLs?

Once the amputee is able to produce a pinch force of at least 3 lb (1.35 kg), functional tasks are taught, including tying shoes, cutting meat, and picking up objects.

O   What is a rigid removable dressing?

The RRD is a socket fabricated with plaster or fiberglass casting bandage over the distal end of the residual limb, typically in the operating room or recovery room as the person is coming out of anesthesia.

O   **When are elastic wraps used?**

Elastic wraps are frequently used to control edema and assist with shaping the residual limb. Though inexpensive, they are labor-intensive and rely on use of proper technique. To ensure proper compression, they should be rewrapped four to six times a day with tension to create a distal to proximal pressure gradient. A herringbone pattern, pulling increased tension when going from posterior to anterior, is commonly used.

O   **What complication can occur with elastic wrapping techniques?**

If applied improperly, an elastic wrap may provide inadequate compression, or if applied too tightly proximally, can create a tourniquet effect resulting in more edema.

O   **What are the major components of lower extremity (LE) prosthesis?**

The major components of a prosthesis are the socket, a skin-socket interface such as socks or a liner, a suspension system, articulating joints if needed, the pylon, and a foot.

O   **How are prosthetic feet classified?**

Prosthetic feet are broadly classified as energy storing or not energy storing and are made of a multitude of materials such as wood, foam, rubber, metal alloys, graphite, plastic polymers, and silicones.

O   **What are liners?**

Liners vary from semirigid to flexible and are made from a large number of different materials, such as a dense foam, multi density layered foam, multidurometer rubber, silicones, plastics, or a composite of several materials.

O   **What are suspension systems?**

Suspension systems to secure the prosthesis to the residual limb can be straps, wedges, sleeves, suction, or a combination.

O   **What is the socket?**

The socket provides the weight bearing interface between the patient's residual limb and the prosthesis. It must contain and protect the tissues of the residual limb while simultaneously controlling and transmitting the forces involved in standing and ambulation.

O   **What is the difference between a provisional and definitive socket?**

The provisional (temporary or preparatory) socket will need to be modified to accommodate changes in volume and shape as postsurgical edema resolves, atrophy occurs, or the patient's weight fluctuates. The definitive (permanent) prosthetic socket is made when the shaping and shrinking process is complete and the residual limb volume has stabilized.

O   **What is an exoskeletal system?**

The socket is attached to joints or the foot via an endoskeletal or exoskeletal system. The exoskeletal system can be conceptualized as a hollow column. It consists of a shank made of a light weight rigid foam that is shaped to match the patient's natural limb, then laminated with a hard resin or plastic shell. The laminated load-bearing shell is highly durable and transmits the patient's weight to the prosthetic foot.

O   **What is an endoskeletal system?**

The endoskeletal system can be thought of as an internal weight bearing pipe with a cosmetic non-load-bearing outer shell. It uses a lightweight metal or plastic pylon covered with soft, shaped foam for cosmesis. The endoskeletal systems are very modular in design, allowing easy interchangeability of components and alignment.

○   **What are the three main types of AK sockets?**

There are three main AK socket designs: the quadrilateral, the NSNA (normal shape, normal alignment) or CATCAM (contoured adducted trochanteric controlled alignment method), and the flexible socket.

○   **What is the basic function of an AK socket?**

The socket is designed to contain the soft tissues and effectively control the movement and force of the residual femur during standing and ambulation.

○   **What is the quadrilateral AK socket?**

It is a relatively square socket with narrow anterior posterior and wide medial lateral dimensions. The posterior brim contains a broad flat posterior seat for weight bearing on the ischial tuberosity region. It does not cup or contain the ischial tuberosity.

○   **What is a disadvantage of the quadrilateral socket?**

In the 1980s, observation and x-ray studies confirmed that the wide medial lateral dimension allowed the proximal part of the residual femur to shift laterally, distally compressing the medial soft tissue of the residual limb and resulting in a lateral shift of the person's body relative to the socket during the stance phase.

○   **What are the distinguishing features of the other AK sockets?**

The NSNA, CATCAM, and ischial-containment hard socket have wide anterior-posterior and narrow medial-lateral dimensions, providing medial-lateral compression of the soft tissues, which limits the lateral shift of the femur within the socket during the stance phase. This maintains a more anatomic alignment of the residual femur. The posterior brim ischial seat includes a high posterior medial wall that cups the ischial tuberosity, creating a bony lock of the socket to the ischium during the stance phase, further limiting lateral socket shift.

○   **What is the flexible AK socket?**

The flexible socket is a two piece socket that has a hard, usually windowed, outer frame with a semiflexible plastic or silicon polymer socket inside it. The outer frame is a laminate of resin and a high strength material such graphite braid. The unit can be fabricated utilizing the same design contours of the quadrilateral or NSNA type socket. The inner liner can be made of a relatively clear, low temperature polymer that becomes more flexible as warms from body heat. Depending on the properties of the chosen polymer, this can improve comfort, owing to the ability of the liner to change shape with the changes weight-bearing forces or muscle activity, or to accommodate mild increased residual limb volume.

○   **What is the PTB socket?**

The PTB socket is designed to put more force over pressure tolerant areas. These typically are the patella tendon, the medial flare and shaft of the tibia, the soft tissues of the anterior compartment between the tibia and the fibula, the lateral shaft of the fibula, and the posterior compartment. This is accomplished by taking away material over these areas on the positive mold of the residual limb, resulting in an smaller dimension or tighter fit when the socket is casted. All other areas in the PTB socket receive partial contact but are not designed to transfer any significant force to the residual limb.

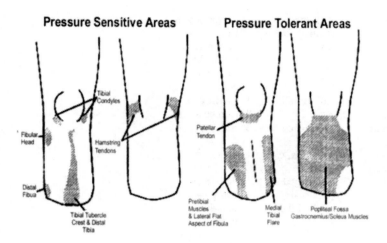

Pressure Sensitive Areas

- Tibial Condyles
- Fibular Head
- Hamstring Tendons
- Distal Fibula
- Tibial Tubercle Crest & Distal Tibia

Pressure Tolerant Areas

- Patellar Tendon
- Pretibial Muscles & Lateral Flat Aspect of Fibula
- Medial Tibial Flare
- Popliteal Fossa Gastrocnemius/Soleus Muscles

○ **What is the Syme amputation?**

The Syme amputation is a surgical disarticulation of the ankle, with shaving of the malleoli, slight trimming of the tibia, preservation of the weight bearing distal tibial cartilage, and reattachment of the heel pad.

○ **How are partial foot amputations classified?**

Partial foot amputations are categorized as toe amputation, transmetatarsal amputation, disarticulation at the proximal metatarsal midfoot level (Lisfranc), disarticulation at the midfoot-hindfoot level (Chopart), and removal of the foot except for preservation of the calcaneus and a large portion of the talus (Boyd).

○ **What is the function of the great toe in gait?**

The great toe aids in slowing down the transition from the foot flat to the toe off phase as well as imparting energy for forward propulsion. Without the great toe, there is the tendency to roll over the front of the foot too quickly, as well as having decreased push off.

○ **How can a prosthetist normalize gait mechanics in great toe amputation?**

To normalize gait mechanics and provide some energy return during toe off, a great toe amputation is best dealt with by adding a spring steel shank to the sole of the shoe or inserting an orthotic foot plate with a foam toe filler. A rocker sole may be needed to create a smooth transition from foot flat to toe off.

○ **What are the different suspension systems available for the lower extremity amputee?**

SUSPENSION	INDICATIONS	CONTRA-INDICATIONS	ACTIONS	ADVANTAGES	DISADVANTAGES
Suction Traditional Modified (gel suspension liners)	1. Smooth residual limb contour	1. Volume fluctuations	1. Precisely fitting socket with air expulsion Valve 2. Socket seals Directly against skin	1. Best proprioception 2. No pistoning 3. Lightweight 4. Easy to maintain	1. Need to maintain precise fit 2. May fall off if suction is lost 3. Need to maintain constant body weight
Anatomic/limb contour	1. Short BK residual limb 2. Knee disarticulation 3. Syme 4. Mild mediolateral	1. Obese or very muscular patient 2. Very long BK residual limb	1. The socket is contoured over some Bony prominence, Normally the femoral	1. Suspension is inherent part of socket 2. Less restrictive to circulation than a cuff strap in BK	1. Requires precise modification 2. High trim lines reduce cosmesis; more damage

	knee instability		condyle or malleoli	3. Aids in knee stability for BK	to clothing in BK 3. May require removable wedge or door.
Straps/belts	1. When other systems have failed 2. Past users 3. Anticipated volume changes	1. Must be careful not to compress blood vessels or bypass grafts	1. SC-cuff strap fits over femoral condyle 2. Waist belt 3. Suspenders	1. Adjustability 2. Axillary suspension for at risk activities, e.g., sports 3. Unlikely that prosthesis could fall off	1. Chafing 2. Cumbersome 3. Bulky
					1. Patient can overpower unit due to air compressing 2. Maintenance, weight, cost
					1. Weight 2. Cost and maintenance

O   What are the indications for a roll on suction suspension system?

The roll on suction suspension works well for AK and BK residual limbs. Its shear-absorbing properties minimize skin breakdown and improve comfort over bony prominences and scar tissue. Custom molded, roll on suction suspension systems can be used for irregularly shaped, excessively bony, or scarred residual limbs.

O   What are the disadvantages of this system?

Disadvantages of this system are cost and hygiene. The airtight seal traps moisture, creating an environment that favors the clogging of pores and the propagation of microorganisms such as bacteria and yeast. The suspension liner and residual limb must be washed daily with low-residue soap.

O   What is a hypobaric sock?

The Hypobaric sock is a standard prosthetic sock with a band of silicone added to provide an airtight seal between the patient's residual limb and the socket wall. The Hypobaric sock has been used for AK and BK residual limbs. The patient dons the sock, lubricates the silicone band, and slides the residual limb and sock into the prosthesis. The air is expelled through a one way air valve. The patient can use multiple Hypobaric socks to accommodate volume changes in the residual limb.

O   What is a flex seal sock?

The Flex seal is a very flexible silicone diaphragm with a hole in the center that is positioned over the proximal part of the socket. The patient dons the prosthesis by inserting the residual limb through the hole against the diaphragm, which conforms to the residual limb shape and creates an airtight seal.

O   What are the suspension systems most commonly used for the AK prosthesis?

The total elastic suspension (TES) belt, Silesian band, and the combined hip joint with pelvic band and waist belt are the nonsuction suspension systems most frequently used for AK suspension. Occasionally a shoulder harness is used.

O   What is the TES belt?

The TES belt, made out of an elastic material such as neoprene, is fastened around the waist. It can be used as a primary suspension, but is mostly utilized as a secondary suspension in tandem with a suction system to help control rotation or provide a backup if suction is lost, to prevent the prosthesis from falling off.

○ **What is the Silesian belt?**

The Silesian belt is the most often used belt system of suspension. Attachment starts near the brim of the posterolateral socket wall. The belt encircles the contralateral side of the patient's pelvis to fasten on the anterior wall of the prosthesis. It provides rotational control and minimizes lateral socket shift with less weight and bulk compared to the combined pelvic band and hip joint.

○ **What is a supracondylar cuff system of suspension?**

The supracondylar cuff strap fits just above the patient's femoral condyles and patella. Tabs attach it to the sides of the prosthesis. It secures the prosthesis during the swing phase and when it is unsupported during knee flexion such as when the patient is sitting on a high stool.

○ **What is a fork strap suspension system?**

A fork strap attached to a waist belt can be used as an additional suspension, in situations where circumferential straps or sleeves are contraindicated or not tolerated. Extension assist is provided when a portion of the strap is elasticized and fastened under tension. It is forked to pass on either side of the patella, to minimize patellar compression when the person sits.

○ **What is the 3S suspension system?**

The polyurethane and silicon gel roll on suction suspension systems (3S) are commonly used with the total contact socket design, since the gel tends to act as a fluid and flows to equalize pressure within the socket.

○ **What kind of prosthetic joints are available in the LE amputee?**

Prosthetic joints are available to replace the loss of anatomic joints at the hip, knee, and ankle. Rotational units, derotational units, and quick-release units are available. Orthotic joints are often modified and incorporated into the prosthetic design to provide additional stability across the remaining joints. Instability may be due to ligamentous factors, weakness, or a short lever arm from a short residual limb. Supplemental orthotic knee joints are used most frequently, followed by hip joints.

○ **What is the function of prosthetic knee joints?**

The prosthetic knee has three functions: support during the stance phase, smooth control during the swing phase, and unrestricted flexion for sitting and kneeling. In the swing phase, the knee controls the speed and timing of knee flexion and extension.

○ **What are the two basic designs of prosthetic knees?**

There are two basic designs of prosthetic knees: the single axis and the polycentric axis. The single axis system involves a simple hinge with a single pivot point. The polycentric axis knee joint is designed to have continually changing instantaneous centers of rotation to mimic human knee function.

○ **What is the polycentric axis knee joint?**

The polycentric axis knee joint is normally designed so that the initial instantaneous center of rotation is posterior to the patient's weight line. This allows the ground force reaction to be anterior to the center of rotation, creating a high degree of knee stability during the stance phase of gait.

○ **What is the single axis foot?**

The single-axis foot controls passive plantarflexion and dorsiflexion by the use of multidurometer rubber bumpers and a single-axis joint. Changing the bumpers determines how fast the forefoot contacts the ground. The faster the forefoot touches the ground, the sooner the ground force reaction line proceeds in front of the knee center of rotation to create a stabilizing extension moment. Stance phase stability is excellent, making this a good choice for the sedentary person who has had an AK amputation.

○   **What is the multi axis foot?**

The multi axis foot is designed to incorporate ankle and foot motions to mimic plantarflexion, dorsiflexion, inversion, eversion, and rotation. Ball and socket joints, U joints, steel tendons, and rubber and polymer bumpers have been utilized to create motion in all three planes. Statically, it may not feel as stable as the single-axis foot. Dynamically, it can reduce shear forces, absorb shock, and adjust to uneven terrain. It is a good choice for the active person who has had an AK or BK amputation and walks on uneven surfaces or needs to control torque and shear over scarred tissue or a bony prominence. The multi axis foot is a good choice for the sedentary to moderately active person who has had an AK or BK amputation.

○   **Compare and contrast the different prosthetic knee joints**

KNEE	INDICATIONS	CONTRA-INDICATIONS	ACTION	STABILITY	ADVANTAGES	DISADVANTAGES
Single-axis constant friction knee	1. Previous user 2. Good hip extensors 3. Long residual limb	1. Weak hip extensors 2. Hip flexion contracture 3. Patient with variable cadence	1. Constant friction 2. Extension aid (optional)	1. TKA alignment 2. Voluntary control (contraction of hip extensors)	1. Low cost 2. Simple design 3. Lightweight 4. Easy to maintain	1. Not cadence responsive (excessive heel rise and terminal impact with increased cadence)
Weight-activated stance-control knee (safety knee)	1. Short residual limb 2. Weak hip extensors 3. Hip flexion contracture 4. Insecure patient (poor balance)	1. Patient with variable cadence 2. Bilateral AK amputation	1. Constant friction in swing 2. Extension aid 3. Weight-activated brake in stance	1. Inherent in stance control 2. TKA alignment 3. Voluntary control (contraction of hip extensors)	1. Increased knee stability even with knee flexed up to 15 degrees	1. Maintenance and noise 2. Increased weight 3. Difficulty in jackknifing on stairs
Polycentric knee (most often 4-bar)	1. Knee disarticulation 2. Weak hip extensors 3. Short residual limb 4. Need for increased stance stability		1. Constant friction, pneumatic, and hydraulic models 2. Inherent shorting of shank in swing phase	1. Instantaneous knee center posterior to GFR line at full extension 2. TKA alignment	1. Shank swings under residual limb in knee disarticulation 2. Good stability	1. Weight (in some older models)
Pneumatic swing-phase control	1. Patient with variable cadence	1. Very active person 2. Inactive, limited ambulation	1. Piston travels in a cylinder forcing air through an adjustable valve, creating resistance 2. Air compressing can act as extension aid	1. TKA alignment 2. 4-bar knee models	1. Simpler, lighter, and less cost than hydraulic	1. Patient can overpower unit due to Air compressing. 2. Weight, maintenance, cost
Hydraulic swing-phase control	1. Patient with variable cadence 2. Medium to long residual limb length 3. Very active	1. Inactive patient	1. Piston travels in a cylinder, forcing a fluid through a set of	1. TKA alignment 2. Voluntary control (contraction of hip extensors)	1. Excellent cadence response 2. Patient with SNS model can descend stairs step	1. Weight 2. Cost and maintenance

patient	orifices and adjustable valves	3. Hydraulic stance-phase control in SNS models		over step and down hills	

○ What is the choke syndrome?

Choke syndrome is a swelling of the tissues that occurs when there is obstruction of venous outflow proximal to a potential space in the prosthetic socket into which the residual limb tissue can swell. Because arterial inflow is unimpeded and outflow is restricted, fluid accumulates in the area of inadequate contact. The obstruction to venous outflow is usually caused by tight proximal contact of the socket with the residual limb Weight gain, edema from trauma or a medical condition, socks with too many plies, and do it yourself prosthetic modifications are the most frequent causes.

○ Compare and contrast the different prosthetic feet available for the LE amputee

FEET	INDICATIONS	CONTRAINDICATIONS	ACTION	ADVANTAGES	DISADVANTAGES
SACH	1. Limited ambulation, such as transfer only 2. Patient with limited funding	1. Active patient	1. Plantarflexion simulated by compression of heel wedge	1. Moderate weight 2. Good durability 3. No moving parts 4. Minimal maintenance	1. Limited plantarflexion and dorsiflexion 2. Heel cushion deteriorates over time 3. Rigid forefoot provides poor shock absorption
Single axis	1. Short AK residual limb	1. Weight of foot 2. Plantarflexion can cause knee hyperextension at heel strike.	1. Plantarflexion simulated by compression of heel bumper and joint	1. Increased knee stability; plantar-flexion reduces knee flexion moment at heel strike 2. Plantarflexion resistance is adjustable	1. High maintenance 2. Increased weight 3. Noise from bumpers
Multi-Axis	1. Uneven terrain 2. Residual limb with scars	1. Patient cannot tolerate added weight 2. Patient does not have access to maintenance	1. Provides motion in all three planes	1. Reduces torque on residual limb 2. Adjustability 3. Good shock absorption	1. Increased weight 2. Increased maintenance and noise
Dynamic response	1. Very active patient	1. Patient relies heavily on an ambulation aid	1. The keel of foot acts like a spring compressing in stance phase (storing energy) and rebounding at toe off (push off)	1. Reduces force at heel strike on contralateral side 2. Some designs are very lightweight	1. High cost

○ What are the features of an acute choke syndrome?

An acute choke syndrome is recognized by indurated red tissues that may have an orange-peel appearance, prominent skin pores, and skin changes that appear eczematous with open or weeping skin blisters may be present, especially on old scars. The skin eventually may macerate and leave an open, superficial ulcer if the constriction is allowed to continue. Pain may be the major complaint, especially after the prosthesis has been off for a brief time. The presence of choke syndrome does not exclude the possibility of a superimposed infection or carcinoma. Increased warmth, proximal advancement of the erythema, diffuse redness, foul odor, purulence, and constitutional symptoms suggest infection.

O   **What features characterize the chronic choke syndrome?**

As the choke syndrome becomes chronic, the skin may take on a verrucose appearance with serous crusting. In the case of a chronic choke syndrome, the skin color may become brownish-orange from deposition of hemosiderin pigment in the skin. This latter change is a permanent condition. Venous stasis ulceration from the chronic venous hypertension can occur.

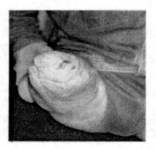

O   **What are the most common dermatological problems in the LE amputee?**

Dermatologic problems occur in about one third of **amputees** wearing prostheses and are responsible for significant impairment of function. Several easily recognizable patterns of physical dermatosis resulting from suboptimal prosthesis fit are predominant. Acute contact dermatitis (ACD) is common, and some patients with stump dermatitis may require patch testing. A thorough history is essential in uncovering relevant positive reactions.

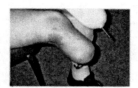

O   **Where are sebaceous (epidermoid) cysts likely to occur in the LE amputee?**

Folliculitis and sebaceous cyst formation are found in areas of increased repeated shear or excessive weightbearing contact Excessive sweating and poor hygiene can exacerbate this The medial tibial flare, popliteal fossa, and groin are common areas of involvement.

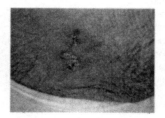

ORTHOTICS

O   **What is the difference between static and dynamic orthosis?**

Static orthoses: As the word static implies, these devices do not allow motion. They serve as a rigid support in fractures, inflammatory conditions of tendons and soft tissue, and nerve injuries.

Dynamic/functional orthoses: In contrast to static orthoses, these devices do permit motion on which its own effectiveness depends. These types of upper extremity orthoses are used primarily to assist movement of weak muscles.

O   What are the functions of upper extremity orthoses?

Increase range of motion (ROM).
Immobilize an extremity to help promote tissue healing.
Apply traction either to correct or prevent contractures.
Assist in providing enhanced function.
Serve as an attachment for assistive devices.
Help correct deformities.
Block unwanted movement of a joint.

O   What is the static wrist hand orthosis (WHO)?

The static wrist-hand orthosis supports the wrist joint, maintains the functional architecture of the hand, and prevents wrist hand deformities. Occasionally the static wrist hand orthosis is used as a platform for other therapeutic attachments (e.g., MCP extension stop, IP extension assist, thumb extension assist).

O   What are common attachments used in the static WHO?

Two of the most common attachments used with the static wrist-hand orthosis are the MCP extension stop and the IP extension assist. If there is a loss of range in flexion at the MCP joints and a loss of range in extension at the proximal IP joints, then these two attachments can help prevent a claw hand deformity by preventing hyperextension of the MCP joints while simultaneously encouraging extension of the IP joints of the second through fifth fingers.

O   What is a swivel thumb?

The thumb can be maintained in opposition with a limited range of motion by the addition of a "swivel thumb". The swivel thumb acts as a carpal metacarpal (CM) abduction/flexion assist for the thumb and consists of a custom-contoured metal band over the proximal phalanx of the thumb that is secured to the radial extension of the palmar piece with a simple cantilevered wire spring.

O   What are elbow orthosis often used for?

Elbow orthoses designed for reducing soft-tissue contracture must be custom-designed and fabricated with structural plastic (e.g., polypropylene) bands, totally contacting flexible plastic (e.g., polyethylene) cuffs and straps, and incorporate at least one of a variety of mechanisms for increasing the range of motion.

O   What is the gunslinger?

It is a dynamic arm and shoulder support called the *gunslinger*. The patient's arm is strapped to a forearm trough, which is mechanically coupled to a plastic interface anchored on the patient's pelvis (iliac crest). The coupling between the forearm trough and iliac cap can be customized to permit a variety of motions including internal and external rotation, flexion extension, and horizontal flexion and extension at the glenohumeral joint, and flexion and extension at the elbow joint. The arm and hand are held in a cosmetically pleasing pose, and the hand is available for use, enabling early recovery while allowing limited functional activities.

O   Which patient population can benefit form the gunslinger?

The patient with an injured brachial plexus can benefit from the application of the gunslinger shoulder elbow orthosis both for the prevention of further stretch injury during the healing process and for positioning of the hand in a useful location for functional activities.

O   **What is an airplane splint?**

This shoulder-elbow-wrist orthosis transmits the weight of the upper limb to the ipsilateral side of the pelvis and the system is stabilized with trunk straps. This type of shoulder-elbow-wrist orthosis is often used for patients with an axillary burn, the objective being to provide as much contact as possible while keeping the glenohumeral joint in maximum abduction. The anatomic elbow joint may be restricted or left with free motion. Generally, the wrist is supported in extension to protect the associated soft tissues against the forces of gravity.

O   **What are the indications for an airplane splint?**

The airplane shoulder-elbow-wrist orthosis is an excellent orthosis to prescribe after rotator cuff repairs, after anterior or posterior capsular repairs, after manipulation, and in conjunction with Bankart procedures. This orthosis is also frequently prescribed for axillary burns to prevent contracture, and alternatively, to help reduce soft tissue contractures resulting from a variety of causes (e.g., long-term immobility).

O   **What is the ratchet-hand orthosis?**

The ratchet wrist hand orthosis is a functional prehension orthosis that enables the patient to grasp and release objects by utilizing external power The ratchet wrist-hand orthosis is manually controlled and substitutes for finger flexor and extensor muscles that are less than grade 3 (fair) in strength. The wrist is stabilized for function, but the position can be changed for different activities.

O   **What is the unique feature of the ratchet system?**

A ratchet system is employed so that the hand can be closed in discrete increments. Pinch is achieved by applying distally directed force on the proximal end of the ratchet bar (black knob) or by using the patient's own chin, other arm, or any stationary object to flex the second and third fingers toward the thumb to form a three-jaw chuck.

O   **Which patients are candidates for the ratchet WHO?**

The ratchet wrist hand orthosis is appropriate for patients with paralysis or severe weakness of the hand and wrist musculature. Some functional proximal strength is required to use the ratchet wrist hand orthosis For optimal use the patient should have at least grade 3+ (fair+) strength in shoulder flexion, abduction, external rotation, and internal rotation.

O   **What is the wrist driven wrist hand orthosis?**

The wrist driven wrist hand orthosis (flexor hinge wrist hand orthosis) is a dynamic prehension orthosis utilizing a transfer of power from the wrist extensors to the fingers. Active wrist extension provides grasp and gravity assisted wrist flexion enables the patient to open the hand.

O   **Which patients are candidates for the wrist driven WHO?**

The wrist driven wrist-hand orthosis is an appropriate orthosis for the patient with paralysis or severe weakness of the hand. Wrist extensor strength must be at least grade 3+ (fair+) and proximal strength must be functional. For patients with wrist extensor strength of less than grade 3+ who are improving or with grade 3+ (fair+) strength with poor endurance, a rubber band wrist extension assist is indicated. Candidates for the wrist driven wrist hand orthosis are patients with C5 functional level with some return of C6 functional level (wrist extensors), C6, or C7 tetraplegia. By using active wrist extension, a patient can achieve functional three-point pinch.

O   **What are mobile arm supports?**

Mobile arm support (MAS) is a shoulder-elbow orthosis that supports the weight of the arm and provides assistance to the shoulder and elbow motions through a linkage of mechanical joints. This orthosis performs a wide range of useful purposes.

O   **What are the basic components of a MAS?**

The basic components of the MAS are the wheelchair mounting bracket, the proximal arm, the distal arm, and the forearm trough. The elevating proximal arm is an available option with an elevating feature to counterbalance the weight of the patient's. In addition, an optional standard wheelchair mounting upper bracket is available with a pivot type of adjustment for tilting the axis of the proximal arm.

○   Which patients are candidates for an MAS?

The MAS can increase upper-limb function for patients who have severe arm paralysis due to such disabilities as muscular dystrophy, poliomyelitis, cervical spinal cord lesion, Guillain Barré syndrome, and amyotrophic lateral sclerosis. Patients should have sufficient muscle weakness or limited endurance to warrant use of the support.

○   What muscle groups allow the MAS to function?

The patient must have adequate muscular strength to move the MAS. The neck, trunk, shoulder girdle, shoulder, and elbow may serve alone or in combination as power sources. The deltoid, elbow flexors, and external rotators are the most significant muscles to evaluate because of their importance in arm function.

○   What are the criteria for MAS use?

1.   Absent or weak elbow flexion (poor to fair).
2.   Absent or weak shoulder flexion and abduction (poor to fair).
3.   Absent or weak external rotation (poor to fair).
4.   Limited endurance for sustained upper limb activity.

○   What is the Long opponens thumb spica splint?

The splint covers two thirds of the distal radial forearm up to the interphalangeal (IP) joint of the thumb.
The wrist should be placed in 15-30° of dorsiflexion while maintaining motion of digits 2-5.
The thumb should be maintained in an abducted position to achieve a 3-point jaw chuck prehension.

○   What are the indications for this orthosis?

1.   Used for maintaining the thumb ROM in patients who have had burns.
2.   Used to restrict motion in patients with arthritis.
3.   Used for serial static stretching, such as in contractures and burns.
4.   Used to stabilize the thumb in opposition for 3-point chuck pinch in patients with peripheral nerve, cerebrovascular diseases, C5 level of SCI, and other upper motor neuron lesions.
5.   Used in patients who have had tendon transfers/repairs, arthroplasty, and DeQuervain tenosynovitis.

○   What is the PIP orthosis?

The proximal interphalangeal (PIP) orthosis is used to immobilize the PIP joint hyperflexion deformities in patients with Boutonniere deformities or to prevent hyperextension of the PIP joint in swan-neck deformities, both of which are found in patients with rheumatoid arthritis.

○   What is the DIP orthosis?

The distal interphalangeal (DIP) orthosis is used to immobilize the DIP joints in extensor tendon and collateral ligament repairs.

○   What is the MP orthosis?

The MP orthosis is used to maintain a functional position for the distal phalanges, while preventing hyperextension of the MP joints These devices are used in patients with burns, scleroderma, or nerve injuries.

○   What is the static thumb orthosis (short opponens)?

The static thumb orthosis is used to support the carpometacarpal joint, the interphalangeal joint, or the metacarpophalangeal joint in patients with traumatic or arthritic conditions, and in patients with thenar muscle weakness by providing static support for the thumb.

O   **What are dynamic hand orthoses?**

Dynamic hand orthoses are used to maintain support, while at the same time to provide dynamic corrective force in positioning the fingers, assisting weak motor finger extensor function. These devices are used with outrigger supports, cuffs, elastic threads, rubber bands, and hook applications for their function of providing dynamic assistance.

O   **What is the MP joint dynamic orthosis?**

The MP joint dynamic orthosis is used to assist with flexion of the DIP joint in swan-neck deformities and to act as a substitute for weakness of the flexor digitorum superficialis muscle. The MP joint dynamic orthosis also can be used in correcting or maintaining contractures of the MP joints The MP extension splint has the same mechanism as the MP flexion splint; however, it is placed on the dorsal side and serves mainly as a splint in patients with weak wrist extensors and for traction of MP flexion contractures.

O   **What are dynamic PIP orthoses used for?**

A dynamic PIP joint extension with MP extension stop device is comprised of a bar placed across the dorsum of the hand and is used in patients with ulnar nerve palsy with claw hand deformity by allowing extension while resisting flexor deformity pull.

O   **What are thumb PIP orthoses used for?**

A thumb interphalangeal dynamic orthosis is used to assist in interphalangeal joint extension of the thumb, while maintaining the position of the other hand joints. This device is used to substitute for weakness of the extensor pollicis longus muscle.

O   **What are dynamic WHO used for?**

A reciprocal wrist-extension finger-flexion orthosis is used in patients with C6 tetraplegia who, given their level of injury, can extend their wrists but cannot flex their fingers. By using the wrist extension force, finger flexion at the MP joints of the second and third digits is attained. Wrist extension is used to flex the MP joints of digits 2 and 3 through tenodesis Preservation of extensor carpi radialis longus and brevis normally is observed in C6 level SCI. Use of this device allows for a 3-point pinch.

O   **What is the soft collar?**

The soft collar is a common orthotic device made of lightweight material, polyurethane foam rubber, with a stockinette cover. It has Velcro closure strap for easy donning and doffing. Patients find the collar comfortable to wear, but it is soiled easily with long-term use.

O   **What are the indications and benefits of the soft collar for the patient?**

Warmth
Psychological comfort
Support to the head during acute neck pain
Relief with minor muscle spasm associated with spondylolysis
Relief in cervical strains

O   **Does the soft cervical collar provide restrictions of motion?**

Limits full flexion and extension by 5°
Limits full lateral bending by 5°

Limits full rotation by 10°	

○   **What are hard cervical collars (HCO)?**

The hard cervical collars are similar in shape to a soft collar but are made of Plastizote, a rigid polyethylene material shaped like a ring with padding. Height can be adjusted in certain designs to fit patients better Velcro straps are used for easy donning and doffing. The hard collar is more durable than a soft collar with long-term use. Several problems can be alleviated with use of a hard collar.

○   **What are indications for hard cervical collars?**

Support to the head during acute neck pain
Relief of minor muscle spasm associated with spondylosis
Psychological comfort
Interim stability and protection during halo application

○   **What are the motion restrictions for the hard cervical collars?**

Limits full flexion and extension by 20-25%
Less effective in restricting rotation and lateral bending
Better than a soft collar in motion restriction

○   **What is the Philadelphia collar?**

The Philadelphia collar is a semirigid HCO with a 2-piece system of Plastizote foam. Plastic struts on the anterior and posterior sides are used for support. The upper portion of the orthosis supports the lower jaw and occiput, while the lower portion covers the upper thoracic region. The Philadelphia collar comes in various sizes and is comfortable to wear, improving patient compliance. Velcro straps are used for easy donning and doffing. The Philadelphia collar is difficult to clean and becomes soiled very easily. An anterior hole for a tracheostomy is available. A thoracic extension can be added to increase motion restriction and treat C6-T2 injuries.

○   **What are the motion restrictions provided by this collar?**

Limits flexion and extension by 65°
Limits rotation by 60°
Limits lateral bending by 30°

○   **What are the indications for this collar?**

Anterior cervical fusion
Halo removal
Dens type I cervical fracture of C2
Anterior diskectomy
Suspected cervical trauma in unconscious patients
Tear drop fracture of the vertebral body (Note: Some teardrop fractures require anterior decompression and fusion.)
Cervical strain

○   **What is the Miami J collar?**

The Miami J collar is another cervical orthotic device in common use. The Miami J collar has a 2-piece system made of polyethylene and a soft washable lining. The anterior piece has a tracheostomy opening similar to that in the Philadelphia collar. Velcro straps provide easy donning and doffing. The Miami J collar is a semi-rigid HCO. A thoracic extension can be added to increase support and treat C6-T2 injuries The Miami J collar is available in various sizes and can be heated and molded to a contoured fit.

○   **What motion restrictions does it provide?**

| Limits flexion and extension by 55-75% |
| Limits rotation by 70% |
| Limits lateral bending by 60% |

○   **What are the indications for the Miami J collar?**

Indications for use of a Miami J collar are the same as the Philadelphia collar.

○   **What is the Malibu collar?**

The Malibu collar is similar to the Philadelphia collar as it is a semi-rigid orthosis designed in a 2-piece system with an anterior opening for a tracheostomy. The Malibu collar comes in only one size, but it is adjustable in multiple planes to ensure proper fit. Anterior chin support height is also adjustable. Straps around the chin, occiput, and lower cervical area provide for tightening. Padding around the chin can be trimmed to ensure proper fit Thoracic extension can be added to increase support and treat C6-T2 injuries.

○   **What motion restrictions does it provide?**

| Limits flexion and extension by 55-60% |
| Limits rotation by 60% |
| Limits lateral bending by 60% |

○   **What are the indications for the use of a Malibu collar?**

Indications for use of a Malibu collar are similar to those for the Miami J and Philadelphia collars.

○   **What is the Aspen collar?**

The Aspen Collar has a 2-piece system made of polyethylene with soft foam liner with an anterior opening for a tracheostomy. The Aspen collar is a semi-rigid HCO with Velcro straps for easy donning and doffing.

○   **What motion restrictions are provided by this collar?**

| Limits flexion and extension by 55-60% |
| Limits rotation by 60% |
| Limits lateral bending by 60% |

○   **What are the indications for this collar?**

Indications for use of the Aspen collar include the same as the orthoses discussed above.

○   **What is the SOMI?**

The Sternal Occipital Mandibular Immobilizer (SOMI) is a rigid three-poster CTO with anterior chest plate that extends to the xiphoid process and has metal or plastic bars that curve over the shoulder Straps from the metal bars go over the shoulder and cross to the opposite side of the anterior plate for fixation. A removable chin piece attaches to the chest plate with an optional headpiece that can be used when the chin piece is removed for eating. The two-poster CTOs start from the chest plate and attach to the occipital component.

○   **What are the indications for the SOMI?**

The SOMI is ideal for bedridden patients since it has no posterior rods. It is indicated for immobilization in atlantoaxial instability because of rheumatoid arthritis and immobilization for neural arch fractures of C2 since flexion causes instability

○   **What are the motion restrictions provided by the SOMI?**

Proper adjustment is crucial for motion restriction; in fact, motion restriction may be compromised with incorrect application. The SOMI is less effective compared to other braces in controlling extension, but it is very effective in controlling flexion at the atlantoaxial and C2-C3 segments. The SOMI is better than the cervicothoracic brace in controlling flexion in the C1-C3 segments. It limits cervical flexion and extension by 70%-75%, limits lateral bending by 35% and limits rotation by 60-65%.

○   **What is the Yale orthosis?**

The Yale orthosis is a modified Philadelphia collar with thoracic extension made of fiberglass extending anteriorly and posteriorly with mid-thoracic straps on the sides connecting the two thoracic extensions. The thoracic component helps to treat C6-T2 injuries. The occipital piece extends higher up on the skull posteriorly. Increased contact surface area improves stability of the brace. Patients find the Yale orthosis comfortable to wear.

○   **What are the indications for this orthosis?**

Immobilization to C1 fractures with intact transverse ligament
Immobilization after surgical fixation of Dens Type III fractures
Immobilization to Dens type I fractures
Immobilization to Hangman fractures (traumatic spondylolisthesis of C2)
Immobilization to Jefferson fractures (multiple fractures of C1 ring with spreading due to axial loading)
Provide immobilization to postoperative fixation

○   **What motion is restricted by this orthosis?**

Limits flexion and extension by 85%
Limits rotation by 70% to 75%
Limits lateral bending by 60%

○   **What is the four poster brace?**

The four-poster brace is a rigid orthosis with anterior and posterior chest pads connected by a leather strap Molded occipital and mandibular support pieces connect to the chest pads and have adjustable struts. Straps connect the occipital and mandibular support pieces. The mandibular plate can interfere with eating. This brace uses shoulder straps, but it has no underarm support. Open design allows heat loss from the neck. The brace is as effective as the cervicothoracic brace in controlling flexion in the mid-cervical area and is better than the Philadelphia collar. The four-poster design limits lateral bending and rotation better than the two poster brace.

○   **What are the motion restrictions provided by this brace?**

Motion restrictions provided by the four-poster orthosis include the following:

Limits flexion and extension by 80%
Limits lateral bending by 55%-80%
Limits rotation by 70%

○   **What is the Guilford brace?**

The Guilford brace is a rigid CTO with a two-poster design with anterior chest plate and shoulder straps that connect to the posterior plate. Chin plate and occipital piece connect to the anterior and posterior struts. Underarm straps circle the lower chest wall for stability. The brace has poor control of flexion, extension, rotation, and lateral bending at C1-C2.

○   **What are its motion restrictions?**

Motion restrictions afforded by the Guilford brace include limitation of flexion and extension from C3-T2.

O   **What are the indications for this orthosis?**

1   Immobilization to minimally unstable fractures from C3-T2
2.   Immobilization after postoperative internal fixation from C3-T2

O   **What is the Halo device?**

The halo device is the most common device for treatment of unstable cervical and upper thoracic fractures and dislocations as low as T3. The halo provides maximum motion restriction of all cervical orthotics. The halo ring is made of graphite or metal with pin fixation on the frontal and parietal occipital areas of the skull. Development of lightweight composite material led to design of radiolucent rings compatible with magnetic resonance imaging (MRI). The halo ring attaches to the vest anteriorly and posteriorly via four posters The halo vest has shoulder and underarm straps for tightening and usually is made of rigid polyethylene and extends down to the umbilicus.

O   **What are the limitations of the HALO device?**

Restriction in cervical motion depends on the fit of the halo vest since improper fit can allow 31% of normal spine motion. The halo vest is the weak link in terms of motion control. Compressive and distractive force can occur with variable fit of the vest. Multidirectional shear forces can cause increased pinhole size with crater like enlargement. Pin loosening occurs twice as frequently with a heavier halo vest. Generally, upper cervical spine injuries are treated best with a full-length vest to the iliac crest.

O   **What are the indications for the Halo vest?**

Dens type I, II, and III fractures of C2 (Note: Dens type III fractures of C2 are treated more successfully with surgery.)
C1 fractures with rupture of the transverse ligament
Atlantoaxial instability from rheumatoid arthritis with ligamentous disruption and erosion of the dens
C2 neural arch fracture and disc disruption between C2 and C3 (Note: Some patients may need surgery for stabilization.)
Bony single column cervical fractures
Following cervical arthrodesis
Following cervical tumor resection in an unstable spine
Following debridement and drainage of infection in an unstable spine
Following spinal cord injury (SCI)

O   **What are the contraindications for the halo vest?**

1.   Concomitant skull fracture with cervical injury
2.   Damaged or infected skin over pin insertion sites

O   **What are the relative contraindications for the halo vest?**

1.   Cervical instability with ligamentous disruption
2.   Cervical instability with 2 or 3 column injury
3.   Cervical instability with rotational injury involving facet joints

O   **What are the pin settings in the adult and child?**

In adults, pin insertion requires a torque wrench set at 8 inches per pound since this lowers incidence of pin infection and loosening. In children, set the torque wrench between 2-5 inches per pound since the skull is too weak to sustain heavier forces. Use multiple pin sites in children because of the weaker skull.

O   **What motion restrictions are provided by the halo vest?**

Limits flexion and extension by 90
Limits lateral bending by 92
Limits rotation by 98

O **What complications occur with halo placement?**

Neck pain or stiffness 80%
Pin loosening 60%
Pin site infection 22%
Scars 30%
Pain at pin sites 18%
Pressure sores 11%
Redislocation 10%
Restricted ventilation 8%
Dysphagia 2%
Nerve injury 2%
Dural puncture 1%
Neurological deterioration 1%
Avascular necrosis of the dens
Ring migration

O **What are the strengths and limitations of the different cervical devices on immobilization of the cervical spine?**

All orthotics tend to control flexion better than extension.
The halo is the most effective in controlling flexion and extension at C1-C3, followed by the four-poster brace, and then the cervicothoracic orthotics.
The cervicothoracic orthotics are best at controlling flexion and extension at C3-T1, while the SOMI brace is best at controlling flexion from C1-C5.
The SOMI is less effective in controlling extension compared to other orthotics.
The halo is the best at controlling rotation and lateral bending from C1-C3.
The cervicothoracic brace is second best at controlling rotation and lateral bending in the cervical spine.
The four-poster brace is slightly better at controlling lateral bending compared to the cervicothoracic brace in the cervical spine.

O **What is the CASH brace?**

The cruciform anterior spinal hyperextension (CASH) brace features anterior sternal and pubic pads to produce force opposed by the posterior pad and strap around the thoracolumbar region. Sternal and pelvic pads attach to the anterior metal cross shaped bar, which can be bent to reduce excess pressure on the chest and pelvis. The brace is easy to don and doff, but it is difficult to adjust. Compared to the Jewett brace, it provides greater breast and axillary pressure relief. Two round upper chest pads can be used instead of the sternal pad to decrease discomfort around the breast area.

O **What are the indications for the CASH brace?**

1. Flexion immobilization to treat thoracic and lumbar vertebral body fractures
2. Reduction of kyphosis in patients with osteoporosis

O **What are the motion restrictions provided by the CASH brace?**

1. Limits flexion and extension from T6-L1
2. Ineffective in limiting lateral bending and rotation of the upper lumbar spine

O **What are the contraindications for the CASH brace?**

1) Three-column spine fractures involving anterior, middle, and posterior spinal structures

2) Compression fractures due to osteoporosis

O   **What is the Jewett hyperextension brace?**

The Jewett hyperextension brace employs a 3-point pressure system with 1 posterior and 2 anterior pads. The anterior pads place pressure over the sternum and pubic symphysis. The posterior pad places opposing pressure in the mid-thoracic region. The posterior pad keeps the spine in an extended position, and it has a lightweight design that is more comfortable than the CASH brace. Pelvic and sternal pads can be adjusted from the lateral axillary bar where they attach. The pads can cause discomfort from pressure applied to small surface area. No abdominal support is provided with this device. When the patient is seated, the sternal pad should be half an inch inferior to the sternal notch, and the pubic pad should be half an inch superior to the pubic symphysis.

O   **What are the indications for the Jewett brace?**

1.   Symptomatic relief of compression fractures not due to osteoporosis
2.   Immobilization after surgical stabilization of thoracolumbar fractures

O   **What motion restrictions are provided by the Jewett brace?**

1.   Limits flexion and extension between T6-L1
2.   Ineffective in limiting lateral bending and rotation of the upper lumbar spine

O   **What are contraindications to the Jewett brace?**

Three column spine fractures involving anterior, middle, and posterior spinal structures
Compression fractures above T6 since segmental motion increases above the sternal pad
Compression fractures due to osteoporosis

O   **What is the Knight Taylor brace?**

The Knight Taylor brace features a corset type front with lateral and posterior uprights and shoulder straps to help reduce lateral bending, flexion, and extension. Shoulder straps may cause discomfort in some patients. The brace can be prefabricated and made with polyvinyl chloride or aluminum the posterior portion of the brace has added cross supports below the inferior angle of the scapula and a pelvic band fitted at the sacrococcygeal junction. The anterior corset is made of canvas and provides intracavitary pressure. The anterior corset is laced to the lateral uprights The brace is indicated to provide flexion immobilization to treat thoracic and lumbar vertebral body fractures.

O   **What are the motion restrictions of the Knight Taylor brace?**

1.   Poor rotation control
2.   Limits flexion, extension, and lateral bending

O   **What is the custom molded TLSO?**

Custom molded plastic body jacket, or thoracolumbosacral orthosis (TLSO), is fabricated from polypropylene or plastic, offers best control in all planes of motion, and increases intracavitary pressure. This orthosis has a lightweight design and is easy to don and doff. The material is easy to clean and comfortable to wear. This brace sometimes is referred to as the clamshell. The TLSO provides efficient force transmission as pressure is distributed over wide surface area, which is ideal for use in patients with neurologic injuries. The brace may have a tendency to ride up on the patient in a supine position. Plastic retains heat, so an undershirt helps to absorb perspiration and protect the skin. Frequent checks to ensure proper fit help prevent pressure ulcers. Velcro straps are used to tighten the brace.

O   **What are the indications for a TLSO?**

Immobilization for compression fractures from osteoporosis
Immobilization after surgical stabilization for spinal fractures

Bracing for idiopathic scoliosis
Immobilization for unstable spinal disorders for T3 to L3

○ **What are the motion restrictions for a custom molded TLSO?**

Limits sidebending
Limits flexion and extension
Limits rotation to some extent

○ **Can the TLSO be used for idiopathic scoliosis management?**

Clinical information on the custom molded TLSO suggests that it is more effective in preventing idiopathic scoliosis curve progression than the Milwaukee and Charleston braces. The mean curve progression with TLSO is less than 2 degrees while the Charleston and Milwaukee braces have a curve progression greater than 6 degrees. Fewer than 18% of patients treated with TLSO brace required surgery for scoliosis compared to 23% for patients treated with a Milwaukee brace.

○ **What is the chair back brace?**

The chairback brace is a rigid short lumbosacral orthotic (LSO) with 2 posterior uprights with thoracic and pelvic bands. The abdominal apron has straps in front for adjustment to increase intracavitary pressure. The thoracic band is located 1 inch below the inferior angle of scapula. The thoracic band extends laterally to the mid-axillary line, and the pelvic band extends laterally to the mid-trochanteric line. Place the pelvic band as low as possible without interfering with sitting comfort. Position the posterior uprights over the paraspinal muscles. Uprights can be made from metal or plastic The brace employs a 3 point pressure system and can be custom molded to improve the fit for each individual patient.

○ **What are the indications for the chair back brace?**

Unloading of the intervertebral discs and transmit pressure to soft tissue areas
Relief for low back pain (LBP)
Immobilization after lumbar laminectomy
Kinesthetic reminder to patient following surgery

○ **What are the motion restrictions for the chair back brace?**

Limits flexion and extension at the L1-L4 level
Limits rotation minimally
Limits lateral bending by 45% in the thoracolumbar spine

○ **What is the Williams brace?**

The Williams brace is a short LSO with an anterior elastic apron to allow for forward flexion. Lateral uprights attach to the thoracic band, and oblique bars are used to connect the pelvic band to the lateral uprights. The abdominal apron is laced to the lateral uprights. The brace limits extension and lateral trunk movement but allows forward flexion. The brace is indicated to provide motion restriction during extension to treat spondylolysis and spondylolisthesis The device is contraindicated in spinal compression fractures.

○ **What are the motion restrictions of the Williams Brace?**

1. Limits extension
2. Limits side bending at terminal ends only

○ **What is the standard LSO corset?**

The Standard LSO corset has metal bars within the cloth material posteriorly that can be removed and adjusted to fit the patient. The anterior abdominal apron has pull-up laces from the back to tighten. The abdominal apron can come with

Velcro closure for easy donning and doffing. The Standard LSO corset has a lightweight design and is comfortable to wear. The corset increases intracavitary pressure. Anteriorly, the brace covers the area between the xiphoid process and pubic symphysis. Posteriorly, the brace covers the area between the lower scapula and gluteal fold.

O   **What are the indications for the standard LSO?**

1.   Treatment of LBP
2.   Immobilization after lumbar laminectomy

O   **What pattern of motion restrictions are provided by the standard LSO?**

Motion restrictions of the Standard LSO corset include limitation of flexion and extension.

O   **What is the rigid LSO?**

The rigid LSO is a custom-made orthosis molded over the iliac crest for improved fit. Plastic anterior and posterior shells overlap for a tight fit. Velcro closure in the front is designed for easy donning and doffing. Multiple holes can be made for aeration to help decrease moisture and limit skin maceration. The rigid LSO can be trimmed easily to make adjustments for patient comfort and may be used in the shower if needed.

O   **What are the indications for the rigid LSO?**

1.   Post-surgical lumbar immobilization
2.   Treatment of lumbar compression fractures

O   **What are the motion restrictions for the rigid LSO?**

1.   Limits flexion and extension
2.   Limits some rotation and side bending

O   **What are the features of a hip spica?**

Rigid LSO with hip spica uses a thigh piece on the symptomatic side and extends to 5 cm above the patella. The hip is held in 20 degrees of flexion to allow sitting and walking. Some patients require a cane for ambulation after application.

O   **What are the indications for a hip spica?**

1.   Immobilization to treat lumbar instability from L3-S1
2.   Immobilization after lumbosacral fusion with anchoring to the sacrum

O   **What are the motion restrictions imposed by the hip spica?**

1.   Limits flexion and extension
2.   Limits some rotation and side bending

O   **What is the Milwaukee brace?**

The Milwaukee brace is a CTLSO originally designed by Blount and Schmidt to help maintain postoperative correction in patients with scoliosis secondary to polio. The brace is designed to stimulate corrective forces from the patient. When the patient has been fitted properly with a brace, the trunk muscles are in constant use; therefore, disuse atrophy does not occur. The brace has an open design with constant force provided by the plastic pelvic mold. The pelvic portion helps reduce lordosis, derotates the spine, and corrects frontal deformity.

O   **What are the key design elements in the Milwaukee brace?**

Uprights have localized pads to apply transverse force, which is effective for small curves. The main corrective force is the thoracic pad, which attaches to the 2 posterior uprights and 1 anterior upright. Discomfort from the thoracic pad creates a righting response to an upright posture. The lumbar pads play a passive role compared to the thoracic pads. The uprights are perpendicular to the pelvic section, so any leg length discrepancy should be corrected to level the pelvis. The neck ring is another corrective force and is designed to give longitudinal traction. Jaw deformity is a potential complication of the neck ring. The throat mold, instead of a mandibular mold, allows use of distractive force without jaw deformity.

○ **What are the indications for the Milwaukee brace?**

1. Patients with Risser score of I-II and curves greater than 20-30 degrees that progress by 5 degrees over 1 year need application of brace.
2. Curves between 30-40 degrees need bracing, but not curves less than 20 degrees.
3. Curves of 20-30 degrees, with no year-over-year progression, require observation every 4-6 months. The Milwaukee brace is used for curves with apex above T7.

○ **What are adverse effects of using the Milwaukee brace?**

Jaw deformity
Pain
Skin breakdown
Unsightly appearance
Difficulty with mobility
Difficulty with transfers
Increased energy expenditure with ambulation

○ **What is the Boston brace?**

The Boston brace is a prefabricated symmetric thoracolumbar-pelvic mold with built-in lumbar flexion that can be worn under clothes. Lumbar flexion is achieved through posterior flattening of the brace and extending of the mold distally to the buttock. Braces with superstructures have a curve apex above T7. Curves with an apex at or below T7 do not require superstructures to immobilize cervical spine movement. This brace, unlike the Milwaukee brace, cannot be adjusted if the patient grows in height. Both braces need to be changed if pelvic size increases.

○ **What are the indications for the Boston brace?**

Curves 20-25 degrees with 10-degree progression over 1 year
Curves 25-30 degrees with 5-degree progression over 1 year
Skeletally immature patients with curves 30 degrees or greater

○ **What are the adverse effects of the Boston brace?**

Local discomfort
Hip flexion contracture
Trunk weakness
Increased abdominal pressure
Skin breakdown
Accentuation of hypokyphosis above brace in the thoracic spine

○ **What is the Charleston brace?**

The Charleston bending brace is a rigid custom-made orthosis designed to correct scoliosis at nighttime to improve patient compliance. This brace holds the patient in maximum side-bending correction. The Charleston brace is less effective at treating single thoracolumbar or lumbar curves, but the figures are not statistically significant compared to those for the Boston brace.

○   **What are the Indications for use of this particular brace?**

Curves 20-25 degrees with 10-degree progression over 1 year
Curves 25-30 degrees with 5-degree progression over 1 year
Skeletally immature patients with curves 30 degrees or greater

○   **What is a cushioned heel?**

A wedge of compressible rubber is inserted into the heel to absorb impact at heel strike. This cushion often is used with a rigid ankle to reduce the knee flexion moment by allowing for more rapid ankle plantar flexion.

○   **What is a heel flare?**

A medial flare is used to resist inversion, and a lateral flare is used to resist eversion. Both flares are used to provide heel stability.

○   **What is a heel wedge?**

A medial wedge is used to promote inversion, and a lateral wedge is used to promote eversion. The heel counter should be strong enough to prevent the hindfoot from sliding down the incline created by the wedge.

○   **What is an extended heel?**

Extended heel: The Thomas heel projects anteriorly on the medial side to provide support to the medial longitudinal arch. The reverse Thomas heel projects anteriorly on the lateral side to provide stability to the lateral longitudinal arch.

○   **What is a heel elevation?**

A shoe lift is used to compensate for fixed equinus deformity or for any leg-length discrepancy of more than one quarter of an inch.

○   **What is a rocker bar?**

It is a convex structure placed posterior to the metatarsal head. The rocker bar is used to shift the rollover point from metatarsal head to metatarsal shaft to avoid irritation of ulcers along the metatarsal head in patients with diabetes mellitus (DM).

○   **What is a metatarsal bar?**

It is a bar with a flat surface placed posterior to the metatarsal head. The metatarsal bar is used to relieve the pressure from the metatarsal heads.

○   **What is a sole wedge?**

A medial wedge is used to promote supination, and a lateral wedge is used to provide pronation.

○   **What is a sole flare?**

A medial flare is used to resist inversion, and a lateral flare is used to resist eversion. Both flares promote great stability.

○   **What is a steel bar?**

The steel bar is placed between the inner sole and outer sole. This bar is used to reduce forefoot motion to reduce the stress from phalanges and metatarsals.

○ **What are common internal heel modifications?**

A heel cushion relief is a soft pad with excavation is placed under the painful point of the heel.
A heel wedge can be applied medially or laterally A medial heel wedge can rotate the hindfoot into inversion. A lateral heel wedge can evert the hindfoot to avoid pressure on the cuboid.

○ **What is a metatarsal pad?**

This domed pad is designed to reduce the stress from metatarsal heads by transferring the load to metatarsal shafts in metatarsalgia.

○ **What is inner sole excavation?**

A soft pad filled with compressible material is placed under one or more metatarsal heads.

○ **What is a scaphoid pad?**

This type of pad extends from one half-inch posterior to the first metatarsal head to the anterior tubercle of the calcaneus. The apex of the scaphoid pad is between the talonavicular joint and the navicular tuberosity. The scaphoid pad is used for medial arch support.

○ **What is a toe crest?**

A crescent-shaped pad is placed behind the second through fourth phalanges. The toe crest fills the void under the proximal phalanges and reduces the stress

○ **What are thermoplastic AFOs?**

These devices are plastic molded AFOs, consisting of the following 3 parts: (1) a shoe insert, (2) a calf shell, and (3) a calf strap attached proximally The rigidity depends on the thickness and composition of the plastic, as well as the trim line and shape. Thermoplastic AFOs are contraindicated in cases of fluctuating edema and insensation.

○ **What is a Posterior leaf spring (PLS)?**

The PLS is the most common form of AFO with a narrow calf shell and a narrow ankle trim line behind the malleoli. The PLS is used for compensating for weak ankle dorsiflexors by resisting ankle plantar flexion at heel strike and during swing phase with no mediolateral control.

○ **What is a Spiral AFO?**

This AFO consists of a shoe insert; a spiral that starts medially, passes around the leg posteriorly, and then passes anteriorly to terminate at the medial tibial flare where a calf band is attached The spiral AFO allows for rotation in the transverse plane while controlling ankle dorsiflexion and plantar flexion, as well as eversion and inversion.

○ **What is a Hemispiral AFO?**

This AFO consists of a shoe insert with a spiral starting on the lateral side of the shoe insert, passing up the posterior leg, and terminating at the medial tibial flare where the calf band is attached This design is used for achieving better control of equinovarus than the spiral AFO can.

○ **What is a Solid AFO?**

The solid AFO has a wider calf shell with trim line anterior to the malleoli. This AFO prevents ankle dorsiflexion and plantar flexion, as well as varus and valgus deviation.

○   **What is an AFO with a flange?**

This AFO has an extension (flange) that projects from the calf shell medially for maximum valgus control and laterally for maximum varus control.

○   **What is a Hinged AFO?**

The adjustable ankle hinges can be set to the desired range of ankle dorsiflexion or plantar flexion.

○   **What is a tone-reducing AFO (TRAFO)?**

The broad footplate is used to provide support around most of the foot, extending distally under the toes and up over the foot medially and laterally to maintain the subtalar joint in normal alignment. The TRAFO is indicated for patients with spastic hemiplegia.

○   **What are the basic features of metal AFOs?**

This type of AFO consists of a shoe or foot attachment, ankle joint, two metal uprights (medial and lateral), with a calf band (application of force) connected proximally. The stirrup anchors the uprights to the shoes between the sole and the heel. The caliper is a round tube placed in the heel of the shoe, which connects to the uprights and allows for easy detachability of the uprights. A molded shoe insert is another alternative to fit the stirrup into the shoe, which also allows maximum control of the foot and aligns the anatomic and mechanical ankles.

○   **What are the basic properties of ankle joints in AFOs?**

The mechanical ankle joints can control or assist ankle dorsiflexion or plantar flexion by means of stops (pins) or assists (springs). The mechanical ankle joint also controls mediolateral stability. Knee extension moment is promoted by ankle plantar flexion, and knee flexion moment is promoted by ankle dorsiflexion.

○   **What is a Free motion ankle joint?**

The stirrup has a completely circular top, which allows free ankle motion and provides only mediolateral stability.

○   **What is a Plantar flexion ankle joint stop?**

This ankle joint stop is produced by a pin inserted in the posterior channel of the ankle joint or by flattening the posterior lip of the stirrup's circular stop. The plantar flexion stop has a posterior angulation at the top of the stirrup that restricts plantar flexion but allows unlimited dorsiflexion and promotes knee flexion moment. This design is used in patients with weakness of dorsiflexion during swing phase and flexible pes equinus.

○   **What is a Dorsiflexion ankle joint stop?**

The stirrup has a pin inserted in the anterior channel of the ankle joint or by flattening the anterior lip of the stirrup's circular stop. The dorsiflexion stop has an anterior angulation at the top of the stirrup that restricts dorsiflexion but allows unlimited plantar flexion and promotes a knee extension moment in the meantime. This design is used in patients with weakness of plantar flexion during late stance.

○   **What is a Limited motion ankle joint stop?**

This ankle joint stop has anterior and posterior angulations at the top of the stirrup with restricted dorsiflexion and plantar flexion ankle motion. The limited motion ankle joint stop has a pin in the anterior and the posterior channel, and it is used in ankle weakness affecting all muscle groups.

○   **What is a Dorsiflexion assist spring joint?**

This joint has a coil spring in the posterior channel and helps to aid dorsiflexion during swing phase.

○   **What is a Varus or valgus correction straps (T-straps):**

A T strap attached medially and circling the ankle until buckling on the outside of the lateral upright is used for valgus correction. A T strap attached laterally and buckling around the medial upright is used for varus correction.

○   **What are the basic features of KAFOs?**

KAFO: This orthosis can be made of metal leather and metal plastic or plastic and plastic metal. The metal design includes double upright metal KAFO (most common), single upright metal KAFO (lateral upright only), and Scott Craig metal KAFO. The plastic designs are indicated for closer fit and maximum control of the foot, including supracondylar plastic KAFO, supracondylar plastic-metal KAFO, and plastic shells with metal uprights KAFO.

○   **What is a double upright metal KAFO?**

This is an AFO with 2 metal uprights extending proximally to the thigh to control knee motion and alignment This orthosis consists of a mechanical knee joint and 2 thigh bands between 2 uprights.

○   **What is a Scott-Craig orthosis?**

It consists of a cushioned heel with a T shaped foot plate for mediolateral stability, ankle joint with anterior and posterior adjustable stops, double uprights, a pretibial band, a posterior thigh band, and knee joint with pawl locks and bail control. Hyperextension of the hip allows the center of gravity falling behind the hip joint and in front of the locked knee and ankle joint With 10° of ankle dorsiflexion alignment; it allows a swing-to or swing-through gait with crutches. This orthosis is used for standing and ambulation in patients with paraplegia due to spinal cord injury (SCI).

○   **What is a supracondylar plastic orthosis?**

The supracondylar plastic orthosis uses immobilized ankle in slight plantar flexion to produce a knee extension moment in stance to help eliminate the need for a mechanical knee lock. This orthosis also resists genu recurvatum and provides mediolateral knee stability.

○   **What are the basic features of knee joints in KAFOs?**

The mechanical knee joint can be polycentric or single axis. Polycentric is used for significant knee motion, and a single axis is more common and is used for knee stabilization.

○   **What is a free motion knee joint?**

This joint has unrestricted knee flexion and extension with a stop to prevent hyperextension. The free motion knee joint is used for patients with recurvatum but good strength of the quadriceps to control knee motion.

○   **What is an offset knee joint?**

The hinge is located posterior to the knee joint and ground reaction force; thus, it extends the knee and provides great stability during early stance phase of the gait cycle. This joint flexes the knee freely during swing phase and is contraindicated with knee or hip flexion contracture and ankle plantar flexion stop.

○   **What is a drop ring lock knee joint?**

The drop ring lock is the most commonly used knee lock to control knee flexion. The rings drop to unlock over the knee joint while the knee is in extension by gravity or manual assistance. This type of joint is stable, but gait is stiff without knee motion. A ball bearing on a spring can be added just above the drop lock to keep it from slipping up as the patient ambulates. Patients over 120 pounds usually feel more secure with both medial and lateral drop locks.

○   **What is a pawl lock with bail release knee joint?**

The semicircular bail attaches to the knee joint posteriorly, and it can unlock both joints easily by pulling up the bail or backing up to sit down in a chair. A major drawback is the accidental unlocking while the patient is pulling his or her pants up or bumping into a chair.

○ What is an adjustable knee lock joint (dial lock)?

The serrated adjustable knee joint allows knee locking at different degrees of flexion. This type of knee joint is used in patients with knee flexion contractures that are improving gradually with stretching.

○ What is an ischial weight bearing KAFO?

Most individuals in a KAFO sit partially on the upper thigh band unless the cuff is brought up above the ischium.

○ What are the basic features of a HKAFO?

A hip-knee-ankle-foot orthosis (HKAFO) consists of a hip joint and pelvic band in addition to a KAFO. The orthotic hip joint is positioned with the patient sitting upright at 90°, while the orthotic knee joint is centered over the medial femoral condyle. Pelvic bands complicate dressing after toileting unless the orthosis is worn under all clothing. Pelvic bands increase the energy demands for ambulation.

○ What are the different types of pelvic bands?

1. Bilateral pelvic band: This band is used more commonly with its posterior metal ends located anterior to the lateral midline of the pelvis and is interconnected by a flexible belt.
2. Unilateral pelvic band: This band rarely is used because most conditions requiring a HKAFO have bilateral involvement.
3. Pelvic girdle: The pelvic girdle is made of molded thermoplastic materials, providing a maximum degree of control in patients with bilateral involvement.
4. Silesian belt: This belt has no metal or rigid band and offers mild resistance to abduction and rotation of the hip. The Silesian belt attaches to the lateral upright and encircles the pelvis.

○ What are the different types of hip joints and locks used in HKAFOs?

1. Single axis hip joint with lock: This joint is the most common hip joint with flexion and extension. The single axis hip joint with lock may include an adjustable stop to control hyperextension.
2. Two-position lock hip joint: This hip joint can be locked at full extension and 90° of flexion and is used for hip spasticity control in a patient who has difficulty maintaining a seated position.
3. Double axis hip joint: This hip joint has a flexion-extension axis and abduction-adduction axis to control these motions.

○ What is the reciprocating gait orthosis?

Reciprocating gait orthosis (RGO): An RGO consists of bilateral KAFOs with posteriorly offset locking knee joints, hip joints, and a custom-molded pelvic girdle with a thoracic extension. The hip joints are coupled with cables preventing bilateral hip flexion simultaneously The hip extension on one side coupling hip flexion on the other side through the cables produces reciprocal walking gait pattern. The RGO combined with functional electronic stimulation (FES) can be used for 2-point or 4-point gait patterns in ambulatory paraplegic or tetraplegic (C8) patients. Using the RGO with FES can double the patient's optimum gait speed, lower blood pressure and heart rate, and increase oxygen uptake as compared to ambulating with the RGO without FES.

○ What is the para walker?

This device is a hip guidance orthosis, which consists of bilateral KAFOs with a ball bearing hip joint and a body brace. Ambulation is performed through trunk motion transmitted to the lower extremities with hip flexion and extension via the brace Hip flexion is restricted by a stop, and hip extension may be free or limited by a stop. The para walker is developed for patients with SCI. A study of 5 paraplegic patients found an average reduction in oxygen consumption of 27%, with 33% faster ambulatory rate compared to the RGO.

O   **What is the parapodium?**

This device is developed for pediatric myelodysplastic patients to allow them to stand without crutches for functional activities with their upper limbs free The parapodium consists of a shoe clamp, aluminum uprights, a foam knee block, and back and chest panels. Hip and knee may be locked for standing and unlocked for sitting A torque converter under the base allows side-to-side rocking to be translated into forward propulsion.

O   **What is the standing frame?**

Standing frame: This allows standing but does not permit hip and knee flexion. The standing frame is used for children to learn standing balance and achieve a swing-through gait.

WHEELCHAIRS

O   **What are the wheelchair categories according to medicare?**

- Standard (K0001)
- Standard Hemi (K0002)
- Lightweight (K0003)
- High Strength Lightweight (K0004)
- Ultra Lightweight (K0005)
- Rigid "Sport" UltraLite
- Reclining
- Tilt in Space

O   **What are the standard wheelchair dimensions?**

- Weight: <36lbs.
- Seat Width: 16″ or 18″
- Arm Style: fixed or detachable
- Seat Depth: 16″
- Seat Height: >19″ & 21″
- Back Height: nonadjustable 16″-17″
- Footplate Extension: 16″ to 21″
- Footrests: fixed or detached

O   **What are the high strength light weight wheelchair dimensions?**

- Lifetime Warranty on frame
- Weight: <34lbs.
- Seat Width: 14″, 16″, or 18″
- Arm Style: fixed or detachable
- Seat Depth: 14″ or 16″
- Seat Height: >17″ & 21″
- Back Height: sectional or adjustable 15″ to 19″
- Footrests: fixed or detached

O   **What are the ultra lightweight wheelchair dimensions?**

- Lifetime Warranty on frame
- Weight: <30lbs.

- Seat Width: 14", 16", or 18"
- Arm Style: fixed or detachable
- Seat Depth: 14" or 16"
- Seat Height: >17" & 21"
- Back Height: sectional or adjustable 15" to 19"
- Footplate extension: 16" to 21"
- Footrests: fixed or detached

O   What is the amputee wheelchair?

The amputee chair is designed to compensate for the change in the location of the center of gravity brought about by the absence of the legs. Persons with other types of disability who need the additional stability afforded by the approximately 2-inch longer wheelbase sometimes use it. Accessories are selected according to whether or not prostheses are to be worn, and according to any other disabilities the amputee may have, such as an upper-limb amputation.

O   What is the one arm drive chair?

The one-hand drive chair has been designed for persons such as hemiplegics and unilateral arm amputees, who have use of only one arm The driving wheels are interconnected so that either or both can be controlled through a dual set of hand rims. When one hand rim is moved independently of the other, only one wheel is driven. When both hand rims are grasped in the hand and moved together, both wheels are driven.

O   What is the reclining wheelchair?

The reclining wheelchair is needed by individuals that have limited control of the head and/or the torso, with or without spasticity, or when push-ups cannot be carried out to achieve pressure relief, or where a change of position helps respiration Two types are available: semi-reclining and full reclining.

O   What are the differences of desk arms and full length arms?

The desk models are foreshortened to permit the user to get closer to a desk or table top. The removable desk arm is by far the most popular type. The full-length models are indicated when the forepart is needed to support the arms of the user in rising from the chair; or when lordosis, obesity, or some other physical factor make it necessary to use the front part of the arm for support while the patient is in the sitting position. The standard removable desk model can be turned end-for-end to provide this feature.

O   What is a disadvantage of desk arms?

The simplest type of removable arm design adds nearly 2 inches to the overall width of the basic chair.

O   What is the front rigging?

It is the collective term for the foot and leg rests. Elevating front riggings consisting of adjustable footrests and leg rests are available for those patients with conditions such as edema, arthrodesed knee, and leg in a cast, which require that one or both legs be elevated.

O   What does the leg rest consist of?

Leg rests consist of an elevating support bracket with swing-away mechanism, pivot and slide tube with footplate, and calf pad to support the back of the leg when elevated.

O   What are the foot rest options?

Footrests can be fixed or can be detached from the wheelchair for those occasions when their presence is restrictive, such as maneuvering in a small bathroom. Detachable foot rests and front rigging are available that can be pivoted about the vertical axis to aid entry and exit and to permit the chair and occupant to get closer to a desk or counter.

O   **What are the standard dimensions for the rear and front wheels?**

The standard chair uses two 24 inch-diameter rear wheels and two 8-inch-diameter front caster wheels. Rear wheels with a diameter of 20 and 22 inches are available as well as caster wheels of dimensions less than the standard 8 inches.

O   **What are the three kinds of tires used with wheelchairs?**

Three types of tires are available for use with either the wire spoke or one-piece wheel: solid, pneumatic, and semi-pneumatic

O   **What are the indications for indoor use?**

Solid tires with a smooth tread are recommended when the wheelchair is to be used mostly indoors, because their resistance to rolling is the lowest and the cushioning provided by pneumatic tires is not required for indoor use.

O   **What are the advantages of pneumatic tires?**

Pneumatic tires provide the cushioning needed for outdoor use, not only to make the ride more comfortable but also to reduce the wear and tear on the wheelchair when used under normal outside conditions. Several types of pneumatic tires are available. The standard pneumatic tire has a tread to provide better traction and is sometimes called a "clincher" tire. The "all-terrain" tire is similar but has a wider and different tread. Both use standard inner tubes. A special high performance tire is the "sew-up" tire, which is lighter than the others. It uses a Latex tube that is literally sewn to the inside of a smooth tread tire The price for high performance here is that a puncture means replacement of the tire.

O   **What are hand rims?**

Hand rims are attached to the driving wheels of wheelchairs to permit control without soiling the hands. The standard hand rim is a circular steel tube. For users who have problems gripping the smooth surface of a metal ring, vinyl-coated rings are available as well as a variety of knobs and projections that can be added to the ring, making it easier for patients with hand deformities to propel the driving wheels.

O   **What are casters?**

Casters make steering possible and are available in two diameters: 8 inches and 5 inches. Pneumatic, semi pneumatic, and solid tires are available. The 8-inch-diameter wheel with solid rubber tires is standard on the basic chair, and is suitable for use on smooth surfaces and indoors. The semi pneumatic and pneumatic tires provide shock absorption, and thus are more suitable for rough surfaces and outdoor use. The 5-inch model is available only with solid tires, and is used on children's chairs and in special circumstances on adult chairs and basketball chairs, when more maneuverability is desired. The larger diameter caster wheels make it easier to climb curbs, but are more susceptible to shimmy, or flutter.

O   **What kinds of locks are available for the wheelchair?**

Most users need some means of securing one or more wheels to keep the chair from rolling down inclines or to provide stability during transfer to and from the chair. Two types of parking locks are available for the large wheel: toggle and lever. Selection depends upon user preference, which is usually based on the residual function of the upper limb and hand. These devices are designed strictly as locks to hold the chair in place and should never be used to slow down a chair because the abrupt stop that would result could cause the chair to overturn Pin type locks are available for retaining a caster in the trail position and to prevent swiveling during lateral transfer. Extensions are available so that users with limited function can operate the locks.

O   **What other accessories are available for the wheelchair?**

Lap trays, boards and anti-tipping devices

O   **What are the dimensions of the patient required for determination of critical wheelchair dimensions?**

| Length of leg from bottom of heel to popliteal fold. This distance determines height of seat from floor. |
| Distance from bottom of buttocks to olecranon, with elbow flexed to 90 degrees. This distance deter-mines the height of the arm. |
| Distance from bottom of buttocks to level of scapulae. This distance determines height of back. |
| Widest distance across shoulders and hips This distance determines width of seat and back. |
| Distance between popliteal and back of buttocks. This distance determines seat depth |

O   **What are the indications for a power wheelchair?**

They are indicated for patients with physical limitations not compatible with manual wheelchair propulsion, i.e., those who cannot propel a WC using either the hands or feet because of limb absence, paralysis, deformity, or other neuromusculoskeletal problems and those with poor endurance (because of cardiopulmonary or neuromusculoskeletal conditions) who must conserve their energy for other functions (e.g., vocational work).

O   **What are some common conditions indicated for a power wheelchair?**

Some common conditions that might warrant powered WCs include high-level spinal cord injury (e.g., C4 and above); advanced muscle weakness because of amyotrophic lateral sclerosis, multiple sclerosis, or muscular dystrophy; and poor coordination in all limbs (e.g., cerebral palsy). Powered WCs are usually indicated for outdoor use (rarely for indoor use) in patients of all ages who have to travel long distances (usually without help) and who tire easily. Patients with powered WCs generally need standard WCs for indoor use and as backups when their powered WCs are being repaired or cannot be transported.

O   **What are the user requirements for power wheelchairs?**

To safely use a powered WC, patients must have at least one reproducible movement (using the upper limb or other part of the body) to access the control system; a basic understanding of cause and effect and directionality; sufficient vision, perceptual ability, and judgment to permit movement through the environment; and proper motivation. Even children as young as 2 to 3 years old can be taught to safely operate a powered WC.

O   **What are the basic principles of power wheelchair prescription?**

Prescription guidelines: a powered WC is based on the same general WC prescription principles described above but with greater emphasis on the safety (of the user and of others) and performance of the powered WC. Although it uses the same seating and positioning principles as those described for manual WCs, the positioning of the upper limbs or other body parts is critical for placement of the WC control system.

O   **What are the main factors to consider in power wheelchair prescription?**

| Primary use: usually for outdoor use; consider the type of terrain and the need for "all-terrain WCs"; |
| Stability: lower seat and wider WC base have more stability; |
| Overall weight and portability: ease of assembly and disassembly, if appropriate; the weight, size, and transportability of each disassembled part; |
| Availability of adapted vehicles for WC transportation: vans with ramps or hydraulic lifts; |
| Environmental barriers: need for extensive environmental modifications; dimensions required for turning (in small spaces, short-based WCs are easier to maneuver); |
| Battery life: the range (or distance capability) of the powered WCs based on a single battery charge. |
| Power adjustability: speed, acceleration |

O   **What is a direct drive system?**

Direct-drive powered WCs (or power-base WCs) consist of a rigid mainframe (that contains the batteries and drive mechanisms); a seat, which is positioned directly above the power base on a pedestal attached to the rigid mainframe; and four small balloon tires (diameter of 8-10 inches or 20-25 cm and width of 3 inches or 7.6 cm; some newer models have slightly larger wheels in the rear) They are durable and better suited for rough terrain (because of their low center of gravity and wider tires). However, they are less maneuverable indoors or on carpets, and the large caster wheels have a tendency to wrinkle and roll carpeting, especially small rugs.

O   **What is the belt driven system?**

Belt driven powered WCs have comparable rigid mainframe and seating system as direct drive WCs but usually have two large rear wheels and two small front casters (the wheels of belt-driven powered WCs look almost like those of manual WCs). They are more versatile (i.e., their frames are better suited to modification and the addition of different components), more stable, and are generally capable of reaching greater speeds than direct drive WCs; however, they tend to be less durable.

O   **What are control systems?**

Control systems can be activated by any reproducible movement of the body such as those involving the upper extremity (i.e., hand, wrist, arm, fingertip, or upper limb residual limb) or non-upper limb body parts (e.g., head, chin, mouth, lips, tongue, and lower limbs). In general, the controls have a high and low range as well as options to increase power (e.g., when negotiating carpeted floor, grassy ground, or rough terrain). If possible, the control system of the powered WC should be compatible with the patient's environmental control unit.

O   **What are the activating devices commonly used?**

These include joysticks (i.e., a small pressure-sensitive stem attached to a control box; joystick-stem modifications include T bar handles, knobs, long extension handles, mouthstick, etc.), chin or head pressure controls, and pneumatic controls (e.g., Sip-and-Puff, which uses soft or intense inspiration [sip] or expiration [puff]).

O   **What are other special controls?**

These include the leaf switch, touch plate, toggle switch, voice-activated switch, myoelectric control switch, proximity sensing system, and scanning system (i.e., a control option that presents grouped or single choices one at a time until the user selects it by activating a switch).

ASSISTIVE DEVICES

O   **What are the basic effects of canes on gait and weight bearing?**

Canes widen the base of support and decreases stress on the opposite hip. They can unload the lower limb weight by bearing up to 25% of body weight. Canes are made of wood or aluminum. Tubular aluminum is lighter than wood. Aluminum canes are adjustable, which facilitates their use by patients of all sizes.

O   **How are canes measured?**

With the patient in an upright position, measure from the tip of the cane to the level of the greater trochanter The elbow should be flexed approximately 20°.
An incorrectly fitted cane produces an inefficient gait pattern.
A short cane reduces support during the stance phase, and it tends to keep the elbow in complete extension.
A long cane causes excess elbow flexion, which leads to increased muscle fatigue on the triceps and shoulder muscles.

O   **What are the 3 types of canes in general use?**

The C cane is the most common. Other names used for this device include the crook top cane, J cane, and single point cane.

O   **What is the functional grip cane?**

Provides better grip and controlled balance for patients
Grip is more comfortable than with a C cane
Ortho cane is an example.

○   **What is the quad cane?**

Additional support compared with other canes
Narrow- versus wide-based forms
Especially helpful for hemiplegics patients
Slow gait is one disadvantage.

○   **What is the walk-cane or hemi-walker?**

Combines the features of a walker and quad cane
Usually made of tubular aluminum, is adjustable, and can be folded
Provides wider base and lateral support than the regular quad cane

○   **What are the indications?**

Patients with hemiplegia or as an intermediate step during ambulation training for the period after parallel bars and before ambulation with less restrictive assistive devices

○   **What is the biomechanical advantage offered by a cane?**

The cane usually is used on the side opposite the supporting lower limb. The cane helps decrease the force generated across the affected hip joint by decreasing the work of the gluteus medius-minimus complex. The force is exerted by the upper extremity through the cane to help minimize pelvic drop on the side opposite the weight-bearing lower limb If the cane is held on the affected side, the affected hip in turn experiences an increased load of 4 times the body weight during ambulation.

○   **How is the cane used during ambulation on level surfaces?**

The cane usually is held on the patient's unaffected side and provides support to the opposite lower limb. The cane is advanced simultaneously with the opposite affected lower limb. The weight is borne through the arm as needed.

○   **How is the cane used on stairs?**

The pneumonic "up with the good and down with the bad" can help patients recall the appropriate pattern for stair climbing. Advance the unaffected lower limb first when going up and advance the affected lower limb first when coming down. The patient always should have the "good" lower limb assume the first full weight-bearing step on level surfaces.

○   **What is an axillary crutch?**

An axillary crutch is a type of orthosis made of wood or aluminum that provides support from the axilla to the floor. Both wood and aluminum crutches are made to be adjustable. The extension crutch (i.e., the length can be adjusted) is heavier than the regular crutch because of the one extra piece of wood. Standard axillary crutches have double uprights with a shoulder piece and handgrip or bar.

○   **What are the advantages of axillary crutches?**

The primary advantage of an axillary crutch is that it allows transfer of 80% of the individual's body weight. Axillary crutches provide better trunk support than non-axillary or forearm crutches, and patients can free their hands for activities by leaning on the shoulder piece. However, the patient should be advised of the possibility of sustaining compressive brachial neuropathies with the use of axillary crutches the axillary crutch is not designed for the patient to rest for body support. Patients should avoid resting their body weight on the axillary area. Providing extra padding to the axillary area should be discouraged for this reason.

○   **How are axillary crutches measured?**

Determine the crutch length by measuring the distance from the anterior axillary fold to a point 6 inches lateral to the fifth toe with the patient standing.
With the proper crutch length determined and the crutch then placed 3 inches lateral to the foot, proper hand piece location can be measured The patient's elbow should be flexed 30°, the wrist in maximal extension, and the fingers in a fist.
The patient should be able to raise the body 1-2 inches by performing complete elbow extension

○   **What are non-axillary crutches?**

Non-axillary crutches allow transfer of 40-50% of the patient's body weight. Also called forearm or arm canes or forearm or arm orthoses, these devices require good trunk control. The patient needs confidence in his/her ambulation skills.

○   **What are Lofstrand crutches?**

Most popular non-axillary crutches
Most useful substitute for canes
Most often used bilaterally
Made of tubular aluminum
Padded hand bar
Forearm cuff

○   **How are they measured?**

With the proper crutch length determined and the crutch then placed 3 inches lateral to the foot, proper hand piece location can be measured The patient's elbow should be flexed 20°, the wrist in maximal extension, and the fingers in a fist. The open end of the cuff is placed on the lateral aspect of the forearm to permit elbow flexion and grasping without dropping the orthosis The proximal portion of the orthosis is angled at 20° to provide a comfortable stable fit.

○   **What are the advantages and disadvantages of Lofstrand crutches?**

1.   Safer and easier ambulation
2.   A good substitution for the cane because the forearm support stabilizes the wrist during weight bearing
3.   The patient's hands are free to perform various tasks, while the body weight is supported through the forearm by the forearm cuff pivots. The patient does not have to worry about dropping the crutches.
4.   These crutches are shorter than axillary crutches.

○   **What is the Platform forearm orthosis?**

A platform is placed on the top level of the crutch.
A vertical handgrip is placed at the distal end of the platform.
Velcro straps are used to apply around the forearm.
Very helpful for patients with weak hand grip strength

○   **How are they measured?**

With the patient standing upright and the elbow flexed 90°, determine the proper length by measuring from the resting forearm to the ground.

○   **What are the advantages?**

The body weight is borne mostly on the forearm instead of the hand.

○   **What are the indications?**

1. Painful wrist and hand conditions (e.g., arthritis)
2. Weak hand grip because of pain and deformities of the hands and wrists
3. Elbow contractures

○ **What is the four point crutch gait?**

The appropriate sequence is left crutch – right foot – right crutch – left foot. Then repeat.

○ **What are the advantages?**

1. Stability
2. Always have at least 3 points in contact with the ground

○ **What are the disadvantages?**

1. Difficult to learn
2. Relative slow walking gait

○ **What is the indication?**

Patients with weakness in lower limbs or poor coordination (ataxic)

○ **What is the three point crutch gait, its advantages, indications and requirements?**

The appropriate sequence includes first both crutches and the weaker lower limb, then the stronger or unaffected lower limb.
Advantage: Eliminates all weight bearing on the affected lower limb.
Indication: Lower limb fractures, amputations, or pain
Requires good balance and coordination

○ **What is the two-point gait?**

The proper sequence includes the left crutch and right foot, then the right crutch and left foot. Repeat.

○ **What are the advantages?**

1. Provides stability
2. Faster than the 4-point gait
3. Reduces weight bearing to both lower limbs

○ **What is the indication?**

Indication: Patients with weakness in lower limbs or poor coordination (ataxic)

○ **What is the swing through gait?**

The sequence involves both crutches, moving both lower limbs past the crutches.
Advantage: Fastest gait (faster than normal walking gait)
Disadvantage: Very energy-consuming and difficult to learn
Requires strong functional abdominal and upper limb muscles and good trunk balance

○ **What is the swing to gait, advantages and indications?**

The proper sequence includes both crutches; the patient moves both lower limbs almost to the crutches.
Advantage: Easy to learn

Indication: Paraplegic patients

○ **What muscle groups principally involved in the use of crutches?**

Shoulder depressors
Latissimus dorsi
Lower trapezius
Pectoralis minor
Shoulder flexors
Elbow and wrist extensors
Finger flexors
Trunk (deep back) muscles to help improve balance and endurance

○ **How are walkers measured?**

1. Place the front of the walker 12 inches in front of the patient. The walker should partially surround the patient.
2. Measure the proper height of the walker by having the patient stand upright with the elbows flexed 20°.

○ **What are the characteristics of a standard walker?**

Most standard walkers (Pick-up Walker) are lightweight and very durable.
There are adjustable legs, accommodating a large percentage of patients.
The standard walker requires that the patient have upper extremity strength to lift the device up and place it forward to ambulate.

○ **What are the characteristics of a rolling walker (or front wheeled walker) ?**

It has wheels on the front legs, which promote movement of the walker.
It does not require as much strength and balance to maneuver as the standard walker because the patient does not have to lift it from the floor.

○ **What are the advantages of a rolling walker?**

Patients with poor coordination of the upper extremity and trunk who are not able to lift the walker and move it forward may prefer this device.

○ **What are the disadvantages of a rolling walker?**

Instability if proper supervised training session is not carried out to ensure patient safety.

THERAPEUTIC EXERCISE

○ **What are the three stages of energy production in response to exercise?**

During the first few seconds of heavy exercise, energy is obtained anaerobically from the already stored high-energy compounds of phosphocreatine and ATP. This phase may be referred to as the lactic phase. As activity continues over the next 5 to 10 seconds, stored muscle glycogen and glucose are broken down anaerobically to lactate via glycolysis. This is the anaerobic or glycolytic phase. As oxygen becomes available through increased pulmonary ventilation and. circulatory changes, ATP can be generated aerobically through the oxidation of glycogen, glucose, fat, and protein. This is the aerobic phase.

○ **What happens as exercise intensity increases?**

During light exercise, the aerobic supply may be sufficient to sustain activity, but if the exercise is strenuous, the anaerobic contribution may continue and lactic acid accumulates. The major limiting factor to prolonged exercise is intolerance to the accumulation of lactate. During the recovery period, lactate is re oxidized, phosphocreatine and ATP are replenished, and, oxygen consumption gradual) decreases.

○   **What is the cardiovascular response to exercise?**

During exercise with large muscle groups, the cardiovascular system responds with an increase in heart rate and a rise in cardiac output. Simultaneously, blood flow is preferentially increased to the exercising muscles because of local vasodilatation and is shunted away from non-exercising regions such as the splanchnic and renal beds. The pulmonary minute ventilation increases with exercise, allowing increased oxygen uptake and clearance of carbon dioxide.

○   **What is the endocrine response to exercise?**

Catecholamines are released into the circulation in increased quantities during exercise, stimulating glycogenolysis and lipolysis, thus making available glucose and free fatty acids for use as energy sources. Growth hormone levels rise and insulin levels fall, further contributing to the increased availability of glucose. These mechanisms, as well as hepatic gluconeogenesis (synthesis of glucose in the liver), are counterbalanced by increased sensitivity to insulin and increased glucose utilization by muscle cells, the net result being the maintenance of normal serum glucose concentrations.

○   **What is the Hematologic Response to exercise?**

During exercise, there is an acute increase in fibrinolysis as well as an increase in platelets, but platelet function is unchanged. During strenuous exercise circulatory blood volume decreases because of fluid shifts and losses from sweating, but the effect of regular physical exercise is to cause an increase in red cell mass and circulating plasma volume. A disproportionate increase in plasma volume can cause pseudoanemia in athletes.

○   **What is the renal response to exercise?**

During vigorous exercise, acute hemoconcentration occurs, owing to sweating, and decreases renal blood flow and the glomerular filtration rate. Urine output therefore decreases. Serum potassium concentration is transiently increased, owing to release from exercising muscle cells.

○   **What are the psychological effects of exercise?**

Perhaps the best-known acute psychological effect of aerobic exercise is an increase in the plasma level of endorphin, an opiate-like substance associated with mild euphoria. Short-term alleviation of stress is also reported.

○   **What is specificity?**

A key concept in training is that the biophysical adaptations and improved performance of muscle are specific to the training stimulus used, both the type of exercise and the specific muscle groups exercised. The basis for this lies in the differences in the biochemical and morphologic adaptations that result from aerobic (versus anaerobic) training. Furthermore, there is specificity of training, related to motor learning that enhances the skilled performance of a specific task and is best accomplished by practicing that task.

○   **What is overload?**

To continue increasing a patient's strength or endurance, the required training stimulus must be increased periodically, in either intensity or duration of work, to ensure an "overload," or taxing of the musculoskeletal system. As the enzyme systems involved adapt to the increased demand, each task is performed with greater biochemical efficiency. No training effect occurs unless the appropriate systems are stressed beyond the usual daily requirements or beyond the level to which they have become adapted. For any type of training to be effective, a certain minimum amount of exercise (frequency and duration) must be performed at a specified minimum intensity.

○   **What is intensity?**

Intensity refers to the level at which the work will be performed. How intensity is expressed depends on the nature of the exercise being prescribed. When training for endurance (aerobic capacity), intensity may be measured as a percentage of maximum oxygen consumption, maximum heart rate, or perceived rate of exertion. Training for strength may be prescribed in terms of either absolute or relative load.

○   **What is duration?**

Duration may be expressed in units of time for aerobic training or isometric holding, or as the number of repetitions of a dynamic strength or endurance training activity. As a rule, the higher the intensity of an activity, the shorter the duration needed to achieve a training effect, and vice versa, but duration must be long enough at the given intensity to result in overload. For most forms of exercise, there is no generally accepted agreement on minimal or optimal duration.

○   **What is frequency?**

In prescribing exercise, it is important to state the required frequency. Because a training effect often requires overload resulting in a catabolic response in the muscle followed by an anabolic response that overshoots the baseline, daily exercise is not desirable when the goal is high-intensity strength or endurance training. Lower intensity training may require daily doses of exercise to achieve a training response. On the other hand, for neuromuscular reeducation the frequency of training may have to be more than once a day to produce carryover. Stretching exercises usually need to be performed at least once a day to produce a good response. Thus, to decide on the frequency of training required to achieve the desired physiologic response in the patient, the clinician needs to consider the type of exercise, its relative intensity, and the duration.

○   **What is Interval Training?**

Interval training is exercise, performed intermittently; alternating periods of high work intensity with periods of less intense work or rest. This method has several clinical applications. For a very deconditioned person with low exercise tolerance, interval training extends the total time and amount of work that can be done Another application is training for short duration high intensity exercise, such as sprint racing, where anaerobic conditioning is desirable. Anaerobic training occurs if relatively high loads are used during short work intervals, whereas if the exercise stimulus is of submaximal intensity over longer periods, aerobic enzyme systems are utilized and trained. The intensity of the stimulus and duration of the work ultimately determine which system is preferentially trained.

○   **What are the three types of range of motion exercises?**

- Passive
- Active Assistive
- Active

○   What are the three major forms of stretching?

- Ballistic
- Static
- PNF

○   **What is an isotonic contraction?**

By definition, isotonic exercise occurs when the tension or torque generated by the muscle is constant throughout the movement. In practice, this is very difficult to accomplish, and a better term is dynamic contraction, which may be subdivided into several types of contractions: concentric, eccentric, and isokinetic.

○   **What is a concentric contraction?**

Concentric contractions are also known as shortening or positive contractions. As the muscle shortens, less force is generated; thus, the force generated is not uniform throughout the arc of motion. The slower the velocity of shortening, the greater the tension generated.

O   **What are eccentric contractions?**

Eccentric contractions are also referred to as lengthening or negative contractions. At a given velocity, the tension produced by eccentric con- traction is greater than that produced by a concentric contraction. For this reason, eccentric contractions may be used efficiently as part of a strengthening program.

O   **What is the relationship between contraction type and velocity?**

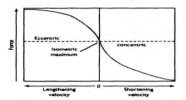

O   **What is delayed onset muscle soreness?**

Delayed onset muscle soreness, which commonly occurs 24 to 48 hours after exercise, is more common with eccentric than with concentric exercise. The possible mechanisms for exercise-induced delayed onset muscle soreness include a model beginning with structural damage in the muscle fiber caused by high tension resulting in disruptive of calcium homeostasis caused by damage to cell membranes. This process leads to necrosis, which peaks about 2 days after exercise. Products of the ensuing macrophage activity and inflammation cause the sensation of soreness.

O   **What is an isokinetic contraction?**

Isokinetic contraction as produced by the Cybex® machine and other devices is performed at a constant angular velocity, torque being generated against a preset device that controls speed of contraction. This form of exercise is defined by the equipment used for the exercise; as such, contractions do not exist in nature.

O   **What is torque?**

Torque is defined as the product of force multiplied by the distance between the center of rotation and the point where the force is applied. to predict function in the real world.

O   **What are the basic principles of isokinetic exercise?**

Most isokinetic devices utilize concentric contraction, but some of the newer machines, such as the KIN-COM®, can produce eccentric isokinetic contractions. These exercise machines are useful for providing a relatively safe dynamic training program after trauma or surgery. Most of them produce elaborate printouts with tabulations of objective data. Such data may be useful for following trends during a rehabilitation program, but caution must be observed in extrapolating from the information

O   **What factors influence isokinetic exercise equipment readings?**

Factors such as positioning in the machine, length of the lever arm, stabilization of the subject, calibration of the machine, speed of contraction, and the effect of gravity are impact. In addition, poor correlation among torque values reported by the various currently available machines makes it impossible to compare norms or data of individual patients when they are obtained on different brands of machines.

O   **What are the problems associated with extrapolating isokinetic testing results?**

Correlations of printout data with patients' functional outcome has been poor, both for orthopedic and neurologic rehabilitation. The principles of specificity of training and testing suggest that it might be difficult to estimate functional work capacity from the results of isokinetic testing.

O   **What is Isometric exercise?**

Isometric, or static, exercise occurs when force is exerted against an immovable or relatively immovable object. Isometric exercise is defined as muscle contraction without movement of the joint(s) crossed by the active muscle(s). The intensity of isometric contraction is usually expressed as a percentage of the maximum force of contraction. Isometric exercise elevates both heart rate and blood pressure. The resulting increase in myocardial oxygen demand may precipitate angina in susceptible person. Isotonic training is the best preparation for isotonic tasks, such as lifting; similarly, isometric training is most appropriate for isometric tasks such as holding or gripping. There is, however, some crossover effect between the two types of training.

O   What are determinants of strength?

1.   Cross-Sectional Area: Strength is proportional to the cross-sectional area of a muscle, which is measured at right angles to the direction of the parallel muscle fibers.

2.   Recruitment: Recruitment of motor fibers in a coordinated, properly sequenced fashion also determines strength. Proper sequencing of agonist and antagonist activity is necessary for maximum voluntary contraction. The degree to which motor units fire simultaneously to produce maximum tension, the synchronization ratio, is one determinant of motor unit recruitment. Another factor in recruitment is the frequency of firing.

O   How do smaller units recruit?

Smaller motor units have a lower threshold for discharge and are recruited with low-force activities As the need for increased force arises, these smaller motor units increase the frequency of discharge and additional (larger) motor units are recruited These larger motor units in turn increase their discharge rate in response to increasing demand. Thus, both recruitment of new motor units and increasing frequency of firing (rate coding) are determinants of maximal strength.

O   How does the length-tension relationship influence strength?

The greatest total tension that a muscle can develop depends on both active and passive tension at any given length. Equilibrium length is defined as the length of a unstimulated, unattached muscle. Maximal force is generated by a muscle at 120% of its equilibrium length, corresponding ultrastructurally with the length at which there is maximum single overlap between actin and myosin. Anatomic limitations of joint motion restrict muscle length to between 70% and 120% of their equilibrium length, allowing the muscle to generate its maximum force at its maximum anatomic length.

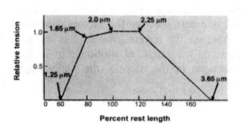
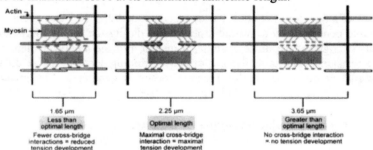

O   How does velocity of contraction influence strength?

The velocity of muscle contraction also affects the maximum strength that can be developed. For a given contractile force, less energy and de-creased muscle activation (as assessed on electromyography) are required during eccentric contraction than during concentric contraction. Rapid concentric contraction produces less tension than slow concentric contraction, whereas rapid eccentric contraction produces more tension than slow eccentric contraction. Accordingly, the greatest force is developed during a rapid eccentric contraction, and the least force with a rapid concentric contraction these characteristics can be used in the design of strengthening programs.

O   What role does fiber type play in strength?

Each human muscle is a mosaic of type I and type II fibers; the relative proportions vary, depending on the general demands made of the muscle. Type I fibers are the slow oxidative fibers and are generally derived from smaller motor neurons, responding to-demands of low, sustained force. The type II fibers (which have two subtypes, IIa and IIb) are recruited later and respond to demands requiring higher forces generated over shorter periods The maximum force generated by a muscle depends on the relative proportions of type I and type II fibers that make up the muscle and how this compares with the task being asked of it.

○ **What is progressive resistance exercise?**

Progressive resistive exercise (PRE) describes dynamic strengthening exercise that involves using weights or resistance for a specified number of repetitions. As training progresses, resistance is increased. Two techniques of PRE have been popularized in the literature: DeLorme and Oxford.

○ **What is a repetition maximum (RM)?**

A repetition maximum is the maximum weight that can be moved through the joint's full range of motion against gravity a given number of times. Thus, a 10 RM is the load that can be lifted 10 times through the full range. Based on a new 10 RM determined each week, the training sessions consist of 10 repetitions each at 50%, 75%, and 100% of the 10 RM. As the patient's strength increases, the 10 RM is increased accordingly. One potential disadvantage of the technique is that the patient may become fatigued toward the end of the session, just when the highest load is to be lifted.

○ **What is the Oxford technique?**

The Oxford technique is similar to the DeLorme technique, except that each session starts with 10 repetitions of 100% 10 RM, followed by 10 reps each of 75% and 50% of 10 RM. The fact that patients report less fatigue with the Oxford method may make this a less effective form of training than the traditional DeLorme technique. Another disadvantage of the Oxford technique is that the muscle is not warmed up before maximal effort is exerted.

○ **What are disadvantages of both techniques?**

Disadvantages of both techniques are that they are time consuming, require assistance from a physical therapist or trainer, and use a constant load. Another issue in designing these programs is the number of repetitions.

○ **What is an effective training schedule for strengthening?**

In review of a number of studies, it may be concluded that the most effective strength training uses a five or six RM schedule. The torque generated by a muscle at any point during the arc of motion varies and is determined by the factors discussed previously-length of the muscle, angle of insertion of the tendon, patient's effort. Because the torque generated is variable but the resistance constant, the net effective training load varies at different points in the range of motion and is thus submaximal at points where the greatest torque is generated. To increase the strength of the muscle, the patient may progressively increase the weight lifted or the rate at which a given weight is lifted.

○ **What is one popular technique for eccentric strengthening?**

One popular technique for eccentric muscle training utilizes equipment manufactured by Nautilus. The Nautilus system of training has as its unique feature a cam that superficially resembles a nautilus shell. This cam variably adjusts the resistance throughout the range of motion to approximate the average torque that is produced for a given muscle group. Because of this specialized cam design, separate devices are necessary to train each muscle group Resistance is provided for both the concentric and eccentric contractions of each muscle group, adding to the efficiency of this strengthening regimen Other machines are also available, including some that provide eccentric isokinetic contractions. Eccentric training can also be accomplished with simple weights, with assistance during the concentric phase provided by an attendant or the other limb, followed by a controlled eccentric contraction to lower the weight.

○ **What are the unique features of isokinetic exercise?**

Isokinetic exercise requires special equipment now produced by a number of manufacturers, to provide a constant velocity (measured in degrees per second) during muscle contraction. The machine allows the individual to exert maximal force throughout the range of motion and provides a corresponding resistance to maintain the velocity of contraction. A particularly useful feature of several of these machines is a printout or graphic documentation of a subject's progress. One unique concern of isokinetic training is the specificity (the velocity of training: velocity chosen for trailing should correspond to the velocity required for the ultimate (functional) activity. The maximum torque for concentric isokinetic contractions decreases with increasing velocity, whereas the reverse is true for eccentric isokinetic contraction. The speeds selected for training should reflect the need to generate an appropriate loading force at the anticipated functional requirements of the patient.

○ **How do isometric exercises contribute to strength?**

Isometric exercise may be performed for strength training; the recommended duration of each contraction is 6 seconds. Muller described an isometric program with a 1-second maximal contraction per muscle per day Although this seems attractive in its simplicity and efficiency; most clinicians find that programs of multiple contractions lasting 6 seconds (to prevent the exaggerated cardiac response) are more effective. The strength gains are specific to the angle at which the exercise is performed, and this limits its general applicability. The major utility of isometric exercise is for patients whose joint range of motion is either very limited or, owing to inflammation or surgery, uncomfortable when the clinician wants to prevent significant atrophy.

○ **What is the major mechanism of strength gains?**

The major mechanisms of strength gains that underlie all strengthening programs are hypertrophy of fibers (cross-sectional area) and neural factors. During the first 1 to 2 weeks of training the major contribution to strength, gain was from neural factors. Hypertrophy becomes the dominant factor in increased strength after 3 to 5 weeks. The mechanisms underlying the early phase of training appear to be better synchronization and more effective recruitment of motor units The relative proportion of type I and II fibers remains constant, but considerable changes can occur within each fiber type (and between type IIa and IIb) with training.

○ **What determines the type of strengthening program selected for a patient?**

Which type of strengthening exercises to prescribe for a patient depends on the desired goal Because the expected results are specific to the training modality, it makes the most sense to tailor the training regimen to the patient's needs and the dynamics of the activity. At all times, it must be remembered that the patient must be "overloaded', and the training tasks must exceed the demands of everyday activity. The clinician must regularly reassess and upgrade the prescription if strength gain is to continue.

○ **What does Training Muscle Endurance imply?**

Muscle endurance must be defined operationally for each situation. It may refer to the holding time for an isometric contraction, the number of repetitions of a brief isometric contraction, or the number of repetitions of a dynamic contraction (concentric, eccentric, or isokinetic). Research shows that isometric and isotonic endurance can be trained preferentially. It is equally important to consider the force of the contraction as a percent-age of the maximal strength of that muscle.

○ **What is the relationship between strength and endurance?**

The graph below demonstrates the relationship between strength and endurance for both dynamic and static work. This relationship clearly indicates that increasing the strength of a muscle increases the endurance for any given absolute submaximal load by making it a smaller percentage of the maximum contraction.

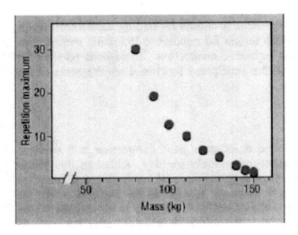

○   **What effect does endurance training have on muscle fiber characteristics?**

Prolonged exercise with lighter loads as well as the muscle training that takes place during aerobic conditioning has a different effect than strength training on histologic and biochemical changes in muscle. With endurance, training there is a decrease in the size of type I fibers instead of the hypertrophy of type II fibers with strength training. This decrease in the cross-sectional area of the type I fibers is accompanied by increases in capillary density and in the myoglobin content of the fibers, thus increasing the cells' ability to transport oxygen to the mitochondria. There is also an accompanying increase in the number and size of the mitochondria and in the concentration of oxidative enzymes within the mitochondria, thus increasing the cells' capacity for aerobic metabolism.

○   **What is the desired effect of aerobic training programs?**

Aerobic training programs increase the maximum oxygen consumption (VO_2max) The changes in the cardiac response to exercise following such a program have been interpreted, as suggesting that there is actually some training or strengthening of the heart itself. This is not the case, however, as is demonstrated by the fact that the cardiac response to exercise only changes for exercise performed by muscle groups involved in the training. Thus, training on a treadmill changes the cardiac response to lower extremity work but has no effect on the cardiac response to upper extremity work, and vice versa.

○   **What are the benefits of aerobic training?**

The benefits of aerobic training are due to a combination of the changes in the type I skeletal muscle fibers noted above and an increase in the blood volume. The peripheral muscle changes reduce the need to shunt blood from other vascular beds to the working muscle, thus reducing the peripheral resistance and, consequently, the afterload on the left ventricle. The muscle changes also make each absolute exercise load a smaller percentage of the maximum capacity, thus reducing the activation of the sympathetic nervous system and reducing the increase in circulating catechol- amines associated with exercise. The increased blood volume that has been demonstrated with these training programs results in increased venous return. This combines with the bradycardia to produce greater diastolic filling, and thus a larger stroke volume, which produces a higher maximum cardiac output, resulting in larger maximum oxygen consumption (aerobic capacity).

○   **What are the prescription parameters for aerobic exercise?**

The usual exercises include walking, running, swimming, rowing, cycling, aerobic calisthenics, and arm ergometry. The intensity of exercise is usually expressed as a percentage of the maximum heart rate, but absolute loads on a calibrated ergometer can also be used. Although training at 75% of any person's age-determined maximum heart rate is usually considered ideal, training can be achieved with intensities in the range of 40% to 60% of maximum, if a wider margin of safety is needed because of coronary artery disease or if the patient is too debilitated to tolerate a more strenuous program.

○   **What are warm up and cool down phases?**

A relatively strenuous program ought to include warm-up and cool-down phases. During a warmup of less intense activity, induction of the aerobic enzymes and stretching of the soft tissues occurs, making the exercise more efficient and less likely to cause injury. A cool-down phase of gradually decreasing intensity exercise reduces the risk of postural hypotension and cardiac arrhythmia. The duration of training is usually 20 to 30 minutes, including the warm-up and cool-down phases.

○   **What is the frequency of training?**

Frequency of training is usually three times a week, though with a very low-intensity program more frequent sessions may be needed to achieve a training effect. A significant increase in aerobic capacity (reflected in lower heart rate at the same submaximal loads) should be evident within 4 to 6 weeks.

MANUAL MEDICINE

○ **What is massage?**

Massage is a therapeutic manipulation of the soft tissues of the body with the goal of achieving normalization of those tissues. Massage can have mechanical, neurological, psychological, and reflexive effects. Massage can be used to reduce pain or adhesions, promote sedation, mobilize fluids, increase muscular relaxation, and facilitate vasodilation. Massage easily can be a preliminary treatment to manipulation; however, it clearly targets the health of soft tissues, while manipulation targets joint segments.

○ **What are the elements of western massage?**

The essence of Western massage is use of the hands to apply mechanical forces to the skeletal muscles and skin, although the intent may be to affect either more superficial or deeper tissues Types of basic Western massage are characterized by whether (1) the focus of pressure is moved by the hands gliding over the skin (i.e., effleurage), (2) soft tissue is compressed between the hands or fingers and thumb (i.e., pétrissage), (3) the skin or muscle is impacted with repetitive compressive blows (i.e., tapotement), or (4) shearing stresses are created at tissue interfaces below the skin (i.e., deep friction massage).

○ **What is Effleurage?**

In this approach, the practitioner's hands glide across the skin overlying the skeletal muscle being treated. Oil or powder is incorporated to reduce friction; hand-to-skin contact is maintained throughout the massage strokes. Effleurage can be superficial or deep. Light strokes energize cutaneous receptors and act by neuroreflexive or vascular reflexive mechanisms, whereas deep stroke techniques mechanically mobilize fluids in the deeper soft tissue structures. Deep stroking massage is performed in the direction of venous or lymphatic flow, whereas light stroking can be in any direction desired. The main mechanical effect of effleurage is to apply sequential pressure over contiguous soft a tissue so that fluid is displaced ahead of the hands as tissue compression is accomplished.

○ **What are the indications for effleurage?**

Effleurage may be used to gain initial relaxation and patient confidence, occasionally to diagnose muscle spasm and tightness, and to provide contact of the practitioner's hands from one area of the body to another.

○ **What is Pétrissage?**

Pétrissage involves compression of underlying skin and muscle between the fingers and thumb of one hand or between the two hands. Tissue is squeezed gently as the hands move in a circular motion perpendicular to the direction of compression. The main mechanical effects are compression and subsequent release of soft tissues, reactive blood flow, and neuroreflexive response to flow.

○ **What is Tapotement?**

This percussion-oriented massage involves striking soft tissue with repetitive blows, using both hands in a rhythmic, gentle, and rapid fashion. Numerous variations can be defined by the part of the hands making an impact with the body. The therapeutic effect of tapotement may result from compression of trapped air that occurs on impact. The overall effect of tapotement may be stimulatory; therefore, healthy persons with increased tolerance for this approach are more likely to find this type of massage useful.

○ **What is deep friction massage?**

Pressure is applied with the ball of the practitioner's thumb or fingers to the patient's skin and muscle.
The main effect of deep friction massage is to apply shear forces to underlying tissues, particularly at the interface between two tissue types (eg, dermis-fascia, fascia-muscle, muscle-bone) Deep pressure keeps superficial tissues from shearing so that shear and force are directed at the deeper tissue surface interface. Deep friction massage frequently is used to prevent or slow adhesions of scar tissue.

○   **What are the therapeutic benefits of massage?**

Massage may be used as primary therapeutic intervention or as an adjunct to other therapeutic techniques. Uses can include, but are not limited to, (1) mobilization of inter tissue fluids, (2) reduction or modification of edema, (3) increase of local blood flow, (4) decrease of muscle soreness and stiffness, (5) moderation of pain, (6) facilitation of relaxation, and (7) prevention or elimination of adhesions. Massage may be used to alter pathophysiology of a primary condition (eg, contracture) or to prevent or modify deleterious effects of a previously used treatment modality.

○   **What are contraindications to massage?**

Massage is contraindicated when it could cause worsening of a particular condition, unwanted tissue destruction, or spread of disease. Malignancy, thrombi, atherosclerotic plaques, and infected tissue could be spread by massage. Absolute contraindications to massage include (1) DVT because of the fact that increased blood flow in a limb could cause thrombus to detach from the vessel wall creating an embolism, (2) acute infection, (3) bleeding, and (4) new open wound. Relative contraindications include (1) incompletely healed scar tissue, (2) fragile skin, (3) calcified soft tissue, (4) skin grafts, (5) atrophic skin, (6) inflamed tissue, (7) malignancy, (8) inflammatory muscle disease, and (9) pregnancy.

○   **What is traction?**

Traction is the act of drawing or pulling and relates to forces applied to the body to stretch a given part or to separate two or more parts. Currently, traction is used effectively in treatment of fractures. In physiatric practice, use of traction often is limited to the cervical or lumbar spine with the goal of relieving pain in, or originating from, those areas.

○   **What are the physiological effects of cervical traction?**

In the cervical spine, the most reproducible result of traction is elongation. Studies have shown that optimum weight for cervical traction to accomplish vertebral separation is 25 pounds. Additionally, 2-20 mm elongation of the cervical spine has been shown to be achievable with 25 or more pounds of traction force. Studies have shown that anterior intervertebral space shows the most increase in cervical flexion of 30°.

○   **What are the physiological effects of lumbar traction?**

In a classic study, Cyriax reported applying force of 300 pounds manually, with a resultant 1 cm increase in cumulative lumbar spine interspace distance. Once friction is overcome in the lumbar spine, the major physiologic effect of traction is elongation. Investigators have reported widening of lumbar interspaces requiring between 70-300 pounds of pull. This widening averaged up to slightly more than 3 mm at one intervertebral level. The length of time that the separation persists remains indeterminate with studies documenting distraction durations of 10-30 minutes after treatment.

○   **What are the indications for traction?**

The literature does not give clear indications what types of neck or low back pain (LBP) may improve from traction. Studies strongly suggest that traction does not produce significant influence on long-term outcome of neck pain or LBP. Practitioners who rely on sound scientific advice may use traction rarely. Practitioners who are receptive to empirical treatments may be amenable to the concept that traction may separate vertebrae and decrease the size of herniated discs, thereby benefiting radiculopathy; however, no consensus has been reached among clinicians or researchers in this area.

○   **What is the definition of manipulation?**

A consensus definition of manipulation is the use of the hands applied to the patient incorporating the use of instructions and maneuvers to achieve maximal painless movement and posture of the musculoskeletal system. Most common types of manipulation involve passive mechanical forces applied to specific vertebral segments, regions, or other joint segments of the musculoskeletal system with a primary goal of restoration of diminished ROM.

○   **What are the different categories of manual maneuvers?**

Direct thrust, articulatory technique, indirect positional technique, counterstrain, muscle energy techniques, soft tissue techniques, and myofascial release

O   **What are indications for manipulation?**

Manipulation is appropriate for a variety of musculoskeletal problems, especially those of the thorax, rib cage, upper and lower extremities, back, pelvis, and neck. It is also useful when loss of motion or function is encountered or when localized tenderness or pain is noted on induced motion

O   **What are contraindications to manipulation?**

Articulatory techniques are contraindicated for patients with vertebral malignancy, infection or inflammation, myelopathy, multiple adjacent radiculopathies, cauda equina syndrome, vertebral bone disease, bony joint instability, and cervical rheumatoid disease. Direct manipulation (eg, high velocity/low amplitude) is contraindicated in those cases and, additionally, in the presence of (1) spinal deformity, (2) systemic anticoagulation treatment, (3) severe diabetes or atherosclerotic disease, (4) degenerative joint disease, (5) vertebral basilar disease or insufficiency, (6) spondyloarthropathies, (7) ligamentous joint instability or congenital joint laxity, (8) aseptic necrosis, (9) local aneurysm, (10) osteoporosis, (11) acute disc herniation, and (12) osteomalacia.

BIBLIOGRAPHY

Cardiopulmonary:
American Association of Cardiovascular & Pulmonary Rehabilitation., Ed. (third) (2004). Guidelines for pulmonary rehabilitation programs, Human Kinetics. 0736055738.

American Association of Cardiovascular & Pulmonary; Rehabilitation. Ed. (fourth) (2004). Guidelines for cardiac rehabilitation and secondary prevention programs, Human Kinetics. 0736048642.

Lymphedema:

Zuther, Joachim E. (2005) Lymphedema Management: The Comprehensive Guide for Practitioners. THIEME NEW YORK. 1588902846

Musculoskeletal:

Sheon, R. R. M., Victor Goldberg, Ed. (third) (1996). Soft tissue rheumatic pain, William & Wilkins. 0-683-07678-7.

AMA; (fifth) (2001). Guidelines to the evaluation of permanent impairment AMA. 0-89970-553-7.

Borenstein, D. S. W., Boden, Scott, Ed. (third) (2004). Low Back and Neck Pain: Comprehensive Diagnosis and Management, W. B.Saunders. 072169277X

Sataloff, T. R. A. B., Richard Lederman, Ed. (second) (1998). Performing Arts Medicine, Singular Publishing. 1-56593-982-4.

Clark, Charles R.; Benzel, Edward C. ; Currier, Bradford L.; (fourth) (2004). The Cervical Spine Lippincott-Raven. 0-397-51535-9.

Herkowitz, Harry N.; Dvorak, Jiri ; Bell, Gordon R. Ed. (third) (2004). The Lumbar Spine, W.B. Saunders Co. 0-7216-6942-5.

Wadell, G., Ed. (second) (2004). The Back Pain Revolution, Churchill-Livingstone. 0-443-06039-8.
An evidence based medicine type reference for the spine and its disorders.

Andrews, J. G. H., Kevin Wilk, Ed. (third) (2004). Physical Rehabilitation of the injured athlete, W.B. Saunders Co. 0-7216-6549-7.

DeLee, Jesse C.; Drez, David ; Miller, Mark D. Ed. (second) (2003). DeLee & Drez's Orthopaedic Sports Medicine: Principles and Practice (2-Volume Set), SAUNDERS W B CO. 0721688454

Loeser, John D.; Butler, Stephen H. ; Chapman, C. Richard Ed. (third) (2001). Bonica's The management of pain, LIPPINCOTT WILLIAMS & WILKINS. 0683304623

Rachlin, E., Ed. (second) (2002). Myofascial pain and fibromyalgia, Mosby. 0-8016-6817-4.

Waldman, S. A. W., Ed. (second) (2001). Interventional Pain Management, W. B. Saunders. 0-7216-5874-1.
Hoppenfeld, Stanley; Murthy, Vasantha L. (2000). Treatment and Rehabilitation of Fractures, LIPPINCOTT WILLIAMS & WILKINS. 0781721970.

Bladder and Bowel:

Getliffe, Kathryn; Dolman, Mary (Eds.) (second) (2003). Promoting Continence: A Clinical and Research Resource, BAILLIERE TINDALL.

0702026379

Amputee:

Lusardi, Michelle M. ; Nielsen, Caroline C. Ed. (2000). Orthotics and Prosthetics in Rehabilitation, BUTTERWORTH HEINEMANN. 0750698071

Stroke:

Losseff, Nick Ed. (2004). Neurological Rehabilitation of Stroke, MARTIN DUNITZ LTD. 1841843229

Spinal Cord Injury:

Kirshblum, Steven ; Campagnolo, Denise I. ; DeLisa, Joel A. Ed. (2002). Spinal Cord Medicine, LIPPINCOTT WILLIAMS & WILKINS. 078172869X

Tator, Charles H.; Benzel, Edward C. Ed. (2000). Contemporary Management of Spinal Cord Injury: From Impact to Rehabilitation, AMER. ASSN. OF NEUROLOGICAL SURG. 1879284723.

Traumatic brain injury:

Rosenthal, M. E. G., Ed. (third) (1999). Rehabilitation of the adult and child with TBI, F.A. Davis. 0391-6.
A standard reference in TBI rehabilitation.

Multiple sclerosis and Parkinson's disease:

Good, D. J. R. C., Ed. (1994). Handbook of Neuro rehabilitation, Marcel Dekker. 0-8247-8822-2.
    Addresses acquired CNS disorders and their rehabilitation from a neurologists perspective.

Lazar, R., Ed. (1998). Principles of neurologic rehabilitation, McGraw Hill. 0-07-036794-9.

Greenwood, Richard J.; Barnes, Michael P.; Macmillan, Thomas M. Ed (second) (2003). Handbook of Neurological Rehabilitation, PSYCHOLOGY PRESS. 02068204

Umphred, D. A., Ed. (fourth) (2001). Neurological Rehabilitation, Mosby. 0-8016-7925-7.

Cerebral Palsy and Myelomeningocele:

Molnar, G., Ed. (third) (1999). Pediatric Rehabilitation, William & Wilkins. 0-683-06118-6.

Motor neuron and neuromuscular disorders:

Swash, M. M. S.; (third) (1997). Neuromuscular Diseases, Springer. 3-540-76025-3.

Dyck, P. J., Ed. (third) (1993). Peripheral Neuropathy, W.B. Saunders Co. 0-7216-3242-4.

Dawson, D. M. H., Asaj. Wilbourn, Ed. (third) (1999). Entrapment Neuropathies. LIPPINCOTT WILLIAMS & WILKINS. 0-316-17733-4.

Bach, J., Ed. (1999). Guide to the evaluation and management of neuromuscular disease, Hanley Belfus. 1-56053-301-3.

Rehabilitation technology and techniques:

Frontera, Walter R.; Dawson, David M.; Slovik, David M. Ed. (1999). Exercise in Rehabilitation Medicine, HUMAN KINETICS PUBLISHERS. 0880118393

Cameron, M., Ed. (second) (2002). Physical Agents in Rehabilitation, W.B. Saunders Co. 0-7216-6244-7.

Greenman, P., Ed. (third) (2003). Principles of Manual Medicine, William & Wilkins. 0-683-03558-4.

medicine, A. C. o. s., Ed. (fourth) (2001). Guidelines or exercise testing and prescription, William & Wilkins. 0-683-00026-8.

Bowker, J. M., Ed. (1992). Atlas of limb prosthetics, AAOS.

Goldberg, Bertram; J. H., Ed. (1997). Atlas of orthoses and assistive devices, AAOS/Mosby.

NOTES

NOTES

NOTES

NOTES

NOTES